Roitt's
Essential
Immunology

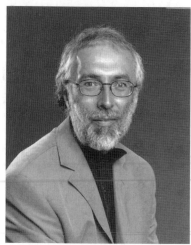

Peter J. Delves

Dr Delves obtained his PhD from the University of London in 1986 and is currently a Reader in Immunology at University College London. His research focuses on molecular aspects of antigen recognition. He has authored and edited a number of immunology books, and teaches the subject at a broad range of levels.

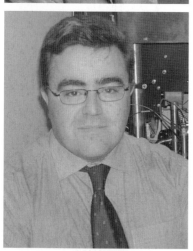

Seamus J. Martin

Professor Martin received his PhD from The National University of Ireland in 1990 and trained as a post-doctoral fellow at University College London (with Ivan Roitt) and The La Jolla Institute for Allergy and Immunology, California, USA (with Doug Green). Since 1999, he is the holder of the Smurfit Chair of Medical Genetics at Trinity College Dublin and is also a Science Foundation Ireland Principal Investigator. His research is focused on various aspects of programmed cell death (apoptosis) in the immune system and in cancer and he has received several awards for his work in this area. He has previously edited two books on apoptosis and was elected as a Member of The Royal Irish Academy in 2006.

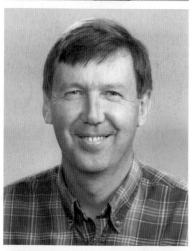

Dennis R. Burton

Professor Burton obtained his BA in Chemistry from the University of Oxford in 1974 and his PhD in Physical Biochemistry from the University of Lund in Sweden in 1978. After a period at the University of Sheffield, he moved to the Scripps Research Institute in La Jolla, California in 1989 where he is Professor of Immunology and Molecular Biology. His research interests include antibodies, antibody responses to pathogens and vaccine design, particularly in relation to HIV.

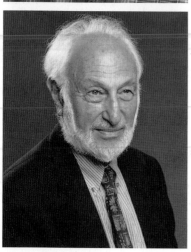

Ivan M. Roitt

Professor Roitt was born in 1927 and educated at King Edward's School, Birmingham and Balliol College, Oxford. In 1956, together with Deborah Doniach and Peter Campbell, he made the classic discovery of thyroglobulin autoantibodies in Hashimoto's thyroiditis which helped to open the whole concept of a relationship between autoimmunity and human disease. The work was extended to an intensive study of autoimmune phenomena in pernicious anaemia and primary biliary cirrhosis. In 1983 he was elected a Fellow of The Royal Society, and has been elected to Honorary Membership of the Royal College of Physicians and appointed Honorary Fellow of The Royal Society of Medicine.

ELEVENTH EDITION

Roitt's Essential Immunology

Peter J. Delves
PhD
Department of Immunology and Molecular Pathology
University College London
London, U.K.

Seamus J. Martin
PhD, FTCD, MRIA
The Smurfit Institute of Genetics
Trinity College
Dublin 2, Ireland

Dennis R. Burton
PhD
Department of Immunology and Molecular Biology
The Scripps Research Institute
California, USA

Ivan M. Roitt
MA, DSc(Oxon), FRDPath, Hon FRCP (Lond), FRS
Emeritus Professor, Department of Immunology and Molecular Pathology
University College London
London

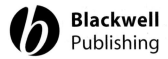
Blackwell
Publishing

© 2006 Peter J Delves, Seamus J. Martin, Dennis R. Burton, Ivan M. Roitt
Published by Blackwell Publishing Ltd
Blackwell Publishing, Inc., 350 Main Street, Malden, Massachusetts 02148-5020, USA
Blackwell Publishing Ltd, 9600 Garsington Road, Oxford OX4 2DQ, UK
Blackwell Publishing Asia Pty Ltd, 550 Swanston Street, Carlton, Victoria 3053, Australia

First published 1971
Reprinted 1972 (twice), 1973 (twice)
Second edition 1974, Reprinted 1975
Third edition 1977, Reprinted 1978, 1979
Fourth edition 1980, Reprinted 1982, 1983
Fifth edition 1984
Sixth edition 1988, Reprinted 1988, 1989
Seventh edition 1991
Eighth edition 1994, Reprinted 1996
Ninth edition 1997, Reprinted 1999
Tenth edition 2001, Reprinted 2003
Spanish editions 1972, 1975, 1978, 1982, 1988, 1989, 1993
Italian editions 1973, 1975, 1979, 1986, 1988, 1990, 1993, 1995
Eleventh Edition 2006

Portuguese editions 1973, 1979, 1983
French editions 1975, 1979, 1990
Dutch editions 1975, 1978, 1982
Japanese editions 1976, 1978, 1982, 1986, 1988
German editions 1977, 1984, 1988, 1993
Polish edition 1977
Greek editions 1978, 1989, 1992
Turkish edition 1979
Slovak edition 1981
Indonesian editions 1985, 1991
Russian edition 1988
Korean edition 1991
ELBS editions 1977, 1982, 1988, Reprinted 1991

Chinese (Taiwan) editions 1991, 1994

3   2008

Library of Congress Cataloging-in-Publication Data

Data available

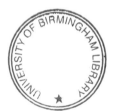

ISBN 978-1-4051-3603-7

A catalogue record for this title is available from the British Library

Set in 9.75/12.5pt Palatino by SNP Best-set Typesetter Ltd., Hong Kong
Printed and bound in Singapore by Markono Print Media Pte Ltd

2366188)

Commissioning Editor: Martin Sugden
Editorial Assistant: Caroline Boyd
Development Editor: Mirjana Misina
Production Controller: Kate Charman

Website: Meg Barton, Shaun Embury, Jake Farr

For further information on Blackwell Publishing, visit our website:
http://www.blackwellpublishing.com

Contents

Companion website: www.roitt.com

Acknowledgements

The input of the editorial team of Martin Sugden, Mirjana Misina and Meg Barton at Blackwell Publishing, and the illustrators Anthea Carter and Graeme Chambers is warmly acknowledged. We are much indebted to the co-editors of *Immunology*, J. Brostoff and D. Male, together with the publishers, Mosby, and the following individuals for permission to utilize or modify their figures: J. Brostoff and A. Hall for figures 1.15 and 15.10; J. Horton for figure 11.20; G. Rook for figures 12.5 and 12.11; and J. Taverne for figure 12.22 and table 12.2.

IMR would like to acknowledge the indefatigable secretarial assistance of Christine Griffin. DRB wishes to particularly acknowledge the invaluable contributions of Amandeep Gakhal, Erin Scherer, Rena Astronomo and Wendelien Oswald. He is grateful to Jenny Woof, Ann Feeney, Beatrice Hahn, Jim Marks, Don Mosier, Paul Sharp, Robyn Stanfield, James Stevens and Mario Stevenson for many very helpful comments. PJD would particularly like to thank Per Brandtzaeg, Volker Brinkmann and Peter Lydyard.

Every effort has been made by the authors and the publisher to contact all the copyright holders to obtain their permission to reproduce copyright material. However, if any have been inadvertently overlooked, the publisher will be pleased to make the necessary arrangements at the first opportunity.

A number of scientists very generously provided illustrations for inclusion in this edition, and we have acknowledged our gratitude to them in the relevant figure legends.

Preface

In view of the ever-increasing intensity and scope of the subject of Immunology and global differences in the curricula, it was decided that the authorship of the 10th edition be broadened to include notable scientists from other countries. Accordingly, Professor Seamus Martin of Trinity College, Dublin and Professor Dennis Burton of the Scripps Research Institute, California were invited to contribute to the current edition. We feel sure that the reader will find that their contributions will make a powerful impact and yet still maintain the reader-friendly character of earlier editions.

Many subjects have been thoroughly updated and sometimes expanded. These include sections on HIV AIDS, regulatory T-cells, chemokines, cell signaling, T-cell development, vaccines and therapies involving lymphocyte ablation.

Dear reader, we hope you will enjoy this new edition and find the content attractive and rewarding.

Peter J. Delves
Seamus J. Martin
Dennis R. Burton
Ivan M. Roitt

Abbreviations

AAV	adeno-associated virus	CEA	carcinoembryonic antigen
Ab	antibody	CFA	complete Freund's adjuvant
ACh-R	acetylcholine receptor	cGMP	cyclic guanosine monophosphate
ACT	adoptive cell transfer	CHIP	chemotaxis inhibitory protein
ACTH	adrenocorticotropic hormone	$C_{H(L)}$	constant part of Ig heavy (light) chain
ADA	adenosine deaminase	CLA	cutaneous lymphocyte antigen
ADCC	antibody-dependent cellular cytotoxicity	CLIP	class II-associated invariant chain peptide
AEP	asparagine endopeptidase	CMI	cell-mediated immunity
Ag	antigen	CML	cell-mediated lympholysis
AID	activation-induced cytidine deaminase	CMV	cytomegalovirus
AIDS	acquired immunodeficiency syndrome	Cn	complement component 'n'
AIRE	autoimmune regulator	C̄n	activated complement component 'n'
ANCA	antineutrophil cytoplasmic antibodies	iCn	inactivated complement component 'n'
APC	antigen-presenting cell	Cna	small peptide derived by proteolytic
ARRE-1	antigen receptor response element-1		activation of Cn
ARRE-2	antigen receptor response element-2	CpG	cytosine phosphate-guanosine dinucleotide
ART	antiretroviral therapy		motif
ASFV	African swine fever virus	CR(n)	complement receptor 'n'
AZT	zidovudine (3'-azido-3'-deoxythymidine)	CRP	C-reactive protein
		CsA	cyclosporin A
BAFF	B-cell-activating factor of the tumor necrosis	CSF	cerebrospinal fluid
	factor family	CSR	class switch recombination
B-cell	lymphocyte which matures in bone marrow	CTLR	C-type lectin receptors
BCG	bacille Calmette–Guérin attenuated form of		
	tuberculosis	D gene	diversity minigene joining V and J segments to
BCR	B-cell receptor		form variable region
BM	bone marrow	DAF	decay accelerating factor
BSA	bovine serum albumin	DAG	diacylglycerol
BSE	bovine spongiform encephalopathy	DC	dendritic cells
Btk	Bruton's tyrosine kinase	DMARD	disease-modifying antirheumatic drug
BUDR	bromodeoxyuridine	DNP	dinitrophenyl
		DTH	delayed-type hypersensitivity
C	complement	DTP	diphtheria, tetanus, pertussis triple
$C\alpha(\beta/\gamma/\delta)$	constant part of TCR $\alpha(\beta/\gamma/\delta)$ chain		vaccine
CALLA	common acute lymphoblastic leukemia		
	antigen	EAE	experimental allergic encephalomyelitis
cAMP	cyclic adenosine monophosphate	EBV	Epstein–Barr virus
CCP	complement control protein repeat	ELISA	enzyme-linked immunosorbent assay
CD	cluster of differentiation	EM	electron microscope
CDR	complementarity determining regions of Ig or	Eφ	eosinophil
	TCR variable portion	EPO	erythropoietin

ER	endoplasmic reticulum
ES	embryonic stem (cell)
ET	exfoliative toxins
F(B)	factor (B, etc.)
Fab	monovalent Ig antigen-binding fragment after papain digestion
F(ab')$_2$	divalent antigen-binding fragment after pepsin digestion
FasL	Fas-ligand
FACS	fluorescence-activated cell sorter
Fc	Ig crystallisable-fragment originally; now non-Fab part of Ig
FcγR	receptor for IgG Fc fragment
FDC	follicular dendritic cell
flt-3	flk-2 ligand
(sc)Fv	(single chain) V_H–V_L antigen binding fragment
GADS	GRB2-related adapter protein
g.b.m.	glomerular basement membrane
G-CSF	granulocyte colony-stimulating factor
GEFs	guanine-nucleotide exchange factors
GM-CSF	granulocyte–macrophage colony-stimulating factor
gp$n$	nkDa glycoprotein
GRB2	growth factor receptor-binding protein 2
GSK3	glycogen synthase kinase 3
g.v.h.	graft versus host
H-2	the mouse major histocompatibility complex
H-2D/K/L	main loci for classical class I (class II)
(A/E)	murine MHC molecules
HAMA	human antimouse antibodies
HATA	human anti-toxin antibody
HBsAg	hepatitis B surface antigen
hCG	human chorionic gonadotropin
HCMV	human cytomegalovirus
HEL	hen egg lysozyme
HEV	high-walled endothelium of post capillary venule
Hi	high
HIV-1(2)	human immunodeficiency virus-1 (2)
HLA	the human major histocompatibility complex
HLA-A/B/C	main loci for classical class I (class II)
(DP/DQ/DR)	human MHC molecules
HMG	high mobility group
HR	hypersensitive response
HRF	homologous restriction factor
HSA	heat-stable antigen
HSC	hematopoietic stem cell
hsp	heat-shock protein
5HT	5-hydroxytryptamine
HTLV	human T-cell leukemia virus
H-Y	male transplantation antigen
IBD	inflammatory bowel disease
ICAM-1	intercellular adhesion molecule-1
Id (αId)	idiotype (anti-idiotype)
IDC	interdigitating dendritic cells

IDDM	insulin-dependent diabetes mellitus
IDO	indoleamine 2,3-dioxygenase
IEL	intraepithelial lymphocyte
IFNα	α-interferon (also IFNβ, IFNγ)
Ig	immunoglobulin
IgG	immunoglobulin G (also IgM, IgA, IgD, IgE)
sIg	surface immunoglobulin
Ig-α/Ig-β	membrane peptide chains associated with sIg B-cell receptor
IgSF	immunoglobulin superfamily
IL-1	interleukin-1 (also IL-2, IL-3, etc.)
iNOS	inducible nitric oxide synthase
IP$_3$	inositol triphosphate
ISCOM	immunostimulating complex
ITAM	immunoreceptor tyrosine-based activation motif
ITIM	immunoreceptor tyrosine-based inhibitory motif
ITP	idiopathic thrombocytopenic purpura
IVIg	intravenous immunoglobulin
JAK	Janus kinases
J chain	peptide chain in IgA dimer and IgM
J gene	joining gene linking V or D segment to constant region
Ka(d)	association (dissociation) affinity constant (usually Ag–Ab reactions)
kDa	units of molecular mass in kilo Daltons
KIR	killer immunoglobulin-like receptors
KLH	keyhole limpet hemocyanin
LAK	lymphokine activated killer cell
LAMP	lysosomal-associated membrane proteins
LAT	linker for activation of T cells
LATS	long-acting thyroid stimulator
LBP	LPS binding protein
LCM	lymphocytic choriomeningitis virus
Le$^{a/b/x}$	Lewis$^{a/b/x}$ blood group antigens
LFA-1	lymphocyte functional antigen-1
LGL	large granular lymphocyte
LHRH	luteinizing hormone releasing hormone
LIF	leukemia inhibiting factor
Lo	low
LT(B)	leukotriene (B etc.)
LPS	lipopolysaccharide (endotoxin)
Mϕ	macrophage
mAb	monoclonal antibody
MAC	membrane attack complex
MAdCAM	mucosal addressin cell adhesion molecule
MALT	mucosa-associated lymphoid tissue
MAM	*Mycoplasma arthritidis* mitogen
MAP kinase	mitogen-activated protein kinase
MAPKKK	mitogen-associated protein kinase kinase kinase
MBL	mannose binding lectin
MBP	major basic protein of eosinophils (also myelin basic protein)

MCP	membrane cofactor protein (C′ regulation)
MCP-1	monocyte chemotactic protein-1
M-CSF	macrophage colony-stimulating factor
MDP	muramyl dipeptide
MHC	major histocompatibility complex
MICA	MHC class I chain-related A chain
MIDAS	metal ion-dependent adhesion site
MIF	macrophage migration inhibitory factor
MIIC	MHC class II-enriched compartments
MLA	monophosphoryl lipid A
MLR	mixed lymphocyte reaction
MMTV	mouse mammary tumor virus
MRSA	methicillin-resistant *Staphylococcus aureus*
MS	multiple sclerosis
MSC	mesenchymal stem cell
MSH	melanocyte stimulating hormone
MTP	microsomal triglyceride-transfer protein
MuLV	murine leukemia virus
NADP	nicotinamide adenine dinucleotide phosphate
NAP	neutrophil activating peptide
NBT	nitro blue tetrazolium
NCF	neutrophil chemotactic factor
NFAT	nuclear factor of activated T-cells
NFκB	nuclear transcription factor
NK	natural killer cell
NO·	nitric oxide
NOD	Nonobese diabetic mouse
NZB	New Zealand Black mouse
NZB × W	New Zealand Black mouse × NZ White F1 hybrid
·O$^-_2$	superoxide anion
OD	optical density
ORF	open reading frame
OS	obese strain chicken
Ova	ovalbumin
PAF(-R)	platelet activating factor (-receptor)
PAGE	polyacrylamide gel electrophoresis
PAMP	pathogen-associated molecular pattern
PBSCs	peripheral blood stem cells
PCA	passive cutaneous anaphylaxis
PCR	polymerase chain reaction
PERV	porcine endogenous retroviruses
PG(E)	prostaglandin (E etc.)
PHA	phytohemagglutinin
phox	phagocyte oxidase
PI3K	phosphatidylinositol 3-kinase
PIAS	protein inhibitor of activated STAT
pIgR	poly-Ig receptor
PIP$_2$	phosphatidylinositol diphosphate
PKC	protein kinase C
PKR	RNA-dependent protein kinase
PLC	phospholipase C
PLCγ2	phospholipase Cγ2
PMN	polymorphonuclear neutrophil
PMT	photomultiplier tube
PNH	paroxysmal nocturnal hemoglobinuria

PPAR	peroxisome proliferator-activated receptor
PPD	purified protein derivative from *Mycobacterium tuberculosis*
PRR	pattern recognition receptors
PTFE	polytetrafluroethylene
PTK	protein tyrosine kinase
PWM	pokeweed mitogen
RA	rheumatoid arthritis
RANTES	regulated upon *a*ctivation *n*ormal *T*-cell *e*xpressed and *s*ecreted chemokine
RAST	radioallergosorbent test
RF	rheumatoid factor
Rh(D)	rhesus blood group (D)
RIP	rat insulin promoter
RNAi	RNA interference
ROI	reactive oxygen intermediates
RSS	recombination signal sequence
SAP	serum amyloid P
SAP	sphingolipid activator protein
SAR	systemic acquired resistance
SARS	severe acute respiratory syndrome
SARS-CoV	SARS-associated coronavirus
SC	Ig secretory component
SCF	stem cell factor
scFv	single chain variable region antibody fragment (V$_H$ + V$_L$ joined by a flexible linker)
SCG	sodium cromoglycate
SCID	severe combined immunodeficiency
SDF	stromal-derived factor
SDS	sodium dodecyl sulfate
SDS-PAGE	sodium dodecylsulfate–polyacrylamide gel electrophoresis
SEA(B etc.)	*Staphylococcus aureus* enterotoxin A (B etc.)
SEREX	serological analysis of recombinant cDNA expression libraries
siRNA	short-interfering RNA
SIV	Simian immunodeficiency virus
SLE	systemic lupus erythematosus
SLIT	sublingual allergen immunotherapy
SLP76	SH2-domain containing leukocyte protein of 76 kDa
SOCs	*s*uppressor of *c*ytokine signaling
SPE	streptococcal pyogenic exotoxins
SRID	single radial immunodiffusion
SSA	streptococcal superantigen
STAT	signal transducer and activator of transcription
TACI	transmembrane activator and calcium modulator and cyclophilin ligand [CAML] interactor
TAP	transporter for antigen processing
T-ALL	T-acute lymphoblastic leukemia
TB	tubercle bacillus
Tc	cytotoxic T-cell
T-cell	thymus-derived lymphocyte
TCF	T-cell factor

TCR1(2)	T-cell receptor with γ/δ chains (with α/β chains)	TUNEL	TdT-mediated dUTP (deoxyuridine triphosphate) nick end labeling
TdT	terminal deoxynucleotidyl transferase		
TG-A-L	polylysine with polyalanyl side-chains randomly tipped with tyrosine and glutamic acid	$V\alpha(\beta/\gamma/\delta)$	variable part of TCR $\alpha(\beta/\gamma/\delta)$ chain
		vCJD	variant Creutzfeldt–Jakob disease
TGFβ	transforming growth factor-β	VCP	valosin-containing protein
Th(1/2)	T-helper cell (subset 1 or 2)	V gene	variable region gene for immunoglobulin or T-cell receptor
THF	thymic humoral factor		
Thp	T-helper precursor	V_H	variable part of Ig heavy chain
TLI	total lymphoid irradiation	VIP	vasoactive intestinal peptide
TLR	Toll-like receptor	V_L	variable part of light chain
TM	transmembrane	$V_{\kappa/\lambda}$	variable part of $\kappa(\lambda)$ light chain
TNF	tumor necrosis factor	VCAM	vascular cell adhesion molecule
TNP	trinitrophenol	VEGF	vascular endothelial cell growth factor
TPO	thrombopoietin	VIMP	VCP-interacting membrane protein
Treg	regulatory T-cell	VLA	very late antigen
Ts	suppressor T-cell	VLP	virus-like particle
TSAb	thyroid stimulating antibodies	VNTR	variable number of tandem repeats
TSE	transmissible spongiform encephalopathy	VP1	virus-specific peptide 1
TSH(R)	thyroid stimulating hormone (receptor)		
TSLP	thymic stromal lymphopoietin	XL	X-linked
TSST	toxic shock syndrome toxin		
tum–	strongly immunogenic mutant tumors	ZAP-70	zeta chain associated protein of 70 kDa

User guide

Throughout the illustrations standard forms have been used for commonly-occurring cells and pathways. A key to these is given in the figure below.

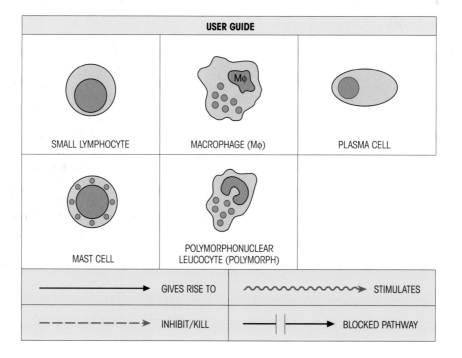

Website: www.roitt.com	
Visit the companion website for this book at:	Includes:
	• Interactive MCQs with feedback
www.roitt.com	• Animations showing key concepts
	• Database of Figures

1 Innate immunity

INTRODUCTION

We live in a potentially hostile world filled with a bewildering array of infectious agents (figure 1.1) of diverse shape, size, composition and subversive character which would very happily use us as rich sanctuaries for propagating their 'selfish genes' had we not also developed a series of defense mechanisms at least their equal in effectiveness and ingenuity (except in the case of many parasitic infections where the situation is best described as an uneasy and often unsatisfactory truce). It is these defense mechanisms which can establish a state of immunity against infection (Latin *immunitas*, freedom from) and whose operation provides the basis for the delightful subject called 'Immunology'.

Aside from ill-understood constitutional factors which make one species innately susceptible and another resistant to certain infections, a number of relatively nonspecific antimicrobial systems (e.g. phagocytosis) have been recognized which are **innate** in the sense that they are not intrinsically affected by prior contact with the infectious agent. We shall discuss these systems and examine how, in the state of **specific acquired immunity**, their effectiveness can be greatly increased.

EXTERNAL BARRIERS AGAINST INFECTION

The simplest way to avoid infection is to prevent the microorganisms from gaining access to the body (figure 1.2). The major line of defense is of course the skin which, when intact, is impermeable to most infectious agents; when there is skin loss, as for example in burns, infection becomes a major problem. Additionally, most bacteria fail to survive for long on the skin because of the direct inhibitory effects of lactic acid and fatty acids in sweat and sebaceous secretions and the low pH which they generate. An exception is *Staphylococcus aureus* which often infects the relatively vulnerable hair follicles and glands.

Mucus, secreted by the membranes lining the inner surfaces of the body, acts as a protective barrier to block the adherence of bacteria to epithelial cells. Microbial and other foreign particles trapped within the adhesive mucus are removed by mechanical stratagems such as ciliary movement, coughing and sneezing. Among other mechanical factors which help protect the epithelial surfaces, one should also include the washing action of tears, saliva and urine. Many of the secreted body fluids contain bactericidal components, such as acid in gastric juice, spermine and zinc in semen, lactoperoxidase in milk and lysozyme in tears, nasal secretions and saliva.

A totally different mechanism is that of microbial antagonism associated with the normal bacterial flora of the body. This suppresses the growth of many potentially pathogenic bacteria and fungi at superficial sites by competition for essential nutrients or by production of inhibitory substances. To give one example, pathogen invasion is limited by lactic acid produced by particular species of commensal bacteria which metabolize glycogen secreted by the vaginal epithelium. When protective commensals are disturbed by antibiotics, susceptibility to opportunistic infections by *Candida* and *Clostridium difficile* is increased. Gut commensals may also produce colicins, a class of bactericidins which bind to the negatively charged surface of susceptible bacteria and insert a hydrophobic helical hairpin into the membrane; the molecule then undergoes a 'Jekyll and Hyde' transformation to become completely hydrophobic and forms a voltage-dependent channel in the membrane

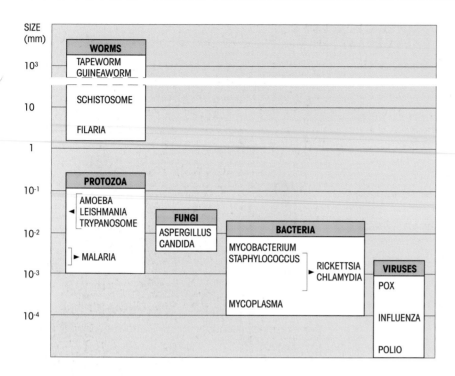

Figure 1.1. **The formidable range of infectious agents which confronts the immune system.** Although not normally classified as such because of their lack of a cell wall, the mycoplasmas are included under bacteria for convenience. Fungi adopt many forms and approximate values for some of the smallest forms are given. ⌐►, range of sizes observed for the organism(s) indicated by the arrow; ◄⌐, the organisms listed have the size denoted by the arrow.

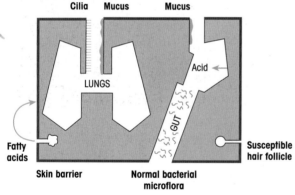

Figure 1.2. **The first lines of defense against infection:** protection at the external body surfaces.

which kills by destroying the cell's energy potential. Even at this level, survival is a tough game.

If microorganisms do penetrate the body, two main defensive operations come into play, the destructive effect of soluble chemical factors such as bactericidal enzymes and the mechanism of **phagocytosis**—literally 'eating' by the cell (Milestone 1.1).

PHAGOCYTIC CELLS KILL MICROORGANISMS

Neutrophils and macrophages are dedicated 'professional' phagocytes

The engulfment and digestion of microorganisms are assigned to two major cell types recognized by Metchnikoff at the turn of the last century as microphages and macrophages.

The polymorphonuclear neutrophil

This cell, the smaller of the two, shares a common hematopoietic stem cell precursor with the other formed elements of the blood and is the dominant white cell in the bloodstream. It is a nondividing short-lived cell with a multilobed nucleus and an array of granules (figure 1.3), which are virtually unstained by histologic dyes such as hematoxylin and eosin, unlike those structures in the closely related eosinophil and basophil (figure 1.4). These neutrophil granules are of two main types: (i) the **primary azurophil granule** which develops early (figure 1.4 e), has the typical lysosomal morphology and contains myeloperoxidase together with most of the nonoxidative antimicrobial effectors including defensins, bactericidal permeability increasing (BPI) protein and cathepsin G (figure 1.3), and (ii) the peroxidase-negative **secondary specific granules** containing lactoferrin, much of the lysozyme, alkaline phosphatase (figure 1.4 d) and membrane-bound cytochrome b_{558} (figure 1.3). The abundant glycogen stores can be utilized by glycolysis enabling the cells to function under anerobic conditions.

The macrophage

These cells derive from bone marrow promonocytes which, after differentiation to blood monocytes, finally settle in the tissues as mature macrophages where they

Milestone 1.1—Phagocytosis

The perceptive Russian zoologist, Elie Metchnikoff (1845–1916), recognized that certain specialized cells mediate defense against microbial infections, so fathering the whole concept of cellular immunity. He was intrigued by the motile cells of transparent starfish larvae and made the critical observation that, a few hours after the introduction of a rose thorn into these larvae, they became surrounded by these motile cells. A year later, in 1883, he observed that fungal spores can be attacked by the blood cells of *Daphnia*, a tiny metazoan which, also being transparent, can be studied directly under the microscope. He went on to extend his investigations to mammalian leukocytes, showing their ability to engulf microorganisms, a process which he termed **phagocytosis**.

Because he found this process to be even more effective in animals recovering from infection, he came to a somewhat polarized view that phagocytosis provided the main, if not the only, defense against infection. He went on to define the existence of two types of circulating phagocytes: the polymorphonuclear leukocyte, which he termed a 'microphage', and the larger 'macrophage'.

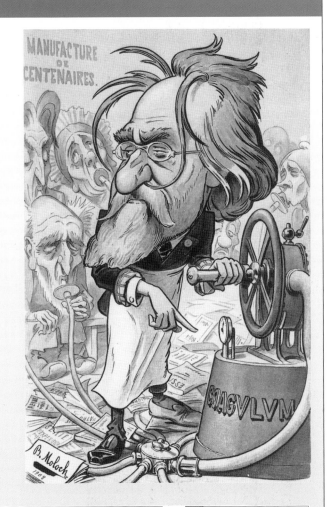

Figure M1.1.1. Caricature of Professor Metchnikoff from *Chanteclair*, 1908, No. 4, p. 7. (Reproduction kindly provided by The Wellcome Institute Library, London.)

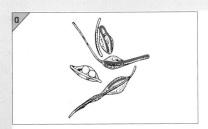 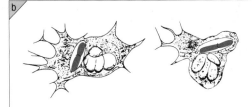 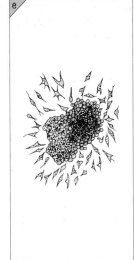

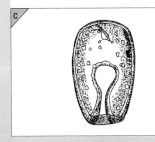 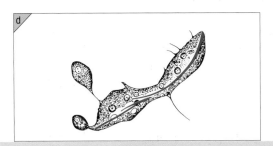

Figure M1.1.2. Reproductions of some of the illustrations in Metchnikoff's book, *Comparative Pathology of Inflammation* (1893). (a) Four leukocytes from the frog, enclosing anthrax bacilli; some are alive and unstained, others which have been killed have taken up the vesuvine dye and have been colored; (b) drawing of an anthrax bacillus, stained by vesuvine, in a leukocyte of the frog; the two figures represent two phases of movement of the same frog leukocyte which contains stained anthrax bacilli within its phagocytic vacuole; (c and d) a foreign body (colored) in a starfish larva surrounded by phagocytes which have fused to form a multinucleate plasmodium shown at higher power in (d); (e) this gives a feel for the dynamic attraction of the mobile mesenchymal phagocytes to a foreign intruder within a starfish larva.

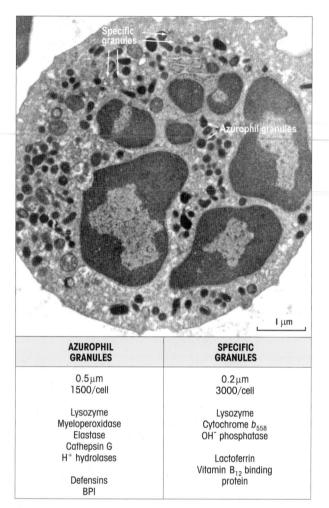

AZUROPHIL GRANULES	SPECIFIC GRANULES
0.5 μm 1500/cell	0.2 μm 3000/cell
Lysozyme Myeloperoxidase Elastase Cathepsin G H⁺ hydrolases Defensins BPI	Lysozyme Cytochrome b_{558} OH⁻ phosphatase Lactoferrin Vitamin B_{12} binding protein

Figure 1.3. Ultrastructure of neutrophil. The multilobed nucleus and two main types of cytoplasmic granules are well displayed. (Courtesy of Dr D. McLaren.)

constitute the **mononuclear phagocyte system** (figure 1.5). They are present throughout the connective tissue and around the basement membrane of small blood vessels and are particularly concentrated in the lung (figure 1.4h; alveolar macrophages), liver (Kupffer cells) and lining of spleen sinusoids and lymph node medullary sinuses where they are strategically placed to filter off foreign material. Other examples are mesangial cells in the kidney glomerulus, brain microglia and osteoclasts in bone. Unlike the polymorphs, they are long-lived cells with significant rough-surfaced endoplasmic reticulum and mitochondria (figure 1.8b) and, whereas the polymorphs provide the major defense against pyogenic (pus-forming) bacteria, as a rough generalization it may be said that macrophages are at their best in combating those bacteria (figure 1.4g), viruses and protozoa which are capable of living within the cells of the host.

Pattern recognition receptors (PRRs) on phagocytic cells recognize and are activated by pathogen-associated molecular patterns (PAMPs)

It hardly needs to be said but the body provides a very complicated internal environment and the phagocytes continuously encounter an extraordinary variety of different cells and soluble molecules. They must have mechanisms to enable them to distinguish these friendly self components from unfriendly and potentially dangerous microbial agents—as Charlie Janeway so aptly put it, they should be able to discriminate between 'noninfectious self and infectious nonself'. Not only must the infection be recognized but it must also generate a signal which, as proposed by Polly Matzinger, betokens 'danger'.

In the interests of host survival, phagocytic cells have evolved a system of receptors capable of recognizing molecular patterns expressed by pathogens (PAMPs) which are conserved (i.e. unlikely to mutate), shared by a large group of infectious agents (sparing the need for too many receptors) and clearly distinguishable from self patterns. Several of these pattern recognition receptors (PRRs) are lectin-like and bind multivalently with considerable specificity to exposed microbial surface sugars with their characteristic rigid three-dimensional geometric configurations (PAMPs). They do not bind appreciably to the array of galactose or sialic acid groups which are commonly the penultimate and ultimate sugars which decorate mammalian surface polysaccharides so providing the molecular basis for discriminating between self and nonself microbial cells.

A major subset of these PRRs belong to the class of so-called **Toll-like receptors (TLRs)** because of their similarity to the Toll receptor in the fruit fly, *Drosophila*, which in the adult triggers an intracellular cascade generating the expression of antimicrobial peptides in response to microbial infection. A series of cell surface TLRs acting as sensors for extracellular infections have been identified (table 1.1) which are activated by microbial elements such as peptidoglycan, lipoproteins, mycobacterial lipoarabinomannan, yeast zymosan and flagellin.

Phagocytes also display another set of PRRs, the cell bound **C-type (calcium-dependent) lectins**, of which the macrophage mannose receptor is an example. These transmembrane proteins possess multiple carbohydrate recognition domains whose engagement with their cognate microbial PAMPs generates an intracellular activation signal. **Scavenger receptors** represent yet a further class of phagocytic receptors which recognize a variety of anionic polymers and acetylated low density

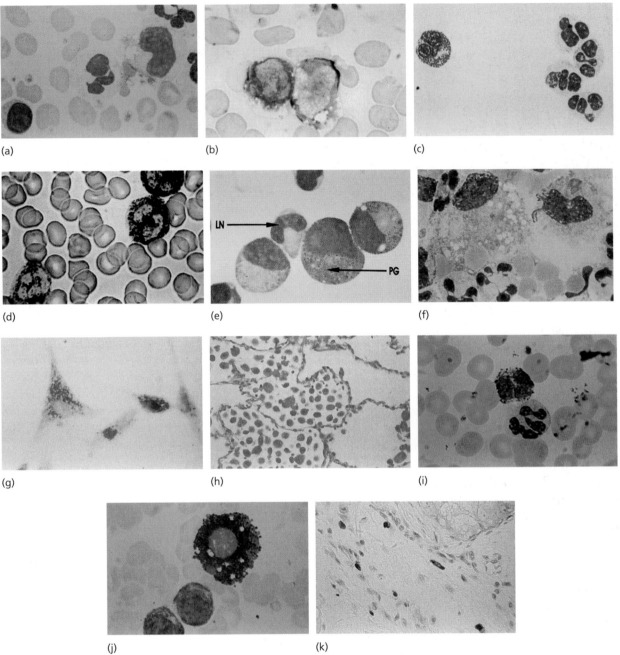

Figure 1.4. Cells involved in innate immunity. (a) Monocyte, showing 'horseshoe-shaped' nucleus and moderately abundant pale cytoplasm. Note the three multilobed polymorphonuclear neutrophils and the small lymphocyte (bottom left). Romanowsky stain. (b) Two monocytes stained for nonspecific esterase with α-naphthyl acetate. Note the vacuolated cytoplasm. The small cell with focal staining at the top is a T-lymphocyte. (c) Four polymorphonuclear neutrophils and one eosinophil. The multilobed nuclei and the cytoplasmic granules are clearly shown, those of the eosinophil being heavily stained. (d) Polymorphonuclear neutrophil showing cytoplasmic granules stained for alkaline phosphatase. (e) Early neutrophils in bone marrow. The primary azurophilic granules (PG), originally clustered near the nucleus, move towards the periphery where the neutrophil-specific granules are generated by the Golgi apparatus as the cell matures. The nucleus gradually becomes lobular (LN). Giemsa. (f) Inflammatory cells from the site of a brain hemorrhage showing the large active macrophage in the center with phagocytosed red cells and prominent vacuoles. To the right is a monocyte with horseshoe-shaped nucleus and cytoplasmic bilirubin crystals (hematoidin). Several multilobed neutrophils are clearly delineated. Giemsa. (g) Macrophages in monolayer cultures after phagocytosis of mycobacteria (stained red). Carbol-Fuchsin counterstained with Malachite Green. (h) Numerous plump alveolar macrophages within air spaces in the lung. (i) Basophil with heavily staining granules compared with a neutrophil (below). (j) Mast cell from bone marrow. Round central nucleus surrounded by large darkly staining granules. Two small red cell precursors are shown at the bottom. Romanowsky stain. (k) Tissue mast cells in skin stained with Toluidine Blue. The intracellular granules are metachromatic and stain reddish purple. Note the clustering in relation to dermal capillaries. (The slides from which illustrations (a), (b), (d), (e), (f), (i) and (j) were reproduced were very kindly provided by Mr M. Watts of the Department of Haematology, Middlesex Hospital Medical School; (c) was kindly supplied by Professor J.J. Owen; (g) by Professors P. Lydyard and G. Rook; (h) by Dr Meryl Griffiths; and (k) by Professor N. Woolf.)

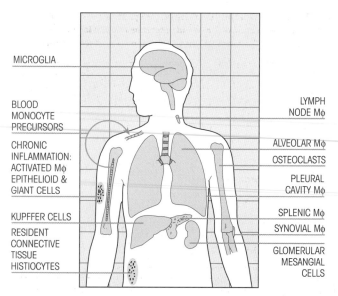

MICROGLIA

BLOOD
MONOCYTE
PRECURSORS

CHRONIC
INFLAMMATION:
ACTIVATED Mφ
EPITHELIOID &
GIANT CELLS

KUPFFER CELLS

RESIDENT
CONNECTIVE
TISSUE
HISTIOCYTES

LYMPH
NODE Mφ

ALVEOLAR Mφ

OSTEOCLASTS

PLEURAL
CAVITY Mφ

SPLENIC Mφ

SYNOVIAL Mφ

GLOMERULAR
MESANGIAL
CELLS

Figure 1.5. The mononuclear phagocyte system. Promonocyte precursors in the bone marrow develop into circulating blood monocytes which eventually become distributed throughout the body as mature macrophages (Mφ) as shown. The other major phagocytic cell, the polymorphonuclear neutrophil, is largely confined to the bloodstream except when recruited into sites of acute inflammation.

proteins. The role of the CD14 scavenger molecule in the handling of Gram-negative LPS (endotoxin) merits some attention, since failure to do so can result in septic shock. The biologically reactive lipid A moiety of LPS is recognized by a plasma LPS-binding protein, and the complex which is captured by the CD14 scavenger molecule on the phagocytic cell then activates TLR4. Like the engagement of the other cell surface TLRs with their cognate microbial PAMPs which alert the cell to danger and initiate the phagocytic process, this in turn unleashes a series of events culminating in the release of NFκB from its inhibitor. The free NFκB translocates to the nucleus, and together with interferon regulatory transcription factors, triggers phagocytosis accompanied by the release of proinflammatory mediators (table 1.1). These include the anti-viral interferons (cf. p. 275), the small protein **cytokines** interleukin-1β (IL-1β), IL-6, IL-12 and TNF (TNFα) (cf. p. 186) which activate other cells through binding to specific receptors, and **chemokines** such as IL-8 which represent a subset of chemoattractant cytokines.

Turning now to the sensing of infectious agents that have succeeded in gaining access to the interior of a cell, microbial nucleotide breakdown products can be recognized by the so-called NOD proteins and the typical CpG DNA motif binds to the endosomal TLR9. Other endosomal Toll-like receptors, TLR3 and TLR7/8, are responsive to intracellular viral RNA sequences.

In addition to activating phagocytosis, binding to PAMPs rapidly releases a group of diverse multifunctional host proteins which recruit and prime macrophages and dendritic cells for interaction with lymphocytes to initiate adaptive immune responses (which will be discussed in the following chapter) through differentiation of immature dendritic cells and upregulation of critical costimulatory molecules B7.1 and B7.2 (cf. p. 172). These potent immunostimulants, including defensins and cathelicidin, which are antimicrobial in their own right, serve as early-warning signals to alert innate and adaptive immune responses.

Programed cell death (apoptosis; see below) is an essential component of embryonic development and the maintenance of the normal physiologic state. The dead cells need to be removed by phagocytosis but since they do not herald any 'danger' this must be done silently without setting off the alarm bells. Accordingly, recognition of apoptotic cells by macrophages directly through the CD14 receptor and indirectly through the binding of C1q to surface nucleosome blebs (see p. 435) proceeds without provoking the release of proinflammatory mediators. In sharp contrast, cells which are injured by infection and become necrotic release endogenous heat-shock protein 60 which acts as a danger signal to the phagocytic cells and establishes a protective inflammatory response.

Microbes are engulfed by activated phagocytic cells

After adherence of the microbe to the surface of the neutrophil or macrophage through recognition of a PAMP (figure 1.6.2), the resulting signal (figure 1.6.3) initiates the ingestion phase by activating an actin–myosin contractile system which extends pseudopods around the particle (figures 1.6.4 and 1.7); as adjacent receptors sequentially attach to the surface of the microbe, the plasma membrane is pulled around the particle just like a 'zipper' until it is completely enclosed in a vacuole (phagosome; figures 1.6.5 and 1.8). Events are now moving smartly and, within 1 minute, the cytoplasmic granules fuse with the phagosome and discharge their contents around the imprisoned microorganism (figures 1.6.7 and 1.8) which is subject to a formidable battery of microbicidal mechanisms.

There is an array of killing mechanisms

Killing by reactive oxygen intermediates
Trouble starts for the invader from the moment phagocytosis is initiated. There is a dramatic increase in activity of the hexose monophosphate shunt generating reduced nicotinamide-adenine-dinucleotide phosphate

Table 1.1. Microbial PAMP 'danger signals' activate macrophages and dendritic cells through Toll-like receptors. Engagement of the PAMP complex with the cellular receptor stimulates intracellular reaction sequences leading to activation of NFκB and other transcription factors. The effector molecules induce phagocytosis and recruit and prime antigen-presenting cells for initiation of adaptive immune responses (cf. Chapter 2).

Toll-like receptor (TLR) — Recognize ⟶	Pathogen-associated molecular pattern (PAMP) — Produce ⟶	Transcription factors — Induce ⟶	Effector molecules
Cell surface TLR1 TLR1/TLR2 TLR2/TLR6	Gram+ve peptidoglycan Lipoproteins Mycobacterial lipoarabinomannan Yeast zymosan	IRF5 NFκB	Inflammatory cytokines
TLR4	Gram-ve LPS	IRF3 NFκB IRF5	IFNβ Inflammatory cytokines
TLR5	Flagellin	NFκB IRF5	Inflammatory cytokines
TLR10	Unknown	NFκB	Inflammatory cytokines
Endosomal TLR3	Viral dsRNA	IRF3 NFκB	IFNβ
TLR7/8	Viral ssRNA Imidazoquinolines (anti-viral drugs)	IRF7	IFNα
TLR9	Bacterial and viral CpG DNA Malarial hemozoin	NFκB IRF5	Inflammatory cytokines

IRF, interferon regulatory transcription factor.

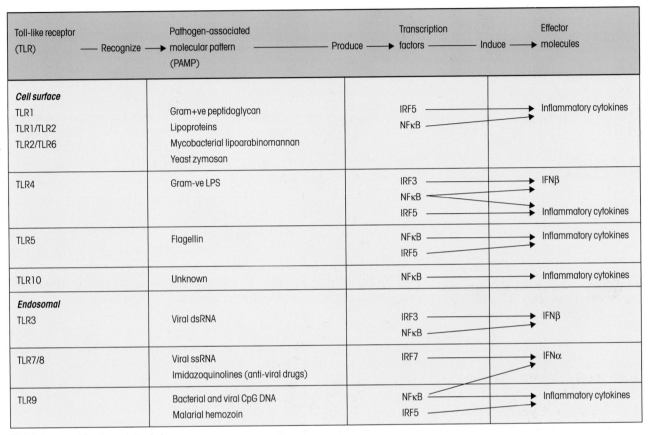

Figure 1.6. Phagocytosis and killing of a bacterium. Stage 3/4, respiratory burst and activation of NADPH oxidase; stage 5, damage by reactive oxygen intermediates; stage 6/7, damage by peroxidase, cationic proteins, antibiotic peptide defensins, lysozyme and lactoferrin.

1. BACTERIUM / PHAGOCYTE — Chemotaxis
2. Adherence through PAMP recognition
3. Membrane activation through 'danger' signal
4. Initiation of phagocytosis
5. GRANULES — Phagosome formation
6. Fusion
7. Killing and digestion
8. Release of degradation products

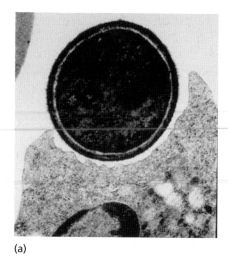

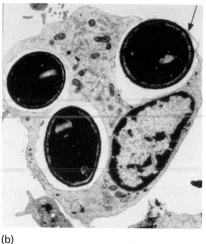

(a) (b)

Figure 1.7. Adherence and phagocytosis. (a) Phagocytosis of *Candida albicans* by a polymorphonuclear leukocyte (neutrophil). Adherence to the yeast wall surface mannan initiates enclosure of the fungal particle within arms of cytoplasm. Lysosomal granules are abundant but mitochondria are rare (×15 000). (b) Phagocytosis of *C. albicans* by a monocyte showing near completion of phagosome formation (arrowed) around one organism and complete ingestion of two others (×5000). (Courtesy of Dr H. Valdimarsson.)

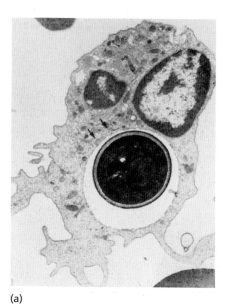

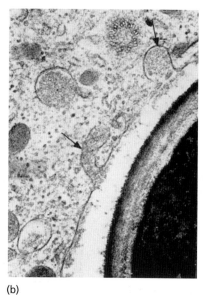

(a) (b)

Figure 1.8. Phagolysosome formation. (a) Neutrophil 30 minutes after ingestion of *C. albicans*. The cytoplasm is already partly degranulated and two lysosomal granules (arrowed) are fusing with the phagocytic vacuole. Two lobes of the nucleus are evident (×5000). (b) Higher magnification of (a) showing fusing granules discharging their contents into the phagocytic vacuole (arrowed) (×33 000). (Courtesy of Dr H. Valdimarsson.)

(NADPH). Electrons pass from the NADPH to a flavine adenine dinucleotide (FAD)-containing membrane flavoprotein and thence to a unique plasma membrane **cytochrome (cyt b_{558})**. This has the very low midpoint redox potential of –245 mV which allows it to reduce molecular oxygen directly to superoxide anion (figure 1.9a). Thus the key reaction catalyzed by this NADPH oxidase, which initiates the formation of reactive oxygen intermediates (ROI), is:

$$NADPH + O_2 \xrightarrow{\text{oxidase}} NADP^+ + \cdot O_2^- \quad \text{(superoxide anion)}$$

The superoxide anion undergoes conversion to hydrogen peroxide under the influence of superoxide dismutase, and subsequently to hydroxyl radicals ($\cdot$OH). Each of these products has remarkable chemical reactivity with a wide range of molecular targets, making them formidable microbicidal agents; $\cdot$OH in particular is one of the most reactive free radicals known. Furthermore, the combination of peroxide, myeloperoxidase and halide ions constitutes a potent halogenating system capable of killing both bacteria and viruses (figure 1.9a). Although H_2O_2 and the halogenated compounds are not as active as the free radicals, they are more stable and therefore diffuse further, making them toxic to microorganisms in the extracellular vicinity.

Killing by reactive nitrogen intermediates
Nitric oxide surfaced prominently as a physiologic mediator when it was shown to be identical with endothelium-derived relaxing factor. This has proved to be just one of its many roles (including the mediation of penile erection, would you believe it!), but of major interest in the present context is its formation by an inducible NO$\cdot$ synthase (iNOS) within most cells, but

particularly macrophages and human neutrophils, thereby generating a powerful antimicrobial system (figure 1.9b). Whereas the NADPH oxidase is dedicated to the killing of extracellular organisms taken up by phagocytosis and cornered within the phagocytic vacuole, the NO· mechanism can operate against microbes which invade the cytosol; so, it is not surprising that the majority of nonphagocytic cells which may be infected by viruses and other parasites are endowed with an iNOS capability. The mechanism of action may be through degradation of the Fe–S prosthetic groups of certain electron transport enzymes, depletion of iron and production of toxic ·ONOO radicals. The *N-ramp* gene linked with resistance to microbes such as bacille Calmette–Guérin (BCG), *Salmonella* and *Leishmania*, which can live within an intracellular habitat, is now known to express a protein forming a transmembrane channel which may be involved in transporting NO· across lysosome membranes.

Killing by preformed antimicrobials (figure 1.9c)
These molecules, contained within the neutrophil granules, contact the ingested microorganism when fusion with the phagosome occurs. The dismutation of superoxide consumes hydrogen ions and raises the pH of the vacuole gently, so allowing the family of cationic proteins and peptides to function optimally. The latter, known as **defensins**, are approximately 3.5–4 kDa and invariably rich in arginine, and reach incredibly high concentrations within the phagosome, of the order of

20–100 mg/ml. Like the bacterial colicins described above, they have an amphipathic structure which allows them to insert into microbial membranes to form destabilizing voltage-regulated ion channels (who copied whom?). These antibiotic peptides, at concentrations of 10–100 µg/ml, act as disinfectants against a wide spectrum of Gram-positive and -negative bacteria, many fungi and a number of enveloped viruses. Many exhibit remarkable selectivity for prokaryotic and eukaryotic microbes relative to host cells, partly dependent upon differential membrane lipid composition. One must be impressed by the ability of this surprisingly simple tool to discriminate large classes of nonself cells, i.e. microbes, from self.

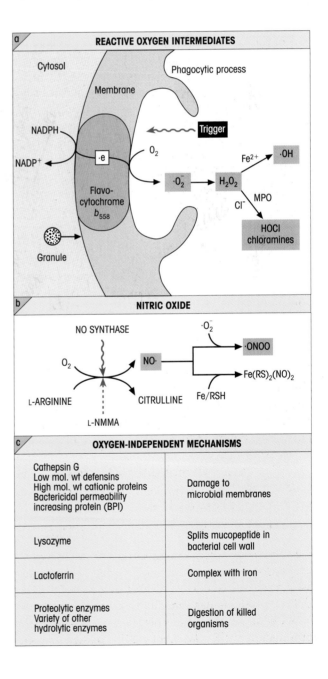

Figure 1.9. Microbicidal mechanisms of phagocytic cells. (a) Production of reactive oxygen intermediates. Electrons from NADPH are transferred by the flavocytochrome oxidase enzyme to molecular oxygen to form the microbicidal molecular species shown in the orange boxes. (*For the more studious*—The phagocytosis triggering agent binds to a classic G-protein-linked seven transmembrane domain receptor which activates an intracellular guanosine triphosphate (GTP)-binding protein. This in turn activates an array of enzymes: phosphoinositol-3 kinase concerned in the cytoskeletal reorganization underlying chemotactic responses (p. 10), phospholipase-Cγ2 mediating events leading to lysosome degranulation and phosphorylation of p47 phox through activation of protein kinase C, and the MEK and MAP kinase systems (cf. figure 8.7) which oversee the assembly of the NADPH oxidase. This is composed of the membrane cytochrome b_{558}, consisting of a p21 heme protein linked to gp91 with binding sites for NADPH and FAD on its intracellular aspect, to which phosphorylated p47 and p67 translocate from the cytosol on activation of the oxidase.) (b) Generation of nitric oxide. The enzyme, which structurally resembles the NADPH oxidase, can be inhibited by the arginine analog *N*-monomethyl-L-arginine (L-NMMA). The combination of NO· with superoxide anion yields the highly toxic peroxynitrite radical ·ONOO which cleaves on protonation to form reactive ·OH and NO_2 molecules. NO· can form mononuclear iron dithioldinitroso complexes leading to iron depletion and inhibition of several enzymes. (c) The basis of oxygen-independent antimicrobial systems.

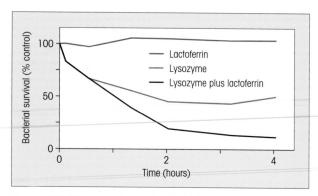

Figure 1.10. The synergistic microbicidal action of lysozyme and lactoferrin. (Reproduced with permission from Singh P.K. *et al.* (2000) *American Journal of Physiology* **279**, L799–L805.)

As if this was not enough, further damage is inflicted on the bacterial membranes both by neutral proteinase (cathepsin G) action and by direct transfer to the microbial surface of BPI, which increases bacterial permeability. Low pH, lysozyme and lactoferrin constitute bactericidal or bacteriostatic factors which are oxygen independent and can function under anaerobic circumstances. Interestingly, lysozyme and lactoferrin are synergistic in their action (figure 1.10). Finally, the killed organisms are digested by hydrolytic enzymes and the degradation products released to the exterior (figure 1.6.8).

By now, the reader may be excused a little smugness as she or he shelters behind the impressive antimicrobial potential of the phagocytic cells. But there are snags to consider; our formidable array of weaponry is useless unless the phagocyte can: (i) 'home onto' the microorganism, (ii) adhere to it, and (iii) respond by the membrane activation which initiates engulfment. Some bacteria do produce chemical substances, such as the peptide formyl.Met.Leu.Phe, which directionally attract leukocytes, a process known as **chemotaxis**; many organisms do adhere to the phagocyte surface and many do spontaneously provide the appropriate membrane initiation signal. However, our teeming microbial adversaries are continually mutating to produce new species which may outwit the defenses by doing none of these. What then? The body has solved these problems with the effortless ease that comes with a few million years of evolution by developing the **complement** system.

COMPLEMENT FACILITATES PHAGOCYTOSIS

Complement and its activation

Complement is the name given to a complex series of

some 20 proteins which, along with blood clotting, fibrinolysis and kinin formation, forms one of the triggered enzyme systems found in plasma. These systems characteristically produce a rapid, highly amplified response to a trigger stimulus mediated by a cascade phenomenon where the product of one reaction is the enzymic catalyst of the next.

Some of the complement components are designated by the letter 'C' followed by a number which is related more to the chronology of its discovery than to its position in the reaction sequence. The most abundant and the most pivotal component is C3 which has a molecular weight of 195 kDa and is present in plasma at a concentration of around 1.2 mg/ml.

C3 undergoes slow spontaneous cleavage

Under normal circumstances, an internal thiolester bond in C3 (figure 1.11) becomes activated spontaneously at a very slow rate, either through reaction with water or with trace amounts of a plasma proteolytic enzyme, to form a reactive intermediate, either the split product C3b, or a functionally similar molecule designated C3i or C3(H_2O). In the presence of Mg^{2+} this can complex with another complement component, factor B, which then undergoes cleavage by a normal plasma enzyme (factor D) to generate $\overline{C3bBb}$. Note that, conventionally, a bar over a complex denotes enzymic activity and that, on cleavage of a complement component, the larger product is generally given the suffix 'b' and the smaller 'a'.

$\overline{C3bBb}$ has an important new enzymic activity: it is a **C3 convertase** which can split C3 to give C3a and C3b. We will shortly discuss the important biological consequences of C3 cleavage in relation to microbial defenses, but under normal conditions there must be some mechanism to restrain this process to a 'tick-over' level since it can also give rise to more $\overline{C3bBb}$, that is, we are dealing with a potentially runaway **positive-feedback loop** (figure 1.12). As with all potentially explosive triggered cascades, there are powerful regulatory mechanisms.

C3b levels are normally tightly controlled

In solution, the $\overline{C3bBb}$ convertase is unstable and factor B is readily displaced by another component, factor H, to form C3bH which is susceptible to attack by the C3b inactivator, factor I (figure 1.12; further discussed on p. 314). The inactivated iC3b is biologically inactive and undergoes further degradation by proteases in the body fluids. Other regulatory mechanisms are discussed at a later stage (see p. 314).

C3 convertase is stabilized on microbial surfaces

A number of microorganisms can activate the $\overline{C3bBb}$

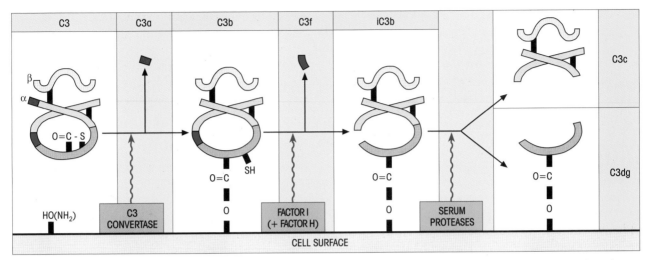

Figure 1.11. Structural basis for the cleavage of C3 by C3 convertase and its covalent binding to ·OH or ·NH₂ groups at the cell surface through exposure of the internal thiolester bonds. Further cleavage leaves the progressively smaller fragments, C3dg and C3d, attached to the membrane. (Based essentially on Law S.H.A. & Reid K.B.M. (1988) *Complement*, figure 2.4. IRL Press, Oxford.)

Figure 1.12. Microbial activation of the alternative complement pathway by stabilization of the C3 convertase (C3bBb), and its control by factors H and I. When bound to the surface of a host cell or in the fluid phase, the C3b in the convertase is said to be 'unprotected' in that its affinity for factor H is much greater than for factor B and is therefore susceptible to breakdown by factors H and I. On a microbial surface, C3b binds factor B more strongly than factor H and is therefore 'protected' from or 'stabilized' against cleavage—even more so when subsequently bound by properdin. Although in phylogenetic terms this is the oldest complement pathway, it was discovered after a separate pathway to be discussed in the next chapter, and so has the confusing designation 'alternative'. ∿➤ represents an activation process. The horizontal bar above a component designates its activation.

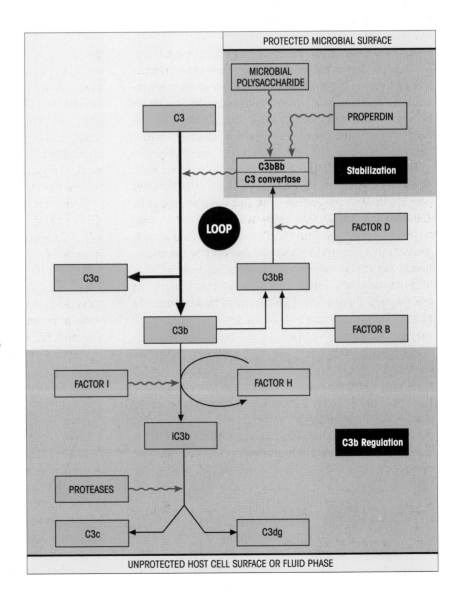

convertase to generate large amounts of C3 cleavage products by stabilizing the enzyme on their (carbohydrate) surfaces, thereby protecting the C3b from factor H. Another protein, properdin, acts subsequently on this bound convertase to stabilize it even further. As C3 is split by the surface membrane-bound enzyme to nascent C3b, it undergoes conformational change and its potentially reactive internal thiolester bond becomes exposed. Since the half-life of nascent C3b is less than 100 μsec, it can only diffuse a short distance before reacting covalently with local hydroxyl or amino groups available at the microbial cell surface (figure 1.11). Each catalytic site thereby leads to the clustering of large numbers of C3b molecules on the microorganism. This series of reactions leading to C3 breakdown provoked directly by microbes has been called **the alternative pathway** of complement activation (figure 1.12).

The post-C3 pathway generates a membrane attack complex

Recruitment of a further C3b molecule into the C3bBb enzymic complex generates a C5 convertase which activates C5 by proteolytic cleavage releasing a small polypeptide, C5a, and leaving the large C5b fragment loosely bound to C3b. Sequential attachment of C6 and C7 to C5b forms a complex with a transient membrane-binding site and an affinity for the β-peptide chain of C8. The C8α chain sits in the membrane and directs the conformational changes in C9 which transform it into an amphipathic molecule capable of insertion into the lipid bilayer (cf. the colicins, p. 1) and polymerization to an annular **membrane attack complex** (MAC; figures 1.13 and 2.4). This forms a transmembrane channel fully permeable to electrolytes and water, and due to the high internal colloid osmotic pressure of cells, there is a net influx of Na⁺ and water frequently leading to lysis.

Complement has a range of defensive biological functions

These can be grouped conveniently under three headings.

1 C3b adheres to complement receptors
Phagocytic cells have receptors for C3b (CR1) and iC3b (CR3) which facilitate the adherence of C3b-coated microorganisms to the cell surface (discussed more fully on p. 265).

2 Biologically active fragments are released
C3a and C5a, the small peptides split from the parent molecules during complement activation, have several

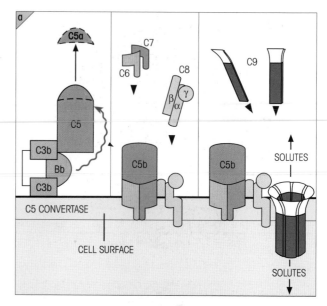

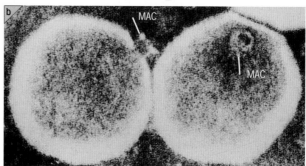

Figure 1.13. Post-C3 pathway generating C5a and the C5b–9 membrane attack complex (MAC). (a) Cartoon of molecular assembly. The conformational change in C9 protein structure which converts it from a hydrophilic to an amphipathic molecule (bearing both hydrophobic and hydrophilic regions) can be interrupted by an antibody raised against linear peptides derived from C9; since the antibody does not react with the soluble or membrane-bound forms of the molecule, it must be detecting an intermediate structure transiently revealed in a deep-seated structural rearrangement. (b) Electron micrograph of a membrane C5b–9 complex incorporated into liposomal membranes clearly showing the annular structure. The cylindrical complex is seen from the side inserted into the membrane of the liposome on the left, and end-on in that on the right. Although in itself a rather splendid structure, formation of the annular C9 cylinder is probably not essential for cytotoxic perturbation of the target cell membrane, since this can be achieved by insertion of amphipathic C9 molecules in numbers too few to form a clearly defined MAC. (Courtesy of Professor J. Tranum-Jensen and Dr S. Bhakdi.)

important actions. Both act directly on phagocytes, especially neutrophils, to stimulate the respiratory burst associated with the production of reactive oxygen intermediates and to enhance the expression of surface receptors for C3b and iC3b. Also, both are **anaphylatoxins** in that they are capable of triggering mediator

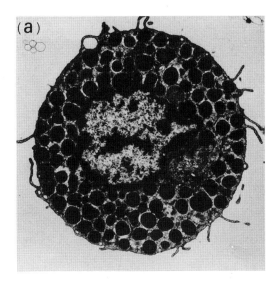

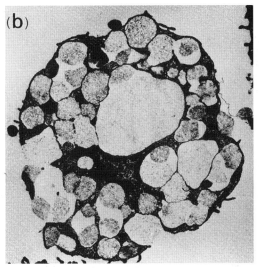

Figure 1.14. The mast cell. (a) A resting cell with many membrane-bound granules containing preformed mediators. (b) A triggered mast cell. Note that the granules have released their contents and are morphologically altered, being larger and less electron dense. Although most of the altered granules remain within the circumference of the cell, they are open to the extracellular space. (Electron micrographs ×5400.) (Courtesy of Drs D. Lawson, C. Fewtrell, B. Gomperts and M.C. Raff from (1975) *Journal of Experimental Medicine* **142**, 391.)

release from mast cells (figures 1.4k and 1.14) and their circulating counterpart, the basophil (figure 1.4i), a phenomenon of such relevance to our present discussion that we have presented details of the mediators and their actions in figure 1.15; note in particular the chemotactic properties of these mediators and their effects on blood vessels. In its own right, C3a is a chemoattractant for eosinophils whilst C5a is a potent neutrophil chemotactic agent and also has a striking ability to act directly on the capillary endothelium to

produce vasodilatation and increased permeability, an effect which seems to be prolonged by leukotriene B_4 released from activated mast cells, neutrophils and macrophages.

3 The terminal complex can induce membrane lesions
As described above, the insertion of the membrane attack complex into a membrane may bring about cell lysis. Providentially, complement is relatively inefficient at lysing the cell membranes of the autologous host due to the presence of control proteins (cf. p. 314).

COMPLEMENT CAN MEDIATE AN ACUTE INFLAMMATORY REACTION

We can now put together an effectively orchestrated defensive scenario initiated by activation of the alternative complement pathway (figure 1.16).

In the first act, $\overline{C3bBb}$ is stabilized on the surface of the microbe and cleaves large amounts of C3. The C3a fragment is released but C3b molecules bind copiously to the microbe. These activate the next step in the sequence to generate C5a and the membrane attack complex (although many organisms will be resistant to its action).

The mast cell plays a central role

The next act sees C3a and C5a, together with the mediators they trigger from the mast cell, acting to recruit polymorphonuclear phagocytes and further plasma complement components to the site of microbial invasion. The relaxation induced in arteriolar walls causes increased blood flow and dilatation of the small vessels, while contraction of capillary endothelial cells allows exudation of plasma proteins. Under the influence of the chemotaxins, neutrophils slow down and the surface adhesion molecules they are stimulated to express cause them to marginate to the walls of the capillaries where they pass through gaps between the endothelial cells (diapedesis) and move up the concentration gradient of chemotactic factors until they come face to face with the C3b-coated microbe. Adherence to the neutrophil C3b receptors then takes place, C3a and C5a at relatively high concentrations in the chemotactic gradient activate the respiratory burst and, hey presto, the slaughter of the last act can begin!

The processes of capillary dilatation (redness), exudation of plasma proteins and also of fluid (edema) due to hydrostatic and osmotic pressure changes, and accumulation of neutrophils are collectively termed the **acute inflammatory response**.

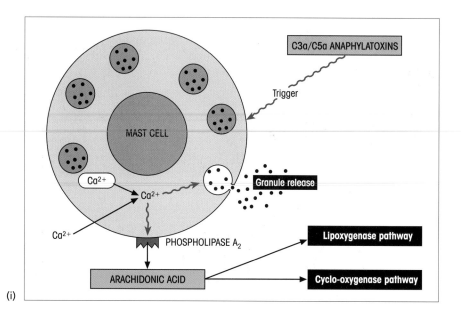

(i)

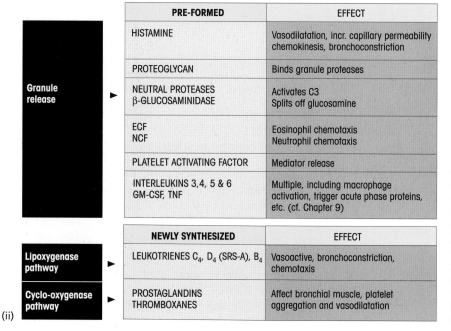

(ii)

Figure 1.15. Mast cell triggering leading to release of mediators by two major pathways: (i) release of preformed mediators present in the granules, and (ii) the metabolism of arachidonic acid produced through activation of a phospholipase. Intracellular Ca^{2+} and cyclic AMP are central to the initiation of these events but details are still unclear. Mast cell triggering may occur through C3a, C5a and even by some microorganisms which can act directly on cell surface receptors. Mast cell heterogeneity is discussed on p. 337. ECF, eosinophil chemotactic factor; GM-CSF, granulocyte–macrophage colony-stimulating factor; NCF, neutrophil chemotactic factor. Chemotaxis refers to directed migration of granulocytes up the pathway concentration gradient of the mediator.

Macrophages can also do it

Although not yet established with the same confidence that surrounds the role of the mast cell in acute inflammation, the concept seems to be emerging that the tissue macrophage may mediate a parallel series of events with the same final end result. Nonspecific phagocytic events and certain bacterial toxins such as the lipopolysaccharides (LPSs) can activate macrophages, but the phagocytosis of C3b-opsonized microbes and the direct action of C5a generated through complement activation are guaranteed to goad the cell into copious secretion of soluble mediators of the acute inflammatory response (figure 1.17).

These upregulate the expression of adhesion molecules for neutrophils on the surface of endothelial cells, increase capillary permeability and promote the chemotaxis and activation of the polymorphonuclear neutrophils themselves. Thus, under the stimulus of complement activation, the macrophage provides a pattern of cellular events which reinforces the mast cell-mediated pathway leading to acute inflammation—yet another of the body's fail-safe redundancy systems (often known as the 'belt and braces' principle).

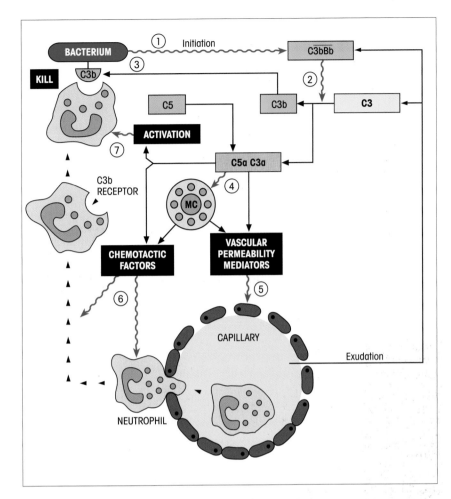

Figure 1.16. The defensive strategy of the acute inflammatory reaction initiated by bacterial activation of the alternative C pathway. Directions: ① start with the activation of the C3bBb C3 convertase by the bacterium, ② notice the generation of C3b (③ which binds to the bacterium), C3a and C5a, ④ which recruit mast cell mediators; ⑤ follow their effect on capillary dilatation and exudation of plasma proteins and ⑥ their chemotactic attraction of neutrophils to the C3b-coated bacterium and triumph in ⑦ the adherence and final activation of neutrophils for the kill.

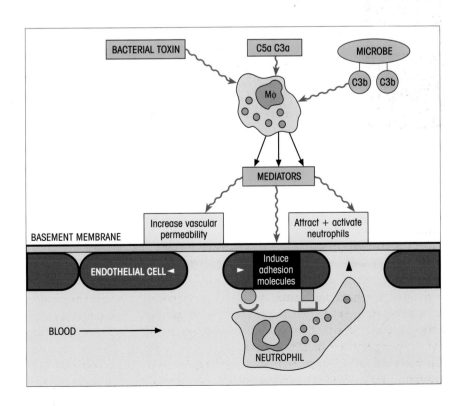

Figure 1.17. Stimulation by complement components and bacterial toxins such as LPS induces macrophage secretion of mediators of an acute inflammatory response. Blood neutrophils stick to the adhesion molecules on the endothelial cell and use this to provide traction as they force their way between the cells, through the basement membrane (with the help of secreted elastase) and up the chemotactic gradient.

HUMORAL MECHANISMS PROVIDE A SECOND DEFENSIVE STRATEGY

Microbicidal factors in secretions

Turning now to those defense systems which are mediated entirely by soluble factors, we recollect that many microbes activate the complement system and may be lysed by the insertion of the membrane attack complex. The spread of infection may be limited by enzymes released through tissue injury which activate the clotting system. Of the soluble bactericidal substances elaborated by the body, perhaps the most abundant and widespread is the enzyme lysozyme, a muramidase which splits the exposed peptidoglycan wall of susceptible bacteria (cf. figure 12.5).

Like the α-defensins of the neutrophil granules, the human β-defensins are peptides derived by proteolytic cleavage from larger precursors; they have β-sheet structures, 29–40 amino acids and three intramolecular disulfide bonds, although they differ from the α-defensins in the placement of their six cysteines. The main human β-defensin, hDB-1, is produced abundantly in the kidney, the female reproductive tract, the oral gingiva and especially the lung airways. Since the word has it that we are all infected every day by tens of thousands of airborne bacteria, this must be an important defense mechanism. This being so, inhibition of hDB-1 and of a second pulmonary defensin, hDB-2, by high ionic strength could account for the susceptibility of cystic fibrosis patients to infection since they have an ion channel mutation which results in an elevated chloride concentration in airway surface fluids. Another airway antimicrobial active against Gram-negative and -positive bacteria is LL-37, a 37-residue α-helical peptide released by proteolysis of a cathelicidin (cathepsin L-inhibitor) precursor.

This theme surfaces again in the stomach where a peptide split from lactoferrin by pepsin could provide the gastric and intestinal secretions with some antimicrobial policing. A rather longer two-domain peptide with 108 residues, termed secretory leukoprotease inhibitor (SLPI), is found in many human secretions. The C-terminal domain is anti-protease but the N-terminal domain is distinctly unpleasant to metabolically active fungal cells and to various skin-associated microorganisms, which makes its production by human keratinocytes particularly appropriate. In passing, it is worth pointing out that many D-amino acid analogs of peptide antibiotics form left-handed helices which retain the ability to induce membrane ion channels and hence their antimicrobial powers and, given their resistance to catabolism within the body, should be attractive candidates for a new breed of synthetic antibiotics.

Lastly, we may mention the two lung surfactant proteins SP-A and SP-D which, in conjunction with various lipids, lower the surface tension of the epithelial lining cells of the lung to keep the airways patent. They belong to a totally different structural group of molecules termed collectins (see below) which contribute to innate immunity through binding of their lectin-like domains to carbohydrates on microbes, and their collagenous stem to cognate receptors on phagocytic cells—thereby facilitating the ingestion and killing of the infectious agents.

Acute phase proteins increase in response to infection

A number of plasma proteins collectively termed acute phase proteins show a dramatic increase in concentration in response to early 'alarm' mediators such as macrophage-derived interleukin-1 (IL-1) released as a result of infection or tissue injury. These include C-reactive protein (CRP), mannose-binding lectin (MBL) and serum amyloid P component (table 1.2). Other acute phase proteins showing a more modest rise in concentration include α₁-antichymotrypsin, fibrinogen, ceruloplasmin, C9 and factor B. Overall, it seems likely that the acute phase response achieves a beneficial effect through enhancing host resistance, minimizing tissue injury and promoting the resolution and repair of the inflammatory lesion.

To take an example, during an infection, microbial products such as endotoxins stimulate the release of

Table 1.2 Acute phase proteins.

Acute phase reactant	Role
Dramatic increases in concentration:	
C-reactive protein	Fixes complement, opsonizes
Mannose binding lectin	Fixes complement, opsonizes
α₁-acid glycoprotein	Transport protein
Serum amyloid P component	Amyloid component precursor
Moderate increases in concentration:	
α₁-proteinase inhibitors	Inhibit bacterial proteases
α₁-antichymotrypsin	Inhibit bacterial proteases
C3, C9, factor B	Increase complement function
Ceruloplasmin	·O₂⁻ scavenger
Fibrinogen	Coagulation
Angiotensin	Blood pressure
Haptoglobin	Bind hemoglobin
Fibronectin	Cell attachment

IL-1, which is an endogenous pyrogen (incidentally capable of improving our general defenses by raising the body temperature), and IL-6. These in turn act on the liver to increase the synthesis and secretion of CRP to such an extent that its plasma concentration may rise 1000-fold.

Human CRP is composed of five identical polypeptide units noncovalently arranged as a cyclic pentamer around a Ca-binding cavity. These protein **pentraxins** have been around in the animal kingdom for some time, since a closely related homolog, limulin, is present in the hemolymph of the horseshoe crab, not exactly a close relative of *Homo sapiens*. A major property of CRP is its ability to bind in a Ca-dependent fashion, as a pattern recognition molecule, to a number of microorganisms which contain phosphorylcholine in their membranes, the complex having the useful property of activating complement (by the classical and not the alternative pathway with which we are at present familiar). This results in the deposition of C3b on the surface of the microbe which thus becomes **opsonized** (i.e. 'made ready for the table') for adherence to phagocytes.

Yet another member of this pentameric family is the serum amyloid P (SAP) component. This protein can complex with chondroitin sulfate, a cell matrix glycosaminoglycan, and subsequently bind lysosomal enzymes such as cathepsin B released within a focus of inflammation. The degraded SAP becomes a component of the amyloid fibrillar deposits which accompany chronic infections—it might even be a key initiator of amyloid deposition (cf. p. 395).

A most important acute phase opsonin is the Ca-dependent **mannose-binding lectin (MBL)** which can react not only with mannose but several other sugars, so enabling it to bind with an exceptionally wide variety of Gram-negative and -positive bacteria, yeasts, viruses and parasites; its subsequent ability to trigger the classical C3 convertase through two novel associated serine proteases (MASP-1 and MASP-2) is the basis of what is known as the **lectin pathway** of complement activation. (Please relax, we unravel the secrets of the classical and lectin pathways in the next chapter.) MBL is a multiple of trimeric complexes, each unit of which contains a collagen-like region joined to a globular lectin-binding domain. This structure places it in the family of **collectins** (**col**lagen + **lectin**) which have the ability to recognize 'foreign' carbohydrate patterns differing from 'self' surface polysaccharides, normally terminal galactose and sialic acid groups, whilst the collagen region can bind to and activate phagocytic cells through complementary receptors on their surface. The collectins, especially MBL and the alveolar surfactant molecules SP-A and SP-D mentioned earlier, have many attributes that qualify them for a first-line role in innate immunity.

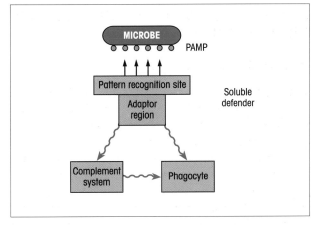

Figure 1.18. A major defensive strategy by soluble factors. The pattern recognition elements (PRRs) link the microorganism to a microbicidal system through the adaptor region. PAMP, pathogen-associated molecular pattern.

These include the ability to differentiate self from nonself, to bind to a variety of microbes, to generate secondary effector mechanisms, and to be widely distributed throughout the body including mucosal secretions. They are of course the soluble counterparts to the cell surface C-type lectins and other pattern recognition receptors described earlier.

Interest in the collectin conglutinin has perked up recently with the demonstration, first, that it is found in humans and not just in cows, and second, that it can bind to *N*-acetylglucosamine; being polyvalent, this implies an ability to coat bacteria with C3b by cross-linking the available sugar residue in the complement fragment with the bacterial proteoglycan. Although it is not clear whether conglutinin is a member of the acute phase protein family, we mention it here because it embellishes the general idea that the evolution of lectin-like molecules which bind to microbial rather than self polysaccharides, and which can then hitch themselves to the complement system or to phagocytic cells, has proved to be such a useful form of protection for the host (figure 1.18).

Interferons inhibit viral replication

These are a family of broad-spectrum antiviral agents present in birds, reptiles and fishes as well as the higher animals, and first recognized by the phenomenon of viral interference in which an animal infected with one virus resists superinfection by a second unrelated virus. Different molecular forms of interferon have been identified, all of which have been gene cloned. There are at least 14 different α-interferons (IFNα) produced by leukocytes, while fibroblasts, and probably all cell types, synthesize IFNβ. We will keep a third type (IFNγ), which is not directly induced by viruses, up our sleeves for the moment.

Cells synthesize interferon when infected by a virus and secrete it into the extracellular fluid where it binds to specific receptors on uninfected neighboring cells. The bound interferon now exerts its antiviral effect in the following way. At least two genes are thought to be derepressed in the interferon-treated cell allowing the synthesis of two new enzymes. The first, a protein kinase, catalyzes the phosphorylation of a ribosomal protein and an initiation factor necessary for protein synthesis, so greatly reducing mRNA translation. The other catalyzes the formation of a short polymer of adenylic acid which activates a latent endonuclease; this in turn degrades both viral and host mRNA.

Whatever the precise mechanism of action ultimately proves to be, the net result is to establish a cordon of uninfectable cells around the site of virus infection so restraining its spread. The effectiveness of interferon *in vivo* may be inferred from experiments in which mice injected with an antiserum to murine interferons could be killed by several hundred times less virus than was needed to kill the controls. However, it must be presumed that interferon plays a significant role in the recovery from, as distinct from the prevention of, viral infections.

As a group, the interferons may prove to have a wider biological role than the control of viral infection. It will be clear, for example, that the induced enzymes described above would act to inhibit host cell division just as effectively as viral replication. The interferons may also modulate the activity of other cells, such as the natural killer cells, to be discussed in the following section.

EXTRACELLULAR KILLING

Natural killer (NK) cells

Viruses lack the apparatus for self renewal and so it is essential for them to penetrate the cells of the infected host in order to take over its replicative machinery. It is clearly in the interest of the host to find a way to kill such infected cells before the virus has had a chance to reproduce. NK cells appear to do just that when studied *in vitro*.

They are large granular leukocytes (figure 2.6a) with a characteristic morphology (figure 2.7b). Killer and target are brought into close opposition (figure 1.19) through recognition by lectin-like (i.e. carbohydrate-binding) and other receptors on the NK cell (cf. p. 27) of structures on high molecular weight glycoproteins on the surface of virally infected cells. Activation of the NK cell ensues and leads to polarization of granules between nucleus and target within minutes and extra-

cellular release of their contents into the space between the two cells followed by target cell death.

One of the most important of the granule components is a **perforin** or cytolysin bearing some structural homology to C9; like that protein, but without any help other than from Ca^{2+}, it can insert itself into the membrane of the target, apparently by binding to phosphorylcholine through its central amphipathic domain. It then polymerizes to form a transmembrane pore with an annular structure, comparable to the complement membrane attack complex (figure 1.19).

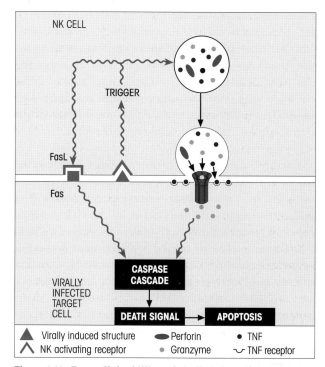

Figure 1.19. **Extracellular killing of virally infected cell by natural killer (NK) cell.** Binding of the NK receptors to the surface of the virally infected cell triggers the extracellular release of perforin molecules from the granules; these polymerize to form transmembrane channels which may facilitate lysis of the target by permitting entry of granzymes which induce apoptotic cell death through activation of the caspase protease cascade and ultimate fragmentation of nuclear DNA. (Model resembling that proposed by Hudig D., Ewoldt G.R. & Woodward S.L. (1993) *Current Opinion in Immunology* **5**, 90.) Another granule component, TNF, activates caspase-dependent apoptosis through the 'death domains' of the surface TNF receptors on the target cell. Engagement of the NK receptor also activates a parallel killing mechanism mediated through the binding of the Fas-ligand (FasL) on the effector to the target cell Fas receptor whose cytoplasmic death domains activate procaspase-8. Because apoptosis is such a fundamental 'default' mechanism in every cell, it is crucial for there to be heavy regulation: thus a large group of regulatory proteins, the Bcl-2 subfamily, inhibit apoptosis while the Bax and BH3 subfamilies promote it. The word 'apoptosis' in ancient Greek describes the falling of leaves from trees or of petals from flowers and aptly illustrates apoptosis in cells where they detach from their extracellular matrix support structures. (See figure 11.8 for morphological appearance of apoptotic cells.)

Target cells are told to commit suicide

Whereas C9-induced cell lysis is brought about through damage to outer membranes followed later by nuclear changes, NK cells kill by activating **apoptosis** (programed cell death), a mechanism present in every cell which leads to self immolation. Apoptosis is mediated by a cascade of proteolytic enzymes termed **caspases**. Like other multicomponent cascades, such as the blood clotting and complement systems, it depends upon the activation by proteolytic cleavage of a proenzyme next in the chain, and so on. The sequence terminates with very rapid nuclear fragmentation effected by a Ca-dependent endonuclease which acts on the vulnerable DNA between nucleosomes to produce the 200 kb 'nucleosome ladder' fragments; only afterwards can one detect release of ^{51}Cr-labeled cytoplasmic proteins through defective cell surface membranes. These nuclear changes are not produced by C9. Thus, although perforin and C9 appear to produce comparable membrane 'pores', there is a dramatic difference in their killing mechanisms.

In addition to perforin, the granules contain tumor necrosis factor (TNFα), lymphotoxin-β, IFNγ and a family of serine proteases termed **granzymes**, one of which, granzyme B, can function as an NK cytotoxic factor by passing through the perforin membrane pore into the cytoplasm where it can split procaspase-8 and activate the apoptotic process. Tumor necrosis factor can induce apoptotic cell death through reaction with cell surface TNF receptors whose cytoplasmic 'death domains' can also activate procaspase-8. Chondroitin sulfate A, a protease-resistant highly negatively charged proteoglycan present in the granules, may subserve the function of protecting the NK cell from autolysis by its own lethal agents.

Killing by NK cells can still occur in perforin-deficient mice, probably through a parallel mechanism involving **Fas** receptor molecules on the target cell surface. Engagement of Fas by the so-called **Fas-ligand (FasL)** on the effector cell provides yet another pathway for the induction of an apoptotic signal in the unlucky target.

The various interferons augment NK cytotoxicity and, since interferons are produced by virally infected cells, we have a nicely integrated feedback defense system.

Eosinophils

Large parasites such as helminths cannot physically be phagocytosed and extracellular killing by eosinophils would seem to have evolved to help cope with this situation. These polymorphonuclear 'cousins' of the neutrophil have distinctive granules which stain avidly with acid dyes (figure 1.4c) and have a characteristic appearance in the electron microscope (figure 12.23). A major basic protein is localized in the core of the granules while an eosinophilic cationic protein together with a peroxidase have been identified in the granule matrix. Other enzymes include arylsulfatase B, phospholipase D and histaminase. They have surface receptors for C3b and on activation produce a particularly impressive respiratory burst with concomitant generation of active oxygen metabolites. Not satisfied with that, nature has also armed the cell with granule proteins capable of producing a transmembrane plug in the target membrane like C9 and the NK perforin. Quite a nasty cell.

Most helminths can activate the alternative complement pathway, but although resistant to C9 attack, their coating with C3b allows adherence of eosinophils through their C3b receptors. If this contact should lead to activation, the eosinophil will launch its extracellular attack which includes the release of the major basic protein and especially the cationic protein which damages the parasite membrane.

SUMMARY

A wide range of innate immune mechanisms operate which do not improve with repeated exposure to infection.

Barriers against infection

• Microorganisms are kept out of the body by the skin, the secretion of mucus, ciliary action, the lavaging action of bactericidal fluids (e.g. tears), gastric acid and microbial antagonism.
• If penetration occurs, bacteria are destroyed by soluble factors such as lysozyme and by phagocytosis with intracellular digestion.

Phagocytic cells kill microorganisms

• The main phagocytic cells are polymorphonuclear neutrophils and macrophages.
• The phagocytic cells use their pattern recognition receptors (PRRs) to recognize and adhere to pathogen-associated molecular patterns (PAMPs) on the microbe surface.

(Continued p.20)

- PRRs include Toll-like, C-type and scavenger receptors.
- Organisms adhering to the phagocyte surface activate the engulfment process and are taken inside the cell where they fuse with cytoplasmic granules.
- A formidable array of microbicidal mechanisms then come into play: the conversion of O_2 to reactive oxygen intermediates, the synthesis of nitric oxide and the release of multiple oxygen-independent factors from the granules.
- Adherence to PRRs on dendritic cells initiates adaptive immune processes (see Chapter 2).

Complement facilitates phagocytosis

- The complement system, a multicomponent triggered enzyme cascade, is used to attract phagocytic cells to the microbes and engulf them.
- In what is known as the alternative complement pathway, the most abundant component, C3, is split by a convertase enzyme formed from its own cleavage product C3b and factor B and stabilized against breakdown caused by factors H and I, through association with the microbial surface. As it is formed, C3b becomes linked covalently to the microorganism and acts as an opsonin.
- The next component, C5, is activated yielding a small peptide, C5a; the residual C5b binds to the surface and assembles the terminal components C6–9 into a membrane attack complex which is freely permeable to solutes and can lead to osmotic lysis.
- C5a is a potent chemotactic agent for neutrophils and greatly increases capillary permeability.
- C3a and C5a act on mast cells causing the release of further mediators, such as histamine, leukotriene B_4 and tumor necrosis factor (TNF), with effects on capillary permeability and adhesiveness, and neutrophil chemotaxis; they also activate neutrophils.

The complement-mediated acute inflammatory reaction

- Following the activation of complement with the ensuing attraction and stimulation of neutrophils, the activated phagocytes bind to the C3b-coated microbes by their surface C3b receptors and may then ingest them. The influx of polymorphs and the increase in vascular permeability constitute the potent antimicrobial **acute inflammatory response** (figure 2.18).
- Inflammation can also be initiated by tissue macrophages which subserve a similar role to the mast cell, since signaling by bacterial toxins, C5a or iC3b-coated bacteria adhering to surface complement receptors causes release of neutrophil chemotactic and activating factors.

Humoral mechanisms provide a second defensive strategy

- In addition to lysozyme, peptide defensins and the complement system, other humoral defenses involve the acute phase proteins, such as C-reactive and mannose-binding proteins, whose synthesis is greatly augmented by infection. Mannose-binding lectin generates a complement pathway which is distinct from the alternative pathway in its early reactions, as will be discussed in chapter 2. It is a member of the collectin family which includes conglutinin and surfactants SP-A and SP-D, notable for their ability to distinguish microbial from 'self' surface carbohydrate groups by their pattern recognition molecules.
- Recovery from viral infections can be effected by the interferons which block viral replication.

Extracellular killing

- Virally infected cells can be killed by natural killer (NK) cells through a perforin/granzyme and a separate Fas-mediated pathway, leading to programed cell death (apoptosis) mediated by activation of the caspase protease cascade which fragments the nuclear DNA.
- Extracellular killing by C3b-bound eosinophils may be responsible for the failure of many large parasites to establish a foothold in potential hosts.

2 Specific acquired immunity

INTRODUCTION

Our microbial adversaries have tremendous opportunities through mutation to evolve strategies which evade our innate immune defenses. For example, most of the *successful* parasites activate the alternative complement pathway and bind C3b, yet eosinophils which adhere are somehow not triggered into offensive action. The same holds true for many bacteria, while some may so shape their exteriors as to avoid complement activation completely. The body obviously needed to 'devise' defense mechanisms which could be dovetailed individually to each of these organisms no matter how many there were. In other words *a very large number* of **specific immune defenses** needed to be at the body's disposal. Quite a tall order!

ANTIBODY — THE SPECIFIC ADAPTOR

Evolutionary processes came up with what can only be described as a brilliant solution. This was to fashion an adaptor molecule which was intrinsically capable not only of activating the complement system *and* of stimulating phagocytic cells, but also of sticking to the offending microbe. The adaptor thus had three main regions, two concerned with communicating with complement and the phagocytes (the biological functions) and one devoted to binding to an individual microorganism (the external recognition function). In most biological systems like hormones and receptors, and enzymes and substrates, recognition usually occurs through fairly accurate complementarity in shape allowing the ligands to approach so close to each other as to permit the normal intermolecular forces to become relatively strong. In the present case, each adaptor would have a recognition portion complementary in shape to some

microorganism to which it could then bind reasonably firmly. The part of the adaptor with biological function would be constant, but for each of hundreds of thousands of different organisms, a special recognition portion would be needed.

Thus the body has to make hundreds of thousands, or even millions, of **adaptors with different recognition sites**. The adaptor is of course the molecule we know affectionately as **antibody** (figure 2.1).

Antibody initiates a new complement pathway ('classical')

Antibody, when bound to a microbe, will link to the first molecule in the so-called **classical complement sequence**, C1q, and trigger the latent proteolytic activity of the C1 complex (figure 2.2). This then dutifully plays its role in the amplifying cascade by acting on components C4 and C2 to generate many molecules of $\overline{\text{C4b2a}}$, a new **C3-splitting enzyme** (figure 2.3).

The molecular events responsible for this seem to be rather clear. C1q is polyvalent with respect to antibody binding and consists of a central collagen-like stem branching into six peptide chains each tipped by an antibody-binding subunit (resembling the blooms on a bouquet of flowers). C1q is associated with two further subunits, C1r and C1s, in a Ca^{2+}-stabilized trimolecular complex (figure 2.2). Both these molecules contain repeats of a 60-amino acid unit folded as a globular domain and referred to as a complement control protein (CCP) repeat since it is a characteristic structural feature of several proteins involved in control of the complement system. Changes in C1q consequent upon binding the antigen–antibody complex bring about the sequential activation of proteolytic activity in C1r and then C1s.

The next component in the chain, C4 (unfortunately components were numbered before the sequence was

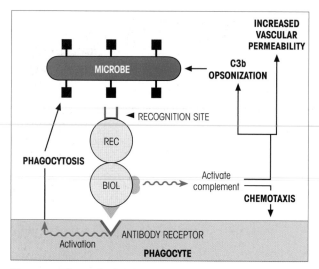

Figure 2.1. The antibody adaptor molecule. The constant part with biological function (BIOL) activates complement and the phagocyte. The portion with the recognition unit for the foreign microbe (REC) varies from one antibody to another.

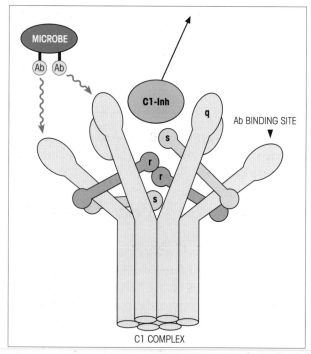

Figure 2.2. Activation of the classical complement pathway. C1 is composed of C1q associated with the flexible rod-like Ca-dependent complex, $C1r_2$–$C1s_2$ (ⓢ—◯◯—ⓡⓡ—◯◯—ⓢ ; s and r indicate potential serine protease active sites), which interdigitates with the six arms of C1q, either as indicated or as 'W' shapes on the outer side of these arms. The C1-inhibitor normally prevents spontaneous activation of $C1r_2$–$C1s_2$. If the complex of a microbe or antigen with antibodies attaches two or more of the globular Ab-binding sites on C1q, the molecule presumably undergoes conformational change which releases the C1–Inh and activates $C1r_2$–$C1s_2$.

established), now binds to C1 through these CCPs and is cleaved enzymically by $C\overline{1s}$. As expected in a multienzyme cascade, several molecules of C4 undergo cleavage, each releasing a small C4a fragment and revealing a nascent labile internal thiolester bond in the residual $C\overline{4b}$ like that in C3 (cf. figure 1.11) which may then bind either to the antibody–C1 complex or the surface of the microbe itself. Note that C4a, like C5a and C3a, has anaphylatoxin activity, although feeble, and C4b resembles C3b in its opsonic activity. In the presence of Mg^{2+}, C2 can complex with the $C\overline{4b}$ to become a new substrate for the $C\overline{1s}$, the resulting product $C\overline{4b2a}$ now has the vital C3 convertase activity required to cleave C3.

This classical pathway C3 convertase has the same specificity as the $C\overline{3bBb}$ generated by the alternative pathway, likewise producing the same C3a and C3b fragments. Activation of a single C1 complex can bring about the proteolysis of literally thousands of C3 molecules. From then on things march along exactly in parallel to the post-C3 pathway with one molecule of C3b added to the $C\overline{4b2a}$ to make it into a C5-splitting enzyme with eventual production of the **membrane attack complex** (figures 1.13 and 2.4). Just as the alternative pathway C3 convertase is controlled by factors H and I, so the breakdown of $C\overline{4b2a}$ is brought about by either a C4-binding protein (C4bp) or a cell surface C3b receptor (CR1) in the presence of factor I.

The mannose-binding lectin and classical complement pathways merge

It is appropriate at this stage to recall the activation of complement by innate immune mechanisms involving mannose-binding lectin (MBL) (cf. p. 17). On complexing with a microbe, MBL associates with and activates the latent proteolytic activity of the serum proteases, MASP-1 and 2, which structurally resemble C1r and C1s respectively. In an entirely parallel fashion, the complex splits C4 and C2 to generate the classical pathway C3 convertase.

The similarities between the pathways are set out in figure 2.3 and show how antibody can supplement and even improve on the ability of the innate immune system to initiate **acute inflammatory reactions** through its ability to recognize a multitude of different microbes. Human antibodies are divided into five main classes: immunoglobulin M (shortened to IgM), IgG, IgA, IgE and IgD, which differ in the specialization of their 'rear ends' for different biological functions such as complement activation or mast cell sensitization. The ability of immunoglobulin E antibodies to sensitize mast cells through binding to their specific surface receptors so that combination with antigen triggers

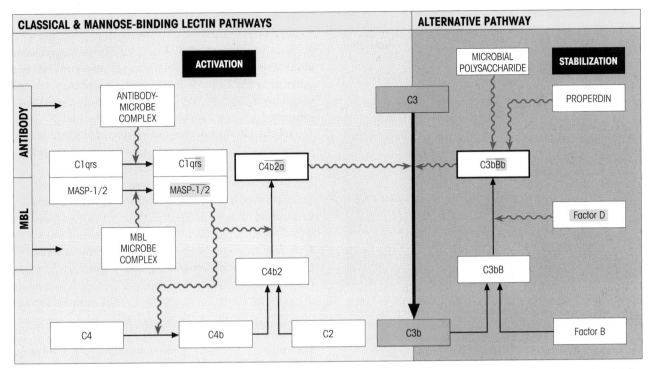

Figure 2.3. Comparison of the alternative, classical and mannose-binding lectin complement pathways. The classical pathway is activated by antibody whereas the alternative and MBL pathways are not. The molecular units with protease activity are highlighted, the enzymic domains showing considerable homology. Beware confusion with nomenclature; the large C2 fragment which forms the C3 conver-tase is designated as C2a, but to be consistent with C4b, C3b and C5b, it would have been more logical to call it C2b. Note that C-reactive protein (p. 17), on binding to microbial phosphorylcholine, can trigger the classical pathway. Mannose-binding lectin, when combined with microbial surface carbohydrate, associates with the serine proteases MASP-1 and 2 (p. 17) which split C4 and C2.

mediator release independently of C3a or C5a (cf. figure 1.15), adds yet more flexibility to our mechanisms for generating inflammatory responses.

Complexed antibody activates phagocytic cells

We drew attention to the fact that some C3b-coated organisms may adhere to phagocytic cells and yet avoid provoking their uptake. If small amounts of antibody are added the phagocyte springs into action. It does so through the recognition of two or more antibody molecules bound to the microbe, using specialized receptors on the cell surface.

A single antibody molecule complexed to the microorganism is not enough because it cannot cause the cross-linking of antibody receptors on the phagocyte surface membrane which is required to activate the cell. There is a further consideration connected with what is often called **the bonus effect of multivalency**; for thermodynamic reasons, which will be touched on in Chapter 5, the association constant of ligands, which use several rather than a single bond to react with receptors, is increased geometrically rather than arithmetically. For example, three antibodies bound close together on a

bacterium could be attracted to a macrophage a thousand times more strongly than a single antibody molecule (figure 2.5).

CELLULAR BASIS OF ANTIBODY PRODUCTION

Antibodies are made by lymphocytes

The majority of resting **lymphocytes** are small cells with a darkly staining nucleus due to condensed chromatin and relatively little cytoplasm containing the odd mitochondrion required for basic energy provision. Figures 2.6 and 2.7 compare the morphology of these cells with that of the minority population of **large granular leukocytes** which includes the natural killer (NK) set referred to in Chapter 1.

The central role of the **small lymphocyte** in the production of antibody was established largely by the work of Gowans. He depleted rats of their lymphocytes by chronic drainage of lymph from the thoracic duct by an indwelling cannula, and showed that they had a grossly impaired ability to mount an antibody response to microbial challenge. The ability to form antibody could be restored by injecting thoracic duct

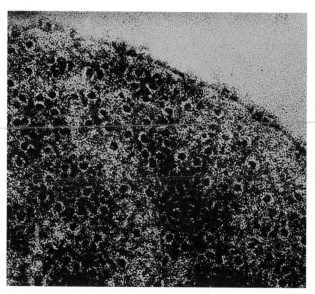

Figure 2.4. Multiple lesions in cell wall of *Escherichia coli* bacterium caused by interaction with IgM antibody and complement. Each lesion is caused by a single IgM molecule and shows as a 'dark pit' due to penetration by the 'negative stain'. This is somewhat of an illusion since in reality these 'pits' are like volcano craters standing proud of the surface, and are each single 'membrane attack' complexes. Comparable results may be obtained in the absence of antibody since the cell wall endotoxin can activate the alternative pathway in the presence of higher concentration of serum (×400 000). (Courtesy of Drs R. Dourmashkin and J.H. Humphrey.)

lymphocytes obtained from another rat. The same effect could be obtained if, before injection, the thoracic duct cells were first incubated at 37°C for 24 hours under conditions which kill off large- and medium-sized cells and leave only the small lymphocytes. This shows that the small lymphocyte is necessary for the **antibody response**.

The small lymphocytes can be labeled if the donor rat is previously injected with tritiated thymidine; it then becomes possible to follow the fate of these lymphocytes when transferred to another rat of the same strain which is then injected with microorganisms to produce an antibody response (figure 2.8). It transpires that after contact with the injected microbes, some of the transferred labeled lymphocytes develop into **plasma cells** (figures 2.6d and 2.9) which can be shown to contain (figure 2.6e) and secrete antibody.

Antigen selects the lymphocytes which make antibody

The molecules in the microorganisms which evoke and react with antibodies are called **antigens** (**gen**erates **anti**bodies). We now know that antibodies are formed before antigen is ever seen and that they are **selected** for by antigen.

It works in the following way. Each lymphocyte of a subset called the **B-lymphocytes**, because they differentiate in the *bone marrow*, is programed to make one, and only one, antibody and it places this antibody on its outer surface to act as a receptor. This can be detected by

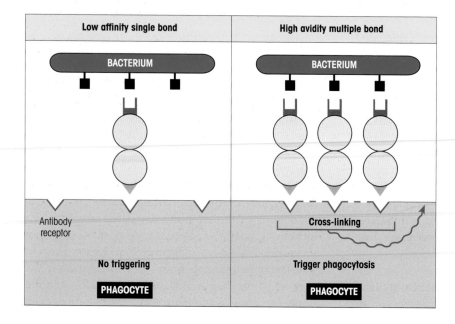

Figure 2.5. Binding of bacterium to phagocyte by multiple antibodies gives strong association forces and triggers phagocytosis by cross-linking the surface receptors for antibody.

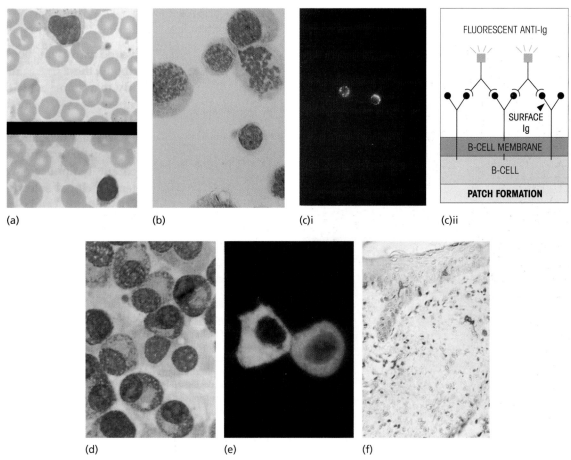

(a)   (b)   (c)i   (c)ii

(d)   (e)   (f)

Figure 2.6. Cells involved in the acquired immune response. (a) Small lymphocytes. Condensed chromatin gives rise to heavy staining of the nucleus. The cell on the bottom is a typical resting agranular T-cell with a thin rim of cytoplasm. The upper nucleated cell is a large granular lymphocyte; it has more cytoplasm and azurophilic granules are evident. Isolated platelets are visible. B-lymphocytes range from small to intermediate in size and lack granules. Giemsa stain. (b) Transformed T-lymphocytes (lymphoblasts) following stimulation of lymphocytes in culture with a polyclonal activator, such as the lectins phytohemagglutinin, concanavalin A and pokeweed mitogen which stimulate a wide range of cells independently of their specificity for antigen. The large lymphoblasts with their relatively high ratio of cytoplasm to nucleus may be compared in size with the isolated small lymphocyte. One cell is in mitosis. May–Grünwald–Giemsa. (c) Immunofluorescent staining of B-lymphocyte surface immunoglobulin using fluorescein-conjugated (■) anti-Ig. Provided the reaction is carried out in the cold to prevent pinocytosis, the labeled antibody cannot penetrate to the interior of the viable lymphocytes and reacts only with surface components. Patches of aggregated surface Ig are seen which are beginning to form a cap in the right-hand lymphocyte. During cap formation, submembranous myosin becomes redistributed in association with the surface Ig and induces locomotion of the previously sessile cell in a direction away from the cap. (d) Plasma cells. The nucleus is eccentric. The cytoplasm is strongly basophilic due to high RNA content. The juxtanuclear lightly stained zone corresponds with the Golgi region. May–Grünwald–Giemsa. (e) Plasma cells stained to show intracellular immunoglobulin using a fluorescein-labeled anti-IgG (green) and a rhodamine-conjugated anti-IgM (red). (f) Langerhans' cells in human epidermis in leprosy, increased in the subepidermal zone, possibly as a consequence of the disease process. Stained red by the immunoperoxidase method with S-100 antibodies. (Material for (a) was kindly supplied by Mr M. Watts of the Department of Haematology, Middlesex Hospital Medical School; (b) and (c) by Professor P. Lydyard; (d) and (e) by Professor C. Grossi; and (f) by Dr Marian Ridley.)

using fluorescent probes and, in figure 2.6c, one can see the molecules of antibody on the surface of a human B-lymphocyte stained with a fluorescent rabbit antiserum raised against a preparation of human antibodies. Each lymphocyte has of the order of 10^5 identical antibody molecules on its surface.

When an antigen enters the body, it is confronted by a dazzling array of lymphocytes all bearing different anti-bodies each with its own individual recognition site. The antigen will only bind to those receptors with which it makes a good fit. Lymphocytes whose receptors have bound antigen receive a triggering signal and develop into antibody-forming plasma cells and, since the lymphocytes are programed to make only one antibody, that secreted by the plasma cell will be identical with that originally acting as the lymphocyte receptor, i.e. it will

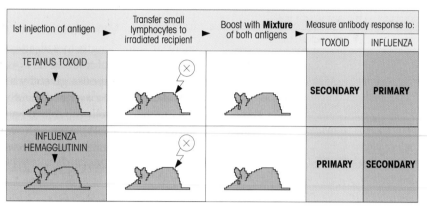

1st injection of antigen	Transfer small lymphocytes to irradiated recipient	Boost with **Mixture** of both antigens	Measure antibody response to:	
			TOXOID	INFLUENZA
TETANUS TOXOID ▼	⊗		**SECONDARY**	**PRIMARY**
INFLUENZA HEMAGGLUTININ ▼	⊗		**PRIMARY**	**SECONDARY**

Figure 2.13. Memory for a primary response can be transferred by small lymphocytes. Recipients are treated with a dose of X-rays which directly kill lymphocytes (highly sensitive to radiation) but only affect other body cells when they divide; the recipient thus functions as a living 'test-tube' which permits the function of the donor cells to be fol-lowed. The reasons for the design of the experiment are given in the text. In practice, because of the possibility of interference between the two antigens, it would be wiser to split each of the primary antigen-injected groups into two, giving a separate boosting antigen to each to avoid using a mixture.

tory to note that Burnet had the sagacity to realize that his clonal selection theory could readily provide the cellular basis for such a mechanism to operate. He argued that if each lymphocyte were preoccupied with making its own individual antibody, those cells programed to express antibodies reacting with circulating self components could be rendered unresponsive without affecting those lymphocytes specific for foreign antigens. In other words, self-reacting lymphocytes could be selectively suppressed or tolerized without undermining the ability of the host to respond immunologically to infectious agents. As we shall see in Chapter 11, these predictions have been amply verified, although we will learn that, as new lymphocytes differentiate throughout life, they will all go through this self-tolerizing screening process. However, self tolerance is not absolute and normally innocuous but potentially harmful anti-self lymphocytes exist in all of us.

VACCINATION DEPENDS ON ACQUIRED MEMORY

Some 200 years ago, Edward Jenner carried out the remarkable studies which mark the beginning of immunology as a systematic subject. Noting the pretty pox-free skin of the milkmaids, he reasoned that deliber-ate exposure to the pox virus of the cow, which is not virulent for the human, might confer protection against the related human smallpox organism. Accordingly, he inoculated a small boy with cowpox and was delighted—and presumably breathed a sigh of relief—to observe that the boy was now protected against a sub-sequent exposure to smallpox (what would today's ethical committees have said about that?!). By injecting a harmless form of a disease organism, Jenner had

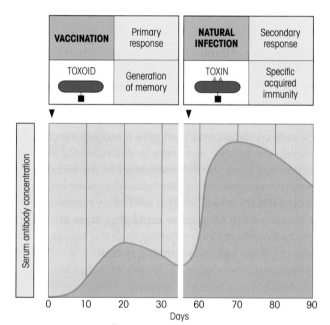

VACCINATION	Primary response	**NATURAL INFECTION**	Secondary response
TOXOID	Generation of memory	TOXIN	Specific acquired immunity

Figure 2.14. The basis of vaccination illustrated by the response to tetanus toxoid. Treatment of the bacterial toxin with formaldehyde destroys its toxicity (associated with ▲▲) but retains antigenicity (asso-ciated with ■). Exposure to toxin in a subsequent natural infection boosts the memory cells, producing high levels of neutralizing anti-body which are protective.

utilized the specificity and memory of the acquired immune response to lay the foundations for modern **vaccination** (Latin *vacca*, cow).

The essential strategy is to prepare an *innocuous* form of the infectious organism or its toxins which still sub-stantially retains the antigens responsible for establish-ing protective immunity. This has been done by using killed or live attenuated organisms, purified microbial components or chemically modified antigens (figure 2.14).

CELL-MEDIATED IMMUNITY PROTECTS AGAINST INTRACELLULAR ORGANISMS

Many microorganisms live inside host cells where it is impossible for humoral antibody to reach them. Obligate intracellular parasites like viruses have to replicate inside cells; facultative intracellular parasites like *Mycobacteria* and *Leishmania* can replicate within cells, particularly macrophages, but do not have to; they like the intracellular life because of the protection it affords. A totally separate acquired immunity system has evolved to deal with this situation based on a distinct lymphocyte subpopulation made up of **T-cells**, designated thus because, unlike the B-lymphocytes, they differentiate within the milieu of the **thymus gland**. Because they are specialized to operate against cells bearing intracellular organisms, T-cells only recognize antigen when it is on the surface of a body cell. Accordingly, the **T-cell surface receptors**, which are different from the antibody molecules used by B-lymphocytes, recognize antigen plus a surface marker which informs the T-lymphocyte that it is making contact with another cell. These cell markers belong to an important group of molecules known as the **major histocompatibility complex (MHC)**, identified originally through their ability to evoke powerful transplantation reactions in other members of the same species. Now naive or virgin T-cells must be introduced to the antigen and MHC by a special dendritic antigen-presenting cell (figures 2.6f and 7.15) before they can be initiated into the rites of a primary response. However, once primed, they are activated by antigen and MHC present on the surface of other cell types such as macrophages as we shall now see.

Cytokine-producing T-cells help macrophages to kill intracellular parasites

These organisms only survive inside macrophages through their ability to subvert the innate killing mechanisms of these cells. Nonetheless, they mostly cannot prevent the macrophage from processing small antigenic fragments (possibly of organisms which have spontaneously died) and placing them on the host cell surface. A subpopulation of T-lymphocytes called **T-helper cells**, if primed to that antigen, will recognize and bind to the combination of antigen with so-called **class II** MHC molecules on the macrophage surface and produce a variety of soluble factors termed **cytokines** which include the interleukins IL-2, etc. (p. 185). Different cytokines can be made by various cell types and generally act at a short range on neighboring cells. Some T-cell cytokines help B-cells to make antibodies, while others such as γ-interferon (IFNγ) act as **macrophage activating factors** which switch on the previously subverted microbicidal mechanisms of the macrophage and bring about the death of the intracellular microorganisms (figure 2.15).

Virally infected cells can be killed by cytotoxic T-cells and ADCC

We have already discussed the advantage to the host of killing virally infected cells before the virus begins to replicate and have seen that natural killer (NK) cells (p. 18) can subserve a cytotoxic function. However, NK cells have a limited range of specificities and, in order to improve their efficacy, this range needs to be expanded.

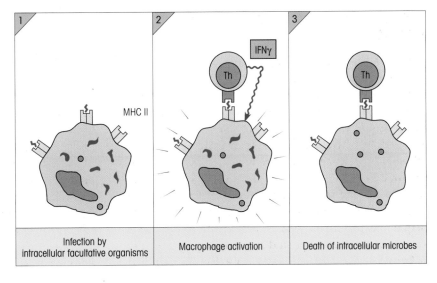

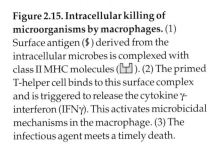

Figure 2.15. Intracellular killing of microorganisms by macrophages. (1) Surface antigen (§) derived from the intracellular microbes is complexed with class II MHC molecules (⊔). (2) The primed T-helper cell binds to this surface complex and is triggered to release the cytokine γ-interferon (IFNγ). This activates microbicidal mechanisms in the macrophage. (3) The infectious agent meets a timely death.

One way in which this can be achieved is by coating the target cell with antibodies specific for the virally coded surface antigens because NK cells have receptors for the constant part of the antibody molecule, rather like phagocytic cells. Thus antibodies will bring the NK cell very close to the target by forming a bridge, and the NK cell being activated by the complexed antibody molecules is able to kill the virally infected cell by its extracellular mechanisms (figure 2.16). This system, termed **antibody-dependent cellular cytotoxicity (ADCC)**, is very impressive when studied *in vitro* but it has proved difficult to establish to what extent it operates within the body.

On the other hand, a **subset** of **T-cells with cytotoxic potential** has evolved for which there is clear evidence of *in vivo* activity. Like the T-helpers, these cells have a very wide range of antigen specificities because they clonally express a large number of different surface receptors similar to, but not identical with, the surface antibody receptors on the B-lymphocytes. Again, each lymphocyte is programed to make only one receptor and, again like the T-helper cell, recognizes antigen only in association with a cell marker, in this case the **class I MHC molecule** (figure 2.16). Through this recognition of surface antigen, the cytotoxic cell comes into intimate contact with its target and administers the 'kiss of apoptotic death'. It also releases **IFNγ** which would help to reduce the spread of virus to adjacent cells, particularly in cases where the virus itself may prove to be a weak inducer of IFNα or β.

In an entirely analogous fashion to the B-cell, T-cells are selected and activated by combination with antigen, expanded by clonal proliferation and mature to give T-helpers and cytotoxic T-effectors, together with an enlarged population of memory cells. Thus both T- and B-cells provide **specific acquired immunity** with a variety of mechanisms, which in most cases operate to extend the range of effectiveness of innate immunity and confer the valuable advantage that a first infection prepares us to withstand further contact with the same microorganism.

IMMUNOPATHOLOGY

The immune system is clearly 'a good thing', but like mercenary armies, it can turn to bite the hand that feeds it, and cause damage to the host (figure 2.17).

Thus where there is an especially heightened response or persistent exposure to exogenous antigens, tissue damaging or **hypersensitivity** reactions may

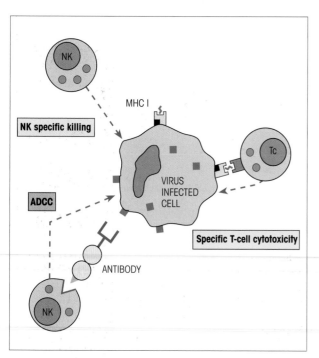

Figure 2.16. Killing virally infected cells. The killing mechanism of the NK cell can be focused on the target by antibody to produce antibody-dependent cellular cytotoxicity (ADCC). The cytotoxic T-cell homes onto its target specifically through receptor recognition of surface antigen in association with MHC class I molecules.

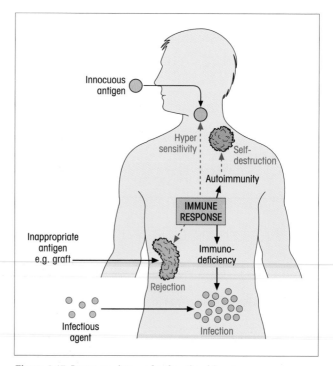

Figure 2.17. Inappropriate and suboptimal immune responses can produce damaging reactions such as the hypersensitivity response to inhaled otherwise innocuous allergens, the destruction of self tissue by autoimmune attack, the rejection of tissue transplants, and the susceptibility to infection in immunodeficient individuals.

result. Examples are allergy to grass pollens, blood dyscrasias associated with certain drugs, immune complex glomerulonephritis occurring after streptococcal infection, and chronic granulomas produced during tuberculosis or schistosomiasis.

In other cases, hypersensitivity to autoantigens may arise through a breakdown in the mechanisms which control self tolerance, and a wide variety of **autoimmune diseases**, such as insulin-dependent diabetes and multiple sclerosis and many of the rheumatologic disorders, have now been recognized.

Another immunopathologic reaction of some consequence is **transplant rejection**, where the MHC antigens on the donor graft may well provoke a fierce reaction. Lastly, one should consider the by no means infrequent occurrence of inadequate functioning of the immune system—**immunodeficiency**. We would like to think that at this stage the reader would have no difficulty in predicting that the major problems in this condition relate to persistent infection, the type of infection being related to the elements of the immune system which are defective.

SUMMARY

Antibody—the specific adaptor

• The antibody molecule evolved as a specific adaptor to attach to microorganisms which either fail to activate the alternative complement pathway or prevent activation of the phagocytic cells.

• The antibody fixes to the antigen by its specific recognition site and its constant structure regions activate complement through the classical pathway (binding C1 and generating a $\overline{C4b2a}$ convertase to split C3) and phagocytes through their antibody receptors.

• This supplementary route into the acute inflammatory reaction is enhanced by antibodies which sensitize mast cells and by immune complexes which stimulate mediator release from tissue macrophages (figure 2.18).

• The innate immune reaction of mannose-binding lectin with microbes activates the MASP-1 and MASP-2 proteases which join the classical complement pathway by splitting C4 and C2.

Cellular basis of antibody production

• Antibodies are made by plasma cells derived from B-lymphocytes, each of which is programed to make antibody of a single specificity which is placed on the cell surface as a receptor.

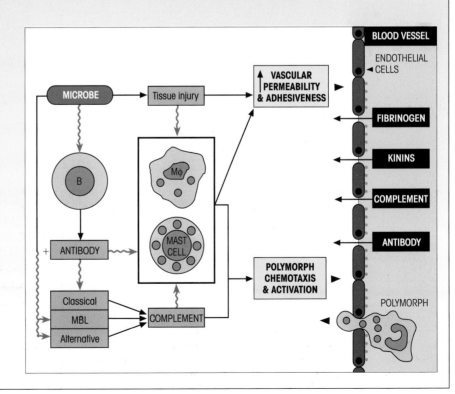

Figure 2.18. Production of a protective acute inflammatory reaction by microbes either: (i) through tissue injury (e.g. bacterial toxin) or direct activation of the alternative complement pathway, or (ii) by antibody-dependent triggering of the classical complement pathway or mast cell degranulation (a special class of antibody, IgE, does this).

(Continued p.34)

• Antigen binds to the cell with a complementary antibody, activates it and causes clonal proliferation and finally maturation to antibody-forming cells and memory cells. Thus the antigen brings about clonal selection of the cells making antibody to itself.

Acquired memory and vaccination

• The increase in memory cells after priming means that the acquired secondary response is faster and greater, providing the basis for vaccination using a harmless form of the infective agent for the initial injection.

Acquired immunity has antigen specificity

• Antibodies differentiate between antigens because recognition is based on molecular shape complementarity. Thus memory induced by one antigen will not extend to another unrelated antigen.

• The immune system differentiates self components from foreign antigens by making immature self-reacting lymphocytes unresponsive through contact with host molecules; lymphocytes reacting with foreign antigens are unaffected since they only make contact after reaching maturity.

Cell-mediated immunity protects against intracellular organisms

• Another class of lymphocyte, the T-cell, is concerned with control of intracellular infections. Like the B-cell, each T-cell has its individual antigen receptor (although it differs structurally from antibody) which recognizes antigen and the cell then undergoes clonal expansion to form effector and memory cells providing specific acquired immunity.

• The T-cell recognizes cell surface antigens in association with molecules of the MHC. Naive T-cells are only stimulated to undergo a primary response by specialized dendritic antigen-presenting cells.

• Primed T-helper cells, which see antigen with class II MHC on the surface of macrophages, release cytokines which in some cases can help B-cells to make antibody and in others activate macrophages and enable them to kill intracellular parasites.

• Cytotoxic T-cells have the ability to recognize specific antigen plus class I MHC on the surface of virally infected cells which are killed before the virus replicates. They also release γ-interferon which can make surrounding cells resistant to viral spread (figure 2.19).

• NK cells have lectin-like 'nonspecific' receptors for cells infected by viruses but do not have antigen-specific receptors; however, they can recognize antibody-coated virally infected cells through their Fcγ receptors and kill the target by antibody-dependent cellular cytotoxicity (ADCC).

• Although the innate mechanisms do not improve with repeated exposure to infection as do the acquired, they play a vital role since they are intimately linked to the acquired systems by **two different pathways** which all but **encapsulate the whole of immunology**. Antibody, complement and polymorphs give protection against most extracellular organisms, while T-cells, soluble cytokines, macrophages and NK cells deal with intracellular infections (figure 2.20).

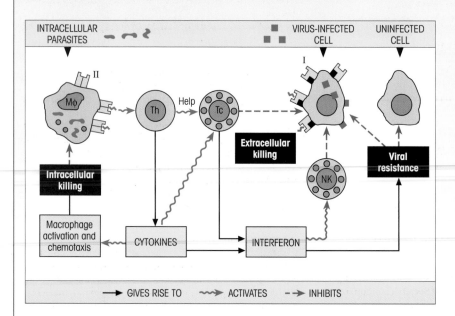

Figure 2.19. T-cells link with the innate immune system to resist intracellular infection. Class I (⊟) and class II (⊟) major histocompatibility molecules are important for T-cell recognition of surface antigen. The T-helper cells (Th) cooperate in the development of cytotoxic T-cells (Tc) from precursors. The macrophage (Mφ) microbicidal mechanisms are switched on by macrophage activating cytokines. Interferon inhibits viral replication and stimulates NK cells which, together with Tc, kill virus-infected cells.

Immunopathology
- Immunopathologically mediated tissue damage to the host can occur as a result of:

inappropriate hypersensitivity reactions to exogenous antigens;

loss of tolerance to self giving rise to autoimmune disease; reaction to foreign grafts.
- Immunodeficiency leaves the individual susceptible to infection.

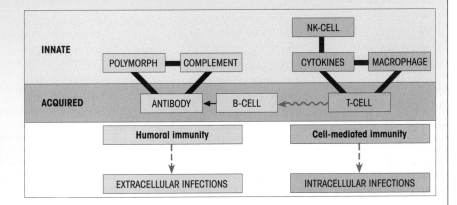

Figure 2.20. The two pathways linking innate and acquired immunity which provide the basis for humoral and cell-mediated immunity, respectively.

FURTHER READING

General reading

Alt F. & Marrack P. (eds) (2001) *Current Opinion in Immunology* **13**. (Appears bimonthly; Issue No. 1 deals with 'Innate Immunity'.) Very valuable critical current reviews.

Kim T. & Kim Y.J. (2005) Overview of innate immunity in Drosophila. *J. Biochem. Mol. Biol.* **38**, 121–127.

Matzinger P. (2005) The danger model: a renewed sense of self. *Science* **296**, 301–305.

Parker L.C. *et al.* (2005) The expression and roles of Toll-like receptors in the biology of the human neutrophil. *J. Leukoc. Biol.* **77**, 886–892.

Reid K.B.M. (1995) The complement system—a major effector mechanism in humoral immunity. *The Immunologist* **3**, 206.

Segal A.W. (2005) How neutrophils kill microbes. *Ann. Rev. Immunol.* **23**, 197–223.

Sinkovics J.G. & Horvath J.C. (2005) Human natural killer cells: a comprehensive review. *Int. J. Oncol.* **27**, 5–47.

Sitaram N. & Nagaraj R. (1999) Interaction of antimicrobial peptides with biological and model membranes: structural and charge requirements for activity. *Biochimica et Biophysica Acta—Biomembranes* **1462**, 29.

Stuart L.M. & Ezekowitz R.A. (2005) Phagocytosis: elegant complexity. *Immunity* **22**, 539–550.

Worthley D.L., Bardy P.G. & Mulligan C.G. (2005) Mannose binding lectin: biology and clinical implications. *Intern. Med. J.* **35**, 538–555.

Historical

Clarke W.R. (1991) *The Experimental Foundations of Modern Immunology*, 4th edn. John Wiley & Sons, New York. (Important for those wishing to appreciate the experiments leading up to many of the major discoveries.)

Ehrlich P. (1890) On immunity with special reference to cell life. In Melchers F. *et al.* (eds) *Progress in Immunology* **VII**. Springer-Verlag, Berlin. (Translation of a lecture to the Royal Society (London) on the side-chain theory of antibody formation, showing this man's perceptive genius. A must!)

Landsteiner K. (1946) *The Specificity of Serological Reactions*. Harvard University Press (reprinted 1962 by Dover Publications, New York).

Mazumdar P.M.M. (ed.) (1989) *Immunology 1930–1980*. Wall & Thompson, Toronto.

Metchnikoff E. (1893) *Comparative Pathology of Inflammation*. Kegan Paul, Trench, Trubner, London (translated by F.A. & E.H. Starling).

Palmer R. (ed.) (1993) *Outstanding Papers in Biology*. Current Biology, London. (A delight to browse through some of the seminal papers which have shaped modern biology; wonderful material for teaching.)

Silverstein A.M. (1989) *A History of Immunology*. Academic Press, San Diego.

Tauber A.I. (1991) *Metchnikoff and the Origins of Immunology*. Oxford University Press, Oxford.

In-depth series for the advanced reader

Advances in Immunology. Elsevier Science Publications.

Advances in Neuroimmunology (edited by G.B. Stefano & E.M. Smith). Pergamon, Oxford.

Annual Review of Immunology. Annual Reviews Inc., California.

Immunological Reviews (edited by P. Parham). Munksgaard, Copenhagen. (Specialized, authoritative and thoughtful.)

Nature Reviews, Nature Publishing Group, London.

Progress in Allergy. Karger, Basle.

Seminars in Immunology. Elsevier Science Publications. (In-depth treatment of single subjects.)

Current information

Current Biology. Current Biology, London. (What the complete biologist needs to know about significant current advances.)

Current Opinion in Immunology. Current Science, London. (Important personal opinions on focused highlights of the advances made in the previous year; most valuable for the serious immunologist.)

Table 2.1. The major immunologic journals and their impact factors.

GENERAL JOURNALS OF PARTICULAR INTEREST TO IMMUNOLOGISTS	*IMPACT FACTOR
Cell	28.4
EMBO J.	10.5
Lancet	21.7
Nature	32.2
Nature Medicine	31.2
New England Journal of Medicine	38.6
Proceedings of the National Academy of Sciences of the USA	10.5
Science	31.9

IMMUNOLOGICAL JOURNALS	*IMPACT FACTOR
AIDS	5.9
Allergy	3.5
Autoimmunity	1.4
Cancer Immunology Immunotherapy	2.3
Cellular Immunology	2.0
Clinical and Experimental Allergy	3.1
Clinical and Experimental Immunology	2.5
Clinical Immunology	3.0
European Journal of Immunology	5.0
Human Immunology	2.7
Immunity	15.5
Immunobiology	2.3
Immunogenetics	2.9
Immunologic Research	2.1
Immunology	3.0
Immunology and Cell Biology	2.6
Immunology Letters	2.1
Infection and Immunity	4.0
International Archives of Allergy and Immunology	2.5
International Immunology	3.5
International Journal of Immunopathology and Pharmacology	3.6
Journal of Allergy and Clinical Immunology	7.2
Journal of Autoimmunity	1.9
Journal of Clinical Immunology	2.4
Journal of Experimental Medicine	14.6
Journal of Immunology	6.5
Journal of Immunological Methods	2.5
Journal of Immunotherapy	3.5
Journal of Leukocyte Biology	4.2
Journal of Reproductive Immunology	2.7
Molecular Immunology	3.2
Nature Immunology	27.6
Parasite Immunology	1.5
Scandinavian Journal of Immunology	1.9
Tissue Antigens	2.0
Transplantation	3.6
Vaccine	2.8

*IMPACT FACTOR = relative frequency with which the journal's 'average article' has been cited in other publications

Trends in Molecular Medicine. Elsevier Science Publications, Amsterdam. (Frequent articles of interest to immunologists with very good perspective.)

The Immunologist. Hogrefe & Huber Publishers, Seattle. (Official organ of the International Union of Immunological Societies— IUIS. Excellent, didactic and compact articles on current trends in immunology.)

Trends in Immunology. Elsevier Science Publications, Amsterdam. (The immunologist's 'newspaper'. Excellent.)

Multiple choice questions

Roitt I.M. & Delves P.J. 400 MCQs each with five annotated learning responses. See **Website**.

Website (linked to Roitt's Essential Immunology) http://www.roitt.com

The website contains:

- 400 multiple-choice revision questions with feedback on each answer selected
- Key concepts illustrated with animations
- Further reading and reference archive
- Image archive with over 400 illustrations from *Essential Immunology*

Major journals

The major journals of interest and their impact factors are noted in table 2.1.

3 Antibodies

INTRODUCTION

In essence, antibody molecules carry out two principal functions in immune defence. The **first function** is to recognize and bind to foreign material (antigen). This generally means binding to molecular structures on the surface of the foreign material (antigenic determinants) that differ from molecular structures made by the cells of the host. These antigenic determinants are usually expressed in multiple copies on the foreign material, e.g. proteins or carbohydrates on a bacterial cell surface or envelope spikes on the surface of a virus. Host antibodies can recognize a huge variety of different molecular structures—a human is capable of producing antibodies against billions of different molecular structures. This is described as antibody diversity and is necessary to respond to the huge diversity of molecular structures associated with (often highly mutable) pathogens.

The simple act of antibody binding may be sufficient to inactivate a pathogen or render harmless a toxin. For instance, antibody coating of a virus can prevent it entering target cells and thereby 'neutralize' the virus. However, in many instances, a **second function** of the antibody molecule is deployed to trigger the elimination of foreign material. In molecular terms, this involves the binding of certain molecules (effector molecules) to antibody-coated foreign material to trigger complex elimination mechanisms, e.g. the complement system of proteins, phagocytosis by host immune cells such as neutrophils and macrophages. The powerful effector systems are generally triggered only by antibody molecules clustered together as on a foreign cell surface and not by free unliganded antibody. This is crucial considering the typically high serum concentrations of antibodies.

THE DIVISION OF LABOR

The requirements imposed on the antibody molecule by the two functions are in a sense quite opposite. The first function requires great antibody diversity. The second function requires that many different antibody molecules share common features, i.e. it is not practical for Nature to devise a different molecular solution for the problem of elimination for each different antibody molecule. The conflicting requirements are elegantly met by the antibody structure shown diagramatically in figure. 3.1. The structure consists of three units. Two of the units are identical and involved in binding to antigen—the **Fab (fragment antigen binding)** arms of the molecule. These units contain regions of sequence which vary greatly from one antibody to another and confer on a given antibody its unique binding specificity. The presence of two identical Fab arms enhances the binding of antibody to antigen in the typical situation where multiple copies of antigenic determinants are presented on foreign material. The third unit—**Fc (fragment crystalline)** is involved in binding to effector molecules. As shown in figure. 3.1, the antibody molecule has a four-chain structure consisting of two identical heavy chains spanning Fab and Fc and two identical light chains associated only with Fab. The relationship between antigen binding, the different units and the four-chain structure of the antibody molecule were revealed by a series of key experiments summarized in Milestone 3.1.

FIVE CLASSES OF IMMUNOGLOBULIN

Antibodies are often referred to as **immunoglobulins** (immune proteins). There are five classes of antibodies or immunoglobulins termed immunoglobulin G (IgG),

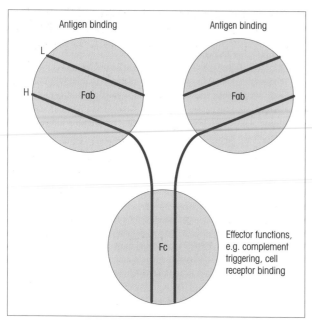

Figure 3.1. Simplified overall layout of the antibody molecule. The structure consists of four polypeptide chains, two identical heavy (H) chains and two identical light (L) chains, arranged to span three structural units as shown. The two identical Fab units bind antigen and the third unit (Fc) binds effector molecules to trigger antigen elimination and to mediate functions such as maternal—fetal transport.

IgM, IgA, IgD and IgE. All these classes have the basic four-chain antibody structure but they differ in their heavy chains termed γ, μ, α, δ and ε, respectively. The differences are most pronounced in the Fc regions of the antibody classes and this leads to the triggering of different effector functions on binding to antigen, e.g. IgM recognition of antigen might lead to complement activation whereas IgE recognition (possibly of the same antigen) might lead to mast cell degranulation and anaphylaxis (increased vascular permeability and smooth muscle contraction). These differences are discussed in greater detail below. Structural differences also lead to differences in the polymerization state of the monomer unit shown in figure 3.1. Thus, IgG and IgE are generally monomeric whereas IgM occurs as a pentamer. IgA occurs predominantly as a monomer in serum and as a dimer in seromucous secretions.

The major antibody in the serum is IgG and, as this is the best-understood antibody in terms of structure and function, we shall consider it first. The other antibody classes will be considered in relation to IgG.

THE IgG MOLECULE

In IgG, the Fab arms are linked to the Fc by an extended region of polypeptide chain known as the hinge. This region tends to be exposed and sensitive to attack by proteases that cleave the molecule in to its distinct func-

tional units arranged around the four-chain structure (Milestone 3.1). This structure is represented in greater detail in figure 3.2a. The light chains exist in two forms known as kappa (κ) and lambda (λ). In humans, κ chains are somewhat more prevalent than λ; in mice, λ chains are rare. The heavy chains can also be grouped into different forms or subclasses, the number depending upon the species under consideration. In humans there are four **subclasses** having heavy chains labeled γ1, γ2, γ3 and γ4 which give rise to the IgG1, IgG2, IgG3 and IgG4 subclasses. In mice, there are again four subclasses denoted IgG1, IgG2a, IgG2b and IgG3. The subclasses—particularly in humans—have very similar primary sequences, the greatest differences being observed in the hinge region. The existence of subclasses is an important feature as they show marked differences in their ability to trigger effector functions. In a single molecule, the two heavy chains are identical as are the two light chains; hybrid molecules have not been described.

The amino acid sequences of heavy and light chains of antibodies have revealed much about their structure and function. However, obtaining the sequences of antibodies is much more challenging than for many other proteins because the population of antibodies in an individual is so incredibly heterogeneous. The opportunity to do this first came from the study of **myeloma proteins**. In the human disease known as multiple myeloma, one cell making one particular individual antibody divides over and over again in the uncontrolled way a cancer cell does, without regard for the overall requirement of the host. The patient then possesses enormous numbers of identical cells derived as a clone from the original cell and they all synthesize the same immunoglobulin—the myeloma protein—which appears in the serum, sometimes in very high concentrations. By purification of myeloma proteins, preparations of a single antibody for sequencing and many other applications can be obtained. An alternative route to single or **monoclonal antibodies** arrived with the development of **hybridoma technology**. Here, fusing individual antibody-forming cells with a B-cell tumor produces a constantly dividing clone of cells dedicated to making the one antibody. Finally, **recombinant antibody technologies**, developed most recently, provide an excellent source of monoclonal antibodies.

Sequence comparison of monoclonal IgG proteins indicates that the carboxy-terminal half of the light chain and roughly three quarters of the heavy chain, again carboxy-terminal, show little sequence variation between different IgG molecules. By contrast, the amino-terminal regions of about 100 amino acid residues show considerable sequence variability in both chains. Within these variable regions there are relatively

Milestone 3.1—Four-polypeptide Structure of Immunoglobulin Monomers

Early studies showed the bulk of the antibody activity in serum to be in the slow electrophoretic fraction termed γ-globulin (subsequently immunoglobulin). The most abundant antibodies were divalent, i.e. had two combining sites for antigen and could thus form a precipitating complex (cf. figure 6.2).

To Rodney Porter and Gerald Edelman must go the credit for unlocking the secrets of the basic structure of the immunoglobulin molecule. If the internal disulfide bonds are reduced, the component polypeptide chains still hang together by strong noncovalent attractions. However, if the reduced molecule is held under acid conditions, these attractive forces are lost as the chains become positively charged and can now be separated by gel filtration into larger so-called heavy chains of approximately 55 000 Da (for IgG, IgA and IgD) or 70 000 Da (for IgM and IgE) and smaller light chains of about 24 000 Da.

The clues to how the chains are assembled to form the IgG molecule came from selective cleavage using proteolytic enzymes. Papain destroyed the precipitating power of the intact molecule but produced two univalent Fab fragments still capable of binding to antigen (Fab = *fragment antigen binding*); the remaining fragment had no affinity for antigen and was termed Fc by Porter (*fragment crystallizable*). After digestion with pepsin a molecule called F(ab')₂ was isolated; it still precipitated antigen and so retained both binding sites, but the Fc portion was further degraded. The structural basis for these observations is clearly evident from figure M3.1.1. In essence, with minor changes, all immunoglobulin molecules are constructed from one or more of the basic four-chain monomer units.

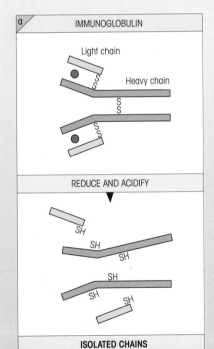
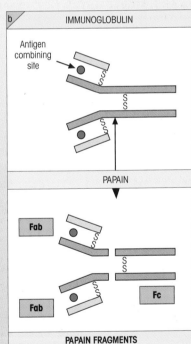
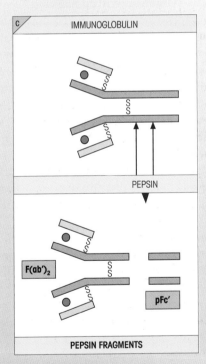

Figure M3.1.1. The antibody basic unit (IgG is represented), consisting of two identical heavy and two identical light chains held together by interchain disulfide bonds, can be broken down into its constituent polypeptide chains and to proteolytic fragments, the pepsin F(ab')₂ retaining two binding sites for antigen and the papain Fab with one. After pepsin digestion the pFc' fragment representing the C-terminal half of the Fc region is formed and is held together by noncovalent bonds. The portion of the heavy chain in the Fab fragment is given the symbol Fd. The N-terminal residue is on the left for each chain.

short sequences which show extreme variation and are designated hypervariable regions. There are three of these regions or 'hot spots' on the light chain and three on the heavy chain. Since the different IgGs in the comparison recognize different antigens, these **hypervariable regions** are expected to be associated with antigen recognition and indeed are often referred to as **complementarity determining regions (CDRs)**. The structural setting for the involvement of the hypervariable regions in antigen recognition and the genetic origins of the constant and variable regions will be discussed shortly.

The comparison of immunoglobulin sequences also reveals the organization of IgG into 12 homology regions or **domains** each possessing an internal disulfide bond. The basic domain structure is central to an understanding of the relation between structure and function in the antibody molecule and will shortly be taken up below. However, the structure in outline form is shown in figure 3.2b,c. It is seen that the light chain consists of two domains, one corresponding to the variable sequence region discussed above and designated the V_L (variable-light) domain and the other corresponding to a constant region and designated the C_L (constant-light) domain. The IgG heavy chain consists of four domains, the V_H and C_H1 domains of the Fab arms being joined to the C_H2 and C_H3 domains of Fc via the hinge. Antigen binding is a combined property of the V_L and V_H domains at the extremities of the Fab arms and effector molecule binding a property of the C_H2 and/or C_H3 domains of Fc.

It is also clear (figure 3.2b,c) that all of the domains except for C_H2 are in close lateral or 'sideways' association with another domain: a phenomenon described as domain pairing. The C_H2 domains have two sugar chains interposed between them. The domains also exhibit weaker *cis*-interactions with neighboring domains on the same polypeptide chain.

Human IgG1 is shown in figure 3.2 as a Y-shaped conformation with the Fab arms roughly in the same plane as the Fc. This is the classical view of the antibody mole-

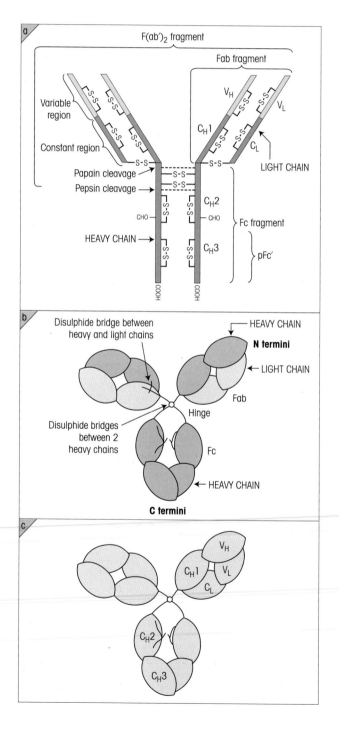

Figure 3.2. The four-chain structure of IgG. (a) Linear representation. Disulfide bridges link the two heavy chains and the light and heavy chains. A regular arrangement of intrachain disulfide bonds is also found. Fragments generated by proteolytic cleavage at the indicated sites are represented. (b) Domain representation. Each heavy chain (shaded) is folded into two domains in the Fab arms, forms a region of extended polypeptide chain in the hinge and is then folded into two domains in the Fc region. The light chain forms two domains associated only with a Fab arm. Domain pairing leads to close interaction of heavy and light chains in the Fab arms supplemented by a disulfide bridge. The two heavy chains are disulfide bridged in the hinge (the number of bridges depending on IgG subclass) and are in close domain-paired interaction at their carboxy-termini. (c) Domain nomenclature. The heavy chain is composed of V_H, C_H1, C_H2 and C_H3 domains. The light chain is composed of V_L and C_L domains. All the domains are paired except for the C_H2 domains, which have two branched N-linked carbohydrate chains interposed between them. Each domain has a molecular weight of approximately 12,000 leading to a molecular weight of ~50,000 for Fc and Fab and 150,000 for the whole IgG molecule. Antigen recognition involves residues from the V_H and V_L domains, complement triggering the C_H2 domain, leukocyte Fc receptor binding the C_H2 domain and the neonatal Fc receptor the C_H2 and C_H3 domains (see text). (Adapted from Burton D.R. Structure and function of antibodies. In: New Comprehensive Biochemistry series, Vol. 17: Molecular genetic of immunoglobulin, F. Calabi and M.S. Neuberger (eds). Elsevier, pp. 1–50, 1987).

cule that has adorned countless meetings ads and appears in many company logos. In reality, this is likely just one of many shapes that the IgG molecule can adopt since it is very **flexible** as illustrated in figure 3.3. It is believed that this flexibility may help IgG function. Thus Fab–Fab flexibility gives the antibody a 'variable reach' allowing it to grasp antigenic determinants of different spacings on a foreign cell surface or to form intricate immune complexes with a toxin (imagine a Y to T shape change). Fc–Fab flexibility may help antibodies in different environments, on foreign cells for example, to interact productively with common effector molecules. Figure 3.4 shows the complete structure of a human IgG1 antibody molecule determined by crystallography. The structure is quite removed from the classical symmetrical Y shape. The Fc is closer to one Fab arm than another and is rotated relative to the Fab arms. This is simply a 'snapshot' of one of the many conformations that the antibody can adopt by virtue of its flexibility.

The structural organization of IgG into domains is clearly evident from figures 3.2–3.4. Each of these domains has a common pattern of polypeptide chain folding (figure 3.5). This pattern, the 'immunoglobulin fold', consists of two twisted stacked β-sheets enclosing an internal volume of tightly packed hydrophobic residues. The arrangement is stabilized by an internal disulfide bond linking the two sheets in a central position (this internal bond is seen in figure 3.2a). One sheet has four and the other three anti-parallel β–strands. These strands or **framework regions** are joined by bends or loops which generally show little secondary structure. Residues involved in the β-sheets tend to be conserved while there is a greater diversity of residues in the loops. The chain folding illustrated in figure 3.5 is for a constant domain. The β-sheets of the variable

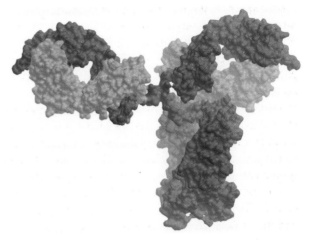

Figure 3.4. The structure of a human IgG molecule. This antibody recognizes the gp120 surface glycoprotein of HIV. The heavy chains are shown in blue and the light chains in green. Relative to the classical cartoon of an IgG molecule as a Y shape, this 'snapshot' of the molecule finds the Fc (bottom) 'side on' to the viewer and much closer to one Fab arm than the other. (Courtesy of Erica Ollmann Saphire.)

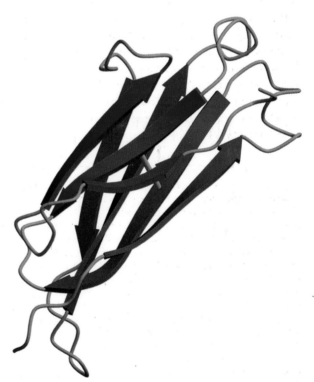

Figure 3.5. The immunoglobulin fold. An anti-parallel three-stranded β-sheet (red) interacts with a four-stranded sheet (blue). The arrangement is stabilized by a disulfide bond linking the two sheets. The β-strands are connected by helices, bends and other structures. This overall structure is the basis of all Ig and Ig-like domains.

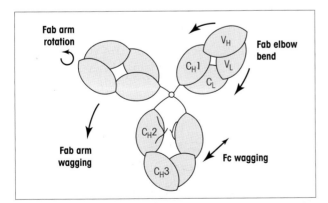

Figure 3.3. Modes of flexibility in the IgG molecule. These modes have been described from electron microscopic studies (see figure 3.10) and biophysical techniques in solution. Flexibility in structure probably facilitates flexibility in antigen recognition and effector function triggering.

domain are more distorted than those of the C domain and the V domain possesses an extra loop.

Structure of Fab fragment

The four individual domains are paired in two ways (figure 3.6). The V_H and V_L domains are paired through the two respective three-strand β-sheet layers (red in figure 3.5). The C_H1 and C_L domains are paired by contact between the two four-strand layers (blue in figure 3.5). The interacting faces of the domains are predominantly hydrophobic and the driving force for domain pairing is thus the removal of these residues from the aqueous environment. The arrangement is further stabilized by a disulfide bond between C_H1 and C_L domains.

In contrast to the 'sideways' interactions, the 'longwise' or *cis* interactions between V_H and C_H1 domains and between V_L and C_L domains are very limited and allow 'elbow bending'. Elbow angles seen in crystal structures vary between about 137° and 180°.

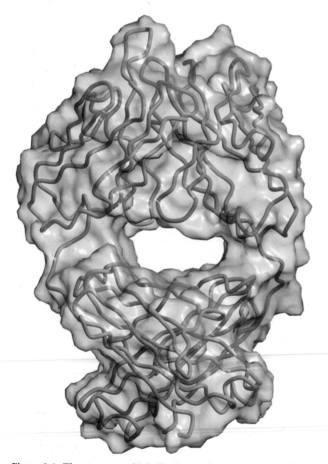

Figure 3.6. The structure of Fab. The heavy chain is shown in yellow and the light chain in green. The V_H and V_L domains (top) are paired by contact between their three-strand faces (red in figure 3.5) and the C_H1 and C_L domains between the four-strand faces (blue in figure 3.5) (Courtsey of Robyn Stanfield).

The antibody combining site

Comparison of antibody sequence and structural data shows how antibodies are able to recognize an enormously diverse range of molecules. Sequence data shows that the variable domains have six hypervariable regions that display great variation in amino acids between different antibody molecules (figure 3.7). Structural data of antibody–antigen complexes reveals that these hypervariable regions, or complementarity determining regions, come together in 3D space to form the antigen binding site, often also termed the **antibody combining site** (figure 3.8). (Courtesy of Robyn Stanfield)

Structure of Fc

For the Fc of IgG (figure 3.9), the two C_H3 domains are classically paired whereas the two C_H2 domains show no close interaction, but have interposed between them two branched N-linked carbohydrate chains that have limited contact with one another. The carbohydrate chains are very heterogeneous. The C_H2 domains contain the binding sites for several important effector molecules, complement C1q and Fc receptors in particular, as shown. The neonatal Fc receptor, which is important in binding to IgG and maintaining its long half-life in serum, binds to a site formed between C_H2 and C_H3 domains. Protein A, much used in purifying IgGs, also binds to this site.

The hinge region and IgG subclasses

The term **'hinge'** arose from electron micrographs of rabbit IgG, which showed Fab arms assuming different angles relative to one another from nearly 0° (acute Y-shaped) to 180° (T-shaped). The Fab was specific for a small chemical group dinitrophenyl (DNP) that could be attached to either end of a hydrocarbon chain. As shown in figures 3.10 and 3.11, different shapes were observed as the Fab arms linked together the bivalent antigen molecule using different Fab–Fab arm angles. Other biophysical techniques have demonstrated hinge flexibility in solution. The function of this flexibility has generally been seen as allowing divalent recognition of variably spaced antigenic determinants. The IgG class of antibody in humans exists as four subclasses and the biggest difference between the subclasses is in the nature and length of the hinge. IgG1 has been shown above. IgG3 has a hinge which if fully extended would be about twice the length of the Fc, thereby potentially placing the Fab arms far removed from the Fc. On the other hand, IgG2 and IgG4 have short compact hinges which probably lead to close approach of Fab and Fc. Interestingly, IgG1 and IgG3 are generally superior at mediating effector functions such as complement activation and ADCC relative to IgG2 and IgG4.

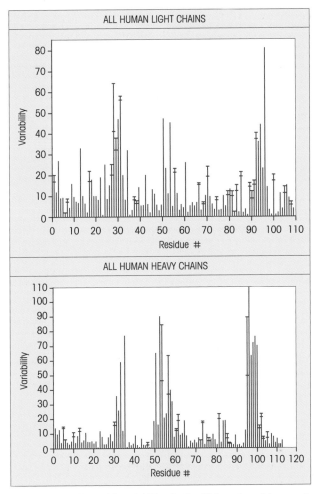

Figure 3.7. **Amino acid variability in the V domains of human Ig heavy and light chains.** Variability, for a given position, is defined as the ratio of the number of different residues found at that position compared to the frequency of the most common amino acid. The CDRs are apparent as peaks in the plot and the frameworks as intervening regions of low variability. (After Dr E.A. Kabat.)

THE STRUCTURE AND FUNCTION OF THE IMMUNOGLOBULIN CLASSES

The immunoglobulin classes (table 3.1) fulfill different roles in immune defence and this can be correlated with differences in their structures organized around the four-chain Ig domain arrangement (figure 3.12). **IgG** is monomeric and the major antibody in serum and non-mucosal tissues, where it inactivates pathogens directly and through interaction with effector triggering molecules such as complement and Fc receptors. **IgM** is pentameric, is found in serum and is highly efficient at complement triggering. A monomeric form of IgM with a membrane-tethering sequence is the major antibody receptor used by B lymphocytes to recognize antigen (cf. figure 2.10). IgM differs from IgG in having an extra pair of constant domains instead of the hinge region. **IgA** exists in three soluble forms. Monomeric and small amounts of dimeric IgA (formed from two monomers linked by an extra polypeptide called J chain) are found in the serum where they can help link pathogens to effector cells via Fc receptors specific for IgA. Secretory IgA (see below) is formed of dimeric IgA and an extra protein known as secretory component and is crucial in protecting the mucosal surfaces of the body against attack by microorganisms. IgA exists as two subclasses in humans. IgA2 has a much shorter hinge than IgA1 and is more resistant to attack by bacterially secreted proteases. **IgE** is a monomeric antibody typically found at very low concentrations in serum. In fact most IgE is probably bound to IgE Fc receptors on mast cells. Antigen binding to IgE cross-links IgE Fc receptors and triggers an acute inflammatory reaction that can assist in immune defence. This can also lead to unwanted allergic symptoms for certain antigens (allergens). IgE, like IgM, has an extra pair of constant domains instead of the hinge region. Finally **IgD** is an antibody primarily found on the surface of B cells as an antigen receptor together with IgM, where it likely serves in the control of lymphocyte activation

(a)   (b)

Figure 3.8. **The proximity of CDRs (variable loops) at the tip of the Fab arms creates the antibody combining site.** The V_H and V_L domains are shown from the side (a) and from above (b). The six CDRs (cf. figure 3.7) are numbered 1–3 as belonging to the heavy (H) or light (L) chain. (Courtesy of Robyn Stanfield).

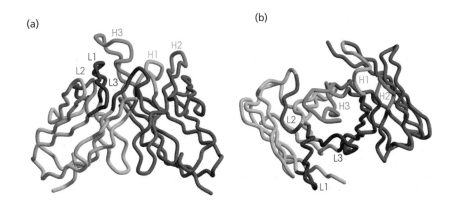

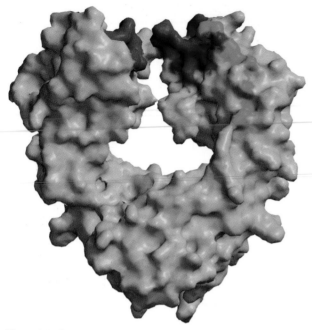

Figure 3.9. Structure of Fc of human IgG. The C_H3 domains (bottom) are paired. The C_H2 domains are not and have two carbohydrate chains filling some of the space between them. Binding sites for the leukocyte as FcγRIII receptor (red), complement C1q (green) and neonatal Fc receptor FcRn (yellow) are shown. The FcγRIII and FcRn sites were determined by crystallographic studies (Sondermann *et al.* (2000) *Nature* **406**, 267; Martin *et al.* (2001) *Molecular Cell* **7**, 867) and the C1q site by mutation analysis (Idusogie *et al.* (2000) *Journal of Immunology* **164**, 4178). (Courtesy of Robyn Stanfield).

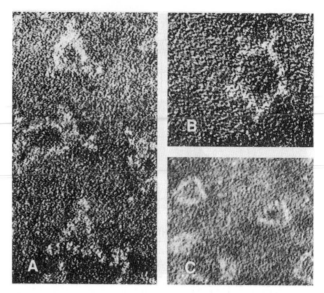

Figure 3.10. (A,B) Electron micrograph (×1000000) of complexes formed on mixing the divalent DNP hapten with rabbit anti-DNP antibodies. The 'negative stain' phosphotungstic acid is an electron-dense solution which penetrates into the spaces between the protein molecules. Thus the protein stands out as a 'light' structure in the electron beam. The hapten links together the Y-shaped antibody molecules to form trimers (A) and pentamers (B). The flexibility of the molecule at the hinge region is evident from the variation in angle of the arms of the 'Y'. (C) As in (A), but the trimers were formed using the F(ab')₂ antibody fragment from which the Fc structures have been digested by pepsin (×500 000). The trimers can be seen to lack the Fc projections at each corner evident in (A). (After Valentine R.C. & Green N.M. (1967) *Journal of Molecular Biology* **27**, 615; courtesy of Dr Green and with the permission of Academic Press, New York.)

and suppression. It is monomeric and has a long hinge region.

The structures of the Fc regions of human IgA1 and IgE (C-terminal domains) have been determined and are compared with IgG1 in figure 3.13. In all three cases, the penultimate domains are unpaired and have carbohydrate chains interposed between them.

Antibodies and complement

The clustering together of IgG molecules, typically on the surface of a pathogen such as a bacterium, leads to the binding of the complement C1 molecule via the hexavalent C1q subcomponent (cf. figure 2.2). This triggers the classical pathway of complement and a number of processes that can lead to pathogen elimination. The subclasses of IgG trigger with different efficiencies. IgG1 and IgG3 trigger best; IgG2 is only triggered by antigens at high density such as carbohydrate antigens on a bacterium; and IgG4 does not trigger. Generally, the nature of the antigen and its environment seems able to influence how well complement is triggered.

IgM triggers by a different mechanism. It is already

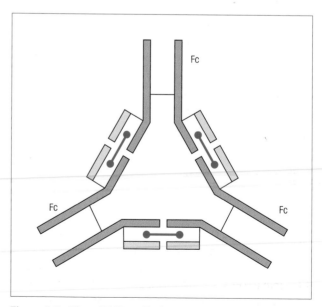

Figure 3.11. Three DNP antibody molecules held together as a trimer by the divalent antigen (●——●). Compare figure 3.10A. When the Fc fragments are first removed by pepsin, the corner pieces are no longer visible (figure 3.10C).

Figure 3.12. Schematic structures of the antibody classes. The two heavy chains are shown in dark and pale blue (two colors to highlight chain pairing; the chains are identical) and the light chains in grey. N-linked carbohydrate chains (branched structures) are shown in blue and O-linked carbohydrates (linear structures) in green. The heavy chain domains are designated according to the class of the heavy chain, e.g. $C\gamma2$ for the C_H2 domain of IgG, etc. For IgG, IgA and IgD, the Fc is connected to the Fab arms via a hinge region; for IgM and IgE an extra pair of domains replaces the hinge. IgA, IgM and IgD have tailpieces at the C termini of the heavy chains. IgA occurs in monomer and dimer forms. IgM occurs as a pentamer. (a) IgG1. The other human IgG subclasses (and IgGs of most other species) have this same basic structure but differ particularly in the nature and length of the hinge. (b) IgA1. The structure resembles IgG1 but with a relatively long hinge bearing O-linked sugar chains. The Fc also shows some differences from IgG1 (see figure 3.13). In IgA2, the hinge is very short and, in the predominant allotype, the light chains are disulfide linked not to the heavy chain but to one another. (c) IgM monomeric unit. This representation relies greatly on comparison of the amino acid sequences of μ and γ heavy chains. (d) IgE. The molecule is similar to the monomeric unit of IgM. (e) IgD. The hinge can be divided into a region rich in charge (possibly helical) and one rich in O-linked sugars. The structure of the hinge may be much less extended in solution than represented schematically here. It is however very sensitive to proteolytic attack so that serum IgD is unstable. Mouse IgD has a structure very different to that of human IgD in contrast to the general similarity in structures for human and mouse Igs. (f) Secretory IgA (see also figure 3.19). (g) Pentameric IgM. The molecule is represented as a planar star shape. One monomer unit is shown shaded as in (c). For clarity the carbohydrate structures have been omitted in (f) and (g). The Fab arms can likely rotate out of the plane about their two-fold axis (see also figure 3.14).

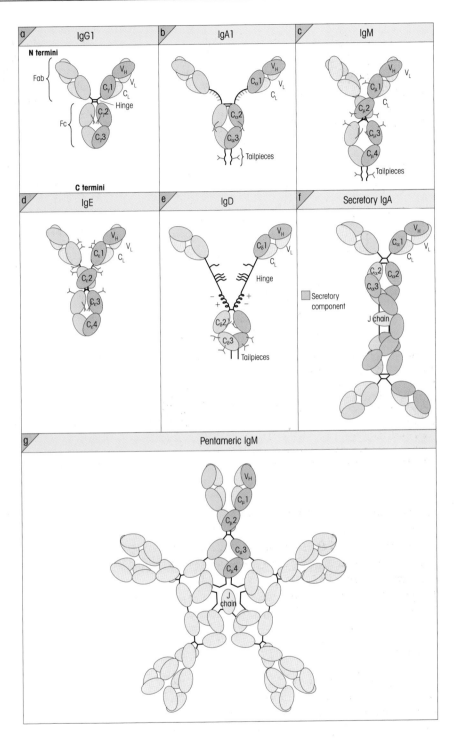

multivalent (pentavalent) but occurs in an inactive form. Binding to multivalent antigen appears to alter the conformation of the IgM molecule to expose binding sites that allow C1q to bind and the classical pathway of complement to be triggered. Electron microscopy studies suggest the conformational change is a 'star' to 'staple' transition, in which the Fab arms move out of the plane of the Fcs (figure 3.14). IgM antibodies tend to be of low affinity as measured in a univalent interaction, e.g. binding of IgM to a soluble monomeric molecule or binding of an isolated Fab from an IgM to an antigen. However, their functional affinity (avidity) can be enhanced by multivalent antibody–antigen interaction (see p. 92) and it is precisely under such circumstances that they are most effective at activating complement.

Table 3.1. The human immunoglobulins.

Class (heavy chain designation)	Human subclasses	Principal molecular forms	Polypeptides	Primary location	Complement activation (pathway)
IgG (γ)	IgG1 IgG2 IgG3 IgG4	Monomer	γ2,L2	Serum (~12 mg/ml), tissues	IgG3 > IgG1 >> IgG2 >> IgG4 (classical)
IgA (α)	IgA1 IgA2	Monomer	α2, L2	Serum (~3 mg/ml): 90% monomer, 10% dimer	Yes (mannose-binding lectin)
		Dimer	(α2,L2)₂, J		
		Secretory	(α2, L2)₂, J, SC	Seromucous secretions, milk, colostrum, tears	
IgM(μ)		Pentamer	(μ2, L2)₅, J	Serum (~1.5 mg/ml)	Yes (classical)
IgE (ε)		Monomer	ε2,L2	Serum (0.05 μg/ml)	No
IgD (δ)		Monomer	δ2,L2	Serum (30 μg/ml)	No

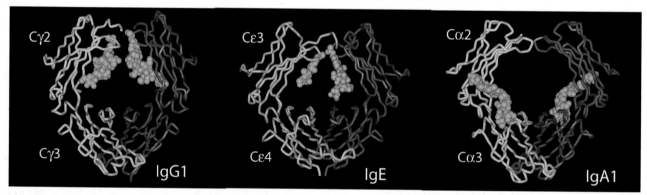

Figure 3.13. The structures of the Fc regions of human IgG1, IgE and IgA1. The structures shown were determined by crystallographic analysis of Fcs in complex with Fc receptors. One heavy chain is shown in red, the other in yellow and the N-linked carbohydrate chains that are interposed between the penultimate domains are shown in blue. For IgE, the structure does not include the Cε2 domains, which form part of the Fc region of this antibody. For IgA1, the N-linked sugars are attached at a position quite distinct from that for IgG1 and IgE. Also the tips of the Cα2 domain are joined by a disulfide bridge (Courtesy of Jenny Woof; after Woof J.M. and Burton D.R. (2004) *Nature Reviews Immunology* **4**, 89–99.)

Antibodies and human leukocyte Fc receptors

Specific human Fc receptors have been described for IgG, IgA and IgE (table 3.2). The receptors differ in their specificities for antibody classes and subclasses, their affinities for different association states of antibodies (monomer vs associated antigen-complexed antibody), their distributions on different leukocyte cell types and their cellular signaling mechanisms. Most of the leukocyte Fc receptors are structurally related, having evolved as members of the Ig gene superfamily. Each comprises a unique ligand binding chain (α chain),

which is often complexed via its transmembrane region with a dimer of the common FcR-γ chain. The latter plays a key role in the **signaling functions** of many of the receptors. FcR-γ chains carry immunoreceptor tyrosine-based activation motifs (ITAMs) in their cytoplasmic regions, critical for initiation of activatory signals. Some receptor α chains carry their own ITAMs in their cytoplasmic regions, while others bear the immunoreceptor tyrosine-based inhibitory motifs (ITIMs).

For IgG, three different classes of human leukocyte FcγRs have been characterized, most with several variant forms. In addition, the neonatal Fc receptor

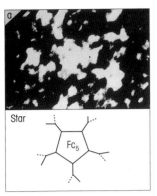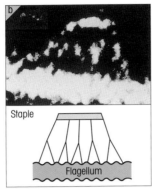

Figure 3.14. Structural changes in IgM associated with complement activation. (a) The 'star' conformation. EM of an uncomplexed IgM protein shows a 'star' shaped conformation (cf. figure 3.12g). (b) The 'staple' conformation. EM of a specific sheep IgM bound to a *Salmonella paratyphi* flagellum as antigen suggests that the 5 F(ab')$_2$ units and Cμ2 domains have been dislocated relative to the plane of the Fcs to produce a 'staple' or 'crab-like' conformation. Complement C1 is activated on binding to antigen-complexed IgM (staple), but interacts only very weakly, yielding no significant activation, with free IgM (star), implying that the dislocation process plays an important role in complement activation. It is suggested that movement of the Fabs exposes a C1q binding site on the Cμ3 domains of IgM. This is supported by observations that an Fc5 molecule, obtained by papain digestion of IgM, can activate complement directly in the absence of antigen. (Electron micrographs are negatively stained preparations of magnification ×2.10^6, i.e. 1 mm represents 0.5 nm; kindly provided by Drs A. Feinstein and E.A. Munn.)

FcRn also binds IgG and will be dealt with later. **FcγRI** (CD64) is characterized by its high affinity for monomeric IgG. It is also unusual in that it has three extracellular Ig-like domains in its ligand-binding chain, while all other Fc receptors have two. FcγRI is constitutively present on monocytes, macrophages and dendritic cells, and is induced on neutrophils and eosinophils following their activation by IFNγ and G-CSF (*g*ranulocyte *c*olony-*s*timulating *f*actor). Conversely, FcγRI can be downregulated in response to IL-4 and IL-13. Structurally, it consists of an IgG-binding α chain and a γ chain homodimer containing ITAMs. It binds monomeric IgG avidly to the surface of the cell thus sensitizing it for subsequent encounter with antigen. Its main roles are probably in facilitating phagocytosis, antigen presentation and in mediating extracellular killing of target cells coated with IgG antibody, a process referred to as *a*ntibody-*d*ependent *c*ellular *c*ytotoxicity (ADCC; p. 32).

FcγRII (CD32) binds very weakly to monomeric IgG but with considerably enhanced affinity to associated IgG as in immune complexes or on an antibody-coated target cell. Therefore cells bearing FcγRII are able to bind antibody-coated targets in the presence of high serum concentrations of monomeric IgG. Unlike the single isoform of FcγRI, there are multiple expressed isoforms of FcγRII which collectively are present on the surface of most types of leukocyte (table 3.2). The binding of IgG complexes to FcγRII triggers phagocytic cells and may provoke thrombosis through their reaction with platelets. The FcγRIIa mediates phagocytosis and ADCC whilst the FcγRIIb2 (and FcγRIII) efficiently mediates endocytosis leading to antigen presentation. FcγRIIb1 on B-cells does not endocytose immune complexes and therefore B-cells principally present only their cognate antigen following ligation and endocytosis of the *B-c*ell *r*eceptor (BCR). In fact, the FcγRIIb molecules have cytoplasmic domains which contain ITIMs and their occupation leads to *downregulation* of cellular responsiveness. In the case of the B-cell this mediates the negative-feedback effect of IgG on antibody production (cf. p. 212). Thus, whereas the isoforms on phagocytic cells are associated with ligand internalization, that on the B-cell fails to internalize but concentrates instead on lymphocyte regulation.

FcγRIII (CD16) also binds rather poorly to monomer IgG but has low to medium affinity for aggregated IgG. The two *FcγRIII* genes encode the isoforms FcγRIIIa and FcγRIIIb which have a medium and low affinity for IgG, respectively. FcγRIIIa is found on most types of leukocyte, whereas FcγRIIIb is restricted mainly to neutrophils and is unique amongst the Fc receptors in being attached to the cell membrane by a glycosylphosphatidylinositol (GPI) anchor rather than a transmembrane segment. FcγRIIIa is known to be associated with the γ chain signaling dimer on monocytes and macrophages, and with either ζ and/or γ chain signaling molecules in NK cells, and its expression is upregulated by transforming growth factor β (TGFβ) and downregulated by IL-4. With respect to their functions, FcγRIIIa is largely responsible for mediating ADCC by NK cells and the clearance of immune complexes from the circulation by macrophages. For example, the clearance of IgG-coated erythrocytes from the blood of chimpanzees was essentially inhibited by the monovalent Fab fragment of a monoclonal anti-FcγRIII. FcγRIIIb cross-linking stimulates the production of superoxide by neutrophils.

For IgE, two different FcεRs have been described. The binding of IgE to its receptor **FcεRI** is characterized by the remarkably high affinity of the interaction, reflecting a very slow dissociation rate (half-life of complex is ~20 hours). FcεRI is a complex comprising a ligand-binding α chain structurally related to those of FcγR, a β chain, and the FcR-γ chain dimer. Contact with antigen leads to degranulation of the mast cells with release of preformed vasoactive amines and cytokines, and the synthesis of a variety of inflammatory mediators derived

Table 3.2. Human leukocyte Fc receptors. (From Woof J.M. & Burton D.R. (2004) *Nature Reviews Immunology* **4**, 89.)

	FcγRI (CD64)	FcγRII (CD32)				FcγRIII (CD16)		FcεRI	FcεRII (CD23)		FcαRI (CD89)
MW (kDa)	50–70	40				50–80		45–65	45–50		50–70
Major isoforms expressed	FcγRIa	FcγRIIa		FcγRIIb	FcγRIIc	FcγRIIIa	FcγRIIIb	FcεRI	FcεRIIa	FcεRIIb	FcαRIa
Allotypes		LR	HR				NA1 and NA2				
Specificity for human Ig*	IgG1 = 3 > 4, IgG2 doesn't bind	IgG3 ≥ 1 = 2, IgG4 doesn't bind	IgG3 ≥ 1 >>> 2	IgG3 ≥ 1 >> 2 > 4	ND	ND	IgG1 = 3 >>> 2 = 4	IgE	IgE		Serum IgA1 = 2, SIgA1 = SIgA2
Affinity for monomer Ig (M^{-1})	High ($10^8 - 10^9$)	Low ($<10^7$)	Low ($<10^7$)	Low ($<10^7$)	Low ($<10^7$)	Medium (10^7)	Low ($<10^7$)	Very high (10^{10})	Low ($<10^7$)		Medium (10^7)
Signaling motif	γ chain ITAM	α chain ITAM		α chain ITIM	α chain ITAM	γ chain ITAM	No signaling motif. Anchored in membrane via glycan phosphatidyl-inositol(GPI) linkage	γ chain ITAM β chain also present but role unclear	C-type lectin	C-type lectin	γ chain ITAM.
Cellular distribution	Monocytes, macrophages, DC, neutrophils (IFNγ stim), eosinophils (IFNγ stim)	Monocytes, macrophages, neutrophils, platelets, Langerhans cells		Monocytes, macrophages, B-cells	Monocytes, macrophages, neutrophils, B-cells	Macrophages, NK cells, γδ T-cells, some monocytes	Neutrophils, eosinophils (IFNγ stim)	Mast cells, basophils, Langerhans cells, activated monocytes	B-cells	B-cells, T-cells, monocytes, eosinophils, macrophages	Neutrophils, monocytes, some macrophages, eosinophils, Kupffer cells, some DC

* Relative affinities of various ligands for each receptor are indicated in decreasing order starting with the isotype with highest affinity. Arrowheads and equal signs are used to show the differences in affinity.

from arachidonic acid (cf. figure 1.15). This process is responsible for the symptoms of hay fever and of extrinsic asthma when patients with atopic allergy come into contact with the allergen, e.g. grass pollen. The main *physiological* role of IgE would appear to be protection of anatomical sites susceptible to trauma and pathogen entry by local recruitment of plasma factors and effector cells through the **triggering of an acute inflammatory reaction**. Infectious agents penetrating the IgA defenses would combine with specific IgE on the mast cell surface and trigger the release of vasoactive agents and factors chemotactic for polymorphs, so leading to an influx of plasma IgG, complement, neutrophils and eosinophils (cf. p. 33). In such a context, the ability of eosinophils to damage IgG-coated helminths and the generous IgE response to such parasites would constitute an effective defense.

The low affinity IgE receptor **FcεRII** (CD23) is a C-type (calcium-dependent) lectin. It is present on many different types of hematopoietic cells (table 3.2). Its primary function appears to be in the regulation of IgE synthesis by B-cells, with a stimulatory role at low concentrations of IgE and an inhibitory role at high concentrations. It can also facilitate phagocytosis of IgE opsonized antigens.

For IgA, **FcαRI** (CD89), is the only well characterized Fc receptor. Its ligand-binding α chain is structurally related to those of the FcγRs and FcεRI but represents a more distantly related member of the family. In fact, it shares closer homology with members of a family including natural killer cell immunoglobulin-like receptors (KIRs), leukocyte Ig-like receptors (LIR/LILR/ILTs) and the platelet-specific collagen receptor (GPVI). FcαRI is present on monocytes, macrophages, neutrophils, eosinophils and Kupffer cells. The cross-linking of FcαRI by antigen can activate endocytosis, phagocytosis, inflammatory mediator release and ADCC. Expression of FcαRI on monocytes is strongly upregulated by bacterial polysaccharide.

Crystal structures are available for FcγRIIa, FcγRIIb, FcγRIIIb, FcεRI and FcαRI (figure 3.15). In all cases, the structures represent the two Ig-like extracellular domains of the receptor α chain, termed D1 (N-terminal, membrane distal) and D2 (C-terminal, membrane proximal). No structure is yet available for the cytoplasmic portions of any receptor. The extracellular regions of FcγRIIa/b, FcγRIII and FcεRI are seen to share the same overall heart-shaped structure and are so similar that they can be readily superimposed. Despite the basic sequence similarity between FcαRI and these receptors, the IgA receptor turns out to have a strikingly different structure. While the two individual domains of the FcαRI extracellular portion fold up in a similar manner to those of the other receptors, the arrangement of the domains relative to each other is very different. The domains are rotated through ~180° from the positions adopted in the other Fc receptors, essentially inverting the D1–D2 orientations.

Crystallographic studies of antibody–Fc receptor complexes have revealed how antibodies interact with leukocyte Fc receptors (figure 3.16). For the IgG–FcγRIII interaction, the D2 membrane-proximal domain of FcγRIII interacts with the top of the C_H2 domains and the bottom of the hinge. This requires the antibody adopt a 'dislocated' conformation in which the Fab arms are rotated out of the plane of the Fc. One consequence of this mode of interaction, recognized many years ago, is that it promotes close approach of the target cell membrane (upwards on the page) to the effector cell membrane. This may favor effector cell activity against the target cell. Given the similiarities between FcγRI, FcγRII and FcγRIII, it is likely that all three FcRs share a common mode of binding to IgG. Indeed, this mode of binding seems also to be shared by IgE binding to the FcεRI receptor although the Cε2–Cε3 domain linker region replaces the hinge contribution to receptor binding. By contrast, IgA binds to the FcαRI receptor at a site between Cα2 and Cα3 domains. This mode of binding permits an IgA:FcR stoichiometry of 2 : 1 whilst the stoichiometry for IgG and IgE in the above complexes is 1 : 1. The significance of these differences in the modes of binding is not understood at this time.

Antibodies and the neonatal Fc receptor

An important Fc receptor for IgG is the neonatal recep-

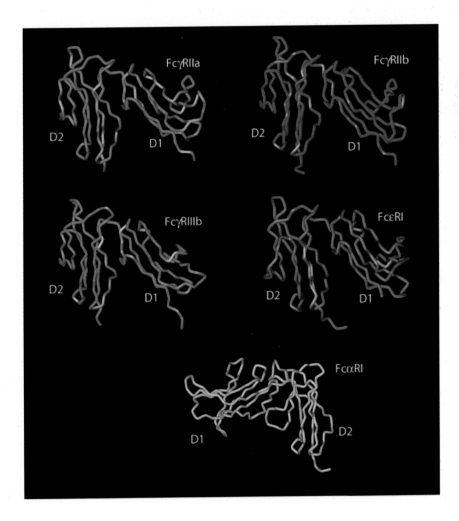

Figure 3.15. Structures of human leukocyte Fc receptors. In each case, a similar view of the receptor is shown, in its uncomplexed state. D1, membrane distal; D2, membrane proximal domain. For the FcγRs and FcεRI, the Fc binding site is present at the 'top' of the D2 domain. For FcαRI, the D1–D2 domain arrangement is reversed and the Fc interaction site is present at the top of the D1 domain. (Courtesy of Jenny Woof.)

tor, FcRn. This receptor mediates **transport of IgG from mother to child** across the placenta (figure 3.17). Such antibody, surviving for some time in the blood of the newborn child, is believed to be important in directly protecting the child from pathogens. Furthermore, the presence of maternal antibody has been proposed to help the development of cellular immunity in the young child by attenuating pathogen challenge rather than stopping it completely. FcRn may also be important in transporting maternal IgG from mother's milk across the intestinal cells of the young infant to the blood. Equally, FcRn is crucial in **maintaining the long half-life of IgG in serum** in adults and children. The receptor binds IgG in acidic vesicles (pH < 6.5) protecting the molecule from degradation, and then releasing the IgG at the higher pH of 7.4 in blood.

Structural studies have revealed the molecular basis for FcRn activity. FcRn is unlike leukocyte Fc receptors and instead has structural similarity to MHC class I molecules. It is a heterodimer composed of a β_2-microglobulin chain noncovalently attached to a membrane-bound chain that includes three extracellular domains. One of these domains, including a carbohydrate chain, together with β_2-microglobulin interacts with a site between the C_H2 and C_H3 domains of Fc (figure 3.18). The interaction includes three salt bridges made to histidine (His) residues on IgG that are positively charged at pH < 6.5. At higher pH, the His residues lose their positive charges, the FcRn–IgG interaction is weakened and IgG dissociates.

Secretory IgA

IgA appears selectively in the seromucous secretions, such as saliva, tears, nasal fluids, sweat, colostrum, milk, and secretions of the lung, genitourinary and gastrointestinal tracts, where it clearly has the job of

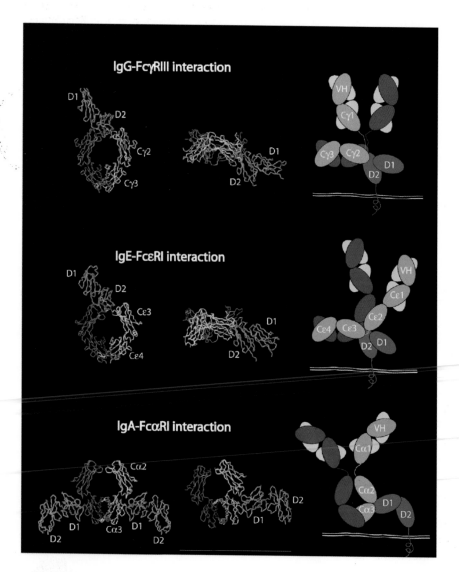

Figure 3.16. Structures of antibody–leukocyte Fc receptor interactions. The left hand side and middle columns show views of the crystal structures of the complexes of the FcRs with their respective Fc ligands. The extracellular domains of the receptors are shown in blue while one heavy chain of each Fc region is shown in red and the other in gold. In the left hand column, each Fc region is viewed face on. The similarity between the IgG-FcγRIII and IgE–FcεRI interaction is striking while the IgA–FcαRI interaction is quite different in terms of the sites involved and the stoichiometry. The middle column shows a view where the D2 domains of each of the receptors are positioned so that their C-termini face downwards. Here the Fc regions of IgG and IgE are seen in a horizontal position from the side. For the IgA interaction only one receptor molecule is shown. The right hand column shows a schematic representation of the receptors and their intact ligands from the same viewpoint as the images in the middle column. Light chains are shown in pale yellow. The necessity for dislocation of IgG and IgE to allow positioning of the Fab tips away from the receptor-bearing cell surface is apparent. (Courtesy of Jenny Woof.)

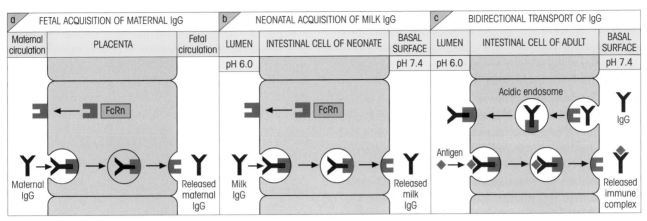

Figure 3.17. Function of the neonatal receptor for IgG (FcRn) on epithelial cells. (a) The FcRn receptor is present in the placenta where it fulfills the important task of transferring maternal IgG to the fetal circulation. This will provide protection prior to the generation of immunocompetence in the fetus. Furthermore, it is self-evident that any infectious agent which might reach the fetus *in utero* will have had to have passed through the mother first, and the fetus will rely upon the mother's immune system to have produced IgG with appropriate binding specificities. This maternal IgG also provides protection for the neonate, because it takes some weeks following birth before the transferred IgG is eventually all catabolized. (b) It has been clearly demonstrated in rodents, although remains speculative in humans, that there is epithelial transport of IgG from maternal milk across the intestinal cells of the newborn. IgG binds to FcRn at pH 6.0, is taken into the cell within a clathrin-coated vesicle and released at the pH of the basal surface. The directional movement of IgG is achieved by the asymmetric pH effect on Ig–receptor interaction. Knockout mice lacking FcRn are incapable of acquiring maternal Ig as neonates. Furthermore, they have a grossly shortened IgG half-life, consistent with the role of FcRn as a protective receptor that prevents degradation of IgG and then recycles it to the circulation. The IgG half-life is unusually long compared with that of IgA and IgM and this enables the response to antigen to be sustained for many months following infection. (c) An additional role of FcRn may be as a bidirectional shuttle receptor. IgG binding on the nonluminal side of the epithelial cell may occur, following endocytosis, within the more favorable pH of acidic endosomes. This receptor may thus provide a mechanism for mucosal immunosurveillance, traveling back and forth across the epithelial cell, delivering IgG to the intestinal lumen and then returning the same antibodies in the form of immune complexes for the stimulation of B-cells by follicular dendritic cells.

defending the exposed external surfaces of the body against attack by microorganisms. This responsibility is clearly taken seriously since approximately 40 mg of secretory IgA/kg body weight is transported daily through the human intestinal crypt epithelium to the mucosal surface as compared with a *total* daily production of IgG of 30 mg/kg.

The IgA is synthesized locally by plasma cells and dimerized intracellularly together with a cysteine-rich polypeptide called J chain, of molecular weight 15 000. Dimeric IgA binds strongly to a receptor for polymeric Ig (**poly-Ig receptor, pIgR**, which also binds polymeric IgM) present in the membrane of mucosal epithelial cells. The complex is then actively endocytosed, transported across the cytoplasm and secreted into the external body fluids after cleavage of the pIgR peptide chain. The fragment of the receptor remaining bound to the IgA is termed secretory component and the whole molecule, **secretory IgA** (figure 3.19).

Isotypes, allotypes and idiotypes: antibody variants

The variability of antibodies is often conveniently divided into three types. **Isotypes** are variants present in all healthy members of a species: immunoglobulin

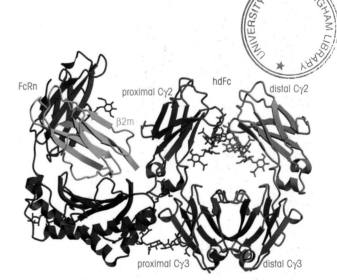

Figure 3.18. Structure of the rat neonatal Fc receptor binding to the Fc of IgG. A heterodimeric Fc (hdFc) is shown with the FcRn binding chain in red and the nonbinding chain in orange. The orange chain has been mutated at several positions to eliminate FcRn binding. If the normal homodimeric molecule is used then oligomeric ribbon structures are created in which FcRn dimers are bridged by Fcs thereby preventing crystallization. The three domains of FcRn are shown in dark blue (two are close together at the bottom of the picture in this view) and β_2-microglobulin in light blue. A portion of the α_2 domain, an N-linked carbohydrate attached to this domain and the C-terminus of β_2-microglobulin form the FcRn side of the interaction site. Residues at the C_H2/C_H3 domain interface form the Fc side of the interaction site. (After Martin W.L. *et al.* (2001) *Molecular Cell* **7**, 867.)

classes and subclasses are examples of isotypic variation involving the constant region of the heavy chain. **Allotypes** are variants that are inherited as alternatives (alleles) and therefore not all healthy members of a species inherit a particular allotype. Allotypes occur mostly as variants of heavy-chain constant-region genes, in man in all four IgG subclasses, IgA2 and IgM. The nomenclature of human immunoglobulin allotypes is based on the isotype on which it is found (e.g. G1m defines allotypes on an IgG1 heavy chain, Km defines allotypes on κ light chains) followed by an accepted WHO numbering system.

The variable region of an antibody can act as an antigen, and the unique determinants of this region that distinguish it from most other antibodies of that species are termed its idiotypic determinants. The **idiotype** of an antibody, therefore, consists of a set of idiotypic determinants which individually are called idiotopes. Polyclonal anti-idiotypic antibodies generally recognize a set of idiotopes whilst a monoclonal anti-idiotype recognizes a single idiotope. Idiotypes are usually specific for an individual antibody clone (private idiotypes) but are sometimes shared between different antibody clones (public, recurrent or cross-reacting idiotypes). An anti-idiotype may react with determinants distant from the antigen binding site, it may fit the binding site and express the image of the antigen or it may react with determinants close to the binding site and interfere with antigen binding. Sequencing of an anti-idiotypic antibody generated against an antibody specific for the polypeptide GAT antigen in mice revealed a CDR3 with an amino acid sequence identical to that of the antigen epitope, i.e. the anti-idiotype contains a true image of the antigen but this is probably the exception rather than the rule.

GENETICS OF ANTIBODY DIVERSITY AND FUNCTION

Antibodies genes are produced by somatic recombination

The immunoglobulin repertoire is encoded for by multiple germline gene segments that undergo somatic diversification in developing B-cells. Hence, although the basic components needed to generate an immunoglobulin repertoire are inherited, an individual's mature antibody repertoire is essentially formed during their lifetime by alteration of the inherited germline genes.

The first evidence that immunoglobulin genes rearrange by **somatic recombination** was reported by Hozumi and Tonegawa in 1976 (Milestone 3.2). Because somatic recombination involves rearrangement of DNA in somatic, in contrast to gamete cells, the newly recombined genes are not inherited. As a result, the primary immunoglobulin repertoire will differ slightly from one individual to the next, and will be further modified during an individual's lifetime by their exposure to different antigens.

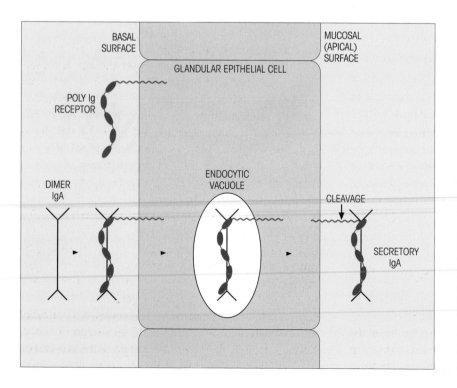

Figure 3.19. IgA secretion at the mucosal surface. The mucosal cell synthesizes a receptor for polymeric Ig (pIgR) which is inserted into the basal membrane. Dimeric IgA binds to this receptor and is transported via an endocytic vacuole to the apical surface. Cleavage of the receptor releases secretory IgA still attached to part of the receptor termed the secretory component. Note how the receptor cleavage introduces an asymmetry, which drives the transport of IgA dimers to the mucosal surface (in quite the opposite direction to the transcytosis of milk IgG in figure 3.17).

Milestone 3.2—The 1987 Nobel Prize in Physiology or Medicine

Susumu Tonegawa was awarded the 1987 Nobel Prize in Physiology or Medicine for 'his discovery of the genetic principle for generation of antibody diversity.' In his 1976 paper, Tonegawa used southern blot analysis of restriction enzyme digested DNA from lymphoid and nonlymphoid cells to show that the immunoglobulin variable and constant genes are distant from each other in the germline genome. Embryo DNA showed two components when hybridized to RNA probes specific for (i) both variable and constant regions and (ii) only the constant region, whereas both probes localized to a single band when hybridized to DNA from an antibody-producing plasmacytoma cell. He proposed that the differential hybridization patterns could be explained if the variable and constant genes were distant from each other in germline DNA, but came together to encode the complete immunoglobulin gene during lymphocyte differentiation.

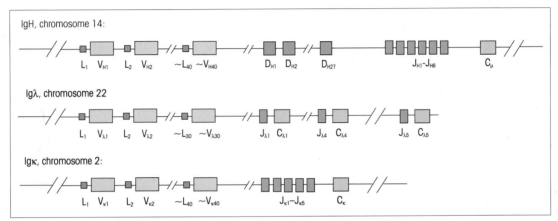

Figure 3.20. The human immunoglobulin loci. Schematics of the human heavy chain (top) and light chain lambda (middle) and kappa (bottom) loci are shown. The human heavy chain locus on chromosome 14 consists of approximately 38–46 functional V_H genes, 27 D_H genes and six J_H genes, which are organized into clusters upstream of the constant regions. The human lambda locus on chromosome 22 consists of approximately 30 functional V_λ genes and five functional J_λ gene segments, with each J segment followed by a constant segment. The human kappa locus on chromosome 2 consists of 34–40 functional V_κ genes and five functional J_κ genes, with the J segments clustered upstream of the constant region. (L, leader sequence.)

The immunoglobulin variable gene segments and loci

The variable light and heavy chain loci in humans contain multiple gene segments which are joined, using somatic recombination, to produce the final V region exon. The human heavy chain variable region is constructed from the joining of three gene segments, **V (variable), D (diversity), and J (joining)**, whereas the light chain variable gene is constructed by the joining of two gene segments, V and J. There are multiple V, D and J segments at the heavy chain and light chain loci, as illustrated in figure 3.20.

The human V_H genes have been mapped to chromosome 14, although orphan IgH genes have also been identified on chromosomes 15 and 16. The human V_H locus is highly polymorphic, and may have evolved through the repeated duplication, deletion and recombination of DNA. Polymorphisms found within the germline repertoire are due to the insertion or deletion of gene segments or the occurrence of different alleles of the same segment. A number of pseudogenes, ranging from those that are more conserved and contain a few point mutations to those that are more divergent with extensive mutations, are also present in immunoglobulin loci. There are approximately one hundred human V_H genes, which can be grouped into seven families based on sequence homology, and these families can be further grouped into three clans. Members of a given family show approximately 80% sequence homology at the nucleotide level. The functional heavy chain repertoire is formed from approximately 38–46 functional V_H genes, 27 D_H genes and six J_H genes. The human lambda locus maps to chromosome 22, with approximately 30 functional V_λ genes and five functional J_λ gene segments. The V_λ genes can be grouped into 10 families, which are further divided into seven clans. The human kappa locus on chromosome 2 is composed of a total of approximately 34–40 functional V_κ genes and five functional J_κ genes. However, the kappa locus contains a large duplication of most of the V_κ genes, and most of the V_κ genes in this distal cluster, although functional are seldom used.

The immunoglobulin loci also contain regulatory elements (figure 3.21), such as a conserved octamer motif and TATA box in the promoter regions. Leader sequences are also found upstream of the variable segments, and enhancer elements are also present within the loci to facilitate productive transcription.

V(D)J recombination and combinatorial diversity

The joining of these gene segments, illustrated in figure 3.22, is known as **V(D)J recombination**. V(D)J recombination is a highly regulated and ordered event. The light chain exon is constructed from a single V-to-J gene segment join. However, at the heavy chain locus, a D-

segment is first joined to a J-segment, and then the V-segment is joined to the combined DJ sequence. The rearranged DNA is transcribed, the RNA transcript is spliced to bring together the V region exon and the C-region exon, and lastly the spliced mRNA is translated to produce the final immunoglobulin protein.

Numerous unique immunoglobulin genes can be made by joining different combinations of the V, D and J segments at the heavy and light chain loci. The creation of diversity in the immunoglobulin repertoire through this joining of various gene segments is known as **combinatorial diversity**. Additional diversity is created by the pairing of different heavy chains with different lambda or kappa light chains. For example, the potential heavy chain repertoire is approximately $40\,V_H \times 27\,D_H \times 6\,J_H = 6.5 \times 10^3$ different combinations. Similarly, there

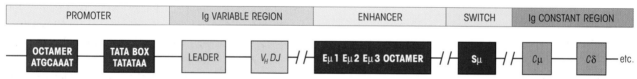

Figure 3.21 Regulatory elements of immunoglobulin loci. Each *VDJ* segment encoding the variable region is associated with a leader sequence. Closely upstream is the TATA box of the promoter, which binds RNA polymerase II and the octamer motif which is one of a number of short sequences which bind transacting regulatory transcription factors. The *V region* promoters are relatively inactive and only association with enhancers, which are also composites of short sequence motifs capable of binding nuclear proteins, will increase the transcription rate to levels typical of actively secreting B-cells. The enhancers are near to the regions that control switching from one Ig class constant region to another, e.g. IgM to IgG (figure 3.27). Primary transcripts are initiated 20 nucleotides downstream of the TATA box and extend beyond the end of the constant region. These are spliced, cleaved at the 3' end and polyadenylated to generate the translatable mRNA.

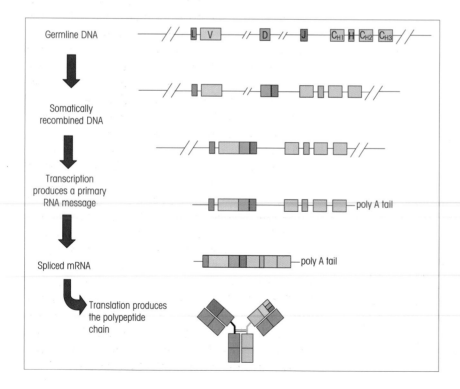

Figure 3.22. Overview of V(D)J recombination. Diversity (D) and joining (J) gene segments in the germline DNA are joined together through somatic recombination at the heavy chain locus. The variable (V) gene segment is then joined to the recombined D-J gene, to produce the fully recombined heavy chain exon. At the light chain loci, somatic recombination occurs with V and J segments only. The recombined DNA is transcribed, and the primary RNA transcript is then spliced, bringing together the variable and constant regions. The spliced mRNA molecule is translated to produce the immunoglobulin protein. The contribution of the different gene segments to the polypeptide sequence is illustrated for one of the heavy chains. H, hinge.

are approximately 165 ($33 \, V_\lambda \times 5 \, J_\lambda$) and 200 ($40 \, V_\kappa \times 5 \, J_\kappa$) different combinations, for a total of 365 light chain combinations. If we consider that each heavy chain could potentially pair with each light chain, then the diversity of the immunoglobulin repertoire is quite large, on the order of 10^6 possible combinations. Additional diversity is also generated during gene segment recombination and by somatic hypermutation, as explained in the following sections. In this manner, although the number of germline gene segments appears limited in size, an incredibly diverse immunoglobulin repertoire can be generated.

Recombination signal sequences

The **recombination signal sequence** (RSS) helps to guide recombination between appropriate gene segments. The RSS (figure 3.23) is a noncoding sequence which flanks coding gene segments. It is made up of a conserved heptamer and nonamer sequences, which are separated by an unconserved 12- or 23-nucleotide spacer. Efficient recombination occurs between segments with a 12-nucleotide spacer and a 23-nucleotide spacer. This **'12/23' rule** helps make certain that appropriate gene segments are joined together.

At the V_H locus, the V and J segments are flanked by RSSs with a 23-nucleotide spacer, whereas the D segments are flanked by RSSs with a 12-nucleotide spacer. At light chain loci, the V_κ segments are flanked by RSSs with 12-nucleotide spacers, J_κ segments are flanked by RSSs with 23-nucleotide spacers, and this arrangement is reversed in the lambda locus.

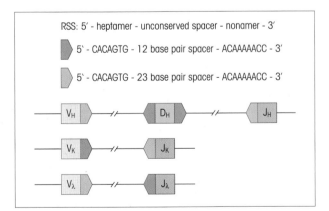

Figure 3.23. The recombination signal sequence. The recombination signal sequence (RSS) is made up of conserved heptamer and nonamer sequences, separated by an unconserved 12- or 23-nucleotide spacer. Efficient recombination occurs between segments with a 12-nucleotide spacer and a 23-nucleotide spacer. RSSs with 23-nucleotide spacers flank the V and J segments of the heavy chain locus, the J segments of the kappa locus and the V segments of the lambda locus, whereas RSSs with 12-nucleotide spacers flank the D segments of the heavy chain locus, the V segments of the kappa locus and the J segments of the lambda locus.

The recombinase machinery

The V(D)J recombinase is a complex of enzymes that mediates somatic recombination of immunoglobulin gene segments (figure 3.24). The gene products of recombination-activating genes 1 and 2, RAG-1 and RAG-2, are lymphocyte-specific enzymes essential for V(D)J recombination. In the initial steps of V(D)J recombination, the RAG complex binds the recombination signal sequences and, in association with high mobility group (HMG) proteins that are involved in DNA bending, the two recombination signal sequences are brought together. In contrast to the lymphoid-specific RAG enzymes, HMG proteins are ubiquitously expressed.

Next, a single-stranded nick is introduced between the 5' heptameric end of the recombination signal sequence and the coding segment. This nick results in a free 3' OH group, that attacks the opposite, anti-parallel DNA strand in a transesterification reaction. This attack gives rise to a double strand DNA break that leads to the formation of covalently sealed hairpins at the two coding ends and the formation of blunt signal ends. At this stage a post-cleavage complex is formed, in which the RAG recombinase remains associated with the DNA ends.

The DNA break is finally repaired by nonhomologous end-joining machinery. The recombination signal sequences are joined precisely to generate the signal joint. By contrast, nucleotides can be lost or added during repair of the coding ends (figure 3.25). **Junctional diversity** is the diversification of variable region exons due to this imprecise joining of the coding ends.

First, a small number of nucleotides are often deleted from the coding end by an unknown exonuclease. Also, junctional diversity involves the potential addition of two types of nucleotides, **N-nucleotides** and **P-nucleotides**. N-nucleotides are generated by the non-templated addition of nucleotides to the coding ends, which is mediated by the enzyme terminal deoxynucleotidyl transferase (TdT). The palindromic sequences that result from the asymmetric cleavage and template mediated fill-in of the coding hairpins are referred to as P-nucleotides. Although N- and P- nucleotides and deletion of the coding end and nucleotides serve to greatly diversify the immunoglobulin repertoire, the addition of these nucleotides may also result in the generation of receptor genes that are out of frame.

Similar to the RAG recombinase complex, the **DNA repair machinery** works as a protein complex. However, unlike the RAG recombinase, the nonhomologous end-joining proteins are ubiquitously expressed. In the first steps of DNA repair, the Ku70 and

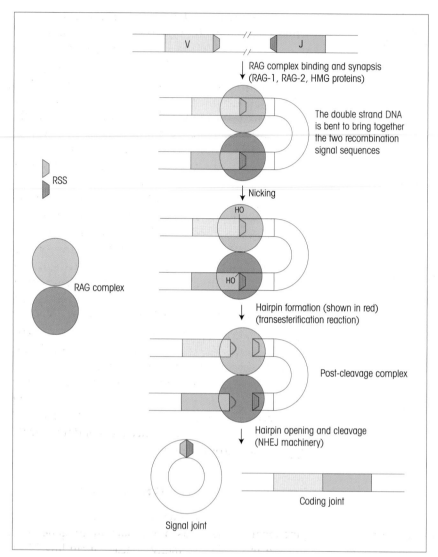

Figure 3.24. The V(D)J recombinase. In the initial steps of V(D)J recombination, the RAG-1 and RAG-2 proteins associate with the recombination signal sequences. A single-stranded nick is then introduced between the 5' heptameric end of the recombination signal sequence and the coding segment, giving rise to a free 3'OH group that mediates a transesterification reaction. This reaction leads to the formation of DNA hairpins at the coding ends. Hairpin cleavage and resolution of the post-cleavage complex by nonhomologous end-joining (NHEJ) proteins results in the formation of separate coding and signal joints, in the final steps of V(D)J recombination.

Ku80 proteins form a heterodimer which bind the broken DNA ends. The Ku complex recruits the catalytic subunit of DNA-dependent protein kinase, DNA-PKcs, a serine-threonine protein kinase. The activated DNA-PKcs then recruits and phosphorylates XRCC4 and Artemis. Artemis is an endonuclease that opens the hairpin coding ends. Finally, DNA ligase IV binds XRCC4 to form an end-ligation complex, and this complex mediates the final ligation and fill-in steps needed to form the coding and signal joints.

Regulating V(D)J recombination

V(D)J recombination and the recombinase machinery must be carefully regulated to avoid wreaking havoc on the cellular genome. For instance, aberrant V(D)J recombination is implicated in certain B-cell lymphomas. V(D)J recombination is largely regulated by controlling expression of the recombination machinery and the accessibility of gene segments and nearby enhancers and promoters. As previously mentioned, RAG-1 and RAG-2 activity is specific to lymphoid cells, and further regulation is imposed by downregulating RAG activity during appropriate stages of B-cell development. Differential accessibility of gene segments to the recombinase machinery, which can be achieved by altering chromatin structure, also plays a role in making certain that appropriate gene segments are recombined in an appropriate order. *Cis*-acting transcriptional control elements, such as enhancers and promoters, also help regulate recombination. Although it is not a hard and fast rule, transcription from certain regulatory elements seems to correlate with rearrangement of the adjacent genes. This **sterile**, or nonproductive, **transcription** may somehow help target required proteins or modulate gene accessibility. Finally, in addition to directing recombination between appropriate gene segments, the precise sequences of the RSS itself, as well as the sequences of the gene segments themselves, can influence the efficiency of the recombination reaction.

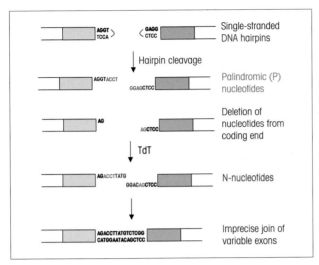

Figure 3.25. Junctional diversity further diversifies the immune repertoire. The immunoglobulin repertoire is further diversified during cleavage and resolution of the coding-end hairpins by deletion of a variable number of coding end nucleotides, the addition of N-nucleotides by terminal deoxynucleotidyl transferase (TdT), and palindromic (P) nucleotides that arise due to template-mediated fill-in of the asymmetrically cleaved coding hairpins. TdT randomly adds nucleotides to the DNA ends (N-nucleotides), and the single-stranded ends pair, possibly but not necessarily, through complementary nucleotides (TG on top strand and AC on bottom strand). Exonuclease trimming, to remove unpaired nucleotides, and the DNA repair machinery act to repair the DNA joint.

Somatic hypermutation

Following antigen activation, the variable regions of immunoglobulin heavy and light chains are further diversified by somatic hypermutation. **Somatic hypermutation** involves the introduction of nontemplated point mutations into V regions of rapidly proliferating B-cells in the germinal centers of lymphoid follicles. Antigen-driven somatic hypermutation of variable immunoglobulin genes can result in an increase in binding affinity of the B-cell receptor for its cognate ligand. As B-cells with higher affinity immunoglobulins can more successfully compete for limited amounts of antigen present, an increase in the average affinity of the antibodies produced during an immune response is observed. This increase in the average affinity of immunoglobulins is known as **affinity maturation**.

Somatic hypermutation occurs at a high rate, thought to be on the order of about 1×10^{-3} mutations per base pair per generation, which is approximately 10^6 times higher than the mutation rate of cellular housekeeping genes. There is a bias for transition mutations, and the 'mutation hotspots' in variable regions map to RGWY motifs (R = purine, Y = pyrimidine, W = A or T). The exact mechanisms by which mutations are introduced

and preferentially targeted to appropriate V regions, while constant regions of the immunoglobulin loci remain protected, is not clearly understood and is the subject of current research. Transcription through the target V region seems required, but is not necessarily sufficient, for somatic hypermutation. Additionally, the enzyme **activation-induced cytidine deaminase (AID)** has been demonstrated to be essential for both somatic hypermutation and class-switch recombination.

AID is a cytidine deaminase capable of carrying out targeted deamination of C to U, and shows strong homology with the RNA-editing enzyme APOBEC-1. Two current hypotheses have been proposed to explain the mechanism by which AID acts, one favoring RNA editing while the second favors DNA deamination. It is possible that AID recognizes and acts on an mRNA precursor, or more likely that AID directly deaminates DNA to produce U : G mismatches. The exact mechanism by which AID can differentially regulate somatic hypermutation and class switch recombination is currently being studied, and may depend on interactions of specific cofactors with specific domains of AID.

Therefore, diversity within the immunoglobulin repertoire is generated by: (i) the combinatorial joining of gene segments; (ii) junctional diversity; (iii) combinatorial pairing of heavy and light chains; and (iv) somatic hypermutation of V regions.

Gene conversion and repertoire diversification

Although mice and humans use combinatorial and junctional diversity as a mechanism to generate a diverse repertoire, in many species, including birds, cattle, swine, sheep, horses and rabbits, V(D)J recombination results in assembly and expression of a single functional gene. Repertoire diversification is then achieved by **gene conversion**, a process in which pseudo-V genes are used as templates to be copied into the assembled variable region exon. Further diversification may be achieved by somatic hypermutation.

The process of gene conversion was originally identified in chickens, in which immature B-cells have the same variable region exon. During B-cell development in the bursa of Fabricius, rapidly proliferating B-cells undergo gene conversion to diversify the immunoglobulin repertoire (figure 3.26). Stretches of sequences from germline variable region pseudogenes, located upstream of the functional V genes, are introduced into the V_L and V_H regions. This process takes place in the ileal Peyer's patches of cattle, swine and horses, and in the appendix of rabbits. These gut-associated lymphoid tissues are the mammalian equivalent of the bursa in these species.

Class switch recombination

Antigen-stimulated IgM expressing B-cells in germinal centers of secondary lymphoid organs, such as the spleen and lymph nodes, undergo class switch recombination. **Class switch recombination (CSR)** allows the IgH constant region exon of a given antibody to be exchanged for an alternative exon, giving rise to the expression of antibodies with the same antigen specificity but of differing isotypes, and therefore of differing effector functions as described above. CSR occurs through a deletional DNA recombination event at the IgH locus (figure 3.27), which has been extensively studied in mice. Constant region exons for IgG, IgA, and

IgE isotypes are located downstream of the IgM ($C\mu$) exon, and CSR occurs between **switch** or **S regions**. S regions are repetitive sequences, which are often G-rich on the nontemplate strand, that are found upstream of each C_H exon. Breaks are introduced into the DNA of two S regions and fusion of the S regions leads to a rearranged C_H locus, in which the variable exon is joined to an exon for a new constant region. The DNA between the two switch regions is excised and forms an episomal circle. Finally, alternative splicing of the primary RNA transcript generated from the rearranged DNA gives rise to either membrane-bound or secreted forms of the immunoglobulin.

Prior to recombination between switch regions, tran-

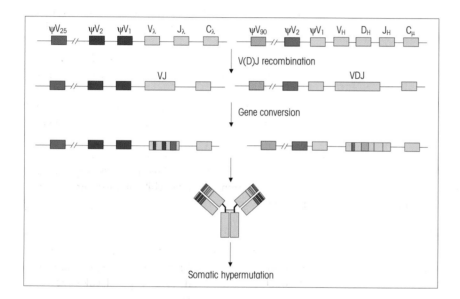

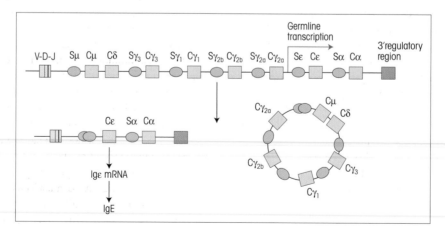

Figure 3.26. Immunoglobulin diversification using gene conversion. V(D)J recombination in chicken B-cells results in assembly of a single variable region exon. In the process of gene conversion, sequences of pseudogenes, located upstream of the functional gene segments, are copied into the recombined variable exons at the light and heavy chain loci in rapidly proliferating B-cells in the bursa of Fabricius. This results in a diversified antibody repertoire.

Figure 3.27. Class switch recombination allows expression of different antibody isotypes. Class switch recombination involves DNA recombination at repetitive sequences termed switch or S regions, and is illustrated here for an IgM to IgE switch, at the mouse heavy chain locus. Switching to an IgE isotype begins with germline transcription from the promoter upstream of the constant region exon and recombination between the $S\mu$ and $S\epsilon$ regions. This DNA recombination reaction brings the IgE constant region exon downstream of the variable region exon. The remaining switch regions and constant region exons are deleted and form an episomal circle. Transcription of the rearranged DNA yields IgE mRNA, which can be translated to give rise to the IgE immunoglobulin protein.

scription is initiated from a promoter found upstream of an exon that precedes all C_H genes capable of undergoing CSR, the intervening (I) exon. These germline transcripts include I, S and C region exons, and do not appear to code for any functional protein. However, this germline transcription is required, although not sufficient, to stimulate CSR. The precise mechanism responsible for CSR is the subject of current study, but work indicates that AID, described previously to be involved

in somatic hypermutation, helps mediate CSR, along with some components of the nonhomologous end-joining pathway and several other DNA repair pathways. The joining of S regions may be mediated by association with transcriptional promoters, enhancers, chromatin factors, DNA repair proteins, AID-associated factors or by interactions involving S region sequences themselves.

SUMMARY

Antibody structure and function

- Antibodies recognize foreign material and trigger its elimination.
- They are Y- or T-shaped molecules in which the arms of the molecule (Fab) recognize foreign material and the stem (Fc) interacts with immune molecules that lead to the elimination of the antibody-decorated foreign material.
- Antibodies are based on a four-chain structure consisting of two identical heavy chains and two identical light chains.
- The N-terminal parts of the heavy chains and the light chains form the two identical Fab arms that are linked to the Fc stem of the molecule consisting of the C-terminal parts of the heavy chains.
- The extremities of the Fab arms consist of regions of variable amino acid sequences that are involved in binding antigen and thereby give each antibody its unique specificity. The human antibody repertoire is vast, allowing the recognition of essentially any molecular shape.
- The Fc stem of the molecule has a more conserved sequence and is involved in binding effector molecules such as complement and Fc receptors.
- Differences in the Fc regions lead to different classes and subclasses of antibodies or immunoglobulins (Igs).
- There are five different classes of Ig—IgG, IgM, IgA, IgD and IgE—which fulfill different roles in immune protection. They also have different polymerization states.
- The structure of antibodies is organized into domains based on a β-sheet arrangement called the immunoglobulin fold.
- For IgG, the Fab arms, consisting of two variable domains and two constant domains, are linked via a flexible hinge region to the Fc, which consists of four constant domains.
- Flexibility is an important feature of antibody structure allowing interaction with antigens and effector molecules in a variety of environments.

Antibody interaction with effector molecules

- IgG triggers complement by binding C1q when clustered on an antigen such as a pathogen. IgM is already multivalent

but, on binding antigen, it undergoes a conformational change to bind C1q.
- Leukocyte receptors have been described for IgG, IgA and IgE that, on binding antigen-associated antibody, trigger effector mechanisms such as phagocytosis, antibody-dependent cellular cytoxicity and acute inflammatory responses. Interaction between antibody and Fc receptors can also be immunoregulatory.
- The structures of IgG Fc receptors and the mast cell IgE Fc receptor and the mode of interaction of the receptors with Ig appear to be quite similar. The IgA receptor has however a distinct structure and mode of interaction with IgA.
- IgG interacts with the neonatal receptor FcRn to promote transport of IgG from mother to child and to maintain the long half-life of IgG in serum.

Overview of the Ig classes

- IgG is monomeric and the major antibody in serum and nonmucosal tissues, where it inactivates pathogens directly and through interaction with triggering molecules such as complement and Fc receptors.
- IgA exists mainly as a monomer in plasma, but in the seromucous secretions, where it is the major Ig concerned in the defense of the external body surfaces, it is present as a dimer linked to a secretory component.
- IgM is most commonly a pentameric molecule although a minor fraction is hexameric. It is essentially intravascular and is produced early in the immune response. Because of its high valency it is a very effective bacterial agglutinator and mediator of complement-dependent cytolysis and is therefore a powerful first-line defense against bacteremia.
- IgD is largely present on the lymphocyte and functions together with IgM as the antigen receptor on naive B-cells.
- IgE binds very tightly to mast cells and contact with antigen leads to local recruitment of antimicrobial agents through degranulation of the mast cells and release of inflammatory mediators. IgE is of importance in certain parasitic infections and is responsible for the symptoms of atopic allergy.

(Continued p.60)

The generation of antibody diversity

• The antibody repertoire of an individual is generated through somatic recombination events from a limited set of germline gene segments.

• The human heavy chain variable region is generated by joining of V_H, D and J gene segments and the light chain variable regions (κ and λ) by joining of V_L and J segments. Joining is imprecise, leading to the generation of further diversity.

• Still further diversification results from somatic mutation events targeted to the variable regions. Somatic mutation and selection allows affinity maturation of antibodies.

• Some species use gene conversion rather than combinatorial and junctional diversity to achieve antibody diversification.

• Class switch recombination events allow the same antibody specificity (variable regions) to be associated with different antibody classes and subclasses (constant regions) and therefore with different functions.

FURTHER READING

Arakawa H. & Buerstedde J. (2004) Immunoglobulin gene conversion: insights from bursal B cells and the DT40 cell line. *Developmental Dynamics* **229**, 458–464.

Chaudhuri J. & Alt F.W. (2004) Class-switch recombination: interplay of transcription, DNA deamination, and DNA repair. *Nature Reviews Immunology* **4**, 541–552.

Cook G.P. & Tomlinson I.M. (1995) The human immunoglobulin V_H repertoire. *Immunology Today* **16**, 237–242.

Dudley D.D., Chaudhuri, J., Bassing, C.H. & Alt, F.W. (2005) Mechanism and control of V(D)J recombination verus class switch recombination: similarities and differences. *Advances in Immunology* **86**, 43–112.

Groner B., Hartmann C. & Wels W. (2004) Therapeutic antibodies. *Current Molecular Medicine* **4**, 539–547.

Honjo T., Nagaoka H., Shinkura R. & Muramatsu M. (2005) AID to overcome the limitations of genomic information. *Nature Immunology* **6**, 655–661.

Hozumi N. & Tonegawa S. (1976) Evidence for somatic rearrangement of immunoglobulin genes coding for variable and constant regions. *Proceedings of the National Academy of Sciences of the USA* **73**, 3628–3632.

Hudson P.J. & Souriau C. (2003) Engineered antibodies. *Nature Medicine* **9**, 129–134.

IMGT database: http://imgt.cines.fr

Jung D. & Alt F.W. (2004) Unraveling V(D)J recombination: insights into gene regulation. *Cell* **116**, 299–311.

Maizels N. (2005) Immunoglobulin gene diversification. *Annual Review of Genetics* **39**, 23–46.

Maki R., Traunecker, A., Sakano, H., Roeder, W. & Tonegawa, S. (1980) Exon shuffling generates an immunoglobulin heavy chain gene. *Proceedings of the National Academy of Sciences of the USA* **77**, 2138–2142.

Martin A. & Scharff M.D. (2002) AID and mismatch repair in antibody diversification. *Nature Reviews Immunology* **2**, 605–614.

Martin W.L., West A.P. Jr, Gan L. & Bjorkman P.J. (2001) Crystal structure at 2.8 Å of an FcRn/heterodimeric Fc complex: mechanism of pH-dependent binding. *Molecular Cell* **7**, 867–877.

Matsuda F. & Honjo T. (1996) Organization of the Human Immunoglobulin Heavy-Chain Locus. *Advances in Immunology* **62**, 1–29.

McCormack W.T., Tjoelker L.W. & Thompson C.B. (1991) Avian B-cell development: generation of an immunoglobulin repertoire by gene conversion. *Annual Review of Immunology* **9**, 219–241.

Metzger H. (2004) The high affinity receptor for IgE, FcεRI. *Novartis Foundation Symposium* **257**, 51–59.

Min I.M. & Selsing E. (2005) Antibody class switch recombination: roles for switch sequences and mismatch repair proteins. *Advances in Immunology* **87**, 297–328.

Neuberger M.S., Harris R.S., Di Noia J. & Petersen-Mahrt S.K. (2003) Immunity through deamination. *Trends in Biochemical Sciences* **28**, 305–312.

Padlan E.A. (1994) Anatomy of the antibody molecule. *Molecular Immunology* **31**, 169–217.

Padlan E.A. (1996) X-ray crystallography of antibodies. *Advances in Protein Chemistry* **49**, 57–133.

Parren P.W. & Burton D.R. (2001) The antiviral activity of antibodies in vitro and in vivo. *Advances in Immunology* **77**, 195–262.

Ravetch J.V. & Bolland S. (2001) IgG Fc receptors. *Annual Review of Immunology* **19**, 275–290.

Roth D.B. (2003) Restraining the V(D)J recombinase. *Nature Reviews Immunology* **3**, 656–666.

Swanson P.C. (2004) The bounty of RAGs: recombination signal complexes and complex outcomes. *Immunological Reviews* **200**, 90–114.

Ward E.S. (2004) Acquiring maternal immunoglobulin; different receptors, similar functions. *Immunity* **20**, 507–508.

Woof J.M. & Burton D.R. (2004) Human antibody-Fc receptor interactions illuminated by crystal structures. *Nature Reviews Immunology* **4**, 89–99.

Woof J.M. & Kerr M.A. (2004) IgA function—variations on a theme. *Immunology* **113**, 175–177.

Yoo E.M. & Morrison S.L. (2005) IgA: an immune glycoprotein. *Clinical Immunology* **116**, 3–10.

Zachau H.G. (2000) The immunoglobulin kappa gene families of human and mouse: a cottage industry approach. *Biological Chemistry* **381**, 951–954.

4 Membrane receptors for antigen

INTRODUCTION

The interaction of lymphocytes with antigen takes place through binding to specialized cell surface antigen-specific receptors functioning as recognition units. In the case of B-cells, the situation is straightforward as membrane-bound immunoglobulin serves as the receptor for antigen. T-cells use distinct antigen receptors, which are also expressed at the plasma membrane, but T-cell receptors (TCRs) differ from B-cell receptors (BCRs) in a very fundamental way; TCRs cannot recognize free antigen as immunoglobulin can. The majority of T-cells can only recognize antigen when presented within the peptide-binding groove of an MHC molecule. While this may seem rather cumbersome, a major advantage that T-cells have over their B-cell brethren is that they can inspect antigens that are largely confined within cells and are therefore inaccessible to Ig. Another leukocyte class, natural killer (NK) cells, can also detect trouble brewing within. NK cells possess their own unique receptors that check for appropriate levels of MHC molecules, as these are normally expressed on practically all nucleated cells within the body; NK receptors can also detect signs of abnormality such as increases in the expression of stress proteins by cells. Here we will focus mainly on the structural aspects of these various receptor types.

THE B-CELL SURFACE RECEPTOR FOR ANTIGEN (BCR)

The B-cell displays a transmembrane immunoglobulin on its surface

In Chapter 2 we discussed the cunning system by which an antigen can be led inexorably to its doom by activating B-cells that are capable of making antibodies complementary in shape to itself through interacting with a copy of the antibody molecule on the lymphocyte surface. It will be recalled that binding of antigen to membrane antibody can activate the B-cell and cause it to proliferate followed by maturation into a clone of plasma cells secreting antibody specific for the inciting antigen (cf. figure 2.11).

Immunofluorescent staining of live B-cells with labeled anti-immunoglobulin (anti-Ig) (e.g. figure 2.6c) reveals the earliest membrane Ig to be of the IgM class. Each individual B-cell is committed to the production of just one antibody specificity and so transcribes its individual rearranged $VJC\kappa$ (or λ) and $VDJC\mu$ genes. Ig can be either secreted or displayed on the B-cell surface through **differential splicing** of the pre-mRNA transcript encoding a particular immunoglobulin. The initial nuclear μ chain RNA transcript includes sequences coding for **hydrophobic transmembrane regions** which enable the IgM to sit in the membrane where it acts as the BCR, but if these are spliced out, the antibody molecules can be secreted in a soluble form (figure 4.1).

As the B-cell matures, it coexpresses a BCR utilizing surface IgD of the same specificity. This surface IgM+surface IgD B-cell phenotype is abundant in the mantle zone lymphocytes of secondary lymphoid follicles (cf. figure 7.8c) and is achieved by differential splicing of a single transcript containing VDJ, $C\mu$ and $C\delta$ segments producing either membrane IgM or IgD (figure 4.2). As the B-cell matures further, other isotypes such as IgG may be utilized in the BCR (cf. p. 247).

Surface immunoglobulin is complexed with associated membrane proteins

Because secreted immunoglobulin is no longer physi-

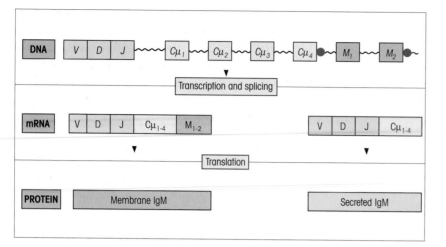

Figure 4.1. Splicing mechanism for the switch from the membrane to the secreted form of IgM. Alternative processing determines whether a secreted or membrane-bound form of the μ heavy chain is produced. If transcription termination or cleavage occurs in the intron between $C\mu_4$ and M_1, the $C\mu_4$ poly-A addition signal (AAUAAA) is used and the secreted form is produced. If transcription continues through the membrane exons, then $C\mu4$ can be spliced to the M sequences resulting in the M_2 poly-A addition signal being utilized. The hydrophobic sequence encoded by the exons M_1 and M_2 then anchors the receptor IgM to the membrane. For simplicity, the leader sequence has been omitted. $\sim\sim$ = introns.

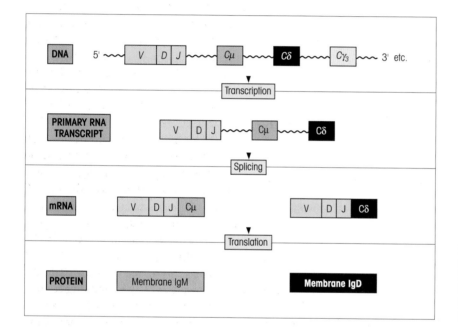

Figure 4.2. Surface membrane IgM and IgD receptors of identical specificity appear on the same cell through differential splicing of the composite primary RNA transcript (leader sequences again omitted for simplicity).

cally connected to the B-cell that generated it, there is no way for the B-cell to know when the secreted Ig has found its target antigen. In the case of membrane-anchored immunoglobulin however, there is a direct link between antibody and the cell making it and this can be exploited to instruct the B-cell to scale-up production. As any budding industrialist knows, one way of increasing production is to open up more manufacturing plants, and another is to increase the rate of productivity in each one. When faced with the prospect of a sudden increase in demand for their particular product, B-cells do both of these things, through clonal expansion and differentiation to plasma cells. So how does the BCR spur the B-cell into action upon encounter with antigen? Unlike many plasma membrane receptors that boast all manner of signaling motifs within their cytoplasmic tails, the corresponding tail region of a membrane-

anchored IgM is a miserable three amino acids long. In no way could this accommodate the structural motifs required for interaction with either adaptor proteins, intracellular protein kinases or phosphatases that typically initiate signal transduction cascades. With some difficulty, it should be said, it eventually proved possible to isolate a disulfide-linked heterodimer, **Ig-α (CD79a) and Ig-β (CD79b)**, which copurifies with membrane Ig and is responsible for transmitting signals from the BCR to the cell interior (figure 4.3). Both Ig-α and Ig-β have an extracellular immunoglobulin-type domain, but it is their C-terminal cytoplasmic domains that are obligatory for signaling and which become phosphorylated upon crosslinking of the BCR by antigen, an event also associated with rapid Ca^{2+} mobilization. Ig-α and Ig-β each contain a single **ITAM (*immunoreceptor tyrosine-based activation motif*)** within their cytoplas-

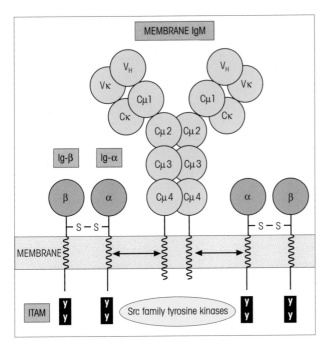

Figure 4.3. Model of B-cell receptor (BCR) complex. The Ig-α/Ig-β heterodimer is encoded by the B-cell-specific genes *mb-1* and *B29*, respectively. Two of these heterodimers are shown with the Ig-α associating with the membrane-spanning region of the IgM μ chain. The Ig-like extracellular domains are colored blue. Each tyrosine (Y)-containing box possesses a sequence of general structure Tyr.X_2.Leu.X_7.Tyr.X_2.Ile (where X is not a conserved residue), referred to as the immunoreceptor tyrosine-based activation motif (ITAM). On activation of the B-cell, these ITAM sequences act as signal transducers through their ability to associate with and be phosphorylated by a series of tyrosine kinases. Note that whilst a κ light chain is illustrated for the surface IgM, some B-cells utilize a λ light chain.

mic tails and this motif contains two precisely spaced tyrosine residues that are central to their signaling role (figure 4.3). Engagement of the BCR with antigen leads to rapid phosphorylation of the tyrosines within each ITAM, by kinases associated with the BCR, and this has the effect of creating binding sites for proteins that have an affinity for phosphorylated tyrosine residues. In this case, a protein kinase called **Syk** becomes associated with the phosphorylated Ig-α/β heterodimer and is instrumental in coordinating events that culminate in entry of the activated B-cell into the cell cycle to commence clonal expansion. We will revisit this topic in Chapter 8 where the details of the BCR signal transduction cascade will be elaborated upon in greater detail (see p. 180).

THE T-CELL SURFACE RECEPTOR FOR ANTIGEN (TCR)

As alluded to earlier, T-cells interact with antigen in a manner that is quite distinct from the way in which B-cells do; the receptors that most T-cells are equipped with cannot directly engage soluble antigens but instead 'see' short fragments of antigen that are immobilized within a narrow groove on the surface of MHC molecules. Moreover, T-cells cannot secrete their receptor molecules in the way that B-cells can switch production of Ig from a membrane-bound form to a secreted form. These differences aside, **T-cell receptors** are structurally quite similar to antibody as they are also built from modules that are based upon the immunoglobulin fold.

The receptor for antigen is a transmembrane heterodimer

Identification of the TCR proved more difficult than initially anticipated (Milestone 4.1), but eventually the receptor was found to be a membrane-bound molecule composed of two disulfide-linked chains, α and β. Each chain folds into two Ig-like domains, one having a relatively invariant structure and the other exhibiting a high degree of variability, so that the αβ TCR has a structure really quite closely resembling an Ig Fab fragment. This analogy stretches even further —each of the two variable regions has three hypervariable regions (or complementarity-determining regions, CDRs) which X-ray diffraction data have defined as incorporating the amino acids which make contact with the peptide–major histocompatibility complex (MHC) ligand. Although the manner in which the TCR makes contact with peptide–MHC is still not fully understood, it appears that CDRs 1 and 2 of the TCR bear much of the responsibility for making contact with the MHC molecule itself, while CDR3 makes contact with the peptide; thus it is here that much of the variability is seen between TCRs, as we shall discuss later.

Both α and β chains are required for antigen specificity as shown by transfection of the T-receptor genes from a cytotoxic T-cell clone specific for fluorescein to another clone of different specificity; when it expressed the new α and β genes, the transfected clone acquired the ability to lyse the fluoresceinated target cells. Another type of experiment utilized T-cell hybridomas formed by fusing single antigen-specific T-cells with T-cell tumors to achieve 'immortality'. One hybridoma recognizing chicken ovalbumin, presented by a macrophage, gave rise spontaneously to two variants, one of which lost the chromosome encoding the α chain, and the other, the β chain. Neither variant recognized antigen but, when they were physically fused together, each supplied the complementary receptor chain and reactivity with antigen was restored.

Milestone 4.1 — The T-cell Receptor

Since T-lymphocytes respond by activation and proliferation when they contact antigen presented by cells such as macrophages, it seemed reasonable to postulate that they do so by receptors on their surface. In any case, it would be difficult to fit T-cells into the clonal selection club if they lacked such receptors. Guided by Ockam's razor (the *Law of Parsimony*, which contends that it is the aim of science to present the facts of nature in the simplest and most economical conceptual formulations), most investigators plumped for the hypothesis that nature would not indulge in the extravagance of evolving two utterly separate molecular recognition species for B- and T-cells, and many fruitless years were spent looking for the Holy Grail of the T-cell receptor with anti-immunoglobulin serums or monoclonal antibodies (cf. p. 112). Success only came when a monoclonal antibody directed to the idiotype of a T-cell was used to block the response to antigen. This was identified by its ability to block one individual T-cell clone out of a large number, and it was

correctly assumed that the structure permitting this selectivity would be the combining site for antigen on the T-cell receptor. Immunoprecipitation with this antibody brought down a disulfide-linked heterodimer composed of 40–44 kDa subunits (figure M4.1.1).

The other approach went directly for the genes, arguing as follows. The T-cell receptor should be an integral membrane protein not present in B-cells. Hence, T-cell polysomal mRNA from the endoplasmic reticulum, which should provide an abundant source of the appropriate transcript, was used to prepare cDNA from which genes common to B- and T-cells were subtracted by hybridization to B-cell mRNA. The resulting T-specific clones were used to probe for a T-cell gene which is rearranged in all functionally mature T-cells but is in its germ-line configuration in all other cell types (figure M4.1.2). In such a way were the genes encoding the β-subunit of the T-cell receptor uncovered.

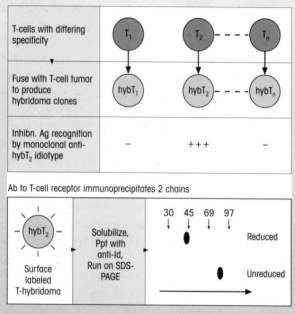

Figure M4.1.1. **Ab to T-cell receptor (anti-idiotype) blocks Ag recognition.** (Based on Haskins K., Kubo R., White J., Pigeon M., Kappler J. & Marack P. (1983) *Journal of Experimental Medicine* **157**, 1149; simplified a little.)

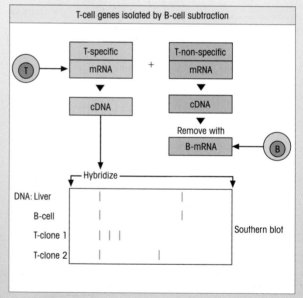

Figure M4.1.2. **Isolation of T-cell receptor genes.** Different sized DNA fragments produced by a restriction enzyme are separated by electrophoresis and probed with the T-cell gene. The T-cells show rearrangement of one of the two germ-line genes found in liver or B-cells. (Based on Hendrick S.M., Cohen D.I., Nielsen E.A. & Davis M.M. (1984) *Nature* **308**, 149.)

CD4 and CD8 molecules act as co-receptors for TCRs

In addition to the TCR, the majority of peripheral T-cells also express one or other of the membrane proteins **CD4 or CD8** that act as co-receptors for MHC molecules (figure 4.4). CD4 is a single chain polypeptide containing four Ig-like domains packed tightly together to form

an extended rod that projects from the T-cell surface. The cytoplasmic tail of the CD4 molecule is important for TCR signaling as this region is constitutively bound by a protein tyrosine kinase, **Lck**, that initiates the signal transduction cascade that follows upon encounter of a T-cell with antigen. CD8 plays a similar role to CD4, as it also binds Lck and recruits this kinase to the TCR

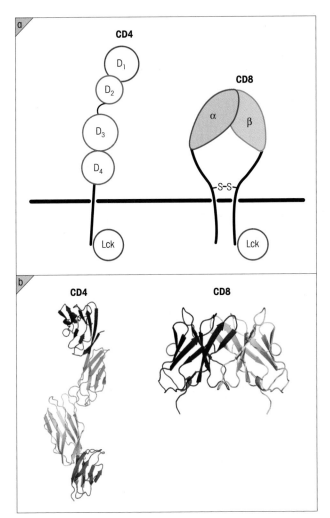

Figure 4.4. CD4 and CD8 act as co-receptors for MHC molecules and define functional subsets of T-cells. (a) Schematic representation of CD4 and CD8 molecules. CD4 is composed of four Ig-like domains (D_1 to D_4, as indicated) and projects from the T-cell surface to interact with MHC class II molecules. CD8 is a disulfide-linked heterodimer composed of Ig-like α and β subunits connected to a heavily glycosylated rod-like region that extends from the plasma membrane. CD8 interacts with MHC class I molecules. The cytoplasmic tails of CD4 and CD8 are associated with the tyrosine kinase Lck. (b) Ribbon diagram representations of the extracellular portions of CD4 and CD8. The Ig-like domains (D_1 to D_4) of CD4 are colored blue, green, yellow and red respectively. A CD8 homodimer of two α subunits is shown. (Structures were kindly provided by Dr Dan Leahy and are based upon coordinates reported in Leahy *et al.* (1992) *Cell* **68**, 1145 and Wu *et al.* (1997) *Nature* **387**, 527.)

MHC molecules that obtain their peptide antigens primarily from intracellular (**MHC class I**), or extracellular (**MHC class II**), sources. This has major functional implications for the T-cell, as those lymphocytes that become activated upon encounter with antigen presented within MHC class I molecules (CD8[+] T-cells) invariably become cytotoxic T-cells, and those that are activated by peptides presented by MHC class II molecules (CD4[+] T-cells) become helper T-cells (see figure 8.1).

There are two classes of T-cell receptors

Not long after the breakthrough in identifying the $\alpha\beta$ TCR, came reports of the existence of a second type of receptor composed of γ and δ chains. Since it appears earlier in thymic ontogeny, the $\gamma\delta$ receptor is sometimes referred to as **TCR1** and the $\alpha\beta$ receptor as **TCR2** (cf. p. 235).

$\gamma\delta$ cells make up only 1–5% of the T-cells that circulate in blood and peripheral organs of most adult animals; however these cells are much more common in epithelial-rich tissues such as the skin, intestine, reproductive tract and the lungs where they can comprise almost 50% of the T-cell population. It cannot be denied that $\gamma\delta$ T-cells are somewhat of an oddity among T-cells; unlike $\alpha\beta$ T-cells, $\gamma\delta$ cells do not appear to require antigen to be presented within the context of MHC molecules and are thought to be able to recognize soluble antigen akin to B-cells. Perhaps because of this lack of dependence on MHC for antigen presentation, the majority of $\gamma\delta$ T-cells do not express either of the MHC co-receptors, CD4 or CD8 (table 4.1).

The mechanism of antigen recognition by $\gamma\delta$ T-cells is still somewhat mysterious but these cells are known to be able to interact with MHC-related molecules, such as the mouse T10 and T22 proteins, in a manner that does not require antigen. Because the latter MHC-like molecules are upregulated upon activation of $\alpha\beta$ T-cells, this has led to the view that $\gamma\delta$ T-cells may have an important immunoregulatory function; by becoming activated by molecules that appear on activated T-cells, $\gamma\delta$ T-cells may help to regulate immune responses in a positive or negative manner. $\gamma\delta$ T-cells can also recognize pathogen-derived lipids, organic phosphoesters, nucleotide conjugates and other nonpeptide ligands.

The encoding of T-cell receptors is similar to that of immunoglobulins

The gene segments encoding the TCR β chains follow a broadly similar arrangement of *V*, *D*, *J* and constant segments to that described for the immunoglobulins (figure

complex, but is structurally quite distinct; CD8 is a disulfide-linked heterodimer of α and β chains, each of which contains a single Ig-like domain connected to an extended and heavily glycosylated polypeptide projecting from the T-cell surface (figure 4.4).

CD4 and CD8 molecules play important roles in antigen recognition by T-cells as these molecules dictate whether a T-cell can recognize antigen presented by

4.5). In a parallel fashion, as an immunocompetent T-cell is formed, rearrangement of V, D and J genes occurs to form a continuous VDJ sequence. The firmest evidence that B- and T-cells use similar recombination mechanisms comes from mice with severe combined immunodeficiency (SCID) which have a single autosomal recessive defect preventing successful recombination of V, D and J segments (cf. p. 54). Homozygous mutants fail to develop immunocompetent B- and T-cells and identical sequence defects in VDJ joint formation are seen in both pre-B- and pre-T-cell lines.

Table 4.1. Comparison between αβ and γδ T-cells.

Characteristic	αβ T-cells	γδ T-cells
Antigen receptor	αβ TCR + CD3 complex	γδ TCR + CD3 complex
Form of antigen recognized	MHC + peptide	MHC-like molecules plus nonprotein ligands
CD4/CD8 expression	Yes	Mainly no
Frequency in blood	60–75%	1–5%
MHC restricted	Yes	Mostly no
Function	Help for lymphocyte and macrophage activation Cytotoxic killing	Immunoregulatory function? Cytotoxic activity

Looking first at the β chain cluster, one of the two $D\beta$ genes rearranges next to one of the $J\beta$ genes. Note that, because of the way the genes are organized, the first $D\beta$ gene, $D\beta_1$, can utilize any of the 13 $J\beta$ genes, but $D\beta_2$ can only choose from the seven $J\beta_2$ genes (figure 4.5). Next one of the 50 or so $V\beta$ genes is rearranged to the preformed $D\beta J\beta$ segment. **Variability in junction formation** and the **random insertion of nucleotides** to create N-region diversity either side of the D segment mirror the same phenomenon seen with Ig gene rearrangements. Sequence analysis emphasizes the analogy with the antibody molecule; each V segment contains two hypervariable regions, while the **DJ** junctional sequence provides the **very hypervariable CDR3** structure, making a total of six potential complementarity determining regions for antigen binding in each TCR (figure 4.6). As in the synthesis of antibody, the intron between VDJ and C is spliced out of the mRNA before translation with the restriction that rearrangements involving genes in the $D\beta_2 J\beta_2$ cluster can only link to $C\beta_2$.

All the other chains of the TCRs are encoded by genes formed through similar translocations. The α chain gene pool lacks D segments but possesses a prodigious number of J segments. The number of $V\gamma$ and $V\delta$ genes is small in comparison with $V\alpha$ and $V\beta$. Like the α chain pool, the γ chain cluster has no D segments. The awkward location of the δ locus embedded within the α gene cluster results in T-cells which have undergone $V\alpha$–$J\alpha$ combination having no δ genes on the rearranged chromosome; in other words, the δ genes are completely excised.

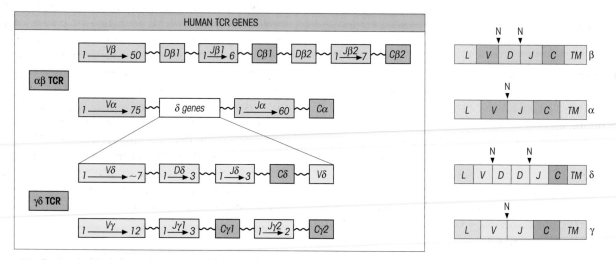

Figure 4.5. **Genes encoding αβ and γδ T-cell receptors.** Genes encoding the δ chains lie between the $V\alpha$ and $J\alpha$ clusters and some V segments in this region can be used in either δ or α chains, i.e. as either $V\alpha$ or $V\delta$. TCR genes rearrange in a manner analogous to that seen with immunoglobulin genes, including N-region diversity at the $V(D)J$ junctions. One of the $V\delta$ genes is found downstream (3′) of the $C\delta$ gene and rearranges by an inversional mechanism.

Figure 4.6. The T-cell receptor/CD3 complex. The TCR resembles the immunoglobulin Fab antigen-binding fragment in structure. The variable and constant segments of the TCR α and β chains (VαCα/VβCβ), and of the corresponding γ and δ chains of the γδ TCR, belong structurally to the immunoglobulin-type domain family. (a) In the model the α chain CDRs are colored magenta (CDR1), purple (CDR2) and yellow (CDR3), whilst the β chain CDRs are cyan (CDR1), navy blue (CDR2) and green (CDR3). The fourth hypervariable region of the β chain (CDR4), which constitutes part of the binding site for some superantigens (cf. p. 7), is colored orange. (Reproduced from Garcia, K. *et al.* (1998) *Science* **279**, 1166, with permission.) The TCR α and β CDR3 loops encoded by *(D)J* genes are both short; the TCR γ CDR3 is also short with a narrow length distribution, but the δ loop is long with a broad length distribution, resembling the Ig light and heavy chain CDR3s, respectively. (b) The TCRs may be expressed in pairs linked to the CD3 complex. Negative charges on transmembrane segments of the invariant chains of the CD3 complex contact the opposite charges on the TCR Cα and Cβ chains conceivably as depicted. (c) The cytoplasmic domains of the CD3 peptide chains contain *i*mmunoreceptor *t*yrosine-based *a*ctivation *m*otifs (ITAM; cf. BCR, figure 4.3) which contact src protein tyrosine kinases. Try not to confuse the TCR γδ and the CD3 γδ chains.

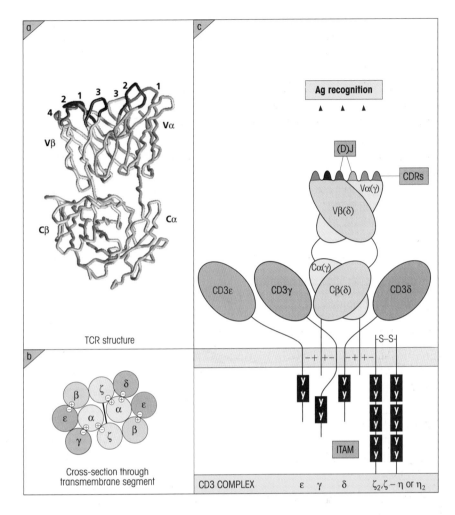

The CD3 complex is an integral part of the T-cell receptor

The T-cell antigen recognition complex and its B-cell counterpart can be likened to army scouts whose job is to let the main battalion know when the enemy has been sighted. When the TCR 'sights the enemy', i.e. ligates antigen, it relays a signal through an associated complex of transmembrane polypeptides (**CD3**) to the interior of the T-lymphocyte, instructing it to awaken from its slumbering G0 state and do something useful—like becoming an effector cell. In all immunocompetent T-cells, the TCR is noncovalently but still intimately linked with CD3 in a complex which, as current wisdom has it, may contain two heterodimeric TCR αβ or γδ recognition units closely apposed to one molecule of the invariant CD3 polypeptide chains γ and δ, two molecules of CD3ε, plus the disulfide-linked ζ–ζ dimer. The total complex therefore has the structure TCR$_2$-CD3γδε$_2$-ζ$_2$ (figure 4.6b).

Similar to the BCR-associated Ig–α/β heterodimer, the CD3 chains also contain one or more ITAMs and these motifs, once again, are instrumental in the propa-gation of activation signals into the lymphocyte. Upon encounter of the TCR with peptide–MHC, the ITAMs within the CD3 complex become phosphorylated at tyrosine residues; these then act as a platform for the recruitment of a veritable multitude of phosphotyrosine-binding proteins that further disseminate the signal throughout the T-cell. It is here that the role of the CD4 and CD8 co-receptors becomes apparent; phosphorylation of the ITAMs within the CD3 ζ chain is accomplished by the Lck tyrosine kinase which, you may recall, is associated with the cytoplasmic tails of CD4 and CD8 (figure 4.4). In mice, either or both of the ζ chains can be replaced by a splice variant from the ζ gene termed η. The ζ chain also associates with the FcγRIIIA receptor in natural killer (NK) cells where it functions as part of the signal transduction mechanism in that context also.

THE GENERATION OF DIVERSITY FOR ANTIGEN RECOGNITION

We know that the immune system has to be capable of

recognizing virtually any pathogen that has arisen or might arise. The awesome genetic solution to this problem of anticipating an unpredictable future involves the generation of millions of different specific antigen receptors, probably vastly more than the lifetime needs of the individual. Since this greatly exceeds the estimated number of 25,000–30,000 genes in the human body, there are some clever ways to generate all this diversity, particularly since the total number of V, D, J and C genes in an individual human coding for antibodies and TCRs is only around 400. Let's revisit the genetics of antibody diversity, and explore the enormous similarities, and occasional differences, seen with the mechanisms employed to generate TCR diversity.

Intrachain amplification of diversity

Random VDJ combination increases diversity geometrically

We saw in Chapter 3 that, just as we can use a relatively small number of different building units in a child's construction set such as Lego to create a rich variety of architectural masterpieces, so the individual receptor gene segments can be viewed as building blocks to fashion a multiplicity of antigen specific receptors for both B- and T-cells. The immunoglobulin light chain variable regions are created from V and J segments, and the heavy chain variable regions from V, D and J segments. Likewise, for both the $\alpha\beta$ and $\gamma\delta$ T-cell receptors the variable region of one of the chains (α or γ) is encoded by a V and a J segment, whereas the variable region of the other chain (β or δ) is additionally encoded by a D segment. As

for immunoglobulin genes, the enzymes RAG-1 and RAG-2 recognize recombination signal sequences (RSSs) adjacent to the coding sequences of the TCR V, D and J gene segments. The RSSs again consist of conserved heptamers and nonamers separated by spacers of either 12 or 23 base pairs (cf. p. 55) and are found at the 3′ of each V segment, on both the 5′ and 3′ sides of each D segment, and at the 5′ of each J segment. Incorporation of a D segment is always included in the rearrangement; $V\beta$ cannot join directly to $J\beta$, nor $V\delta$ directly to $J\delta$. To see how sequence diversity is generated for TCR, let us take the $\alpha\beta$ TCR as an example (table 4.2). Although the precise number of gene segments varies from one individual to another, there are typically around 75 $V\alpha$ gene segments and 60 $J\alpha$ gene segments. If there were entirely **random joining** of any one V to any one J segment, we would have the possibility of generating 4500 VJ combinations (75×60). Regarding the TCR β-chain, there are approximately 50 $V\beta$ genes which lie upstream of two clusters of $D\beta J\beta$ genes each of which is associated with a $C\beta$ gene (figure 4.7). The first cluster, that associated with $C\beta1$, has a single $D\beta1$ gene and 6 $J\beta1$ genes, whereas the second cluster associated with $C\beta2$ again has a single $D\beta$ gene ($D\beta2$) with 7 $J\beta2$ genes. The $D\beta1$ segment can combine with any of the 50 $V\beta$ genes and with any of the 13 $J\beta1$ and $J\beta2$ genes (figure 4.7). $D\beta2$ behaves similarly but can only combine with one of the seven downstream $J\beta2$ genes. This provides 1,000 different possible VDJ combinations for the TCR β-chain. Therefore, although the TCR α and β chain V, D and J genes add up arithmetically to just 200, they produce a vast number of different α and β variable regions by

Table 4.2. Calculations of human V gene diversity. It is known that the precise number of gene segments varies from one individual to another, perhaps 40 or so in the case of the V_H genes for example, so that these calculations represent 'typical' numbers. The number of specificities generated by straightforward random combination of germ-line segments is calculated. These will be increased by the further mechanisms listed: *minimal assumption of approximately 10 variants for chains lacking D segments and 100 for chains with D segments. The calculation for the T-cell receptor β chain requires further explanation. The first of the two D segments, $D\beta_1$, can combine with 50 V genes and with all 13 $J\beta_1$ and $J\beta_2$ genes. $D\beta_2$ behaves similarly but can only combine with the seven downstream $J\beta_2$ genes.

	γδTCR (TCR1)		αβTCR (TCR2)		Ig		
	γ	δ	α	β	H	L	
						κ	λ
V gene segments	12	~8	75	50	40	40	30
D gene segments	-	3	-	1,1	27	-	-
J gene segments	3,2	3	60	6,7	6	5	5
Random combinatorial joining (without junctional diversity)	$V \times J$ 12 × 5	$V \times D \times J$ 8 × 3 × 3	$V \times J$ 75 × 60	$V \times D \times J$ 50(13+7)	$V \times D \times J$ 40 × 27 × 6	$V \times J$ 40 × 5	$V \times J$ 30 × 4
Total	60	72	4500	1000	6480	200	150
Combinatorial heterodimers	60 × 72		4500 × 1000		6480 × 200		6480 × 150
Total (rounded)	4.3×10^3		4.5×10^6		1.3×10^6		1.0×10^6
Other mechanisms: D's in 3 reading frames, junctional diversity, N region insertion;* × 10^3	4.3×10^6		4.5×10^9		1.3×10^9		1.0×10^9
Somatic mutation	-		-		+++		+++

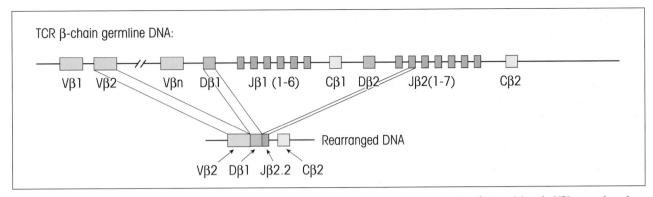

Figure 4.7. Rearrangement of the T-cell receptor β-chain gene locus. In this example Dβ1 has rearranged to Jβ2.2, and then the Vβ2 gene selected out of the 50 or so (Vβn) Vβ genes. If the same V and D segments had been used, but this time Jβ1.4 had been employed, then the Cβ1 gene segment would have been utilized instead of Cβ2.

geometric recombination of the basic elements. But, as with immunoglobulin gene rearrangement, that is only the beginning.

Playing with the junctions

Another ploy to squeeze more variation out of the germ-line repertoire that is used by both the T-cell receptor and the immunoglobulin genes (cf. 3.25) involves variable boundary recombinations of *V, D* and *J* to produce different junctional sequences (figure 4.8).

As discussed in Chapter 3, further diversity results from the generation of palindromic sequences (P-elements) arising from the formation of hairpin structures during the recombination process and from the insertion of nucleotides at the N region between the *V, D* and *J* segments, a process associated with the expression of terminal deoxynucleotidyl transferase. Whilst these mechanisms add nucleotides to the sequence, yet more diversity can be created by nucleases chewing away at the exposed strand ends to remove nucleotides. These maneuvers again greatly increase the repertoire, especially important for the TCR γ and δ genes which are otherwise rather limited in number.

Additional mechanisms relate specifically to the *D*-region sequence: particularly in the case of the TCR δ genes, where the *D* segment can be read in three different reading frames and two *D* segments can join together, such *DD* combinations produce a longer third complementarity determining region (CDR3) than is found in other TCR or antibody molecules.

Since the CDR3 in the various receptor chains is essentially composed of the regions between the *V(D)J* segments, where junctional diversity mechanisms can introduce a very high degree of amino acid variability, one can see why it is that this hypervariable loop usually contributes the most to determining the fine antigen-binding specificity of these molecules.

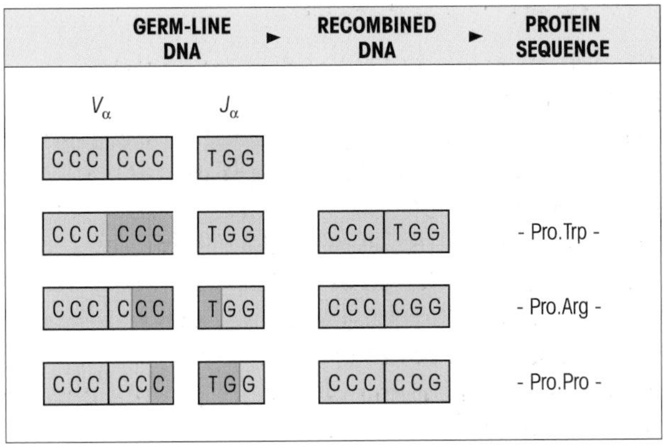

Figure 4.8. Junctional diversity between a TCR Vα and Jα germline segment producing three variant protein sequences. The nucleotide triplet which is spliced out is colored the darker blue. For TCR β-chain and Ig heavy chain genes junctional diversity can apply to *V, D* and *J* segments.

Receptor editing

Recent observations have established that lymphocytes are not necessarily stuck with the antigen receptor they initially make; if they don't like it they can change it. The replacement of an undesired receptor with one which has more acceptable characteristics is referred to as receptor editing. This process has been described for both immunoglobulins and for TCR, allowing the replacement of either nonfunctional rearrangements or autoreactive specificities. Furthermore, receptor editing in the periphery may rescue low affinity B-cells from apoptotic cell death by replacing a low affinity receptor with a selectable one of higher affinity. That this does indeed occur in the periphery is strongly supported by the finding that mature B-cells in germinal centers can express RAG-1 and RAG-2 which mediate the rearrangement process.

But how does this receptor editing work? Well, in the case of the receptor chains which lack *D* gene segments, namely the immunoglobulin light chain and the TCR α chain, a secondary rearrangement may occur by a *V* gene segment upstream of the previously rearranged *VJ* segment recombining to a 3′ *J* gene sequence, both of these segments having intact RSSs that are compatible (figure 4.9a). However, for immunoglobulin heavy chains and TCR β chains the process of *VDJ* rearrangement deletes all of the *D* segment-associated RSSs (figure 4.9b). Because V_H and J_H both have 23 base pair spacers in their RSSs, they cannot recombine: that would break the 12/23 rule. This apparent obstacle to receptor editing of these chains may be overcome by the presence of a sequence near the 3′ end of the *V* coding sequences that can function as a surrogate RSS, such that the new *V* segment would simply replace the previously rearranged *V*, maintaining the same *D* and *J* sequence (figure 4.9b). This is probably a relatively inefficient process and receptor editing may therefore occur more readily in immunoglobulin light chains and TCR α chains than in immunoglobulin heavy chains and TCR β chains. Indeed, it has been suggested that the TCR α chain may undergo a series of rearrangements, continuously deleting previously functionally rearranged *VJ* segments until a selectable TCR is produced.

Interchain amplification

The immune system took an ingenious step forward when two different types of chain were utilized for the recognition molecules because the combination produces not only a larger combining site with potentially greater affinity, but also new variability. Heavy–light chain pairing amongst immunoglobulins appears to be largely random and therefore two B-cells can employ the same heavy chain but different light chains. This route to producing antibodies of differing specificity is easily seen *in vitro* where shuffling different recombinant light chains against the same heavy chain can be used to either fine tune or sometimes even alter the specificity of the final antibody. In general, the available evidence suggests that *in vivo* the major contribution to diversity and specificity comes from the heavy chain, perhaps not unrelated to the fact that the heavy chain CDR3 gets off to a head start in the race for diversity being, as it is, encoded by the junctions between three gene segments: *V*, *D* and *J*.

This random association between TCR γ and δ chains, TCR α and β chains, and Ig heavy and light chains yields a further geometric increase in diversity. From table 4.2 it can be seen that approximately 230 functional TCR and 153 functional Ig germ-line segments can give rise to 4.5 million and 2.3 million different combinations, respectively, by straightforward associations *without* taking into account all of the fancy junctional mechanisms described above. Hats off to evolution!

Somatic hypermutation

As discussed in Chapter 3, there is inescapable evidence that immunoglobulin *V*-region genes can undergo significant **somatic hypermutation**. Analysis of 18 murine λ myelomas revealed 12 with identical structure, four showing just one amino acid change, one with two changes and one with four changes, all within the hypervariable regions and indicative of somatic hypermutation of the single mouse λ germ-line gene. In another study, following immunization with pneumococcal antigen, a single germ-line T15 V_H gene gave rise by mutation to several different V_H genes all encoding phosphorylcholine antibodies (figure 4.10).

A number of features of this somatic diversification phenomenon are worth revisiting. The mutations are the result of single nucleotide substitutions, they are restricted to the variable as distinct from the constant region and occur in both framework and hypervariable regions. The mutation rate is remarkably high, approximately 1×10^{-3} per base pair per generation, which is approximately a million times higher than for other mammalian genes. In addition, the mutational mechanism is bound up in some way with class switch recombination since the enzyme activation-induced cytidine deaminase (AID) is required for both processes and hypermutation is more frequent in IgG and IgA than in IgM antibodies, affecting both heavy (figure 4.10) and light chains. However, V_H genes are on average more mutated than V_L genes. This might be a consequence of receptor editing acting more frequently on light chains, as this would have the effect of wiping the slate clean with respect to light chain *V* gene mutations whilst maintaining already accumulated heavy chain *V* gene point mutations.

Somatic hypermutation does not appear to add significantly to the repertoire available in the early phases of the primary response, but occurs during the generation of memory and is responsible for tuning the response towards higher affinity.

Recently data have been put forward suggesting that there is yet another mechanism for creating further diversity. This involves the insertion or deletion of short stretches of nucleotides within the immunoglobulin *V* gene sequence of both heavy and light chains. This mechanism would have an intermediate effect on antigen recognition, being more dramatic than single

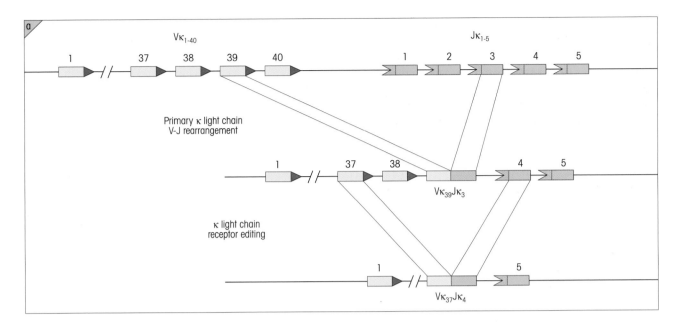

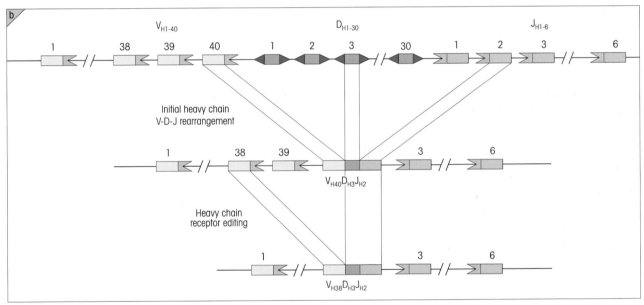

Figure 4.9. Receptor editing. (a) For immunoglobulin light chain or TCR α chain the recombination signal sequences (RSSs; heptamer–nonamer motifs) at the 3′ of each variable (*V*) segment and the 5′ of each joining (*J*) segment are compatible with each other and therefore an entirely new rearrangement can potentially occur as shown. This would result in a receptor with a different light chain variable sequence (in this example $Vk_{37}Jk_4$ replacing $Vk_{39}Jk_3$) together with the original heavy chain. (b) With respect to the immunoglobulin heavy chain or TCR β chain the organization of the heptamer–nonamer sequences in the RSS precludes a *V* segment directly recombining with the *J* segment. This is the so-called 12/23 rule whereby the hep-tamer–nonamer sequences associated with a 23 base pair spacer (colored violet) can only base pair with heptamer–nonamer sequences containing a 12 base pair spacer (colored red). The heavy chain *V* and *J* both have an RSS with a 23 base pair spacer and so this is a nonstarter. Furthermore, all the unrearranged *D* segments have been deleted so that there are no 12 base pair spacers remaining. This apparent bar to secondary rearrangement is probably overcome by the presence of an RSS-like sequence near the 3′ end of the *V* gene coding sequences, so that only the *V* gene segment is replaced (in the example shown, the sequence $V_{H38}D_{H3}J_{H2}$ replaces $V_{H40}D_{H3}J_{H2}$).

point mutation, but considerably more subtle than receptor editing. In one study, a *r*everse *t*ranscriptase-*p*olymerase *c*hain *r*eaction (RT-PCR) was employed to amplify the expressed V_H and V_L genes from 365 IgG+ B-cells and it was shown that 6.5% of the cells contained nucleotide insertions or deletions. The transcripts were left in-frame and no stop codons were introduced by these modifications. The percentage of cells containing these alterations is likely to be an underestimate. All the insertions and deletions were in, or near to, CDR1

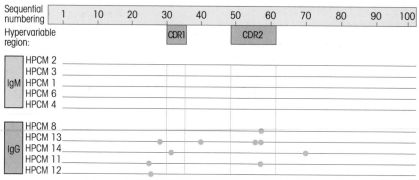

Figure 4.10. Mutations in a germ-line gene. The amino acid sequences of the V_H regions of five IgM and five IgG monoclonal phosphorylcholine antibodies generated during an antipneumococcal response in a single mouse are compared with the primary structure of the T15 germ-line sequence. A line indicates identity with the T15 prototype and an orange circle a single amino acid difference. Mutations have only occurred in the IgG molecules and are seen in both hypervariable and framework segments. (After Gearhart P.J. (1982) *Immunology Today* **3**, 107.) Whilst in some other studies somatic hypermutation has been seen in IgM antibodies, the amount of mutation usually greatly increases following class switching.

and/or CDR2. N-region diversity of the CDR3 meant that it was not possible to analyse the third hypervariable region for insertions/deletions of this type and therefore these would be missed in the analysis. The fact that the alterations were associated with CDRs does suggest that the B-cells had been subjected to selection by antigen. It was also notable that the insertions/deletions occurred at known hot spots for somatic point mutation, and the same error-prone DNA polymerase responsible for somatic hypermutation may also be involved here. The sequences were often a duplication of an adjacent sequence in the case of insertions or a deletion of a known repeated sequence. This type of modification may, like receptor editing, play a major role in eliminating autoreactivity and also in enhancing antibody affinity.

T-cell receptor genes, on the other hand, **do not generally undergo somatic hypermutation**. It has been argued that this would be a useful safety measure since T-cells are positively selected in the thymus for weak reactions with self MHC (cf. p. 234), so that mutations could readily lead to the emergence of high affinity autoreactive receptors and autoimmunity.

One may ask how it is that this array of germ-line genes is protected from genetic drift. With a library of 390 or so functional *V*, *D* and *J* genes, selection would act only weakly on any single gene which had been functionally crippled by mutation and this implies that a major part of the library could be lost before evolutionary forces operated. One idea is that each subfamily of related *V* genes contains a prototype coding for an antibody indispensable for protection against some common pathogen, so that mutation in this gene would put the host at a disadvantage and would therefore be selected against. If any of the other closely related genes in its set became defective through mutation, this indispensable gene could repair them by gene conversion, a mechanism in which it will be remembered that two genes interact in such a way that the nucleotide sequence of part or all of one becomes identical to that of the other. Although gene conversion has been invoked to account for the diversification of MHC genes, it can also act on other families of genes to maintain a degree of sequence homogeneity. Certainly it is used extensively by, for example, chickens and rabbits, in order to generate immunoglobulin diversity. In the rabbit only a single germ-line V_H gene is rearranged in the majority of B-cells; this then becomes a substrate for gene conversion by one of the large number of V_H pseudogenes. There are also large numbers of V_H pseudogenes and orphan genes (genes located outside the gene locus, often on a completely different chromosome) in humans which actually outnumber the functional genes, although there is no evidence to date that these are used in gene conversion processes.

NK RECEPTORS

Natural killer (NK) cells are a population of leukocytes that, like T- and B-cells, employ receptors that can provoke their activation, the consequences of which are the secretion of cytokines, most notably IFN-γ, and/or cytotoxic granules that are capable of killing the cells they target. Unlike the antigen receptors of T- and B-lymphocytes, NK receptors are 'hard-wired' and do not undergo VDJ recombination to generate diversity. NK cells, unlike αβ T-cells, are not **MHC-restricted** in the sense that they do not see antigen only when presented within the groove of MHC class I or MHC class II molecules. On the contrary, one of the main functions of NK cells is to patrol the body looking for cells that have lost expression of the normally ubiquitous MHC class I molecules; a situation that is known as **'missing-self' recognition** (figure 4.11). Such abnormal cells are usually either malignant or infected with a microorganism that interferes with class I expression. Because of the central role that MHC class I molecules play in presenting peptides derived from intracellular pathogens to the immune system, it is relatively easy to understand why these molecules may attract the unwelcome attentions of viruses or other uninvited guests planning to gatecrash their cellular hosts. It is probably for this reason that NK cells co-evolved alongside MHC-restricted T-cells to ensure that pathogens, or other conditions that may interefere with MHC class I expression and hence antigen presentation to αβ T-cells, are given short shrift. Cells that end up in this unfortunate position are likely to soon find themselves looking down the barrel of an activated NK cell. Such an encounter typically results in death of the errant cell as a result of attack by cytotoxic granules, containing a battery of proteases and other destructive enzymes released by the activated NK cell.

NK receptors can be activating or inhibitory

NK cells play an important role in the ongoing battle against viral infection and tumor development and carry out their task using two sets of receptors; **activating receptors**, that recognize molecules collectively present on all cell surfaces, and **inhibitory receptors** that recognize MHC class I molecules. It is the balance between inhibitory and activating stimuli that will dictate whether NK-mediated killing will occur (figure 4.11).

Two structurally distinct families of NK receptors have been identified: the **C-type lectin receptors (CTLRs)** and the **Ig-like receptors**. Both receptor types include inhibitory and activating receptors. Those that are inhibitory contain **ITIMs (*i*mmunoreceptor *t*yrosine-based *i*nhibitory *m*otifs)** within their cytoplasmic tails that exert an inhibitory function within the cell by recruiting phosphatases, such as **SHP-1**, that can antagonize signal transduction events that would otherwise lead to release of NK cytotoxic granules or cytokines (figure 4.12). Activating receptors, on the other hand, are associated with accessory proteins, such as **DAP-12**, that contain positively acting ITAMs within their cytoplasmic tails that can promote events leading to NK-mediated attack. Upon engagement with their cognate ligands (MHC class I molecules), inhibitory receptors

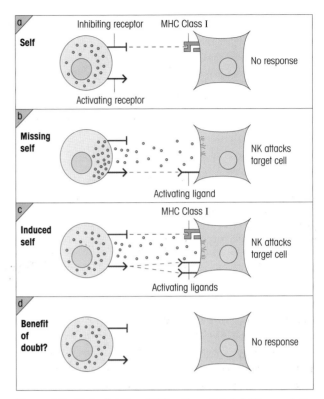

Figure 4.11. Natural killer (NK) cell-mediated killing and the 'missing-self' hypothesis. (a) Upon encounter with a normal autologous MHC class I-expressing cell, NK inhibitory receptors are engaged and activating NK receptors remain unoccupied because no activating ligands are expressed on the target cell. The NK cell does not become activated in this situation. (b) Loss of MHC class I expression ('missing-self'), as well as expression of one or more ligands for activating NK receptors, provokes NK-mediated attack of the cell via NK cytotoxic granules. (c) Upon encountering a target cell expressing MHC class I, but also expressing one or more ligands for activating NK receptors ('induced-self'), the outcome will be determined by the relative strength of the inhibitory and activating signals received by the NK cell. (d) In some cases, cells may not express MHC class I molecules or activating ligands and may be ignored by NK cells possibly due to expression of alternative ligands for inhibitory NK receptors.

suppress signals that would otherwise lead to NK cell activation. Cells that lack MHC class I molecules are therefore unable to engage the inhibitory receptors and are likely to suffer the consequences (figure 4.11).

The main class of MHC class I-monitoring receptors in the mouse is represented by the Ly49 multigene family of receptors that contains approximately 23 distinct genes; Ly49A to W. These receptors are expressed as disulfide-linked homodimers, with each monomer composed of a C-type lectin domain connected to the cell membrane via an α-helical stalk of ~40 amino acids (figure 4.12a); each NK cell expresses from one to four different Ly49 genes. Rather remarkably, humans do not use Ly49-based receptors to carry out the same task, but instead employ a functionally equivalent, but struc-

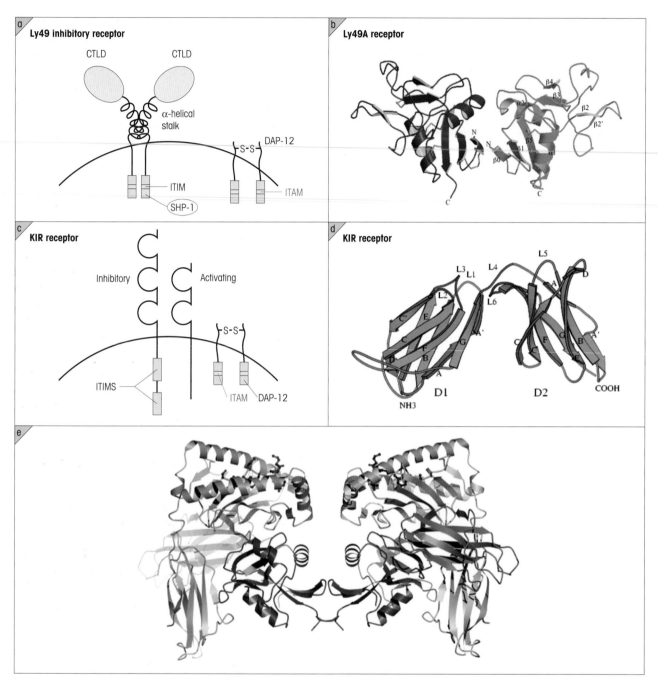

Figure 4.12. NK receptors. (a) Schematic representation of an inhibitory Ly49 receptor dimer composed of two C-type lectin domains (CTLD). The cytoplasmic tails of inhibitory Ly49 receptors contain *i*mmunoreceptor *t*yrosine-based *i*nhibitory *m*otifs (ITIMs) that can recruit phosphatases, such as SHP-1, capable of antagonizing NK activation. Activating Ly49 receptors lack ITIMs and can associate with ITAM-containing accessory proteins such as DAP-12 that can promote NK cell activation. (b) C-type lectin-like domain of the Ly49 NK cell receptors. The three-dimensional structure shown is the dimeric Ly49A (Protein Data Bank entry code 1QO3), the monomer A is colored blue and the monomer B is colored green. For clarity, secondary structural elements α-helices, β-strands, disulfide bonds and N and C termini are labeled only on one monomer. (Kindly provided by Dr Nazzareno Dimasi.) (c) The human KIRs (*k*iller *i*mmunoglobulin-like receptors) are functionally equivalent to the murine Ly49 receptors but remain structurally distinct. These receptors contain two or three Ig-like extracellular domains and can also be inhibitory or activating depending on the presence of an ITIM motif in their cytoplasmic domains, as shown. Activating receptors can associate with the ITAM-bearing DAP-12 accessory complex to propagate activating signals into the NK cell that result in NK-mediated attack. (d) Structure of the extracellular Ig-like domains (D1 and D2) of a KIR receptor. (Kindly provided by Dr Peter Sun and based upon coordinates originally published in Boyington *et al.* (2000) *Nature* **405,** 537.) (e) Ribbon diagram of the crystal structure of the Ly49C/H-2K^b complex. Ly49C, the H-2K^b heavy chain, and β_2M are shown in red, gold and green, respectively. The MHC-bound peptide (gray) is drawn in ball-and-stick representation. (Kindly provided by Dr Lu Deng and Professor Roy A. Mariuzza.)

turally distinct, set of receptors for this purpose, the **killer immunoglobulin-like receptors (KIRs).** This is a good example of **convergent evolution** where unrelated genes have evolved to fulfill the same functional role. Individual Ly49 receptors recognize MHC class I molecules in a manner that is, in most cases, independent of bound peptide. Ly49 dimers make contact with MHC class I molecules at two distinct sites that do not significantly overlap with the TCR binding area on the MHC (figure 4.12e). By contrast, the KIRs make contact with MHC class I molecules in an orientation that resembles the docking mode of the TCR where contact with bound peptide is part of the interaction. However, it is worth emphasizing that although KIRs do make contact with peptide within the MHC class I groove, these receptors do not distinguish between self and nonself peptides as TCRs do.

In addition to recognizing 'missing-self', NK cells also use their receptors to directly recognize pathogen components or MHC class I-like proteins, such as the **MHC class I chain-related A chain (MICA),** that are normally poorly expressed on normal healthy cells. MICA, and related ligands, have a complex pattern of expression but are often upregulated on transformed or infected cells and this may be sufficient to activate NK receptors that are capable of delivering activating signals; a phenomenon that has been termed **'induced-self' recognition** (figure 4.11). Upon ligation, the activating receptors signal the NK cell to kill the target cell and/or to secrete cytokines. The potentially anarchic situation in which the NK cells would attack all cells in the body is normally prevented due to the recognition of MHC class I by the inhibitory receptors.

Another example of an activating NK receptor is CD16, the low-affinity Fc receptor for IgG that is responsible for *antibody-dependent cellular cytotoxicity* (ADCC, cf. p. 32). In this case, the receptor ligand is IgG bound to antigen present on a target cell which is clearly an abnormal situation. The ligands for many of the other NK activating receptors remain obscure at present but this area is one of active investigation and is sure to yield interesting insights in the near future.

Cell stress and DNA damage responses can activate NK cells

Cellular stress can also lead to NK cell activation. The **CD94/NKG2** gene family have been found in human, rat and mouse genomes and belong to the CTLR class of NK receptors. These receptors can exist as CD94/CD94 homodimers or as CD94/NKG2 heterodimers and are expressed on most NK cells as well as γδ T-cells. CD94/NKG2A heterodimers are inhibitory receptors that recognize the MHC class I-related molecules, HLA-

E (human) and Qa1^b (mouse), which are notable for the fact that they mainly bind peptides that are found in the leader sequences of the classical MHC class I molecules. CD94/NKG2 receptors appear to monitor the expression status of MHC class I molecules indirectly because in the absence of the leader sequences from these peptides, HLA-E and Qa1^b are not expressed on the cell surface, thereby triggering NK attack. In the context of cellular stress, heat-shock proteins such as HSP-60 are induced and peptides derived from this heat-shock protein can displace MHC class I-derived peptides; this results in NK activation because CD94/NKG2 heterodimers cannot bind to HLA-E molecules that contain HSP-60 peptides.

Very recent studies also suggest that checkpoint kinases, such as Chk1, that are involved in the **DNA damage response** can induce expression of **NKG2D receptor** ligands when a cell is damaged by γ-irradiation, or after treatment with DNA-damaging drugs. This suggests that cells that have suffered DNA damage may, in addition to activating their DNA repair machinery, also upregulate NK receptor ligands to alert the immune system; such cells are dangerous as they have the potential to escape normal growth controls due to faulty or incomplete DNA repair.

THE MAJOR HISTOCOMPATIBILITY COMPLEX (MHC)

Molecules within this complex were originally defined by their ability to provoke vigorous rejection of grafts exchanged between different members of a species (Milestone 4.2). We have already referred to the necessity for antigens to be associated with class I or class II MHC molecules in order that they may be recognized by T-lymphocytes. Let us now look at these molecules in greater detail.

Class I and class II molecules are membrane-bound heterodimers

MHC class I
Class I molecules consist of a heavy polypeptide chain of 44kDa noncovalently linked to a smaller 12kDa polypeptide called β$_2$**-microglobulin.** The largest part of the heavy chain is organized into three globular domains (α$_1$, α$_2$ and α$_3$; figure 4.13) which protrude from the cell surface; a hydrophobic section anchors the molecule in the membrane and a short hydrophilic sequence carries the C-terminus into the cytoplasm.

The solution of the crystal structure of a human class I molecule provided an exciting leap forwards in our

Milestone 4.2—The Major Histocompatibility Complex

Peter Gorer raised rabbit antiserums to erythrocytes from pure strain mice (resulting from >20 brother–sister matings) and, by careful cross-absorption with red cells from different strains, he identified the strain-specific antigen II, now known as H-2 (table M4.2.1).

He next showed that the rejection of an albino (A) tumor by black (C57) mice was closely linked to the presence of the antigen II (table M4.2.2) and that tumor rejection was associated with the development of antibodies to this antigen.

Subsequently, George Snell introduced the term **histocompatibility (H)** antigen to describe antigens provoking graft rejection and demonstrated that, of all the potential H antigens, differences at the H-2 (i.e. antigen II) locus provoked the strongest graft rejection seen between various mouse strains. *Poco a poco*, the painstaking studies gradually uncovered a remarkably complicated situation. Far from representing a

Table M4.2.1. Identification of H-2 (antigen II).

Rabbit antiserum to:	Antigens detected on Albino red cells		
	I	II	III
Albino (A)	+++	+++	++
Black (C57)	++	–	++

single gene locus, H-2 proved to be a large complex of multiple genes, many of which were highly polymorphic, hence the term **major histocompatibility complex (MHC)**. The major components of the current genetic maps of the human HLA and mouse H-2 MHC are drawn in figure M4.2.1 to give the reader an overall grasp of the complex make-up of this important region (to immunologists we mean!—presumably all highly transcribed regions are important to the host in some way).

Table M4.2.2. Relationship of antigen II to tumor rejection.

Antigen II phenotype of recipient strain	Rejection of tumor inoculum (A strain) by:			
	*Pure strain		**(A x C57) F1 backcross to C57	
	–	+	–	+
Ag II +ve (A)	39	0	17 (19.3)	17 (19.5)
Ag II -ve (C57)	0	45	0	44 (39)

*A tumor inoculum derived from A strain bearing antigen II is rejected by the C57 host (+ = rejection; – = acceptance).

**Offspring of A × C57 mating were backcrossed to the C57 parent and the resulting progeny tested for antigen II (Ag II) and their ability to reject the tumor. The figures in brackets = number expected if tumor growth is influenced by two dominant genes, one of which determines the presence of antigen II.

MAIN GENETIC REGIONS OF THE MAJOR HISTOCOMPATIBILITY COMPLEX											
HUMAN	MHC CLASS		II			III				I	CHROMOSOME 6
	HLA	DP	DQ	DR	C'	HSP	TNF	etc	B	C	A
MOUSE	MHC CLASS	I	II		III				I		CHROMOSOME 17
	H-2	K	A	E	C'	HSP	TNF	etc	D	L	

Figure M4.2.1. Main genetic regions of the major histocompatibility complex.

understanding of MHC function. Both β_2-microglobulin and the α_3 region resemble classic Ig domains in their folding pattern (cf. figure 4.13c). However, the α_1 and α_2 domains, which are most distal to the membrane, form two extended α-helices above a floor created by strands held together in a β-pleated sheet, the whole forming an undeniable **groove** (figure 4.13b,c). The appearance of these domains is so striking, we doubt whether the reader needs the help of gastronomic analogies such as 'two sausages on a barbecue' to prevent any class I structural amnesia. Another curious feature emerged. The groove was occupied by a linear molecule, now known to be a peptide, which had cocrystallized with the class I protein (figure 4.14). How antigenic peptides are processed and selected for presentation within MHC

molecules and how the TCR sees this complex will be revealed in the following chapter.

MHC class II

Class II MHC molecules are also transmembrane glycoproteins, in this case consisting of α and β polypeptide chains of molecular weight 34 kDa and 29 kDa, respectively.

There is considerable sequence homology with class I and structural studies have shown that the α_2 and β_2 domains, the ones nearest to the cell membrane, assume the characteristic Ig fold, while the α_1 and β_1 domains mimic the class I α_1 and α_2 in forming a groove bounded by two α-helices and a β-pleated sheet floor (figures 4.13a and 4.14).

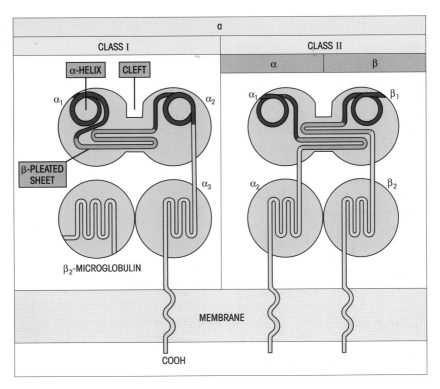

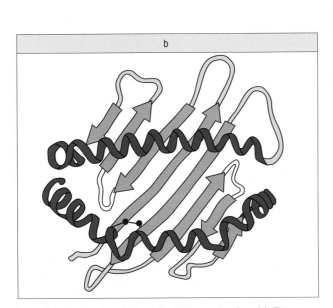

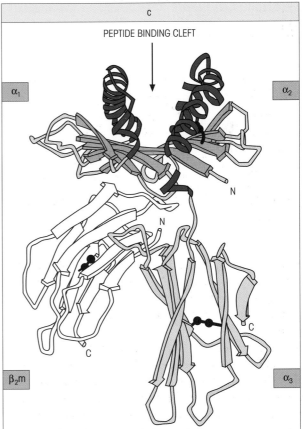

Figure 4.13. Class I and class II MHC molecules. (a) Diagram showing domains and transmembrane segments; the α-helices and β-sheets are viewed end on. (b) Schematic bird's eye representation of the top surface of human class I molecule (HLA-A2) based on the X-ray crystallographic structure. The strands making the β-pleated sheet are shown as thick gray arrows in the amino to carboxy direction; α-helices are represented as dark red helical ribbons. The inside-facing surfaces of the two helices and the upper surface of the β-sheet form a cleft. The two black spheres represent an intrachain disulfide bond. (c) Side view of the same molecule clearly showing the anatomy of the cleft and the typical Ig-type folding of the α$_3$- and β$_2$-microglobulin domains (four antiparallel β-strands on one face and three on the other). (Reproduced from Bjorkman P.J. *et al.* (1987) *Nature* **329**, 506, with permission.)

H-2K^b
SEV9 peptide

I-A^{g7}
GAD65 peptide

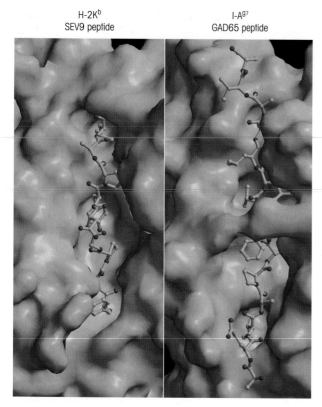

Figure 4.14. Surface view of mouse class I and class II MHC molecules in complex with peptide. Surface solvent-accessible areas of the mouse class I molecule (H-2K^b) in complex with a virus-derived peptide and the mouse class II molecule I-A^{g7} in complex with an endogenous peptide. The views shown here are similar to that schematically depicted in figure 4.13b and look down upon the surface of the MHC molecules. Note that the peptide-binding cleft of class I molecules is more restricted than that of class II molecules with the result that class I-binding peptides are typically shorter than those that bind to class II molecules. (Kindly provided by Dr Robyn Stanfield and Dr Ian Wilson, Department of Molecular Biology, The Scripps Research Institute, La Jolla, California, USA.)

The organization of the genes encoding the α chain of the human class II molecule HLA-DR and the main regulatory sequences which control their transcription are shown in figure 4.15.

MHC class I and class II molecules are polygenic

Several different flavors of MHC class I and class II proteins are expressed by most cells. There are three different class I α-chain genes, referred to as *HLA-A*, *HLA-B* and *HLA-C* in man and *H-2K*, *H-2D* and *H-2L* in the mouse, which can result in the expression of at least three different class I proteins in every cell. This number is doubled if an individual is **heterozygous** for the class I alleles expressed at each locus; indeed, this is often the case due to the **polymorphic** nature of class I genes as we shall discuss later in this chapter.

There are also three different types of MHC class II α- and β-chain genes expressed in humans, *HLA-DQ*, *HLA-DP*, and *HLA-DR*, and two pairs in mice, *H2-A* (I-A) and *H2-E* (I-E). Thus, humans can express a minimum of three different class II molecules, with this number increasing significantly when polymorphisms are considered; this is because different α and β chain combinations can be generated when an individual is heterozygous for a particular class II gene.

The different types of class I and class II molecules all exhibit the same basic structure as depicted in figure 4.13a and all participate in presenting peptides to T-cells but, because of significant differences in their peptide-binding grooves, each presents a different range of peptides to the immune system. This has the highly desirable effect of increasing the range of peptides that

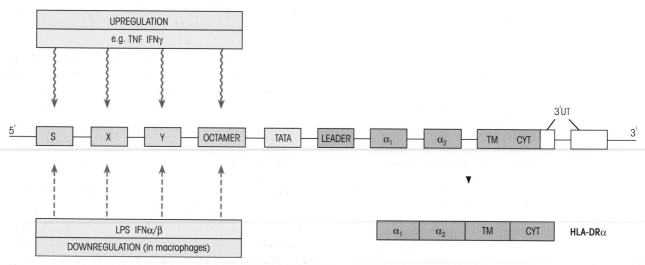

Figure 4.15. Genes encoding human HLA-DRα chain (darker blue) and their controlling elements (regulatory sequences in light blue and TATA box promoter in yellow). α₁/α₂ encode the two extracellular domains; TM and CYT encode the transmembrane and cytoplasmic segments, respectively. 3′ UT represents the 3′ untranslated sequence. Octamer motifs are also found in virtually all heavy and light chain immunoglobulin *V* gene promoters (cf. figure 3.21) and in the promoters of other B-cell-specific genes such as *B29* and *CD20*.

can be presented to T-cells and reduces the likelihood that peptides derived from pathogen proteins will fail to be presented.

Class I and class II MHC molecules probably evolved from a single ancestral gene that underwent serial gene duplications, followed by diversification due to selective pressure, to generate the different class I and class II genes that we see today (figure 4.16). Genes that failed to confer any selective advantage or that suffered deleterious mutations were either deleted from the genome or are still present as pseudogenes (genes that fail to express a functional protein); indeed many pseudogenes are present within the MHC region. This type of gene evolution pattern has been termed the **birth-and-death model** or the accordion model due to the way in which this gene region expanded and contracted during evolution.

Several immune response-related genes contribute to the remaining class III region of the MHC

A variety of other genes which congregate within the MHC chromosome region are grouped under the heading of class III. Broadly, one could say that many are directly or indirectly related to immune defense functions. A notable cluster involves four genes coding for complement components, two of which are for the C4 isotypes C4A and C4B and the other two for C2 and

factor B. The cytokines, tumor necrosis factor (TNF, sometimes referred to as TNFα) and lymphotoxin (LTα and LTβ), are encoded under the class III umbrella as are three members of the human 70 kDa heat-shock proteins. As ever, things don't quite fit into the nice little boxes we would like to put them in. Even if it were crystal clear where one region of the MHC ends and another begins (and it isn't), some genes located in the middle of the 'classical' (cf. figure 4.17) class I or II regions should more correctly be classified as part of the class III cohort. For example, the *LMP* and *TAP* genes concerned with the intracellular processing and transport of T-cell epitope peptides are found in the class II region (see below), but do not have the classical class II structure nor are they expressed on the cell surface.

Gene map of the MHC

The complete sequence of a human MHC was published at the very end of the last millennium after a gargantuan collaborative effort involving groups in England, France, Japan and the USA. The entire sequence, which represents a composite of several MHC haplotypes, comprises 224 gene loci. Of the 128 of these genes which are predicted to be expressed, it is estimated that about 40% of them have functions related to the immune system. It is not clear why so many immune response-related genes are clustered within this relatively small region, although this phenomenon has also been observed with housekeeping genes that share related functions. Because the location of a gene within chromatin can profoundly influence its transcriptional activity, perhaps it has something to do with ensuring that the genes within this region are expressed at similar levels. Genes found within condensed regions of chromatin are often expressed at relatively low levels and in some cases may not be expressed at all. The region between class II and class I in the human contains 60 or so class III genes. An overall view of the main clusters of class I, II and III genes in the MHC of the mouse and human may be gained from figure M4.2.1 in Milestone 4.2. More detailed maps of each region are provided in figures 4.17–4.19. A number of pseudogenes have been omitted from these gene maps in the interest of simplicity.

The cell surface class I molecule, based on a transmembrane chain with three extracellular domains associated with β_2-microglobulin, has clearly proved to be a highly useful structure judging by the number of variants on this theme that have arisen during evolution. It is helpful to subdivide them, first into the **classical class I molecules** (sometimes referred to as class Ia), HLA-A, -B and -C in the human and H-2K, -D and -L in the

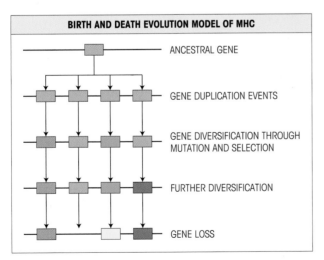

Figure 4.16. Birth and death model of MHC evolution. Different MHC genes most likely arose though duplication events that resulted in diversification of the duplicated genes as a result of selective pressure. Genes that confer no selective advantage can suffer deleterious mutations resulting in pseudogenes or may be deleted from the genome altogether. Different environments impose distinct selective pressures, due to different pathogens for example, resulting in a high degree of polymorphism within this gene family. MHC polymorphism is seen primarily within the peptide-binding regions of MHC class I and class II molecules.

mouse. These were defined serologically by the antibodies arising in grafted individuals using methods developed from Gorer's pioneering studies (Milestone 4.2). Other molecules, sometimes referred to as class Ib, have related structures and are either encoded within the MHC locus itself ('**nonclassical**' MHC molecules, for example the human HLA-E, -F and -G, HFE, MICA and MICB, the murine H-2T, -Q and -M), or elsewhere in the genome ('**class I chain-related**', including the CD1 family and FcRn). Nonclassical MHC genes are far less

HUMAN	HLA GENE	MICB	MICA	B	C	E	A	G	F
	GENE PRODUCT	MICB	MICA	HLA-B	HLA-C	HLA-E	HLA-A	HLA-G	HLA-F

MOUSE	H-2 GENE	TAPASIN	K	D	L	Q	T	M
	GENE PRODUCT	TAPASIN	H-2K	H-2D	H-2L	Q	T	H-2M

Figure 4.17. MHC class I gene map. The 'classical' polymorphic class I genes, *HLA-A, -B, -C* in humans and *H-2K, -D, -L* in mice, are highlighted with orange shading and encode peptide chains which, together with β₂-microglobulin, form the complete class I molecules originally identified in earlier studies as antigens by the antibodies they evoked on grafting into another member of the same species. Note that only some strains of mice possess an *H-2L* gene. The genes expressed most abundantly are *HLA-A* and *-B* in the human and *H-2K* and *-D* in the mouse. The other class I genes ('class Ib') are termed 'non-classical' or 'class I chain-related'. They are oligo- rather than polymorphic or sometimes invariant, and many are silent or pseudogenes. In the mouse there are approximately 15 *Q* (also referred to as *Qa*) genes, 25 *T* (also referred to as *TL* or *Tla*) genes and 10 *M* genes. MICA and MICB are ligands for NK cell receptors. Tapasin is involved in peptide transport (cf. p. 97). The gene encoding this molecule is at the centromeric end of the MHC region and therefore is shown in this gene map with respect to the mouse, but in figure 4.18, the class II gene map with respect to the human — look at figure M4.2.1 to see why.

HUMAN	HLA GENE	TAPASIN	DPB	DPA	DOA	DMA	DMB	LMP2	TAP1	LMP7	TAP2	DOB	DQB	DQA	DRB	DRA
	GENE PRODUCT	TAPASIN	DPβ	DPα	DOα	DMα	DMβ	PROTEASOME COMPLEX		PEPTIDE TRANSPORTER		DOβ	DQβ	DQα	DRβ	DRα
			HLA-DP		HLA-DO	HLA-DM						HLA-DO	HLA-DQ		HLA-DR	

MOUSE	H-2 GENE	Oa	Ma	Mb2	Mb1	LMP2	TAP2	LMP7	TAP1	Ob	Ab	Aa	Eb	Ea
	GENE PRODUCT	Oα	DMα	DMβ2	DMβ1	PROTEASOME COMPLEX		PEPTIDE TRANSPORTER		β	Aβ	Aα	Eβ	Eα
		H-2O	H-2DM							H-2O	H-2A		H-2E	

Figure 4.18. MHC class II gene map with 'classical' *HLA-DP, -DQ, -DR* in the human and *H-2A (I-A)* and *H-2E (I-E)* in mice more heavily shaded. Both α and β chains of the class II heterodimer are transcribed from closely located genes. There are usually two expressed *DRB* genes, *DRB1* and one of either *DRB3, DRB4* or *DRB5*. A similar situation of a single α chain pairing with different β chains is found in the mouse I-E molecule. The *LMP2* and *LMP7* genes encode part of the proteasome complex which cleaves cytosolic proteins into small peptides which are transported by the *TAP* gene products into the endoplasmic reticulum. *HLA-DMA* and *-DMB* (mouse *H-2DMa, -DMb1* and *-DMb2*) encode the DM αβ heterodimer which removes class II-associated invariant chain peptide (CLIP) from classical class II molecules to permit the binding of high affinity peptides. The mouse H-2DM molecules are often referred to as H-2M1 and H-2M2, although this is a horribly confusing designation because the term *H-2M* is also used for a completely different set of genes which lie distal to the *H-2T* region and encode members of the class Ib family (cf. figure 4.17). The *HLA-DOA* (alternatively called *HLA-DNA*) and *-DOB* genes (*H-2Oa* and *-Ob* in the mouse) also encode an αβ heterodimer which may play a role in peptide selection or exchange with classical class II molecules. (Reproduced with permission from Nature Reviews Immunology Vol. 5, No 10, pp. 783–792 (2005), Macmillan Magazines Ltd.)

HUMAN	CYP21B	C4B	CYP21A	C4A	BF	C2	HSPA1B	HSPA1A	HSPA1L	LTB	TNF	LTA

MOUSE	CYP21A1	C4	CYP21A2	Slp	BF	C2	HSP70-1	HSP70-3	Hsc70t	LTB	TNF	LTA

Figure 4.19. MHC class III gene map. This region is something of a 'rag bag'. Aside from immunologically 'respectable' products like C2, C4, factor B (encoded by the *BF* gene), tumor necrosis factor (*TNF*), lymphotoxin-α and lymphotoxin-β (encoded by *LTA* and *LTB*, respectively) and three 70 kDa heat-shock proteins (the *HSPA1A, HSPA1B* and *HSPA1L* genes in humans, *HSP70-1, HSP70-3* and *Hsc70t* genes in mice), genes not shown in this figure but nonetheless present in this locus include those encoding valyl tRNA synthetase (*G7a*), NOTCH4, which has a number of regulatory activities, and tenascin, an extra-cellular matrix protein. Of course many genes may have drifted to this location during the long passage of evolutionary time without necessarily having to act in concert with their neighbors to subserve some integrated defensive function. The 21-hydroxylases (21OHA and B, encoded by *CYP21A* and *CYP21B*, respectively) are concerned with the hydroxylation of steroids such as cortisone. *Slp* (sex-limited protein) encodes a murine allele of C4, expressed under the influence of testosterone.

polymorphic than the classical MHC, are often invariant, and many are pseudogenes. Many of these nonclassical MHC class I molecules form structures that are very similar to class I molecules and have also been found to serve as antigen-presenting molecules in particular contexts.

The genes of the MHC display remarkable polymorphism

Unlike the immunoglobulin system where, as we have seen, variability is achieved in each individual by a **multigenic** system, the MHC has evolved in terms of variability between individuals with a highly **polymorphic** (literally 'many shaped') system based on **multiple alleles** (i.e. alternative genes at each locus). This has likely arisen through **pathogen-driven selection** to form new alleles that may offer increased 'fitness' for the individual; in this context, fitness could mean increased protection from an infectious organism. The class I and class II genes are the most polymorphic genes in the human genome; for some of these genes over 600 allelic variants have been identified (figure 4.20). This implies that there has been intense selective pressure on the MHC gene region and that genes within this region are mutating at rates much faster than at other gene loci.

As is amply illustrated in figure 4.20, class I HLA-A, -B and -C molecules are highly polymorphic and so are the class II β chains (HLA-DRβ most, -DPβ next and -DQβ third) and, albeit to a lesser extent than the β chains, the α chains of -DP and -DQ. HLA-DRα and β_2-microglobulin are invariant in structure. The amino acid changes responsible for this polymorphism are restricted to the α_1 and α_2 domains of class I and to the α_1 and β_1 domains of class II. It is of enormous significance that they occur essentially in the β-sheet floor and on the inner surfaces of the α-helices which line the central cavity (figure 4.13a) and also on the upper surfaces of the helices; these are the very surfaces that make contact with the peptides which these MHC molecules offer up for inspection by TCRs (figure 4.14). The ongoing drive towards creating new MHC molecules, with slightly altered peptide-binding grooves, is akin to a genetic arms race where the immune system is constantly trying to keep one step ahead of its foe. This genetic one-upmanship has been termed **pathogen-driven balancing selection** because heterozygotes typically have a selective advantage over homozygotes at a given locus.

The MHC region represents an outstanding hotspot with mutation rates two orders of magnitude higher than non-MHC loci. These multiple allelic forms can be generated by a variety of mechanisms: point mutations, recombination, homologous but unequal crossing over and **gene conversion**.

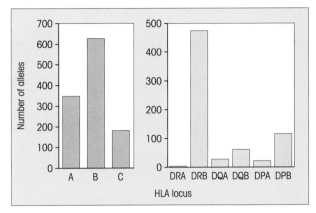

Figure 4.20. Polymorphism within human HLA class I and class II genes. Number of distinct human HLA class I (A, B, C) and class II (DRA, DRB, DQA, DQB, DPA, DPB) alleles at each locus as of January 2005. (Based upon data gathered by the WHO Nomenclature Committee for Factors of the HLA system and published within Marsh *et al.* (2005) *Tissue Antigens* **65**, 301.)

The degree of sequence homology and an increased occurrence of the dinucleotide motif 5'-cytosine-guanine-3' (to produce what are referred to as CpG islands) seem to be important for gene conversion, and it has been suggested that this might involve a DNA-nicking activity which targets CpG-rich DNA sequences. MHC genes that lack these sequences, for example H-2Ea^d and HLA-DRA, do not appear to undergo gene conversion, whereas those that possess CpG islands act as either donors (e.g. H-2Eb^b, H-2Q2^k, H-2Q10^b), acceptors (e.g. H-2A^b) or both (e.g. H-2K^k, HLA-DQB1). The large number of pseudogenes within the MHC may represent a stockpile of genetic information for the generation of polymorphic diversity in the 'working' class I and class II molecules.

Nomenclature

Since much of the experimental work relating to the MHC is based on experiments in our little laboratory friend, the mouse, it may be helpful to explain the nomenclature used to describe the allelic genes and their products. If someone says to you in an obscure language 'we are having free elections', you fail to understand, not because the idea is complicated but because you do not comprehend the language. It is much the same with the shorthand used to describe the H-2 system which looks unnecessarily frightening to the uninitiated. In order to identify and compare allelic genes within the H-2 complex in different strains, it is usual to start with certain pure homozygous inbred strains, obtained by successive brother–sister matings, to provide the prototypes. The collection of genes in the H-2 complex is called the **haplotype** and the haplotype of each prototypic inbred strain will be allotted a given superscript. For example, the DBA strain haplotype is designated H-2^d and the genes constituting the complex are therefore H-$2K^d$, H-$2Aa^d$, H-$2Ab^d$, H-$2D^d$ and so on; their products will be H-2K^d, H-2A^d and H-2D^d and so forth (figure 4.21). When new strains are derived from these by genetic recombination during breeding, they are assigned new haplotypes, but the individual genes are designated by the haplotype of the prototype strain from which they were derived. Thus the A/J strain produced by genetic cross-over during interbreeding between (H-$2^k \times H$-2^d) F1 mice (figure 4.22) is arbitrarily assigned the haplotype H-2^a, but table 4.3 shows that individual genes in the complex are identified by the haplotype symbol of the original parents.

Inheritance of the MHC

Pure strain mice derived by prolonged brother–sister mating are homozygous for each pair of homologous chromosomes. Thus, in the present context, the haplotype of the MHC derived from the mother will be identical to that from the father; animals of the C57BL strain,

for example, will each bear two chromosomes with the H-2^b haplotype (cf. table 4.3).

Let us see how the MHC behaves when we cross two pure strains of haplotypes H-2^k and H-2^d, respectively. We find that the lymphocytes of the offspring (the F1 generation) all display *both* H-2^k and H-2^d molecules on their surface, i.e. there is **codominant expression** (figure 4.22). If we go further and breed F1s together, the progeny have the genotypes k, k/d and d in the proportions to be expected if the **haplotype segregates as a single Mendelian trait**. This happens because the H-2 complex spans 0.5 centimorgans, equivalent to a recombination frequency between the K and D ends of 0.5%, and the haplotype tends to be inherited *en bloc*. Only the relatively infrequent recombinations caused by meiotic cross-over events, as described for the A/J strain above, reveal the complexity of the system.

The tissue distribution of MHC molecules

Essentially, all nucleated cells carry classical class I molecules. These are abundantly expressed on both lymphoid and myeloid cells, less so on liver, lung and

Strain	Haplotype	MHC Designation	I	II					III		I	
C57BL	**b**	H-2^b	K^b	Ab^b	Aa^b	Eb^b	Ea^b	$C4^b$	etc	D^b	etc	
CBA	**k**	H-2^k	K^k	Ab^k	Aa^k	Eb^k	Ea^k	$C4^k$	etc	D^k	etc	

Figure 4.21. How the definition of *H-2* haplotype works. Pure strain mice homozygous for the whole *H-2* region through prolonged brother–sister mating for at least 20 generations are each arbitrarily assigned a **haplotype** designated by a superscript. Thus the particular set of alleles which happens to occur in the strain named C57BL is assigned the haplotype *H-2^b* and the particular nucleotide sequence of each allele in its MHC is labeled as **gene^b**, e.g. **H-2K^b**, etc. It is obviously more convenient to describe a given allele by the haplotype than to trot out its whole nucleotide sequence, and it is easier to follow the reactions of cells of known *H-2* make-up by using the haplotype terminology —see, for example, the interpretation of the experiment in figure 4.22.

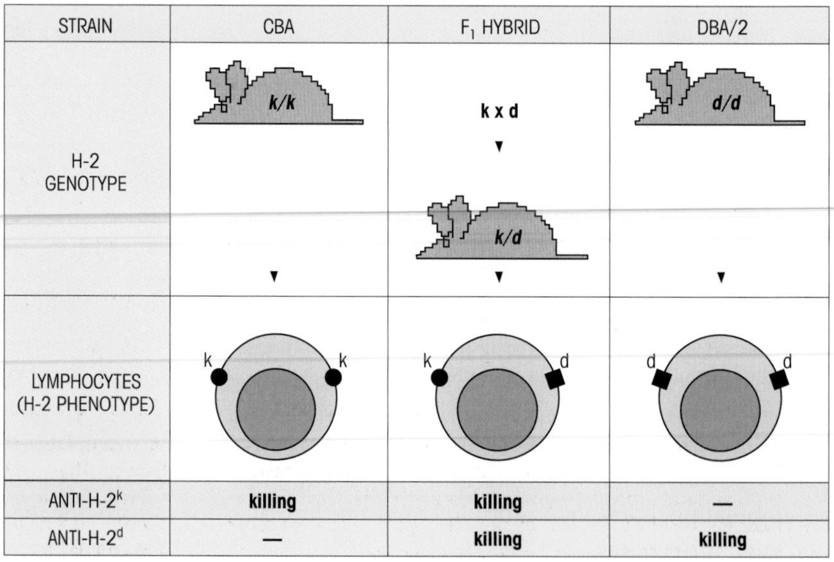

Figure 4.22. Inheritance and codominant expression of MHC genes. Each homozygous (pure) parental strain animal has two identical chromosomes bearing the *H-2* haplotype, one paternal and the other maternal. Thus in the present example we designate a strain which is *H-2^k* as k/k. The first familial generation (F1) obtained by crossing the pure parental strains CBA (*H-2^k*) and DBA/2 (*H-2^d*) has the *H-2* genotype k/d. Since 100% of F1 lymphocytes are killed in the presence of complement by antibodies to H-2^k or to H-2^d (raised by injecting H-2^k lymphocytes into an H-2^d animal and vice versa), the MHC molecules encoded by both parental genes must be expressed on every lymphocyte. The same holds true for other tissues in the body.

STRAIN	CBA	F₁ HYBRID	DBA/2
H-2 GENOTYPE	k/k	k x d → k/d	d/d
LYMPHOCYTES (H-2 PHENOTYPE)	k — k	k — d	d — d
ANTI-H-2^k	killing	killing	—
ANTI-H-2^d	—	killing	killing

kidney and only sparsely on brain and skeletal muscle. In the human, the surface of the placental extravillous cytotrophoblast lacks HLA-A and -B, although there is now some evidence that it may express HLA-C. What is well established is that the extravillous cytotrophoblast and other placental tissues bear HLA-G, a molecule which generally lacks allodeterminants and which does not appear on most other body cells, except for medullary and subcapsular epithelium in the thymus, and on blood monocytes following activation with γ-interferon. The role of HLA-G in the placenta is unclear, but it may function as a replacement for allodeterminant-bearing classical class I molecules and/or may play a role in shifting potentially harmful Th1 responses towards a Th2-type response. Class II molecules, on the other hand, are highly restricted in their expression, being present only on B-cells, dendritic cells, macrophages and thymic epithelium. However, when activated by agents such as γ-interferon, capillary endothelia and many epithelial cells in tissues other than the thymus express surface class II and increased levels of class I.

The nonclassical MHC and class I chain-related molecules

These molecules include the **CD1** family which utilize β_2-microglobulin and have a similar overall structure to the classical class I molecules (figure 4.23). They are, however, encoded by a set of genes on a different chromosome to the MHC, namely on chromosome 1 in humans and chromosome 3 in the mouse. Like its true MHC counterparts, CD1 is involved in the presentation of antigens to T-cells, but the antigen-binding groove is to some extent covered over, contains mainly hydrophobic amino acids, and is accessible only through a narrow entrance. Instead of binding peptide antigens, the CD1 molecules generally present lipids or glycolipids. At least four different CD1 molecules are found expressed on human cells; CD1a, b and c are present on cortical thymocytes, dendritic cells and a subset of B-cells, whilst CD1d is expressed on intestinal epithelium, hepatocytes and all lymphoid and myeloid cells. Mice appear to only express two different CD1 molecules

Table 4.3. The haplotypes of the *H-2* complex of some commonly used mouse strains and recombinants derived from them. A/J was derived by interbreeding $(k \times d)$ F1 mice, recombination occurring between E (class II) and S (class III) regions*.

STRAIN	HAPLOTYPE	ORIGIN OF INDIVIDUAL REGIONS				
		K	A	E	S	D
C57BL	b	b	b	b	b	b
CBA	k	k	k	k	k	k
DBA/2	d	d	d	d	d	d
A/J	a	k	k	k*	d	d
B.10A(4R)	h4	k	k	b	b	b

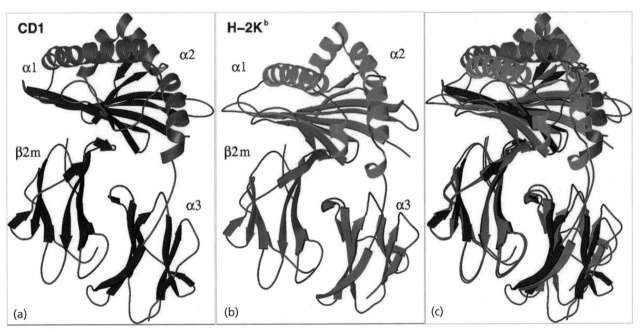

Figure 4.23. Comparison of the crystal structures of CD1 and MHC class I. (a) Backbone ribbon diagram of mouse CD1d1 (red, α-helices; blue, β-strands). (b) Ribbon diagram of the mouse MHC class I molecule H-2K^b (cyan, α-helices; green, β-strands). (c) Superposition using alignment of β_2-microglobulin highlights some of the differences between CD1d1 and H-2K^b. Note in particular the shifting of the α-helices. This produces a deeper and more voluminous groove in CD1d1, which is narrower at its entrance compared with H-2K^b. (Reprinted with permission from Porcelli S.A. *et al.* (1998) *Immunology Today* **19**, 362.)

which are both similar to the human CD1d in structure and tissue distribution and are referred to as CD1d1 and CD1d2 (or CD1.1 and CD1.2).

Genes in the MHC itself which encode nonclassical MHC molecules include the H-2T, -Q and -M loci in mice, each of which encodes a number of different molecules. The T22 and T10 molecules, for example, are induced by cellular activation and are recognized directly by γδ TCR without a requirement for antigen, possibly suggesting that they are involved in triggering immunoregulatory γδ T-cells. Other nonclassical class I molecules do bind peptides, such as H-2M3 which presents *N*-formylated peptides produced either in mitochondria or by bacteria.

In the human, HLA-E binds a nine-amino acid peptide derived from the signal sequence of HLA-A, -B, -C and -G molecules, and is recognized by the CD94/NKG2 receptors on NK cells and cytotoxic T-cells, as well as by the αβ TCR on some cytotoxic T-cells. HLA-E is upregulated when other HLA alleles provide the appropriate leader peptides, thereby perhaps allowing NK cells to monitor the expression of polymorphic

class I molecules using a single receptor. The murine homolog, Qa-1, has a similar function.

The stress-inducible MICA and MICB (*MHC class I chain*-related molecules) have the same domain structure as classical class I and display a relatively high level of polymorphism. They are present on epithelial cells, mainly in the gastrointestinal tract and in the thymic cortex, and are recognized by the NKG2D activating molecule. One possible role for this interaction is in the promotion of NK and T-cell antitumor responses.

The function of HLA-F is unclear. In contrast, although HLA-G shows extremely limited polymorphism, it is known to bind a range of self peptides with a defined binding motif and there is evidence for HLA-G restricted T-cells.

HFE, previously referred to as HLA-H, possesses an extremely narrow groove which is unable to bind peptides, and it may serve no role in immune defense. However, it binds to the transferrin receptor and appears to be involved in iron uptake. A point mutation (C282Y) in HFE is found in 70–90% of patients with hereditary hemochromatosis.

SUMMARY

The B-cell surface receptor for antigen

- The B-cell inserts its Ig gene product containing a transmembrane segment into its surface where it acts as a specific receptor for antigen.
- The surface Ig is complexed with the membrane proteins Ig-α and Ig-β which become phosphorylated on cell activation and transduce signals received through the Ig antigen receptor.
- The cytoplasmic tails of the Ig-α and Ig-β *i*mmunorecep*t*or *t*yrosine-based *a*ctivation *m*otifs (ITAMs) that, upon phosphorylation, can recruit phosphotyrosine-binding proteins that play important roles in signal transduction from the BCR.

The T-cell surface receptor for antigen

- The receptor for antigen is a transmembrane dimer, each chain consisting of two Ig-like domains.
- The outer domains are variable in structure, the inner ones constant, rather like a membrane-bound Fab.
- Both chains are required for antigen recognition.
- CD4 and CD8 act as co-receptors, along with the TCR, for MHC molecules. CD4 acts as a co-receptor for MHC class II molecules and CD8 recognizes MHC class I molecules.
- Most T-cells express a receptor (TCR) with α and β chains (TCR2). A separate lineage (TCR1) bearing γδ receptors is transcribed strongly in early thymic ontogeny but is associated mainly with epithelial tissues in the adult.
- The encoding of the TCR is similar to that of immunoglo-

bulins. The variable region coding sequence in the differentiating T-cell is formed by random translocation from clusters of *V*, *D* (for β and δ chains) and *J* segments to give a single recombinant *V(D)J* sequence for each chain.

- Like the Ig chains, each variable region has three hypervariable sequences which function in antigen recognition.
- The CD3 complex, composed of γ, δ, ε and either ζ, ζη or η, covalently linked dimers, forms an intimate part of the receptor and has a signal transducing role following ligand binding by the TCR.

The generation of antibody diversity for antigen recognition

- Ig heavy and light chains and TCR α and β chains generally are represented in the germ-line by between 33 and 75 variable region genes, between 2 and 27 *D* segment minigenes (Ig heavy and TCR β and δ only) and 3–60 short *J* segments.
- TCR γ and δ chains are encoded by far fewer genes.
- Random recombination of any single *V*, *D* and *J* from each gene cluster generates approximately 6.5×10^3 Ig heavy chain *VDJ* sequences, 350 light chains, 4.5×10^3 TCR α, 1×10^3 TCR β, but only 60 TCR γ and 72 TCR δ.
- Random interchain combination produces roughly 2.4×10^6 Ig, 4.5×10^6 TCR αβ and 4.3×10^3 TCR γδ receptors.
- Further diversity is introduced at the junctions between *V*, *D* and *J* segments by variable combination as they are spliced together by recombinase enzymes and by the N-region insertion of random nontemplated nucleotide

sequences. These mechanisms may be particularly important in augmenting the number of specificities which can be squeezed out of the relatively small γδ pool.

- Useless or self-reactive receptors can be replaced by receptor editing.
- In addition, after a primary response, B-cells but not T-cells undergo high rate somatic mutation affecting the *V* regions.

NK receptors

- NK cells bear a number of receptors with Ig-type domains and other receptors with C-type lectin domains. Members of both types of receptor family can function as inhibitory or activating receptors to determine whether the target cell should be killed.
- Loss of MHC class I molecules can provoke attack by NK cells.
- NK cells can also recognize ligands that are upregulated by cells that suffer stress or DNA damage.

MHC

- MHC molecules act as receptors for antigen and present antigen-derived peptides to T-cells.
- Each vertebrate species has an MHC identified originally through its ability to evoke very powerful transplantation rejection.
- Each contains three classes of genes. Class I encodes 44 kDa transmembrane polypeptides associated at the cell surface with β_2-microglobulin. Class II molecules are transmembrane heterodimers. Class III products are heterogeneous but include complement components linked to the formation of C3 convertases, heat-shock proteins and tumor necrosis factors.

- Several different types of MHC class I and class II molecules are expressed by all cells. MHC genes also display remarkable polymorphism. A given MHC gene cluster is referred to as a 'haplotype' and is usually inherited *en bloc* as a single Mendelian trait, although its constituent genes have been revealed by crossover recombination events.
- Classical class I molecules are present on virtually all cells in the body and present peptides to CD8[+] cytotoxic T-cells.
- Class II molecules are particularly associated with B-cells, dendritic cells and macrophages but can be induced on capillary endothelial cells and epithelial cells by γ-interferon. Class II molecules present peptides to CD4[+] T-helpers for B-cells and macrophages.
- The two domains distal to the cell membrane form a peptide binding cavity bounded by two parallel α-helices sitting on a floor of β-sheet strands; the walls and floor of the cavity and the upper surface of the helices are the sites of maximum polymorphic amino acid substitutions.
- Silent class I genes may increase polymorphism by gene conversion mechanisms.
- Nonclassical MHC molecules and MHC-like molecules have a number of functions, and include CD1 which presents lipid and glycolipid antigens to T-cells, and HLA-E which presents signal sequence peptides from classical class I molecules to the CD94/NKG2 receptor of NK cells.

FURTHER READING

Braud V.M., Allan D.S.J. & McMichael A.J. (1999) Functions of nonclassical MHC and non-MHC-encoded class I molecules. *Current Opinion in Immunology* **11**, 100–108.

Call M.E. & Wucherpfennig K.W. (2005) The T cell receptor: critical role of the membrane environment in receptor assembly and function. *Annual Review of Immunology* **23**, 101–125.

Carding S.R. & Egan P.J. (2002) γδ T cells: functional plasticity and heterogeneity. *Nature Reviews Immunology* **2**, 336–345.

Clark D.A. (1999) Human leukocyte antigen-G: new roles for old? *American Journal of Reproductive Immunology* **41**, 117–120.

Garcia K.C. & Adams E.J. (2005) How the T cell receptor sees antigen—a structural view. *Cell* **122**, 333–336.

Gleimer M. & Parham P. (2003) Stress management: MHC class I and class II molecules as receptors of cellular stress. *Immunity* **19**, 469–477.

Grawunder U. & Harfst E. (2001) How to make ends meet in V(D)J recombination. *Current Opinion in Immunology* **13**, 186–194.

Kelsoe G. (1999) V(D)J hypermutation and receptor revision: coloring outside the lines. *Current Opinion in Immunology* **11**, 70–75.

Kumanovics A. *et al.* (2003) Genomic organization of the mammalian MHC. *Annual Review of Immunology* **21**, 629–657.

Kumar V. & McNerney M.E. (2005) A new self: MHC class I-independent natural-killer cell self-tolerence. *Nature Reviews Immunology* **5**, 363–374.

Lanier L.L. (2005) NK cell recognition. *Annual Review of Immunology* **23**, 225–274.

Mak T.W. (1998) T-cell receptor, αβ. In Delves P.J. & Roitt I.M. (eds) *Encyclopedia of Immunology*, 2nd edn, pp. 2264–2268. Academic Press, London. (See also article by Hayday A. & Pao W. on the γδ TCR; *ibid.*, pp. 2268–2278.)

Matsuda F. *et al.* (1998) The complete nucleotide sequence of the human immunoglobulin heavy chain variable region locus. *Journal of Experimental Medicine* **188**, 2151–2162.

MHC Sequencing Consortium (1999) Complete sequence and gene map of a human major histocompatibility complex. *Nature* **401**, 921–923.

Moody D.B., Zajonc D.M. & Wilson I.A. (2005) Anatomy of CD1–lipid antigen complexes. *Nature Reviews Immunology* **5**, 387–399.

Nemazee D. (2000) Receptor editing in B cells. *Advances in Immunology* **74**, 89–126.

Parham P. (ed.) (1999) Genomic organisation of the MHC: structure, origin and function. *Immunological Reviews* **167**.

Porcelli S.A. & Modlin R.L. (1999) The CD1 system: antigen-presenting molecules for T cell recognition of lipids and glycolipids. *Annual Review of Immunology* **17**, 297–329.

Prugnolle F. *et al.* (2005) Pathogen-driven selection and worldwide HLA class I diversity. *Current Biology* **15**, 1022–1027.

Raulet D.H. (2004) Interplay of natural killer cells and their receptors with the adaptive immune response. *Nature Immunology* **5**, 996–1002.

de Wildt R.M.T. *et al.* (1999) Somatic insertions and deletions shape the human antibody repertoire. *Journal of Molecular Biology* **294**, 701–710.

CHAPTER 5

5 The primary interaction with antigen

INTRODUCTION

In adaptive immunity, antigens are recognized by two classes of molecules: (i) antibodies, present either as soluble proteins or membrane-bound on the surface of B-cells; (ii) T-cell receptors present on the surface of T-cells. Antibodies recognize antigens on the surface of pathogens or as soluble foreign material such as toxins. T-cell receptors recognize peptides or glycolipids in the context of MHC molecules on the surface of host cells. Antibodies can thus be thought of as scanning for foreign material directly. T-cells are scanning for cells that are infected with pathogens.

WHAT ANTIBODIES SEE

Antibodies recognize molecular shapes (epitopes) on antigens. Generally, the better the fit of the epitope (in terms of geometry and chemical character) to the antibody combining site, the more favorable the interactions that will be formed between the antibody and antigen and the higher the affinity of the antibody for antigen. The affinity of the antibody for the antigen is one of the most important factors in determining how effective the antibody the efficacy of *in vivo*.

Epitopes come in a huge variety of different shapes, as do antibody combining sites. Protein surfaces are typically recognized by a complementary surface in the antibody combining site, as illustrated in figure 5.1 which shows how an antibody recognizes an epitope on the human epidermal growth factor receptor, HER-2. The extent of complementarity of the interacting surfaces is readily appreciated.

The area of antigen that contacts antibody is referred to as a footprint and is typically between about 400 and 1000 Å^2. Footprints are of different sizes and irregular,

but a rough appreciation can be gained by projecting a 25 Å × 25 Å square on to the protein (figure 5.2).

Antibodies recognize a topographic surface of a protein antigen. Most usually, key residues in the epitope will arise from widely different positions in the linear amino acid sequence of the protein (figure 5.3). This follows because of the manner in which proteins are folded; the linear sequence typically snakes from one side of the protein to the other a number of times. Such epitopes are described as **discontinuous**. Occasionally, key residues arise from a linear amino acid sequence. In such cases, the antibody may bind with relatively high affinity to a peptide incorporating the appropriate linear sequence from the antigen. Furthermore, the peptide may inhibit the antigen binding to the antibody. The epitope in such cases is described as **continuous**. An example of a continuous epitope would be a loop on the surface of the protein for which an antibody recognized successive residues in the loop. It should be noted, however, that an antibody that recognizes a continuous epitope does not bind a random or disordered structure. Rather it recognizes a defined structure that is found in the complete protein but can readily be adopted by the shorter peptide. The structure of an antibody that recognizes a linear epitope in complex with a peptide that contains the epitope is shown in figure 5.4; note that the structure of the peptide is largely helical in this example.

The antibody complementarity determining regions (CDRs) contact the epitope

The antibody combining site can vary greatly in shape and character depending upon the length and characteristics of the CDRs. Generally most or all of the CDRs

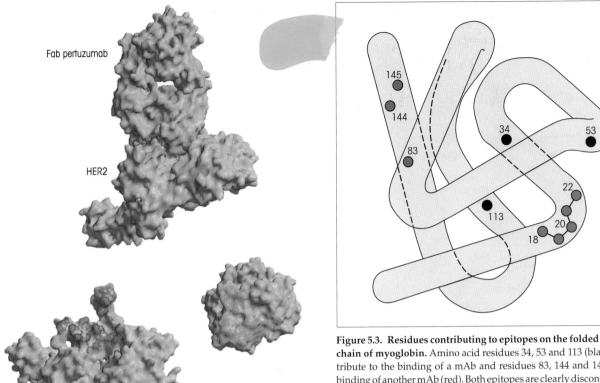

Fab pertuzumab

HER2

Figure 5.3. Residues contributing to epitopes on the folded peptide chain of myoglobin. Amino acid residues 34, 53 and 113 (black) contribute to the binding of a mAb and residues 83, 144 and 145 to the binding of another mAb (red). Both epitopes are clearly discontinuous. By contrast, a third mAb binds to residues 18–22 (green). The mAb binds to isolated peptides containing the sequence corresponding to residues 18-22. The epitope is described as continuous. Much of the myoglobin structure is in α-helical conformation. (Based on Benjamin D.C. *et al.* (1986) *Annual Review of Immunology* **2**, 67.)

Figure 5.1. Complementarity of the antibody combining site and the epitope recognized on the antigen. The structure of the complex of the Fab of the antibody pertuzumab and its antigen HER2 is shown. HER2, the human epidermal growth factor receptor, is overexpressed on some breast cancer cells and pertuzumab is an antibody, similar to Herceptin, with potential as a therapeutic against breast cancer. Below, the two molecules are shown separately with the interaction footprint shown on each. (Courtesy of Robyn Stanfield.)

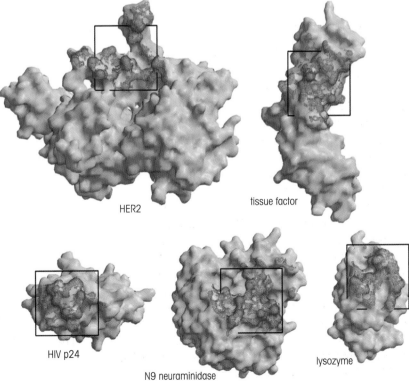

HER2

tissue factor

HIV p24

N9 neuraminidase

lysozyme

Figure 5.2. Antibody footprints (red) on a range of antigens. These footprints are determined from crystal structures of the antigens with antibody bound. The footprints are irregular but can be very roughly represented as a square of dimensions 25 Å × 25 Å as shown. (Courtesy of Robyn Stanfield.)

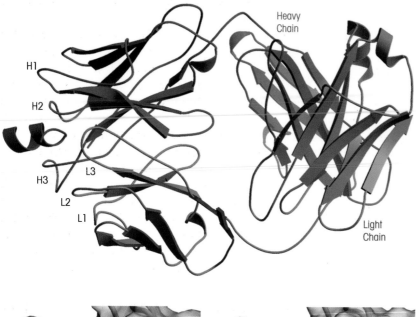

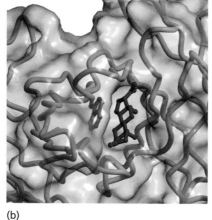

Figure 5.4. **The structure of an antibody bound to a peptide corresponding to a linear epitope.** The antibody 4E10 neutralizes HIV by binding to a linear epitope on the glycoprotein gp41 on the surface of the virus. The antibody binds to peptides containing the amino acid sequence NWFDIT and peptides containing this sequence can inhibit the binding of 4E10 to gp41. The structure of the Fab fragment of 4E10 bound to a peptide (gold) containing the NWFDIT sequence shows the peptide adopts a helical conformation. It is likely that the antibody recognizes its epitope in a helical conformation on the virus. (Courtesy of Rosa Cardoso.)

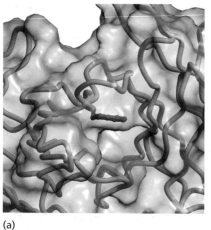

(a)   (b)

Figure 5.5. **Conformational change in an antibody combining site.** (a) An anti-progesterone antibody has a very hydrophobic pocket that is filled by a tryptophan residue (colored red) in the free antibody. (b) To bind progesterone (dark blue), the tryptophan residue swings out of the pocket and the antigen gains access. (Courtesy of Robyn Stanfield.)

contribute to antigen binding but their relative contributions vary. The heavy chain CDRs, and particularly CDR H3, tend to contribute disproportionately to antigen binding. The CDR H3 in human antibodies can be quite long and has a finger-like appearance that could be used to bind into cavities on the antigen. The combining site of antibodies against smaller molecules such as carbohydrates and organic groups (haptens) are often more obviously grooves or pockets rather than the extended surfaces typically found in anti-protein antibodies.

Structural changes and conformational rearrangements can occur in antibodies or antigens on interaction. In other words, on some occasions, the relationship between antibody and antigen will be like a 'lock and key' but on other occasions the lock or key or both can be deformed to make a good fit. For the antibody, possible conformational changes include side chain rearrangements, segmental movements of CDRs or of the main-chain backbone, and rotation of the V_L–V_H domain upon antigen binding. Large changes in the conformation of the CDR H3 have been documented in crystal structures of Fab complexes. As shown in figure 5.5, an antibody to progesterone has a very hydrophobic combining pocket, which is normally filled with a tryptophan from the CDR H3. Antigen binding involves this residue moving out of the pocket, the antigen molecule moving in and the trytophan stabilizing the antigen binding.

As more and more structures have been solved it has become clear that antibody–antigen interactions come in all shapes and sizes with few general rules. It is important to bear in mind that high-affinity antibodies evolve in each individual following rounds of mutation and selection. There are multiple ways in which high-affinity recognition of an antigen can be achieved, and indeed no two antibody–antigen interactions are exactly the same.

Antigens vs immunogens

An epitope on an antigen may bind very tightly to a given antibody but it may elicit such antibodies infrequently when the antigen is used to immunize an animal. In other words, there may be a perfectly good site on a pathogen for antibody binding but the antibody response to that site is so poor it cannot contribute to antibody protection against the pathogen. We say that the site has low immunogenicity and the consequences can clearly be great.

An extreme example of the distinction between the ability to be recognized by an antibody (which we will term antigenicity) and the ability to elicit antibodies when used to immunize an animal (which we will term immunogenicity) is provided by experiments using small molecules known as haptens such as *m*-aminobenzene sulfonate. Immunization with free hapten produces no antibodies to the hapten (figure 5.6). However immunization with hapten groups linked to a protein carrier generates antibodies that react with high affinity to hapten alone or linked to a molecule other than the carrier. It is logical to refer to the hapten as the antigen and the hapten–protein complex as the immunogen, although strictly the word 'antigen' is derived from '*anti*body *gen*erating' substance.

IDENTIFYING B-CELL EPITOPES ON A PROTEIN

How many epitopes are there on a single protein? This depends upon how one defines an epitope. For the small protein lysozyme (molecular weight ~14 300 daltons), the structures of three noncompeting monoclonal antibodies in complex with the protein antigen have been determined. They have minimally overlapping footprints that cover just under half of the surface of the protein (figure 5.7). One could extrapolate that a small protein such as this could have of the order of between three and six nonoverlapping epitopes recognized by noncompeting antibodies. The specificity of a given antibody could then be defined by its ability to compete with the three to six 'prototype' antibodies. In practice,

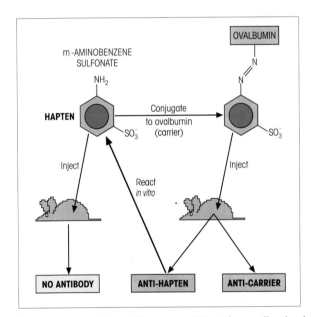

Figure 5.6. Antigenicity and immunogenicity. A free small molecule hapten will not induce antibodies if injected in to an animal. However, high affinity antibodies specific for the free hapten can be obtained by injecting the hapten conjugated to a protein carrier molecule such as ovalbumin.

Figure 5.7. Three epitopes on the small protein lysozyme. The crystal structures of lysozyme bound to three antibodies (HyHEL-5, HyHEL-10 and D1.3) have been determined. In the figure, the Fv fragment of each antibody is shown separated from lysozyme to reveal the footprint of interaction in each case. The three epitopes are nearly nonoverlapping with only a small overlap between HyHEL-10 and D1.3. (After Davies *et al.* (1990) *Annual Review of Biochemistry* **59**, 439.)

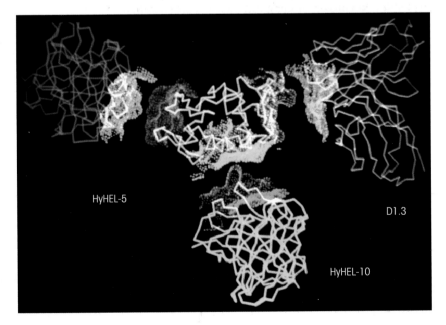

Milestone 5.1 —MHC Restriction of T-cell Reactivity

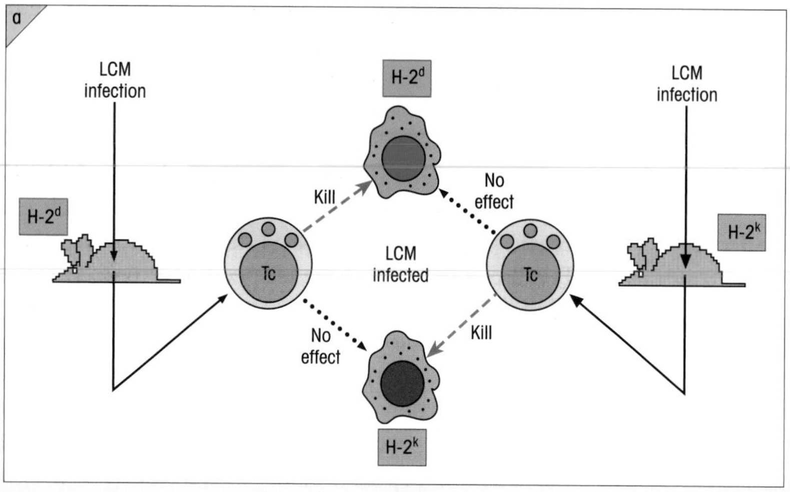

a

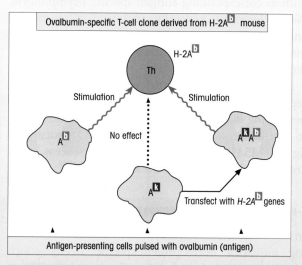

			% KILLING OF TARGET BY NP-SPECIFIC T-CELLS
Infected	Haplotype	Ab added	
−	HLA-A2	−	
+	HLA-A2	−	
+	HLA-A1	−	
+	HLA-A2	anti-HLA-A2	
+	HLA-A2	anti-HLA-A1	
+	HLA-A2	anti-HLA-DR	
+	HLA-A2	anti-NP	

Figure M5.1.1. T-cell killing is restricted by the MHC haplotype of the virus-infected target cells. (a) Haplotype-restricted killing of lymphocytic choriomeningitis (LCM) virus-infected target cells by cytotoxic T-cells. Killer cells from H-2^d hosts only killed H-2^d-infected targets, not those of H-2^k haplotype and vice versa. (b)

The realization that the MHC, which had figured for so long as a dominant controlling element in tissue graft rejection, should come to occupy the center stage in T-cell reactions has been a source of fascination and great pleasure to immunologists—almost as though a great universal plan had been slowly unfolding.

One of the seminal observations which helped to elevate the MHC to this lordly position was the dramatic Nobel prize-winning revelation by Doherty and Zinkernagel that cytotoxic T-cells taken from an individual recovering from a viral infection will only kill virally infected cells which share an MHC haplotype with the host. They found that cytotoxic T-cells from mice of the H-2^d haplotype infected with lymphocytic choriomeningitis virus could kill virally infected cells derived from any H-2^d strain but not cells of H-2^k or other H-2 haplotypes. The reciprocal experiment with H-2^k mice shows that this is not just a special property associated with H-2^d (figure M5.1.1a). Studies with recombinant strains (cf. table 4.3) pin-pointed class I MHC as the restricting element and this was confirmed by showing that antibodies to class I MHC block the killing reaction.

The same phenomenon has been repeatedly observed in the human. HLA-A2 individuals recovering from influenza have cytotoxic T-cells which kill HLA-A2 target cells infected with influenza virus, but not cells of a different HLA-A tissue-type specificity (figure M5.1.1b). Note how cytotoxicity could be inhibited by antiserum specific for the donor HLA-A type, but not by antisera to the allelic form HLA-A1 or the HLA-DR class II framework. Of striking significance is the inability of antibodies to the nucleoprotein to block T-cell recognition even though the T-cell specificity in these studies was known to be directed towards this antigen. Since the antibodies react with nucleoprotein in its native form, the conformation of the antigen as presented to the T-cell must be quite different.

Killing of influenza-infected target cells by influenza nucleoprotein (NP)-specific T-cells from an HLA-A2 donor (cf. p. 371 for human MHC nomenclature). Killing was restricted to HLA-A2 targets and only inhibited by antibodies to A2, not to A1, nor to the class II HLA-DR framework or native NP antigen.

Ovalbumin-specific T-cell clone derived from H-2A^b mouse

Figure M5.1.2. The T-cell clone only responds by proliferation *in vitro* when the antigen-presenting cells (e.g. macrophages) pulsed with ovalbumin express the same class II MHC.

In parallel, an entirely comparable series of experiments has established the role of MHC class II molecules in antigen presentation to helper T-cells. Initially, it was shown by Shevach and Rosenthal that lymphocyte proliferation to antigen *in vitro* could be blocked by antisera raised between two strains of guinea-pig which would have included antibodies to the MHC of the responding lymphocytes. More stringent evidence comes from the type of experiment in which a T-cell clone proliferating in response to ovalbumin on antigen-presenting cells with the H-2A^b phenotype fails to respond if antigen is presented in the context of H-2A^k. However, if the H-2A^k antigen-presenting cells are transfected with the genes encoding H-2A^b, they now communicate effectively with the T-cells (figure M5.1.2).

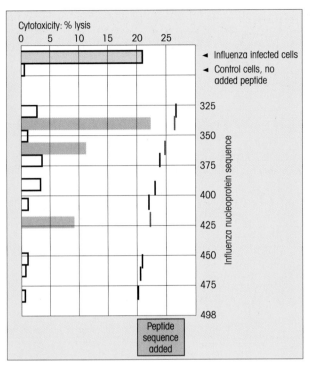

Figure 5.13. Cytotoxic T-cells, from a human donor, kill uninfected target cells in the presence of short influenza nucleoprotein peptides. The peptides indicated were added to ^{51}Cr-labeled syngeneic (i.e. same as T-cell donor) mitogen-activated lymphoblasts and cytotoxicity was assessed by ^{51}Cr release with a killer to target ratio of 50:1. The three peptides indicated in red induced good killing. Blasts infected with influenza virus of a different strain served as a positive control. (Reproduced from Townsend A.R.M. *et al.* (1986) *Cell* **44**, 959–968, with permission. Copyright ©1986 by Cell Press.)

somes are the optimal length (octamers or nonamers) to fit into the MHC class I groove; about 70% are likely to be too small to function in antigen presentation, and the remaining 20% would require further trimming by, for example, cytosolic aminopeptidases. The cytokine IFNγ increases the production of three specialized catalytic proteosomal subunits, the polymorphic LMP2 (β_1i) and LMP7 (β_5i) and the nonpolymorphic MECL1 (β_2i). These molecules replace the homologous catalytic subunits (β_1, β_5 and β_2, respectively) in the housekeeping proteasome to produce what has been termed the **immunoproteasome**, a process which modifies the cleavage specificity in order to tailor peptide production for class I binding.

Both proteasome- and immunoproteasome-generated peptides are translocated into the ER by the *t*ransporters *a*ssociated with *a*ntigen *p*rocessing (TAP1 and TAP2) (figure 5.15), a process which might also involve heat-shock protein family members. The newly synthesized class I heavy chain is retained in the ER by the molecular chaperone calnexin, which is thought to assist in folding, disulfide bond formation and promotion of assembly with β_2-microglobulin. In the human,

but not in the mouse, calnexin is then replaced by calreticulin. The ER-resident protein, Erp57, which has thiol reductase, cysteine protease and chaperone functions, becomes associated with the complex of calreticulin–calnexin and class I heavy chain which now folds together with β_2-microglobulin. The empty class I molecule bound to these chaperones becomes linked to TAP1/2 by tapasin. Upon peptide loading, the class I molecule can dissociate from the various accessory molecules, and the now stable peptide–class I heavy chain–β_2-microglobulin complex traverses the Golgi stack and reaches the surface where it is a sitting target for the cytotoxic T-cell.

PROCESSING OF ANTIGEN FOR CLASS II MHC PRESENTATION FOLLOWS A DIFFERENT PATHWAY

Class II MHC complexes with antigenic peptide are generated by a fundamentally different intracellular mechanism, since the antigen-presenting cells which interact with T-helper cells need to sample the antigen from both the *extra*cellular and *intra*cellular compartments. In essence, a trans-Golgi vesicle containing class II has to intersect with a late endosome containing exogenous protein antigen taken into the cell by an endocytic mechanism.

Regarding the class II molecules themselves, these are assembled from α and β chains in the ER in association with the transmembrane **invariant chain (Ii)** (figure 5.16) which trimerizes to recruit three MHC class II molecules into a nonameric complex. Ii has several functions. First, it acts as a dedicated chaperone to ensure correct folding of the nascent class II molecule. Second, an internal sequence of the luminal portion of Ii sits in the MHC groove to inhibit the precocious binding of peptides in the ER before the class II molecule reaches the endocytic compartment containing antigen. Additionally, combination of Ii with the αβ class II heterodimer inactivates a retention signal and allows transport to the Golgi. Finally, targeting motifs in the N-terminal cytoplasmic region of Ii ensure delivery of the class II-containing vesicle to the endocytic pathway.

Meanwhile, exogenous protein is taken up by endocytosis and, as the early endosome undergoes progressive acidification, is processed into peptides by endopeptidases, exopeptidases and GILT (interferon-γ-induced lysosomal thiol reductase). Particularly implicated are the cysteine proteases cathepsin S, L, B, F, H and (in humans) V, and asparagine endopeptidase (AEP). Most of these enzymes have broad specificity. The late endosomes characteristically acquire

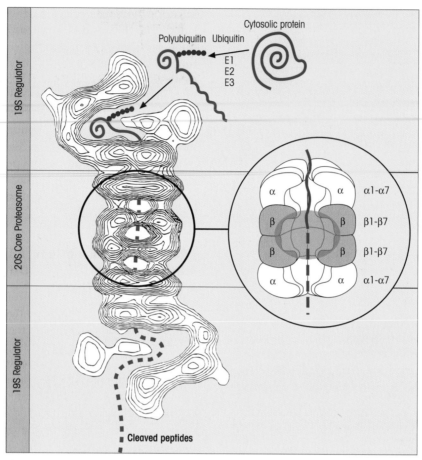

Figure 5.14. Cleavage of cytosolic proteins by the proteasome. Cytosolic proteins become polyubiquitinated in an ATP-dependent reaction in which the enzyme E1 forms a thiolester with the C-terminus of ubiquitin and then transfers the ubiquitin to one of a number of E2 ubiquitin-carrier proteins. The C-terminus of the ubiquitin is then conjugated by one of several E3 ubiquitin-protein ligase enzymes to a lysine residue on the polypeptide. There is specificity in these processes in that the individual E2 and E3 enzymes have preferences for different proteins. The ubiquitinated cytosolic protein binds to the ATPase-containing 19S regulator where ATP drives the unfolded protein chain into the cylindrical structure of the 20S core proteasome which is made up of 28 subunits arranged in four stacked rings. The two outer rings comprise seven different α-subunits (α_1–α_7) whilst the two rings of the central hydrolytic chamber are each made up of seven different β-subunits (β_1–β_7). Within the hydrolytic chamber the protein is exposed to proteolytic activity (red shading). A novel catalytic mechanism is involved in which the nucleophilic residue that attacks the peptide bonds is the hydroxyl group on the N-terminal threonine residue of the β-subunits. Three distinct peptidase activities have been associated with specific β-subunits. One is 'chymotrypsin-like' in that it hydrolyses peptides after large hydrophobic residues, one is 'trypsin-like' and cleaves after basic residues, and one hydrolyses after acidic residues. The *low molecular weight proteins* LMP2 (β_1i), LMP7 (β_5i), and MECL1 (*multicatalytic endopeptidase complex like 1*, (β_2i)) immunoproteasome-associated molecules show similar specificities but have enhanced chymotrypsin and trypsin activity and reduced postacidic cleavage compared to their counterparts in the housekeeping proteasome. (Based on Peters J.-M. *et al.* (1993) *Journal of Molecular Biology* **234**, 932–937 and Rubin D.M. & Finley D. (1995) *Current Biology* **5**, 854–858.)

lysosomal-associated membrane proteins (LAMPs), which are implicated in enzyme targeting, autophagy (the enveloping of cellular organelles into an autophagosome for subsequent degradation) and lysosomal biogenesis. These late endosomes fuse with the vacuole containing the class II–Ii complex. Under the acidic conditions within these *MHC class II*-enriched *compartments* (MIICs), AEP and cathepsins S and L degrade Ii except for the part sitting in the MHC groove which, for the time being, remains there as a peptide referred to as CLIP (*class II-associated invariant chain peptide*). An MHC-related dimeric molecule, DM, then catalyzes the removal of CLIP and keeps the groove open so that peptides generated in the endosome can be inserted (figure 5.17). Initial peptide binding is determined by the concentration of the peptide and its on-rate, but DM may subsequently assist in the removal of lower affinity peptides to allow their replacement by high affinity peptides, i.e. act as a peptide editor permitting the incorporation of peptides with the most stable binding characteristics, namely those with a slow off-rate. Particularly in B-cells an additional MHC-related molecule, DO, associates with DM bound to class II and modifies its function in a pH-dependent fashion. Its

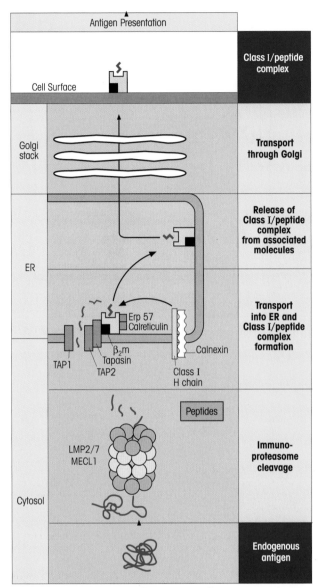

Figure 5.15. Processing and presentation of endogenous antigen by class I MHC. Cytosolic proteins are degraded by the proteasome complex into peptides which are transported into the endoplasmic reticulum (ER). TAP1 and TAP2 are members of the ABC family of ATP-dependent transport proteins and, under the influence of these transporters, the peptides are loaded into the groove of the membrane-bound class I MHC. The peptide–MHC complex is then released from all its associated transporters and chaperones, traverses the Golgi system, and appears on the cell surface ready for presentation to the T-cell receptor. Mutant cells deficient in TAP1/2 do not deliver peptides to class I and cannot function as cytotoxic T-cell targets.

effect may be to favor the presentation of antigens internalized via the BCR over those taken up by fluid phase endocytosis. The tetraspanin family member CD82 is also present in the MIIC, though its role is unclear at present. The class II–peptide complexes are eventually transported to the membrane for presentation to T-helper cells.

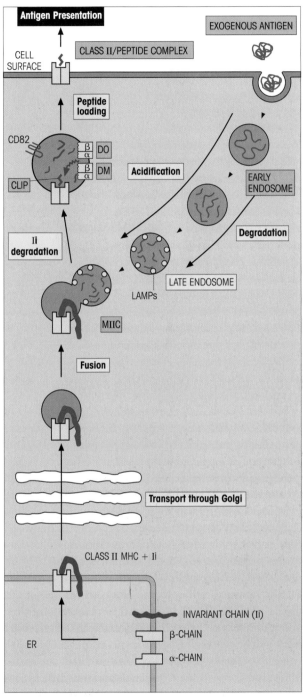

Figure 5.16. Processing and presentation of exogenous antigen by class II MHC. Class II molecules with Ii are assembled in the endoplasmic reticulum (ER) and transported through the Golgi to the trans-Golgi reticulum (actually as a nonamer consisting of three invariant, three α and three β chains—not shown). There it is sorted to a late endosomal vesicle with lysosomal characteristics known as MIIC (meaning MHC class II-enriched compartment) containing partially degraded protein derived from the endocytic uptake of exogenous antigen. Degradation of the invariant chain leaves the CLIP (*cl*ass II-associated *i*nvariant chain *p*eptide) lying in the groove but, under the influence of the DM molecule, this is replaced by other peptides in the vesicle including those derived from exogenous antigen, and the complexes are transported to the cell surface for presentation to T-helper cells. This version of events is supported by the finding of high concentrations of invariant chain CLIP associated with class II in the MIIC vacuoles of DM-deficient mutant mice which are poor presenters of antigen to T-cells.

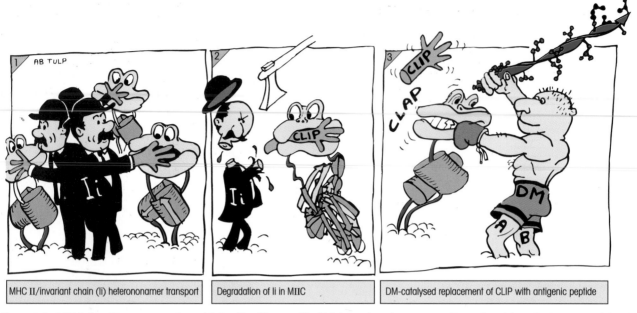

Figure 5.17. **MHC class II transport and peptide loading** illustrated by Tulp's gently vulgar cartoon. (Reproduced from Benham A. *et al.* (1995) *Immunology Today* **16**, 359–362, with permission of the authors and Elsevier Science Ltd.)

CROSS-PRESENTATION FOR ACTIVATION OF NAIVE CD8⁺ T-CELLS

We have just seen how, in general, MHC class I presents endogenous antigen whilst MHC class II presents exogenous antigen. However, given that naive T-cells require dendritic cells for their activation, how can cytotoxic T-cells specific for peptides presented by MHC class I become aroused to destroy virus-infected cells? After all, most viruses are not tropic for dendritic cells and therefore not naturally present in the cytosol of the professional APCs. The answer to this conundrum lies in the phenomenon of 'cross-presentation'. Phagocytosed or endocytosed antigens can sneak out of the vacuole into which they have been engulfed and gain entry to the cytosol (figure 5.18). The escape route may involve the Sec61 multimolecular channel. Once they enter the cytosol they are fair game for ubiquitination and subsequent degradation by the proteasome, TAP-mediated transfer into the ER, and presentation by MHC class I. It is also possible that some endocytosed antigens can be loaded directly into recycling MHC class I molecules within the endosome without the need to be first processed in the cytosol. In addition to dendritic cells, macrophages also seem to be able to play the cross-presentation game, albeit less efficiently.

Conversely, proteins and peptides within the ER are also potential clients for the class II groove and could make the journey to the MIIC. This may occur by chaperone-mediated autophagy involving various heat-

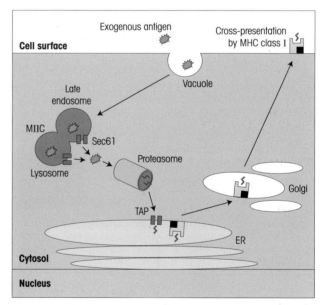

Figure 5.18. Cross-presentation of exogenous antigens. Engulfed exogenous antigens are able to access the class I processing pathway by entering the cytosol from the MHC class II compartments (MIIC), perhaps through Sec61 channels. Other routes for the presentation of peptides derived from exogenous antigens on MHC class I may include peptide exchange with MHC class I molecules recycling from the cell membrane. Cross-presentation can also work the 'other way round' with endogenous antigens gaining entry into the class II processing and presentation pathway.

shock proteins which bind to the protein to be processed. The protein complex is then recognized by LAMP-2a and dragged into the lumen of the lysosome for subsequent processing.

THE NATURE OF THE 'GROOVY' PEPTIDE

The MHC grooves impose some well-defined restrictions on the nature and length of the peptides they accommodate and the pattern varies with different MHC alleles. Otherwise, at the majority of positions in the peptide ligand, a surprising degree of redundancy is permitted and this relates in part to residues interacting with the T-cell receptor rather than the MHC.

Binding to MHC class I

X-ray analysis reveals the peptides to be tightly mounted along the length of the groove in an extended configuration with no breathing space for α-helical structures (figure 5.19). The N- and C-termini are tightly H bonded to conserved residues at each end of the groove, independently of the MHC allele.

The naturally occurring peptides can be extracted from purified MHC class I and sequenced. They are predominantly eight or nine residues long; longer peptides bulge upwards out of the cleft. Analysis of the peptide pool sequences usually gives strong amino acid signals at certain key positions (table 5.1). These are called **anchor positions** and represent the preferred amino acid side-chains which fit into allele-specific pockets in the MHC groove (figure 5.20a). There are usually two, sometimes three, such major anchor positions for class I-binding peptides, one at the C-terminal end (peptide position 8 or 9) and the other frequently at peptide position 2 (P2), but they may also occur at P3, P5 or P7. For example, the highly prevalent HLA-A*0201 has pockets for leucine or methionine at peptide position P2 and for valine or leucine at P9. Sometimes, a major anchor pocket may be replaced by two or three more weakly binding secondary pockets. Even with the constraints of two or three anchor motifs, each MHC class I allele can accommodate a considerable number of different peptides.

Except in the case of viral infection, the natural class I ligands will be self peptides derived from proteins endogenously synthesized by the cell, histones, heat-shock proteins, enzymes, leader signal sequences, and so on. It turns out that 75% or so of these peptides originate in the cytosol (figure 5.21) and most of them will be in low abundance, say 100–400 copies per cell. Thus proteins expressed with unusual abundance, such as oncofetal proteins in tumors and viral antigens in infected cells, should be readily detected by resting T-cells.

Binding to MHC class II

Unlike class I, where the allele-independent H bonding

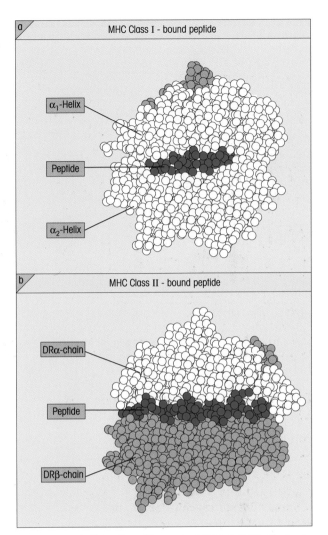

Figure 5.19. Binding of peptides to the MHC cleft. T-cell receptor 'view' looking down on the α-helices lining the cleft (cf. figure 4.13b) represented in space-filling models. (a) Peptide 309–317 from HIV-1 reverse transcriptase bound tightly within the class I HLA-A2 cleft. In general, one to four of the peptide side-chains point towards the TCR, giving a solvent accessibility of 17–27%. (b) Influenza hemagglutinin 306–318 lying in the class II HLA-DR1 cleft. In contrast with class I, the peptide extends out of both ends of the binding groove and from four to six out of an average of 13 side-chains point towards the TCR, increasing solvent accessibility to 35%. (Based on Vignali D.A.A. & Strominger J.L. (1994) *The Immunologist* **2**, 112, with permission of the authors and publisher.)

to the peptide is focused at the N- and C-termini, the class II groove residues H bond along the entire length of the peptide with links to the atoms forming the main chain. With respect to class II allele-specific binding pockets for peptide side-chains, motifs based on three or four major anchor residues seem to be the order of the day (figure 5.20b). Secondary binding pockets with less strict preference for individual side-chains can still modify the affinity of the peptide–MHC complex, while 'nonpockets' may also influence preferences for particular peptide sequences, especially if steric hindrance

Table 5.1. Natural MHC class I peptide ligands contain two allele-specific anchor residues. (Based on Rammensee H.G., Friede T. & Stevanovic S. (1995) *Immunogenetics* **41**, 178.) Letters represent the Dayhoff code for amino acids; where more than one residue predominates at a given position, the alternative(s) is given; • = any residue.

Class I allele	Amino acid position								
	1	2	3	4	5	6	7	8	9
H-2K^d	•	Y	•	•	•	•	•	•	I/L
H-2K^b	•	•	•	•	Y/F	•	•	L/M	
H-2D^b	•	•	•	•	N	•	•	•	L/M/I
HLA-A*0201	•	L/M/I	•	•	•	•	•	•	L/V/I/M
HLA-B*2705	•	R	•	•	•	•	•	•	R/K/L/F

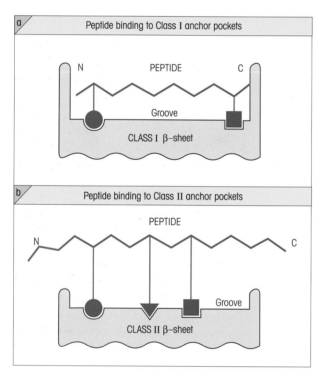

Figure 5.20. Allele-specific pockets in the MHC-binding grooves bind the major anchor residue motifs of the peptide ligands. Cross-section through the longitudinal axis of the MHC groove. The two α-helices forming the lateral walls of the groove lie horizontally above and below the plane of the paper. (a) The class I groove is closed at both ends. The anchor at the carboxy terminus is invariant but the second anchor very often at P2 may also be at P3, P5 or P7 depending on the MHC allele (cf. table 5.1). (b) By contrast, the class II groove is open at both ends and does not constrain the length of the peptide. There are usually three major anchor pockets at P1, P4, P6, P7 or P9 with P1 being the most important.

becomes a factor. Unfortunately, we cannot establish these preferences for the individual residues within a given peptide because the open nature of the class II groove places no constraint on the length of the peptide, which can dangle nonchalantly from each end of the

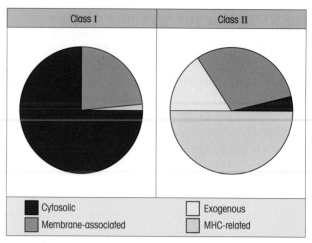

Figure 5.21. The origins of class I- and class II-bound peptides. The majority of class I peptides are derived from endogenous self proteins and, during infection, cell-resident pathogens such as viruses. Processing in the endosomal compartments ensures that proteins of endogenous origin and those derived from membranes constitute over 90% of the peptides bound to the class II grooves. (Reproduced from Vignali D.A.A. & Strominger J.L. (1994) *The Immunologist* **2**, 112, with permission of the authors and publisher.)

groove, quite unlike the strait-jacket of the class I ligand site (figures 5.19 and 5.20). Thus, as noted earlier, each class II molecule binds a collection of peptides with a spectrum of lengths ranging from eight to 30 amino acid residues, and analysis of such a naturally occurring pool isolated from the MHC would not establish which amino acid side-chains were binding preferentially to the nine available sites within the groove. One modern approach to get around this problem is to study the binding of soluble class II molecules to very large libraries of random-sequence nonapeptides expressed on the surface of bacteriophages (cf. the combinatorial phage libraries, p. 115). The idea is emerging that each amino acid in a peptide contributes independently of the others to the total binding strength, and it should be possible to compute each contribution quantitatively from this random binding data, so that ultimately we could predict which sequences in a given protein antigen would bind to a given class II allele.

Because of the accessible nature of the groove, as the native molecule is unfolded and reduced, but before any degradation need occur, the high affinity epitopes could immediately bury themselves in the class II-binding groove where they are protected from proteolysis. At least for the HLA-DR1 molecule it has been shown that peptide binding leads to a transition from a more open conformation to one with a more compact structure extending throughout the peptide-binding groove. Trimming can take place after peptide binding, leaving peptides from eight to 30 amino acids long. Several factors will influence the relative concentration of peptide–MHC complex formed: the affinity for the groove as determined by the fit of the anchors, enhancement or hindrance by internal residues (sequences outside the binding residues have little or no effect on peptide-binding specificity), sensitivity to proteases and disulfide reduction, and downstream competition from determinants of higher affinity.

The range of concentration of the different peptide complexes which result will engender a hierarchy of epitopes with respect to their ability to interact with T-cells; the most effective will be **dominant**, the less so **subdominant**. Dominant, and presumably subdominant, **self** epitopes will generally induce tolerance during T-cell ontogeny in the thymus (see p. 238). Complexes with some self peptides which are of relatively low abundance will not tolerize their T-cell counterparts and these autoreactive T-cells constantly pose an underlying threat of potential autoimmunity. Sercarz has labeled these **cryptic** epitopes, and we will discuss their possible relationship to autoimmune disease in Chapter 18.

THE αβ T-CELL RECEPTOR FORMS A TERNARY COMPLEX WITH MHC AND ANTIGENIC PEPTIDE

The forces involved in peptide binding to MHC and in TCR binding to peptide–MHC are similar to those seen between antibody and antigen, i.e. noncovalent. When soluble TCR preparations produced using recombinant DNA technology are immobilized on a sensor chip, they can bind MHC–peptide complex specifically with rather low affinities (K_a) in the 10^4 to 10^7 M^{-1} range. This low affinity and the relatively small number of atomic contacts formed between the TCRs and their MHC–peptide ligands when T-cells contact their target cell make the contribution of TCR recognition to the binding energy of this cellular interaction fairly trivial. The brunt of the attraction rests on the antigen-independent major adhesion molecules, such as ICAM-1/2, LFA-1/2 and CD2, but any subsequent triggering of the T-cell by MHC–peptide antigen must involve signaling through the T-cell receptor.

Topology of the ternary complex

Of the three complementarity determining regions present in each TCR chain, CDR1 and CDR2 are much less variable than CDR3 which, like its immunoglobulin counterpart, has (D)J sequences which result from a multiplicity of combinatorial and nucleotide insertion mechanisms (cf. p. 68). Since the MHC elements in a given individual are fixed, but great variability is expected in the antigenic peptide, a logical model would have CDR1 and CDR2 of each TCR chain contacting the α-helices of the MHC, and the CDR3 concerned in binding to the peptide. In accord with this view, several studies have shown that T-cells which recognize small variations in a peptide in the context of a given MHC restriction element differ only in their CDR3 hypervariable regions.

The combining sites of the TCRs which have been crystallized to date are relatively flat (figure 5.22), which would be expected given the need for complementarity to the gently undulating surface of the peptide–MHC combination (figure 5.23a). In nearly all the structures so far solved, recognition involves the TCR lying either diagonally or orthogonally (figure 5.23b,c) across the peptide–MHC with the TCR Vα domain overlying the MHC class I α$_2$-helix, or class II β$_1$-helix, and the Vβ domain overlying the α$_1$-helix. As suggested above, the

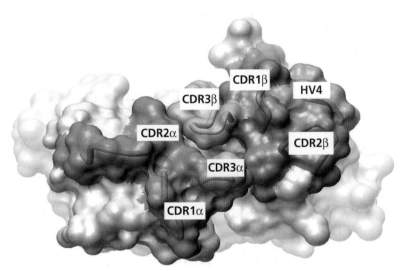

Figure 5.22. T-cell receptor antigen combining site. Although the surface is relatively flat, there is a clearly visible cleft between the CDR3α and CDR3β which can accommodate a central upfacing side-chain of the peptide bound into the groove of an MHC molecule. The surface and loop traces of the Vα CDR1 and CDR2 are colored magenta, Vβ CDR1 and CDR2 blue, Vα CDR3 and Vβ CDR3 yellow, and the Vβ fourth hypervariable region, which makes contact with some superantigens, orange. (Reproduced from Garcia K.C. *et al.* (1996) *Science* **274**, 209–219, with permission.)

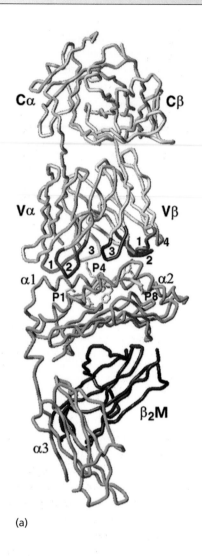

(a)

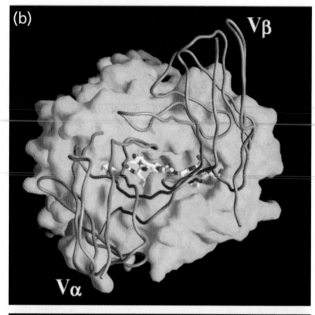

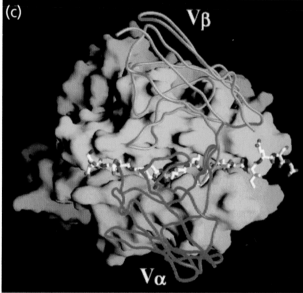

Figure 5.23. Complementarity between MHC–peptide and T-cell receptor. (a) Backbone structure of a TCR (designated 2C) recognizing a peptide (dEV8) presented by the MHC class I molecule H-2K[b]. The TCR is in the top half of the picture, with the α chain in pink and its CDR1 colored magenta, CDR2 purple and CDR3 yellow. The β chain is colored light blue with its CDR1 cyan, CDR2 navy blue, CDR3 green and the fourth hypervariable loop orange. Below the TCR is the MHC α chain in green and β2-microglobulin in dark green. The peptide with its side-chains is colored yellow. (Reproduced from Garcia K.C. *et al.* (1998) *Science* **279**, 1166-1172, with permission.) (b) The same complex looking down onto a molecular surface representation of the H-2K[b] in yellow, with the diagonal docking mode of the TCR in a backbone worm representation colored pink. The dEV8 peptide is drawn in a ball and stick format. (c) By contrast, here we see the orthogonal docking mode of a TCR recognizing a peptide presented by MHC class II. The TCR (scD10) backbone worm representation shows the Vα in green and Vβ in blue, and the I-A[k] class II molecular surface representation has the α chain in light green and the β chain in orange, holding its conalbumin-derived peptide. (Reproduced from Reinherz E.L. *et al.* (1999) *Science* **286**, 1913–1921, with permission.)

CDR1 and CDR2 regions of both the TCR chains do indeed mainly bind to the α-helices of the MHC whilst the more variable CDR3 regions make contact with the peptide, particularly focusing in on the middle residues (P4 to P6). There is evidence to suggest that the TCR initially binds to the MHC in a fairly peptide-independent fashion, followed by significant conformational changes in the CDR loops of the TCR and in the peptide–MHC to permit further contacts with the peptide. Activation through the TCR can operate if these adjustments permit more stable and multimeric binding.

T-CELLS WITH A DIFFERENT OUTLOOK

Nonclassical class I molecules can also present antigen

MHC class I-like molecules

In addition to the highly polymorphic classical MHC class I molecules (HLA-A, -B and -C in the human and H-2K, D and L in the mouse), there are other loci encoding MHC molecules containing β_2-microglobulin with relatively nonpolymorphic heavy chains. These are **H-2M**, **Q** and **T** in mice, and **HLA-E**, **F** and **G** in *Homo sapiens*.

The **H-2M3** molecule encoded by the H-2M locus is unusual in its ability to present bacterial *N*-formyl methionine peptides to T-cells. Expression of H-2M3 is limited by the availability of these peptides so that high levels are only seen during prokaryotic infections. The demonstration of H-2M3-restricted CD8$^+$ $\alpha\beta$ T-cells specific for *Listeria monocytogenes* encourages the view that this class I-like molecule could underwrite a physiological function in infection. Discussion of the role of HLA-G expression in the human syncytiotrophoblast will arise in Chapter 16 (see p. 381).

The family of CD1 non-MHC but class I-like molecules presents lipid antigens

After MHC class I and class II, the CD1 family (see p. 83) represents a third lineage of antigen-presenting molecules recognized by T-lymphocytes. The CD1 polypeptide chain associates with β_2-microglobulin as becomes an honest class I-like moiety, and the overall structure is similar to that of classical class I molecules, although the topology of the binding groove is altered (see figure 4.23).

CD1 molecules can present a broad range of **lipid, glycolipid** and **lipopeptide** antigens, and even certain small organic molecules, to clonally diverse $\alpha\beta$ and $\gamma\delta$ T-cells. A common structural motif facilitates CD1-mediated antigen presentation and comprises a hydrophobic region of a branched or dual acyl chain and a hydrophilic portion formed by the polar or charged groups of the lipid and/or its associated carbohydrate or peptide. The hydrophobic regions are buried in the deep binding groove of CD1, whilst the hydrophilic regions, such as the carbohydrate structures, are recognized by the TCR (figure 5.24). One major group of ligands for CD1b are glycophosphatidylinositols, such as the mycobacterial cell wall component lipoarabinomannan.

Both endogenous and exogenous lipids can be presented by CD1 and, like MHC class I, the CD1 heavy chain complexes with calnexin and calreticulin in the endoplasmic reticulum. Erp57 is then recruited into the

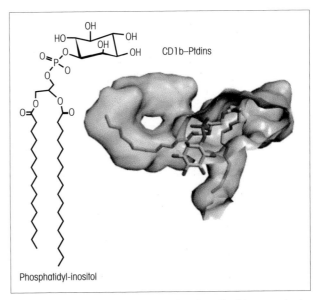

Figure 5.24. Antigen presentation by CD1. In this example the binding of phosphatidylinositol (Ptdins) to CD1b is shown with the binding pocket represented from a top view, looking directly into the groove. Aliphatic backbones are in green, phosphor atom in blue and oxygen atoms in red. (Reproduced with permission from Hava D.L. *et al.* (2005) *Current Opinion in Immunology* **17**, 88–94).

complex. Subsequent dissociation of the complex permits the binding of β_2-microglobulin and, in a step that may involve the *microsomal triglyceride-transfer protein* (MTP), the insertion of endogenous lipid antigens into the CD1 antigen-binding region. Just like their proteinaceous colleagues, exogenously derived lipid and glycolipid antigens are delivered to the acidic endosomal compartment. Localization of CD1b, c and d molecules to the endocytic pathway is mediated by a tyrosine-based cytosolic targeting sequence in the cytoplasmic tail. CD1a, which lacks this targeting motif, traffics through early recyling endosomes. Both humans and mice deficient in prosaposin, a precursor molecule of the sphingolipid activator proteins (SAPs) saposin A–D, are defective in the presentation of lipid antigens to T-cells. Various lines of enquiry indicate that these molecules are probably involved in the transfer of lipid antigens to CD1 in the endosomes.

Some T-cells have NK markers

NKT-cells possess the NK1.1 marker, characteristic of NK cells, together with a T-cell receptor. However, the TCR bears an invariant α chain (Vα14Jα18 in mice, Vα24Jα18 in humans) with no N-region modifications and an extremely limited β chain repertoire based upon Vβ11 in the human and Vβ8 in the mouse. They recognize lipid antigens such as α-galactosylceramide and isoglobosides presented by CD1d and constitute a major component of the T-cell compartment, accounting for 20–30% of T-cells in bone marrow and liver in mice, and up to 1% of spleen cells. The ability of NKT-cells to rapidly secrete IL-4 and IFNγ following stimulation suggests they may have important regulatory functions.

γδ TCRs have some features of antibody

Unlike αβ T-cells, γδ T-cells recognize antigens directly without a requirement for antigen processing. In the mouse, γδ T-cells have been isolated which directly recognize the MHC class I molecule I-E^k and the non-classical MHC molecules T10 and T22. Neither the polymorphic residues associated with peptide binding to classical MHC molecules nor the peptide itself are involved. T10 and T22 are expressed by αβ T-cells following their activation, and it has been suggested that γδ T-cells specific for these nonclassical MHC molecules may exert a regulatory function. Stressed or damaged cells appear to be powerful activators of γδ cells, and there is evidence for molecules such as heat-shock proteins as stimulators of γδ T-cells. Low molecular weight **phosphate-containing nonproteinaceous** antigens, such as isopentenyl pyrophosphate and ethyl phosphate, which occur in a range of microbial and mammalian cells, have also been identified as potent stimulators.

Evidence for direct recognition of antigen by γδ T-cells came from experiments such as those involving a γδ T-cell clone specific for the herpes simplex virus glycoprotein-1. This clone could be stimulated by the native protein bound to plastic, suggesting that the cells are triggered by cross-linking of their receptors by antigen which they recognize in the intact native state just as antibodies do. There are structural arguments to give weight to this view. The CDR3 loops, which are critical for foreign antigen recognition by T-cells and antibodies, are comparable in length and relatively constrained with respect to size in the α and β chains of the αβ TCR, reflecting a relative constancy in the size of the MHC–peptide complexes to which they bind. CDR3 regions in the immunoglobulin light chains are short and similarly constrained in length, but in the heavy chains they are longer on average and more variable in length, related perhaps to their need to recognize a wide range of epitopes. Quite strikingly, the γδ TCRs resemble antibodies in that the γ chain CDR3 loops are short with a narrow length distribution, while in the δ chain they are long with a broad length distribution. Therefore, in this respect, the γδ **TCR resembles antibody** more than the αβ TCR. The X-ray crystallographic structure of a γδ

TCR bound to its ligand, the nonclassical MHC molecule T22 mentioned above, has recently been solved. In this example the extended CDR3 loop of the δ chain, particularly the Dδ2 segment encoded by a nonmutated (germline) sequence, mediates most of the binding with a minor contribution also made by the CDR3 of the γ chain. Whilst structural determinations of additional γδTCR–antigen complexes will reveal whether this type of interaction is representative of other γδ TCRs, the broad length distribution of the different CDR3 Vδ loops suggests that γδ TCRs will generally have topographically more adventurous binding sites than the TCRs of αβ T-cells, thereby facilitating the ability of γδ T-cells to interact with intact rather than processed antigen.

A particular subset of γδ cells, which possess a diverse range of TCRs utilizing different *D* and *J* gene segments but always using the same *V* gene segments, *V*γ9 (*V*γ2 in an alternative nomenclature system) and *V*δ2, expand *in vivo* to comprise a large proportion (8–60%) of all peripheral blood T-cells during a diverse range of infections. These Vγ9Vδ2 T-cells recognize alkylamines and organophosphates. Indeed, individual Vγ9Vδ2 T-cells can recognize **both** positively charged alkylamines **and** negatively charged molecules such as ethyl phosphate. However, this should be fairly straightforward for the receptor given the small hapten-like size of these antigens. A number of alkylamine antigens are produced by human pathogens, including *Salmonella typhimurium*, *Listeria monocytogenes*, *Yersinia enterocolitica* and *Escherichia coli*.

The above characteristics provide the γδ cells with a distinctive role complementary to that of the αβ population and enable them to function in the direct recognition of microbial pathogens and of damaged or stressed host cells. Recent evidence also suggests that they can express MHC class II and may be able to act as professional antigen-presenting cells for the activation of αβ T-cells.

SUPERANTIGENS STIMULATE WHOLE FAMILIES OF LYMPHOCYTE RECEPTORS

Bacterial toxins represent one major group of T-cell superantigens

Whereas an individual peptide complexed to MHC will react with antigen-specific T-cells which represent a relatively small percentage of the T-cell pool because of the requirement for specific binding to particular CDR3 regions, a special class of molecule has been identified which stimulates the 5–20% of the total T-cell population expressing the same TCR Vβ family structure.

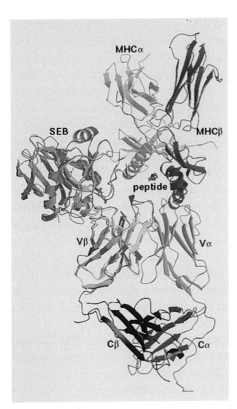

Figure 5.25. Interaction of superantigen with MHC and TCR. In this composite model, the interaction with the superantigen staphylococcal enterotoxin B (SEB) involves SEB wedging itself between the TCR Vβ chain and the MHC, effectively preventing interaction between the TCR and the peptide in the groove, and between the TCR β chain and the MHC. Thus direct contact between the TCR and the MHC is limited to Vα amino acid residues. (Reproduced from Li H. *et al.* (1999) *Annual Review of Immunology* **17**, 435–466, with permission.) Other superantigens disrupt direct TCR interactions with peptide–MHC to varying extents.

These molecules do this irrespective of the antigen specificity of the receptor. They have been described as **superantigens** by Kappler and Marrack.

The pyogenic toxin superantigen family can cause food poisoning, vomiting and diarrhea and includes *Staphylococcus aureus* enterotoxins (SEA, SEB and several others), staphylococcal toxic shock syndrome toxin-1 (TSST-1), streptococcal superantigen (SSA) and several streptococcal pyogenic exotoxins (SPEs). Although these molecules all have a similar structure, they stimulate T-cells bearing different Vβ sequences. They are strongly mitogenic for these T-cells in the presence of MHC class II accessory cells. SEA must be one of the most potent T-cell mitogens known, causing marked proliferation in the concentration range 10^{-13} to 10^{-16} M. Like the other superantigens it can cause the release of copious amounts of cytokines, including IL-2 and lymphotoxin, and of mast cell leukotrienes, which probably form the basis for its ability to produce toxic shock syndrome. Other superantigens which do not belong to the pyogenic toxin superantigen family include staphylococcal exfoliative toxins (ETs), *Mycoplasma arthritidis* mitogen (MAM) and *Yersinia pseudotuberculosis* mitogen.

Superantigens are not processed by the antigen-presenting cell, but cross-link the class II and Vβ independently of direct interaction between MHC and TCR molecules (figure 5.25).

Endogenous mouse mammary tumor viruses (MMTV) act as superantigens

Very many years ago, Festenstein made the curious observation that B-cells from certain mouse strains could produce powerful proliferative responses in roughly 20% of unprimed T-cells from another strain of identical MHC. The so-called Mls gene product responsible for inciting proliferation turned out to be encoded by the open reading frame (ORF) located in the 3′ long terminal repeat of **MMTV**. These are retroviruses which are transmitted as infectious agents in milk and are specific for B-cells. They associate with class II MHC in the B-cell membrane and act as superantigens through their affinity for certain TCR Vβ families in a similar fashion to the bacterial toxins. Other proposed viral superantigens capable of polyclonally activating T-cells include the nucleocapsid protein of rabies virus, and antigens associated with cytomegalovirus and with Epstein–Barr virus.

Microbes can also provide B-cell superantigens

Staphylococcal protein A reacts not only with the Fcγ region of IgG but also with 15–50% of polyclonal IgM, IgA and IgG F(ab′)$_2$, all of which belong to the V$_H$3 family. This superantigen is mitogenic for B-cells through its recognition by a discontinuous binding sequence composed of amino acid residues from FR1, CDR2 and FR3 of the V$_H$ domain. The human immunodeficiency virus (HIV) glycoprotein gp120 also reacts with immunoglobulins which utilize V$_H$3 family members. The binding site partially overlaps with that for protein A and utilizes amino acid residues from FR1, CDR1, CDR2 and FR3.

THE RECOGNITION OF DIFFERENT FORMS OF ANTIGEN BY B- AND T-CELLS IS ADVANTAGEOUS TO THE HOST

It is our conviction that this section deals with a subject of the utmost importance, which is at the epicenter of immunology.

Antibodies combat microbes and their products in the

extracellular body fluids where they exist essentially in their native form (figure 5.26a). Clearly it is to the host's advantage for the B-cell receptor to recognize epitopes on the **native molecules**.

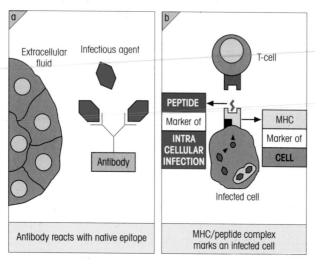

Figure 5.26. (a) Antibodies are formed against the native, not denatured, form of infectious agents which are attacked in the extracellular fluids. (b) Effector T-cells recognize infected cells by two surface markers: the MHC is a signal for the cell, and the foreign peptide is present in the MHC groove since it is derived from the proteins of an intracellular infectious agent. Further microbial cell surface signals can be provided by undegraded antigens and low molecular weight phosphate-containing antigens (seen by γδ T-cells), and lipids and glycolipids presented by CD1 molecules.

αβ T-cells have quite a different job. In the case of cytotoxic T-cells, and the T-cells which secrete cytokines that activate infected macrophages, they have to seek out and bind to the infected cells and carry out their effector function face to face with the target. First, with respect to proteins produced by intracellular infectious agents, the MHC molecules tell the effector T-lymphocyte that it is encountering a cell. Second, the T-cell does not want to attack an uninfected cell on whose surface a native microbial molecule is sitting adventitiously nor would it wish to have its antigenic target on the appropriate cell surface blocked by an excess of circulating antibody. Thus it is of benefit for the infected cell to express the microbial antigen on its surface in a form distinct from that of the native molecule. As will now be more than abundantly clear, the evolutionary solution was to make the T-cell recognize a processed peptide derived from the intracellular antigen and to hold it as a complex with the surface MHC molecules. The single T-cell receptor then recognizes both the **MHC cell marker** and the **peptide infection marker** in one operation (figure 5.26b).

A comparable situation arises when CD1 molecules substitute for MHC in antigen presentation to T-cells, in this case associating with processed microbial lipids and glycolipids. The physiological role of the γδ cells has yet to be fully unraveled.

SUMMARY

Antibody recognition

- Antibodies recognize molecular shapes (epitopes) on antigens.
- Most protein epitopes are discontinuous involving key residues from different parts of the linear sequence of the protein, although some are continuous and can be mimicked by linear peptides.
- The antibody combining site forms a complementary surface to the epitope on the antigen and largely involves the CDRs of the antibody.
- Antibody combining sites come in many shapes and sizes; anti-protein antibodies tend to have more extended recognition surfaces than antibodies to carbohydrates or peptides that are more likely to involve grooves or pockets.
- Both antibody and antigen can sometimes undergo local changes in conformation to permit interaction.

Eliciting antibodies

- Antigenicity (the ability of an antigen to be recognized by antibodies) can be distinguished from immunogenicity (the ability of an antigen (immunogen) to elicit antibodies when used to immunize an animal).
- Small molecule haptens only elicit antibodies when linked to a protein carrier molecule.
- Certain epitopes, usually those with the greatest accessibility on the surface of the protein, e.g. loops, elicit far stronger antibody responses than others.
- Many viruses, such as influenza and HIV, use the tendency of the antibody response to focus on immunodominant epitopes to 'escape' antibody control.

Thermodynamics of antibody–antigen interaction

- Antibody–antigen interaction is reversible and subject to the laws of thermodynamics.
- The tendency of antibody and antigen to interact is reflected in a binding constant (K_a) and a free energy for the interaction (ΔG).
- Physiologically active antibodies mostly have binding constants of the order of 10^9/M ('nM binders').
- The energetics of antibody–antigen interaction is dominated by a few 'hot spots'.

(Continued p.109)

- Multivalency can greatly enhance functional antibody affinity with significant physiological consequences, e.g in toxin inactivation.
- High affinity physiologically active antibodies generally have much lower affinities for antigens other than the target antigen, i.e. they have low cross-reactivity.

T-cell recognition

- $\alpha\beta$ T-cells see antigen in association with MHC molecules.
- The T-cells are restricted to the haplotype of the cell to which they were initially primed.
- Protein antigens are processed by antigen-presenting cells to form small linear peptides which associate with the MHC molecules, binding to the central groove formed by the α-helices and the β-sheet floor.

Processing of antigen for presentation by class I MHC

- Endogenous cytosolic antigens such as viral proteins are cleaved by **immunoproteasomes** and the peptides so formed are **transported** to the ER by the TAP1/2 system.
- The peptide then dissociates from TAP1/2 and forms a stable heterotrimer with newly synthesized class I MHC heavy chain and β_2-microglobulin.
- This **peptide–MHC complex** is then transported to the surface for presentation to cytotoxic T-cells.

Processing of antigen for presentation by class II MHC

- The α and β chains of the **class II molecule** are synthesized in the ER and complex with membrane-bound **invariant chain (Ii)**.
- This facilitates transport of the vesicles containing class II across the Golgi and directs them to an acidified late endosome containing exogenous protein taken into the cell by endocytosis or phagocytosis.
- Proteolytic degradation of Ii in the class II enriched compartments (MIIC) leaves a peptide referred to as CLIP which protects the MHC groove.
- Processing by endosomal proteases degrades the antigen to peptides which replace the CLIP.
- The **class II–peptide** complex now appears on the cell surface for presentation to T-helper cells.

Cross-presentation

- Naive CD8$^+$ cells are activated by dendritic cells which take up viruses by endocytosis and then transfer viral antigens into the cytosol through channels such as that created by the Sec61 multimolecular complex.
- Proteasomal processing generates virus-derived peptides for presentation on the MHC class I molecules of the dendritic cells.
- Autophagy can transfer ER resident proteins to the MIIC for subsequent processing and class II presentation.

The nature of the peptide

- Class I peptides are held in extended conformation within the MHC groove.

- They are usually eight or nine residues in length and have two or three key **anchors**, relatively invariant residues which bind to allele-specific pockets in the MHC.
- Class II peptides are between eight and 30 residues long, extend beyond the groove and usually have three or four anchor residues.
- The other amino acid residues in the peptide are greatly variable and are recognized by the T-cell receptor.

Complex between TCR, MHC and peptide

- The first and second hypervariable regions (CDR1 and CDR2) of each TCR chain mostly contact the MHC α-helices, while the CDR3s, having the greatest variability, interact with the antigenic peptide.

Some T-cells are independent of classical MHC molecules

- MHC class I-like molecules, such as H-2M, are relatively nonpolymorphic and can present antigens such as bacterial N-formyl methionine peptides.
- The CD1 family of non-MHC class I-like molecules can present antigens such as lipid and glycolipid mycobacterial antigens.
- $\gamma\delta$ T-cells resemble antibodies in recognizing whole unprocessed molecules such as low molecular weight phosphate-containing nonproteinaceous molecules.

Superantigens

- These are potent mitogens which stimulate whole lymphocyte subpopulations sharing the same TCR Vβ or immunoglobulin V$_H$ family independently of antigen specificity.
- *Staphylococcus aureus* enterotoxins are powerful human superantigens which cause food poisoning and toxic shock syndrome.
- T-cell superantigens are not processed but cross-link MHC class II and TCR Vβ independently of their direct interaction.
- Mouse mammary tumor viruses are B-cell retroviruses which are superantigens in the mouse.

Recognition of different forms of antigen by B- and T-cells is an advantage

- B-cells recognize epitopes on the native antigen; this is important because antibodies react with native antigen in the extracellular fluid.
- T-cells must contact infected cells and, to avoid confusion between the two systems, the infected cell signals itself to the T-cell by the combination of MHC and degraded antigen.

See the accompanying website (**www.roitt.com**) for multiple choice questions.

FURTHER READING

Burton D.R., Stanfield R.L. & Wilson I.A. (2005) Antibody vs HIV in a clash of evolutionary titans. *Proceedings of the National Academy of Sciences USA* **102**, 14943–14948.

Chapman H.A. (2006) Endosomal proteases in antigen presentation. *Current Opinion in Immunology* **18**, 78–84.

Davies D.R. & Padlan E.A. (1990) Antibody–antigen complexes. *Annual Reviews of Biochemistry* **59**, 439–473.

Davis S.J., Ikemizu S., Evans E.J. *et al.* (2003) The nature of molecular recognition by T-cells. *Nature Immunology* **4**, 217–224.

van den Eynde B.J. & Morel S. (2001) Differential processing of class I-restricted epitopes by the standard proteasome and the immunoproteasome. *Current Opinion in Immunology* **13**, 147–153.

Heath W.R., Belz G.T., Behrens G.M. *et al.* (2004) Cross-presentation, dendritic cell subsets, and the generation of immunity to cellular antigens. *Immunological Reviews* **199**, 9–26.

MacCallum R.M., Martin A.C.R. & Thornton J.M. (1996) Antibody–antigen interactions: contact analysis and binding site topography. *Journal of Molecular Biology* **262**, 732–745.

Moody D.B., Zajonc D.M. & Wilson I.A. (2005) Anatomy of CD1–lipid antigen complexes. *Nature Reviews Immunology* **5**, 387–399.

Nowakowski A., Wang C., Powers D.B. *et al.* (2002) Potent neutralization of botulinum neurotoxin by recombinant oligoclonal antibody. *Proceedings of the National Academy of Sciences USA* **99**, 11346–11350.

Padlan E.A. (1994) Anatomy of the antibody molecule. *Molecular Immunology*, **31**, 169–217.

Rudd P.M., Elliott T., Cresswell P. *et al.* (2001) Glycosylation and the immune system. *Science* **291**, 2370–2376.

Sundberg E.J. & Mariuzza R.A. (2002) Molecular recognition in antibody–antigen complexes. *Advances in Protein Chemistry* **61**, 119–160.

Trombetta E.S. & Mellman I. (2005) Cell biology of antigen processing in vitro and in vivo. *Annual Review of Immunology* **23**, 975–1028.

6 Immunological methods and applications

INTRODUCTION

In addition to being quite handy for protecting our bodies from harmful infectious agents, antibodies are also incredibly useful and exquisitely-specific reagents for detecting and quantitating other proteins, as well as many other substances. Antibodies have, quite literally, numerous practical applications; ranging from the purification of proteins using antibody-based affinity columns, the detection of circulating hormones in blood or urine samples for clinical diagnosis, to the exploration of expression and subcellular localization of proteins.

A variety of experimental approaches are used to explore the composition and function of the immune system. These approaches range from the purely biochemical, to systems where genetic engineering techniques are used to create null mutations ('knockouts') in genes to explore their role in immunity.

MAKING ANTIBODIES TO ORDER

Generation of polyclonal antibodies

Although antibodies can be raised against practically any organic substance, some molecules elicit antibody responses much more readily than others. Proteins usually make excellent immunogens (i.e. substances that can elicit an immune response), although the immune response will typically be concentrated against small regions within the protein (called epitopes or antigenic determinants) spanning approximately 5–8 amino acids. As we discussed earlier (see Chapter 5), an epitope represents the minimal structure required for recognition by antibody and a relatively large molecule, such as a protein, will usually contain multiple epitopes.

Thus, injection of the average antigen into an animal will almost always elicit the production of a mixture of antibodies that are directed against different epitopes within the antigen. It is also quite possible that some of the antibodies within this mixture may be directed towards epitopes that are also found in other antigens. Such antibodies are said to be cross-reactive against the other antigen to which they also bind. Small organic molecules are typically poor immunogens when injected on their own; the immune system appears unable to recognize these structures efficiently. Notwithstanding this, immunologists have found that such molecules can be made visible to the immune system by covalent coupling to a carrier protein (such as albumin) which is itself immunogenic. Such molecules are called haptens (see figure 5.6).

To generate an antibody against a protein of interest, the standard approach is to inject small samples of the protein (in the microgram range) into an animal such as a rabbit. However, administration of antigen alone is rarely sufficient to provoke a robust immune response, even if the antigen is composed of a high proportion of non-self determinants; co-administration of an **adjuvant** is required (figure 6.1). While it is not entirely clear exactly how adjuvants work, one important role they peform is to **activate DCs and APCs** at the site of antigen delivery (see p. 308). Activation of APCs dramatically enhances their ability to provide the costimulatory signals that are required for efficient T- and B-cell activation upon encounter with antigen (see Chapter 8). Potent adjuvants are usually crude preparations of bacterial extracts that contain mixtures of Toll-like receptor (TLR) ligands such as LPS or peptidoglycan. It has been proposed by Janeway that DCs are incapable of providing costimulatory signals unless activated through their TLRs. Therefore, unless an antigen has intrinsic TLR-

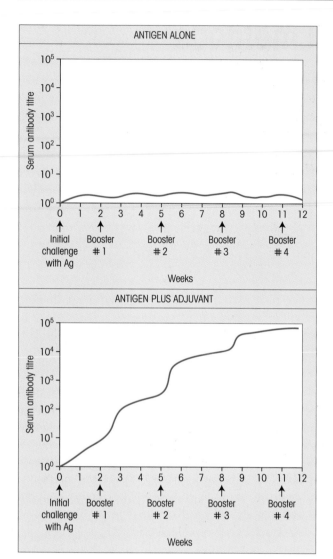

Figure 6.1. Production of polyclonal antibodies. Repeated immunization with antigen plus adjuvant is required to generate efficient antibody responses as immunization with antigen alone is usually ineffective. Polyclonal antisera are generated by immunizing, with a combination of antigen plus adjuvant, several times over a 12-week period. Serum antibody titre (i.e. the highest dilution giving a positive test) frequently increases after each successive boost with antigen.

binding activity, it will fail to activate DCs and therefore fail to elicit a potent immune response on its own.

As we outlined in Chapter 2, because a single dose of antigen usually elicits a relatively modest response (see figure 2.12), the antigen is therefore injected several times over a period of 12 weeks or so. During this time, the concentration of antibodies (what is usually referred to as **antibody titer**) directed against the immunogen will increase (figure 6.1). All going well, we will now have an antiserum that is *enriched* with antibodies against our protein of interest and this can be used as a probe in many different contexts; to localize an antigen

within a cell, to quantify it within a mixture of other antigens, to neutralize its biological activity, and many other applications (these are elaborated upon later in this chapter).

It is important to remind ourselves here that antisera generated in this way will also contain considerable amounts of other antibodies (directed against a variety of determinants) that the animal happens to have made in the recent past. These antibodies will usually be of a significantly lower titer than those directed against the antigen we have repeatedly used for immunization, but they can cause problems and may need to be removed from our antiserum for several applications. Fortunately, this can be achieved by **affinity purification** (see figure 6.6).

Because many antigens contain several distinct epitopes, antisera generated by injection of antigen will typically contain a mixture of antibodies directed against different antigenic determinants on the molecule. Some of these antibodies will bind to the antigen with high avidity, some will not, some will only recognize the native form of the antigen, while others will still recognize the antigen following denaturation to eliminate tertiary structure. Such antisera are said to be **polyclonal** as they contain a mixture of antibodies that are predominantly, although not exclusively, directed against the immunogen to which they were raised.

The monoclonal antibody revolution

First in rodents

A fantastic technological breakthrough was achieved by Köhler and Milstein who devised a technique for the production of 'immortal' clones of cells making single antibody specificities by fusing normal antibody-forming cells with an appropriate B-cell tumor line. These so-called **'hybridomas'** are selected out in a tissue culture medium which fails to support growth of the parental cell types and, by successive dilutions or by plating out, single clones can be established (figure 6.2). These clones can be grown up in the ascitic form in mice when quite prodigious titers of **monoclonal antibody** can be attained, but bearing in mind the imperative to avoid using animals wherever feasible, propagation in large-scale culture is to be preferred. Remember that, even in a good antiserum, over 90% of the Ig molecules have little or no avidity for the antigen, and the 'specific antibodies' themselves represent a whole spectrum of molecules with different avidities directed against different determinants on the antigen. What a contrast is provided by monoclonal antibodies, where all the molecules produced by a given hybridoma are identical: they have the same Ig class and allotype, the same variable

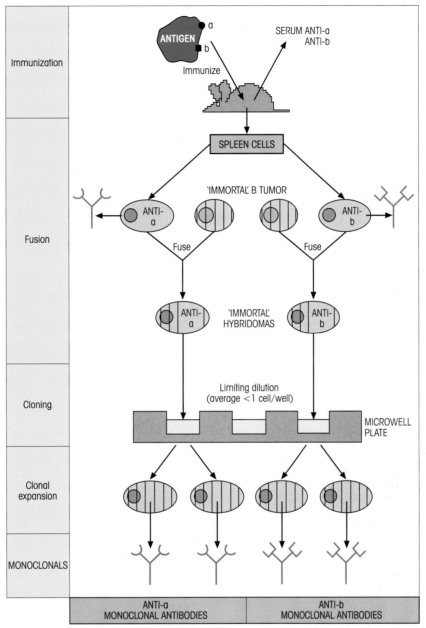

Figure 6.2. Production of monoclonal antibodies. Mice immunized with an antigen bearing (shall we say) two epitopes, a and b, develop spleen cells making anti-a and anti-b which appear as antibodies in the serum. The spleen is removed and the individual cells are fused in polyethylene glycol with constantly dividing (i.e. 'immortal') B-tumor cells selected for a purine enzyme deficiency and usually for their inability to secrete Ig. The resulting cells are distributed into microwell plates in HAT (hypoxanthine, aminopterin, thymidine) medium which kills off the fusion partners. They are seeded at such a dilution that on average each well will contain less than one hybridoma cell. Each hybridoma—the fusion product of a single antibody-forming cell and a tumor cell—will have the ability of the former to secrete a single species of antibody and the immortality of the latter enabling it to proliferate continuously. Thus, clonal progeny can provide an unending supply of antibody with a single specificity—the monoclonal antibody. In this example, we considered the production of hybridomas with specificity for just two epitopes, but the same technique enables monoclonal antibodies to be raised against complex mixtures of multi-epitopic antigens. Fusions using rat cells instead of mouse may have certain advantages in giving a higher proportion of stable hybridomas, and monoclonals which are better at fixing human complement, a useful attribute in the context of therapeutic applications to humans involving cell depletion.

Naturally, for use in the human, the ideal solution is the production of purely human monoclonals. Human myeloma fusion partners have not found wide acceptance since they tend to have low fusion efficiencies, poor growth and secretion of the myeloma Ig which dilutes the desired monoclonal. A nonsecreting heterohybridoma obtained by fusing a mouse myeloma with human B-cells can be used as a productive fusion partner for antibody-producing human B-cells. Other groups have turned to the well-characterized murine fusion partners, and the heterohybridomas so formed grow well, clone easily and are productive. There is some instability from chromosome loss and it appears that antibody production is maintained by translocation of human *Ig* genes to mouse chromosomes. Fusion frequency is even better if Epstein–Barr virus (EBV)-transformed lines are used instead of B-cells.

region, structure, idiotype, affinity and specificity for a given epitope.

The large amount of non-specific, relative to antigen-specific, Ig in a polyclonal antiserum means that background binding to antigen in any given immunological test may be uncomfortably high. This problem is greatly reduced with a monoclonal antibody preparation, since all the antibody is antigen-specific, thus giving a much superior 'signal:noise' ratio. By being directed towards single epitopes on the antigen, monoclonal antibodies frequently show high specificity in terms of their low cross-reactivity with other antigens.

An outstanding advantage of the monoclonal antibody as a reagent is that it provides a single standard material for all laboratories throughout the world to use in an unending supply if the immortality and purity of the cell line are nurtured; antisera raised in different animals, on the other hand, may be as different from each other as chalk and cheese. The monoclonal approach again shows a clean pair of heels relative to conventional strategies in the production of antibodies specific for individual components in a complex mixture of antigens. The uses of monoclonal antibodies are truly legion and include: immunoassay, diagnosis of malignancies, tissue typing, serotyping of microorganisms, the separation of individual cell types with specific surface markers (e.g. lymphocyte subpopulations), therapeutic neutralization of inflammatory cytokines and 'magic bullet' therapy with cytotoxic agents coupled to antitumor-specific antibody—these and many other areas have been transformed by hybridoma technology.

Catalytic antibodies

An especially interesting development with tremendous potential is the recognition that a monoclonal antibody to a stable analog of the transition state of a given reaction can act as an enzyme ('abzyme') in catalyzing that reaction. The possibility of generating enzymes to order promises a very attractive future, and some exceedingly adroit chemical maneuvers have already extended the range of reactions which can be catalyzed in this way. A recent demonstration of sequence-specific peptide cleavage with an antibody which incorporates a metal complex cofactor has raised the pulse rate of the *cognoscenti*, since this is an energetically difficult reaction which has an enormous range of applications. Another innovative approach is to immunize with an antigen which is so highly reactive that a chemical reaction occurs in the antibody combining site. This recruits antibodies which are not only complementary to the active chemical, but are also likely to have some enzymic power over the immunogen–substrate

complex. Thus, using this strategy, an antibody with exceptionally broad substrate specificity for efficient catalysis of aldol and retro-aldol reactions was obtained. A key feature of this antibody is a reactive lysine buried within a hydrophobic pocket in the binding site. The antibody remains catalytically active for several weeks following i.v. injection into mice and has therapeutic potential for a version of antibody-directed enzyme prodrug therapy (see p. 406), here with the enzyme component being a catalytic antibody.

Large combinatorial antibody libraries created by random association between pools of heavy and light chains and expressed on bacteriophages (see below) can be screened for catalytic antibodies by using the substrate in a solid-phase state. Cleavage by the catalytic antibody leaves a solid-phase product which can now be identified by a double antibody system using antibodies specific for the product as distinct from the substrate.

An area of great interest is the presence of catalytic autoantibodies in certain groups of patients, with hydrolytic antibodies against vasoactive intestinal peptide, DNA and thyroglobulin having been described. Catalytic antibodies capable of factor VIII hydrolysis have also recently been discovered in hemophiliacs given this clotting factor, the antibodies preventing the coagulation function of the factor VIII.

Human monoclonals can be made

While scientists were quick to realize that monoclonal antibodies would make powerful and highly-specific therapeutic agents, particularly for the treatment of cancer, this proved to be rather more difficult than originally anticipated. Mouse monoclonals injected into human subjects for therapeutic purposes are frightfully immunogenic and the human anti-mouse antibodies (HAMA in the trade) so formed are a wretched nuisance, accelerating clearance of the monoclonal from the blood and possibly causing hypersensitivity reactions; they also prevent the mouse antibody from reaching its target and, in some cases, block its binding to antigen. In some circumstances it is conceivable that a mouse monoclonal taken up by a tumor cell could be processed and become the MHC-linked target of cytotoxic T-cells or help to boost the response to a weakly immunogenic antigen on the tumor cell surface. In general, however, logic points to removal of the xenogeneic (foreign) portions of the monoclonal antibody and their replacement by human Ig structures using recombinant DNA technology. Chimeric constructs, in which the V_H and V_L mouse domains are spliced onto human C_H and C_L genes (figure 6.3a), are far less immunogenic in humans.

A more refined approach is to graft the six comple-

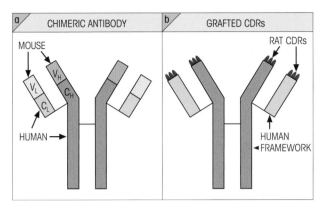

Figure 6.3. Genetically engineering rodent antibody specificities into the human. (a) Chimeric antibody with mouse variable regions fused to human Ig constant regions. (b) 'Humanized' rat monoclonal in which gene segments coding for all six CDRs are grafted onto a human Ig framework.

mentarity determining regions (CDRs) of a high affinity rodent monoclonal onto a completely human Ig framework without loss of specific reactivity (figure 6.3b). This is not a trivial exercise, however, and the objective of fusing human B-cells to make hybridomas is still appealing, taking into account not only the gross reduction in immunogenicity, but also the fact that, within a species, antibodies can be made to subtle differences such as major histocompatibility complex (MHC) polymorphic molecules and tumor-associated antigens on other individuals. In contrast, xenogeneic responses are more directed to immunodominant structures common to most subjects, making the production of variant-specific antibodies more difficult. Notwithstanding the difficulties in finding good fusion partners, large numbers of human monoclonals have been established. A further restriction arises because the peripheral blood B-cells, which are the only B-cells readily available in the human, are not normally regarded as a good source of antibody-forming cells.

Immortalized Epstein–Barr virus-transformed B-cell lines have also been used as a source of human monoclonal antibodies. Although these often produce relatively low affinity IgM antibodies, some useful higher affinity IgG antibodies can occasionally be obtained. The cell lines frequently lose their ability to secrete antibody if cultured for long periods of time, although they can sometimes be rescued by fusion with a myeloma cell line to produce hybridomas, or the genes can be isolated and used to produce a recombinant antibody.

A radically different approach involves the production of transgenic xenomouse strains in which megabase-sized unrearranged human Ig H and κ light chain loci have been introduced into mice whose endogenous murine Ig genes have been inactivated.

Immunization of these mice yields high affinity (10^{-10}–10^{-11} M) human antibodies which can then be isolated using hybridoma or recombinant approaches. Potent anti-inflammatory (anti-IL-8) and anti-tumor (anti-epidermal growth factor receptor) therapeutic agents have already been obtained using such mice.

There is still a snag in that even human antibodies can provoke anti-idiotype responses; these may have to be circumvented by using engineered antibodies bearing different idiotypes for subsequent injections. Even more desirable would be if the prospective recipients could be first made tolerant to the idiotype, perhaps by coadministering the therapeutic antibody together with a nondepleting anti-CD4.

Despite the difficulties involved, a battery of humanized monoclonals have now been approved for therapeutic use. These include: anti-IL-2 (kidney transplant rejection), anti-VEGF (colorectal cancer), anti-TNFα (rheumatoid arthritis), anti-CD11α (psoriasis), anti-CD52 (B-cell chronic lymphocytic leukaemia), anti-CD33 (acute myelogenous leukaemia), anti-HER-2 (a subset of metastatic breast cancers) and several others (cf. table 17.3).

Engineering antibodies

There are other ways around the problems associated with the production of human monoclonals which exploit the wiles of modern molecular biology. Reference has already been made to the 'humanizing' of rodent antibodies (figure 6.3), but an important new strategy based upon bacteriophage expression and **selection** has achieved a prominent position. In essence, mRNA from primed human B-cells is converted to cDNA and the antibody genes, or fragments therefrom, expanded by the polymerase chain reaction (PCR). Single constructs are then made in which the light and heavy chain genes are allowed to combine randomly in tandem with the gene encoding bacteriophage coat protein III (pIII) (figure 6.4). This **combinatorial library** containing most random pairings of heavy and light chain genes encodes a huge repertoire of antibodies (or their fragments) expressed as fusion proteins with pIII on the bacteriophage surface. The extremely high number of phages produced by *E. coli* infection can now be panned on solid-phase antigen to select those bearing the highest affinity antibodies attached to their surface (figure 6.4). Because the genes which encode these highest affinity antibodies are already present within the selected phage, they can readily be cloned and the antibody expressed in bulk. It should be recognized that this **selection** procedure has an enormous advantage over techniques which employ **screening**

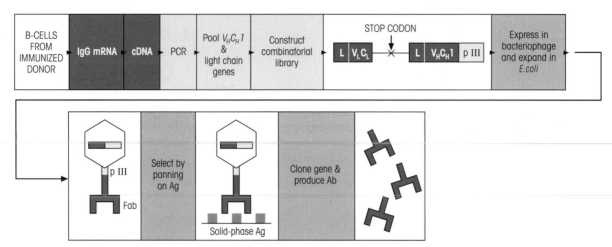

Figure 6.4. Selection of antibody genes from a combinatorial library. B-cells from an immunized donor (in one important experiment, human memory peripheral blood cells were boosted with tetanus toxoid antigen after transfer to SCID mice; Duchosal M.A. *et al.* (1992) *Nature* **355**, 258) are used for the extraction of IgG mRNA and the light chain ($V_L C_L$) and $V_H C_H 1$ genes (encoding Fab) randomly com-bined in constructs fused to the bacteriophage pIII coat protein gene as shown. These were incorporated into phagemids such as pHEN1 and expanded in *E. coli*. After infection with helper phage, the recombinant phages bearing the highest affinity were selected by rounds of panning on solid-phase antigen so that the genes encoding the Fabs could be cloned. L, bacterial leader sequence.

because the number of phages which can be examined is several logs higher.

Combinatorial libraries have also been established using mRNA from **unimmunized** human donors. V_H, V_κ and V_λ genes are expanded by PCR and randomly recombined to form single-chain Fv (scFv) constructs (figure 6.5a) fused to phage pIII. Soluble fragments binding to a variety of antigens have been obtained. Of special interest are those which are autoantibodies to molecules with therapeutic potential such as CD4 and tumor necrosis factor-α (TNFα); lymphocytes express-ing such autoantibodies could not be obtained by normal immunization since they would probably be tolerized, but the random recombination of V_H and V_L can produce entirely new specificities under conditions *in vitro* where tolerance mechanisms do not operate.

Although a 'test-tube' operation, this approach to the generation of specific antibodies does resemble the affinity maturation of the immune response *in vivo* (see pp. 204–206) in the sense that antigen is the determining factor in selecting out the highest affinity responders.

In order to increase the affinities of antibodies pro-duced by these techniques, antigen can be used to select higher affinity mutants produced by random mutagen-esis or even more effectively by site-directed replace-ments at mutational hotspots (figure 6.5b), again mimicking the natural immune response which involves random mutation and antigen selection (see pp. 200–202). Affinity has also been improved by gene 'shuf-fling' in which a V_H gene encoding a reasonable affinity antibody is randomly combined with a pool of V_L genes and subjected to antigen selection. The process can be further extended by mixing the V_L from this combina-tion with a pool of V_H genes. It has also proved possible to shuffle individual CDRs between variable regions of moderate affinity antibodies obtained by panning on antigen, thereby creating antibodies of high affinity from relatively small libraries. The isolation of high affinity llama heavy chain antibody V_{HH} fragments from immunized animals represents yet another approach.

Other novel antibodies have been created. In one con-struct, two scFv fragments associate to form an antibody with two different specificities (figure 6.5c). Another consists of a single heavy chain variable region domain (DAB) whose affinity can be surprisingly high—of the order of 20 nM. If it were possible to overcome the 'stick-iness' of these miniantibodies, their small size could be exploited for tissue penetration. The design of potential 'magic bullets' for immunotherapy can be based on fusion of a toxin (e.g. ricin) to an antibody Fab (figure 6.5d).

Fields of antibodies

Not only can the genes for a monoclonal antibody be expressed in bulk in the milk of lactating animals but plants can also be exploited for this purpose. So-called **'plantibodies'** have been expressed in bananas, pota-toes and tobacco plants. One can imagine a high-tech farmer drawing the attention of a bemused visitor to one field growing anti-tetanus toxoid, another anti-meningococcal polysaccharide, and so on. Multifunc-tional plants might be quite profitable with, say, the root being harvested as a food crop and the leaves expressing

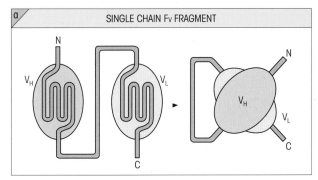

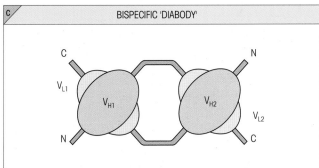

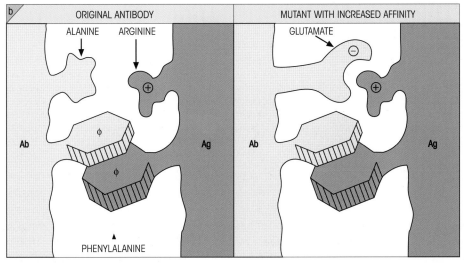

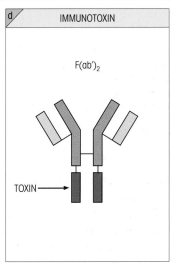

Figure 6.5. Other engineered antibodies. (a) A single gene encoding V_H and V_L joined by a sequence of suitable length gives rise to a single-chain Fv (scFv) antigen-binding fragment. (b) By site-specific mutagenesis of residues in or adjacent to the complementarity determining region (CDR), it is possible to increase the affinity of the antibody. (c) Two scFv constructs expressed simultaneously will associate to form a 'diabody' with two specificities. These bispecific antibodies have a number of uses. Note that such a bispecific antibody directed to two different epitopes on the same antigen will have a much higher affinity due to the 'bonus effect' of cooperation between the two binding sites (cf. p. 94). (d) Potential 'magic bullets' can be constructed by fusing the gene for a toxin (e.g. ricin) to the Fab.

some desirable gene product. At this rate there may not be much left for science fiction authors to write about!

Drugs can be based on the CDRs of minibodies

Millions of **minibodies** composed of a segment of the V_H region containing three β-strands and the H1 and H2 hypervariable loops were generated by randomization of the CDRs and expressed on the bacteriophage pIII coat protein. By panning the library on functionally important ligand-binding sites, such as hormone receptors, useful lead candidates for drug design programs can be identified and their affinity improved by loop optimization, loop shuffling and further selection.

PURIFICATION OF ANTIGENS AND ANTIBODIES BY AFFINITY CHROMATOGRAPHY

The principle is simple and *very* widely applied. Antigen or antibody is bound through its free amino groups to cyanogen bromide-activated Sepharose particles or some other solid support. Insolubilized antibody, for example, can be used to extract the corresponding antigen out of solution, in which it is present as one component of a complex mixture, by absorption to its surface. The uninteresting garbage is washed away and the required ligand released from the affinity absorbent by disruption of the antigen–antibody bonds by changing the pH or adding chaotropic ions such as thiocyanate (figure 6.6). This technique can be used to identify the antigen to which an antibody binds where this is not known; in the case of an autoantibody for example. A very similar approach can also be used to identify **binding partners** for an antigen; such molecules will usually stay attached to the antigen if the immunopurification procedure is carried out under gentle conditions. Many of the proteins that participate in T-cell receptor signal transduction, for instance, were initially identified by using antibodies directed against

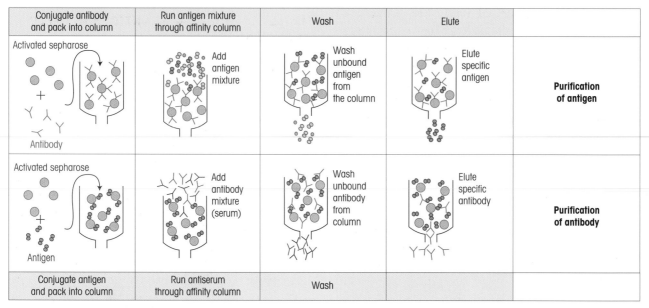

Figure 6.6. Affinity purification of antigen and antibody. Antibody can be immobilized on activated sepharose and used to affinity-purify antigen. Depending on the conditions used to carry out the assay, antigen-associated proteins may also be captured by this procedure. For the purification of specific antibody from a polyclonal antiserum, antigen is immobilized on Sepharose beads and nonspecific unbound antibodies fail to be captured and can be washed away. After capture, specific antibody can be eluted by transiently lowering the pH or increasing the salt concentration of the buffer.

known TCR signalling components to pull out these components from complex protein mixtures, along with their binding-partners. Isolated llama heavy chain (V_{HH}) fragments are proving to be valuable for repeated cycles of antigen purification because of their resistance to denaturation by repeated cycles of exposure to low pH.

In a similar manner, an antigen immunosorbent can be used to absorb out an antibody from a mixture whence it can be purified by elution (figure 6.6). This is especially useful where an antiserum displays high levels of nonspecific reactivity against other antigens rendering it unusable. Affinity-purification of such an antiserum, by means of the antigen that was used to generate it, can often dramatically improve its specificity.

MODULATION OF BIOLOGICAL ACTIVITY BY ANTIBODIES

To detect antibody

A number of biological reactions can be inhibited by addition of specific antibody. Thus the agglutination of red cells by interaction of influenza virus with receptors on the erythrocyte surface can be blocked by antiviral antibodies and this forms the basis for their serological detection. A test for antibodies to *Salmonella* H antigen present on the flagella depends upon their ability to inhibit the motility of the bacteria *in vitro*. Likewise, *Mycoplasma* antibodies can be demonstrated by their inhibitory effect on the metabolism of the organisms in culture.

Using antibody as an inhibitor

The successful treatment of cases of drug overdose with the Fab fragment of specific antibodies has been described and may become a practical proposition if a range of hybridomas can be assembled. Conjugates of cocaine with keyhole limpet hemocyanin (the latter is used as a carrier to elicit efficient Ab production to cocaine) can provoke neutralizing antibodies. Antibodies to hormones such as insulin and thyroid-stimulating hormone (TSH), or to cytokines, can be used to probe the specificity of biological reactions *in vitro*. For example, the specificity of the insulin-like activity of a serum sample on rat epididymal fat pad can be checked by the neutralizing effect of an antiserum. Such antibodies can be effective *in vivo*, and anti-TNF treatment of patients with rheumatoid arthritis has confirmed the role of this cytokine in the disease process. Likewise, as part of the worldwide effort to prevent disastrous overpopulation, attempts are in progress to immunize against chorionic gonadotropin using fragments of the β chain coupled to appropriate carriers, since this hormone is needed to sustain the implanted ovum.

In a totally different context, antibodies raised against myelin-associated neurite growth inhibitory proteins revealed their importance in preventing nerve repair, in that treatment with these antibodies permitted the regeneration of corticospinal axons after a spinal cord lesion had been induced in adult rats. This quite remarkable finding significantly advances our understanding of the processes involved in regeneration and gives ground for cautious optimism concerning the development of treatment for spinal cord damage, although for various reasons this may not ultimately be based on antibody therapy.

Using antibody as an activator

Antibodies can also be used to substitute for natural biological ligands, either because the ligand is unknown, is difficult to purify, or would require a small mortgage to be able to afford it! For example, antibodies can be used instead of ligand to stimulate cell-surface receptors that propagate signals into the cell upon crosslinking. Normally, the natural ligand for the receptor would promote receptor crosslinking but antibodies can be used to mimic this very efficiently. Such an approach has been used to great effect to study intracellular events that take place upon stimulation of T- or B-cell receptor complexes by antibodies directed against these receptors or associated proteins (such as the CD3 complex). In a similar vein, antibodies directed against the Fas (CD95) cell surface receptor can substitute for the natural ligand (FasL/CD95L) in order to stimulate the receptor and study the consequences of this. In the latter case, stimulation of Fas by anti-Fas antibodies induces rapid programmed cell death (apoptosis) in cells bearing this receptor (figure 6.7). Another good example is the induction of histamine release from mast cells by divalent F(ab')$_2$ anti-FcεRI but not by the univalent fragment. Antibody-induced activation can be used to study the signal transduction cascade downstream of receptor engagement by ligand, even where the ligand has not yet been identified.

IMMUNODETECTION OF ANTIGEN IN CELLS AND TISSUES

Immunofluorescence microscopy

Antibodies can be used as highly sensitive probes to explore the subcellular localization of a protein (or other antigenic determinant) within a cell or a tissue. Because fluorescent dyes such as fluorescein and rhodamine can be coupled to antibodies without destroying their specificity, the conjugates can combine with antigen present in a tissue section and be visualized using a microscope equipped with an appropriate light source (typically UV light). Looked at another way, the method can also be used for the detection of antibodies directed against antigens already known to be present in a given tissue section or cell preparation. Before applying the antibody to the cell or tissue preparation, samples require fixation and permeabilization in order to preserve cellular structures and to permit free passage of antibody across the plasma membrane. There are two general ways in which the test is carried out.

Direct test with labeled antibody

The antibody to the tissue antigen is directly conjugated with the fluorochrome and applied to the sample (figure 6.8a). Binding of the antibody to the antigen is betrayed by that part of the cell becoming fluorescent when illuminated using UV light. For example, suppose we wished to show the distribution of a thyroid autoantigen reacting with the autoantibodies present in the serum of a patient with Hashimoto's disease, a type of thyroid autoimmunity. We would isolate IgG from the patient's serum, conjugate it with fluorescein, and apply it to a section of human thyroid on a slide. When viewed

Untreated	anti-Fas
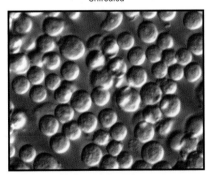	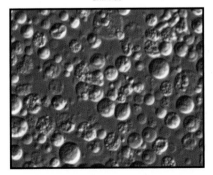

Figure 6.7. Antibody-induced receptor activation. Transformed Jurkat T-cells were either left untreated, or were treated with anti-Fas IgM antibody for 4 hours. Crosslinking of the Fas (CD95) receptor with antibody activates the receptor and results in a signal transduction cascade that culminates in activation of a series of cysteine proteases, called caspases, that provoke apoptosis in the stimulated cell. Apop-

totic cells exhibit plasma membrane blebbing and collapse of the cell into small fragments or vesicles termed 'apoptotic bodies'. Similar effects are also seen when the natural ligand, FasL, is used instead of anti-Fas antibody. (Kindly provided by Dr. Colin Adrain, Dept. of Genetics, Trinity College, Dublin, Ireland.)

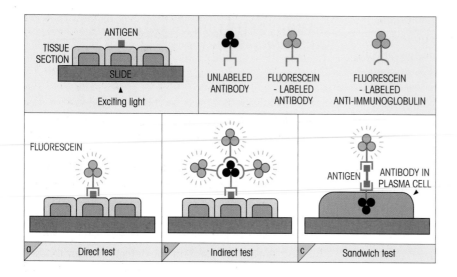

Figure 6.8. The basis of fluorescence antibody tests for identification of tissue antigens or their antibodies. ◉ = fluorescein labeled.

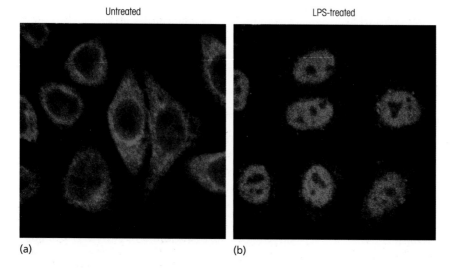

Untreated   LPS-treated

(a)   (b)

Figure 6.9. Immunolocalization of a transcription factor upon receptor stimulation. Transformed human monocytes (THP-1 cells) were either left untreated (a), or were stimulated with bacterial lipopolysaccharide (LPS) for 2 hours (b). Cells were then fixed and immunostained with an anti-NFκB antibody. Note that in unstimulated cells NFκB is abundantly present in the cell cytoplasm but is excluded from the nucleus, whereas the reverse is true in LPS-stimulated cells. (Courtesy of Dr. Lisa Bouchier-Hayes, St. Jude's Hospital, Memphis, USA.)

in the fluorescence microscope we would see that the cytoplasm of the follicular epithelial cells was brightly stained (cf. figure 18.1a).

Let's consider another example to illustrate the versatility of this technique. We have just generated a monoclonal antibody to a transcription factor (NFκB for example) that is known to be important for LPS-induced macrophage activation and IL-1β production. We could compare resting versus LPS-treated macrophages to determine whether the transcription factor does anything 'interesting' upon exposure of macrophages to LPS. In this case we would observe that, whereas resting macrophages contain lots of NFκB, it all appears to be in the cytoplasm. However, we would also certainly note that within minutes of exposure to LPS, practically all of the NFκB had moved to the nucleus (figure 6.9).

By using two (or even three) antisera conjugated to dyes which emit fluorescence at different wavelengths (figure 6.10), several different antigens can be identified

simultaneously in the same preparation. In figure 2.6e, direct staining of fixed plasma cells with a mixture of rhodamine-labeled anti-IgG and fluorescein-conjugated anti-IgM craftily demonstrates that these two classes of antibody are produced by different cells. The technique of coupling biotin to the antiserum and then finally staining with fluorescent avidin is often employed.

Indirect test with labeled secondary antibody

In this double-layer technique, which is the most commonly adopted approach, the unlabeled antibody (the primary antibody) is applied directly to the tissue and visualized by treatment with a fluorochrome-conjugated anti-immunoglobulin serum (the secondary antibody; figure 6.8b). Anti-immunoglobulin antisera are widely available conjugated to different fluorochromes.

This technique has several advantages. In the first place the fluorescence is brighter than with the direct test since several fluorescent anti-immunoglobulins bind on to each of the antibody molecules present in the first layer (figure 6.8b). Second, even when many sera have to be screened for specific antibodies it is only necessary to prepare (or, more usually the case, purchase) a single secondary antibody. Furthermore, the method

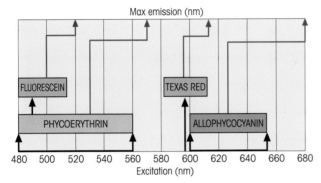

Figure 6.10. Fluorescent labels used in immunofluorescence microscopy and flow cytometry. The fluorescein longer wave emission overlaps with that of Texas Red and is corrected for in the software. The phycobiliproteins of red algae and cyanobacteria effect energy transfer of blue light to chlorophyll for photosynthesis; each molecule has many fluorescent groups giving a broad excitation range, but fluorescence is emitted within a narrow wavelength band with such high quantum efficiency as to obviate the need for a second amplifying antibody.

has great flexibility. For example, by using a mixture of primary antibodies directed against different target antigens, it is possible to compare the relative positions and/or expression of two different antigens within the same cell. Note, however, that in the latter scenario the primary antibodies must not have been generated in the same species or the secondary reagent will not be able to discriminate between them. For example, to simultaneously label cytochrome *c* and tubulin in the same cell, one would need to use anti-tubulin antibody that has been raised in the mouse, in combination with anti-cytochrome *c* antibody that has been raised in rabbit, or visa versa. By using species-specific secondary detection reagents (i.e. anti-mouse and anti-rabbit Ig) that are labeled with different flourochromes, it is a simple matter to detect both proteins within the same cell (figure 6.11).

Further applications of the indirect test may be seen in Chapter 18.

Confocal microscopy

Fluorescent images at high magnification are usually difficult to resolve because of the flare from slightly out of focus planes above and below that of the object. The resulting blurred images are usually of little help

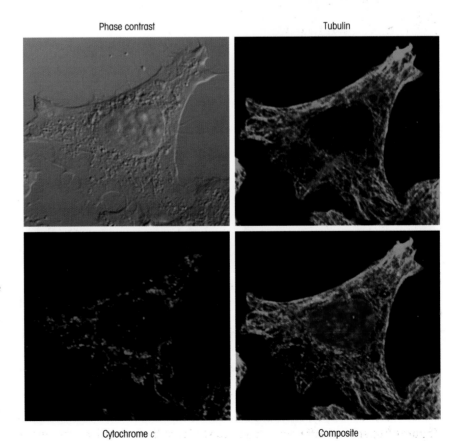

Figure 6.11. Confocal immunofluorescence microscopy. Human HeLa cell immunostained with mouse anti-β-tubulin antibody detected with FITC-labeled anti-mouse Ig (green) and rabbit anti-cytochrome *c* antibody detected with Texas red-labeled anti-rabbit Ig (red). Cells were also stained with the DNA-binding dye, DAPI (blue). A phase contrast image of the same cell is also shown for comparison. Images were acquired on an Olympus Flouroview 1000 confocal microscope. (Courtesy of Petrina Delivani.)

in exploring the finer points of cellular architecture. All that is now a thing of the past, with the advent of commercially available **scanning confocal microscopes** which focus the laser light source on a fine plane within the cell and collect the fluorescence emission in a photomultiplier tube (PMT) with a confocal aperture. Fluorescence from planes above and below the object plane fails to reach the PMT and so the sharpness of the image is dramatically enhanced over conventional immunofluorescence microscopy (figure 6.11). An X–Y scanning unit enables the whole of the specimen plane to be interrogated *quantitatively* and, with suitable optics, three or four different fluorochromes can be used simultaneously. The instrument software can compute three-dimensional fluorescent images from an automatic series of such X–Y scans accumulated in the Z axis (figure 6.12) and rotate them at the whim of the operator. Such Z-stacks can be used to

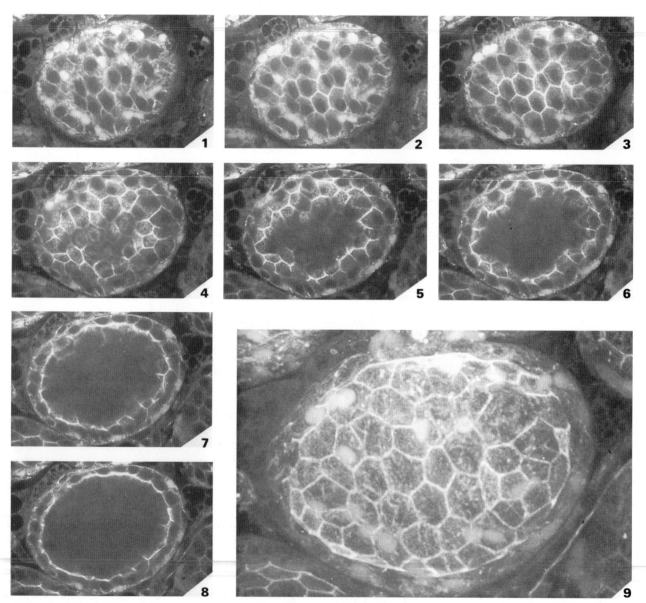

Figure 6.12. Construction of a three-dimensional fluorescent image with the confocal microscope. A spherical thyroid follicle in a thick razor-blade section of rat thyroid fixed in formalin was stained with a rhodamine–phalloidin conjugate which binds F-actin (similar results obtained with antibody conjugates). Although the sample was very thick, the microscope was focused on successive planes at 1-µm intervals from the top of the follicle (image no. 1) to halfway through (image no. 8), the total of the images representing a hemisphere. Note how the fluorescence in one plane does not interfere with that in another and that the composite photograph (image no. 9) of images 1–8 shows all the fluorescent staining in focus throughout the depth of the hemisphere. Clearly the antibody is staining hexagonal structures close to the apical (inner) surface of the follicular epithelial cells. Erythrocytes are visible near the top of the follicle. (Negatives kindly supplied by Dr Anna Smallcombe were taken by Bio-Rad staff on a Bio-Rad MRC-600 confocal imaging system using material provided by Professor V. Herzog and Fr. Brix of Bonn University.)

reconstruct a three-dimensional view of a cell, tissue or organelle, and offer unparalleled insights into cell and molecular structure. Timelapse experiments can also be carried out using the confocal microscope and this often transforms our understanding of events previously only viewed as snapshots in time. Often, seeing really is believing!

Flow cytometry

When a cell population is immunostained for a particular marker (CD4 for example) a subset of the population may express this marker at high levels, a different subset may express the same marker at low levels and the remainder of the population may be negative. To add further complexity, one may wish to examine simultaneously the expression of a different marker (CD8 for example) to determine whether expression of these proteins is mutually exclusive. Assessment of the percentage of cells in a population expressing either CD4 or CD8, or both, would be quite a chore using fluorescence microscopy or confocal microscopy, as this would involve manual counting of several hundred cells to obtain reliable figures. Quite apart from the labor involved, such analyses would also be quite subjective and results may vary depending on the skill of the operator. Fortunately, the **flow cytometer** makes such determinations rather trivial as this instrument can analyze the fluorescence levels associated with thousands of cells per minute in a highly reproducible and quantitative way (figure 6.13).

In its most basic form, the flow cytometer is an instrument equipped with a fluid-handling system capable of moving thousands of cells in **single file** through a narrow chamber illuminated by a laser. The passage of an immunolabeled cell through the chamber (called a **flow cell**) results in excitation of the fluorochrome attached to the cell by the laser. The resulting emission from the fluorochrome is detected by a sensitive photomultiplier-based detector which permits precise quantitation of the fluorescence associated with the cell. Thus it is possible to rapidly discriminate between cells that are negative, slightly positive or highly positive for a given marker or antigen. Most modern flow cytometers are equipped with three or four lasers of different wavelengths (along with associated detectors) and each laser-detector combination can gather signals from different fluorochromes (figure 6.14). As a result, it is possible to immunostain a cell population for four different markers (with a different fluorochrome-labeled antibody used for each one) and to gather data relating to the expression of all four markers as the cell passes through the flow cytometer.

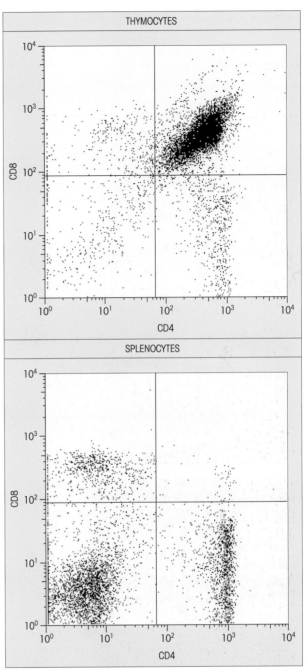

Figure 6.13. Flow cytometric analysis of CD4 and CD8 expression in thymocytes and splenocytes. Mouse thymocytes and splenocytes were stained using FITC-conjugated anti-CD4 and Rhodamine-conjugated anti-CD8 antibodies. Note that the majority of thymocytes are positive for both CD4 and CD8 and are therefore present in the upper right quadrant; thymocytes single-positive for CD4 (bottom right) or CD8 (top left) are also detected, as are double negative cells (bottom left). In the spleen, few double positive cells are found, with the majority of cells (most likely B-cells) negative for CD4 or CD8 along with cells that are single-positive for either marker. (Data kindly provided by Professor Thomas Brunner and Daniela Kassahn.)

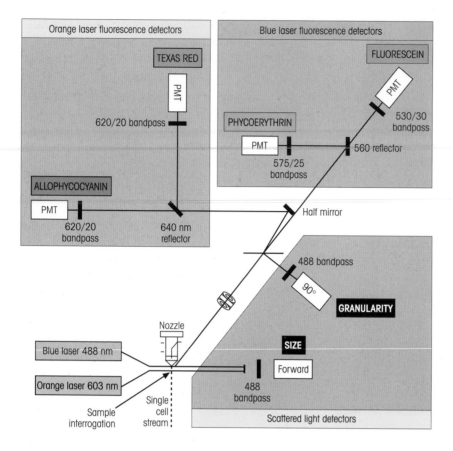

Figure 6.14. Six-parameter flow cytometry optical system for multicolor immunofluorescence analysis. Cell fluorescence excited by the blue laser is divided into green (fluorescein) and orange (phycoerythrin) signals, while fluorescence excited by the orange laser is reflected by a mirror and divided into near red (Texas Red) and far red (allophycocyanin) signals. Blue light scattered at small forward angles and at 90° is also measured in this system, providing information on cell size and internal granularity respectively. PMT, photomultiplier tube. (Based closely on Hardy R.R. (1998) In Delves P.J. & Roitt I.M. (eds) *Encyclopedia of Immunology*, 2nd edn, p. 946. Academic Press, London.) The recent use of three lasers and nine different fluorochromes pushes the system even further, providing 11 parameters!

The good news doesn't end there; the flow cytometer is also capable of providing information relating to **cell size** and **granularity** (organelle density) due to the way in which the laser light is scattered or reflected as it passes through the cell. The latter information (called forward and side scatter) is also very useful as this alone is often enough to permit discrimination between distinct cell types (figure 6.15a).

Thus, the flow cytometer records quantitative data relating to the antigen content and physical nature of each individual cell, with multiple parameters being assessed per cell to give a phenotypic analysis on a single cell rather than a population average. With the impressive number of monoclonal antibodies and of fluorochromes to hand, highly detailed analyses are now feasible, with a notable contribution to the diagnosis of leukemia (cf. p. 394).

We can also probe the cell *interior* in several ways. Permeabilization to allow penetration by fluorescent antibodies (preferably with small Fab or even single-chain Fv fragments) gives a readout of cytokines and other intracellular proteins. Cell cycle analysis can be achieved with DNA-binding dyes such as propidium iodide to measure DNA content (figure 6.15b) and antibody detection of BrdU incorporation to visualize DNA synthesis. In addition, fluorescent probes for intracellu-

lar pH, thiol concentration, Ca^{2+}, Mg^{2+} and Na^+ have been developed.

Other labeled antibody methods

A problem with fluorescent conjugates is that the signals emitted by these probes fade within a relatively short time; photobleaching of the fluorescent label upon exposure to an excitation source (such as UV light) can also occur. In practice, this is not a problem so long as the labeled sample is analyzed in a timely fashion. However, enzymes such as alkaline phosphatase (cf. figure 17.9) or horseradish peroxidase can be coupled to antibodies and then visualized by conventional histochemical methods under the light microscope (figure 6.16). Such stains are relatively stable and are particularly useful for staining tissue sections as opposed to cell suspensions.

Colloidal gold bound to antibody is being widely used as an electron-dense immunolabel by electron microscopists. At least three different antibodies can be applied to the same section by labeling them with gold particles of different size (cf. figure 8.13). A new ultra-small probe consisting of Fab' fragments linked to undecagold clusters allows more accurate spatial localization of antigens and its small size enables it to mark

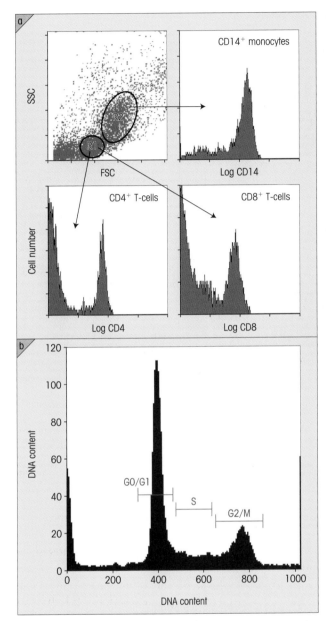

Figure 6.15. Analysis of cell size, granularity and cell cycle position by flow cytometry. (a) Staining of peripheral blood with anti-CD4, anti-CD8, and anti-CD14 antibodies followed by analysis of cells by forward-scatter (FSC) and side-scatter (SSC) characteristics (top left). Cells with low forward- and side-scatter characteristics (lymphocytes, R1) were analyzed for CD4 or CD8 expression, as indicated. Cells with high forward- and side-scatter characteristics (monocytes, R2) were analyzed for CD14 expression. (Data kindly provided by Professor Thomas Brunner.) (b) Cell cycle analysis of transformed Jurkat T-cells by propidium iodide staining. The fluorescent DNA-binding dye, propidium iodide, stains cells in proportion to their DNA content; cells with normal diploid (2N) DNA content appear in the G0/G1 phase of the cell cycle, cells actively synthesizing DNA have greater than 2N DNA content and are therefore assigned to S-phase, whereas cells with 4N (diploid) DNA content are in G2 or mitosis (G2/M). (Courtesy of Dr Colin Adrain.)

sites which are inaccessible to the larger immunolabels. However, clear visualization requires a high-resolution scanning transmission electron microscope.

DETECTION AND QUANTITATION OF ANTIGEN BY ANTIBODY

Immunoassay of antigen by ELISA

The ability to establish the concentration of an analyte (i.e. a substance to be measured) through fractional occupancy of its specific binding reagent is a feature of any ligand-binding system (Milestone 6.1), but because antibodies can be raised to virtually any structure, its application is most versatile in immunoassay.

Large analytes, such as protein hormones, are usually estimated by a noncompetitive two-site assay in which the original ligand binder and the labeled detection reagent are both antibodies (figure M6.1.1). By using monoclonal antibodies directed to two different epitopes on the same analyte, the system has greater power to discriminate between two related analytes; if the fractional cross-reactivity of the first antibody for a related analyte is 0.1 and of the second also 0.1, the final readout for cross-reactivity will be as low as 0.1×0.1, i.e. 1%. Using chemiluminescent and time-resolved fluorescent probes, highly sensitive assays are available for an astonishing range of analytes. For small molecules like drugs or steroid hormones, where two-site binding is impractical, competitive assays (figure M6.1.1) are appropriate.

The **ELISA (Enzyme-Linked Immunosorbent Assay)** is one of the most commonly used techniques for measuring antigens, such as cytokines, from serum or cell culture fluid. The technique is quite straightforward and involves immobilizing antibody to the protein of interest within the plastic wells of a microtiter plate. Unbound protein-binding sites within the plate are then blocked by incubation with an irrelevant protein such as albumin. Samples containing the antigen of interest are then added to the antibody-coated wells and incubated for a couple of hours to allow *capture* of the antigen by antibody. Following washing to remove nonbinding material, the bound antigen is then *detected* by adding a second antibody which is directed against a different binding-site on the antigen to the one recognized by the capture antibody. The antigen is now sandwiched between the two antibodies giving rise to the terms **'sandwich ELISA'** or **antigen-capture assay**. The detection antibody is conjugated to an enzyme such as horseradish peroxidase or alkaline phosphatase which, upon addition of the enzyme substrate, produces a colored or chemiluminescent reaction product. Comparison

H & E   Anti-CD21   Anti-CD68

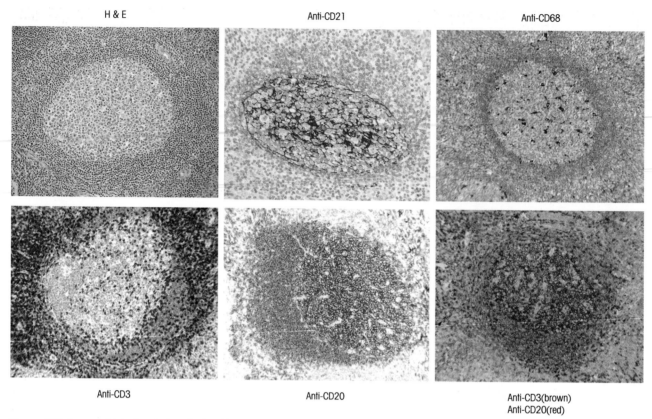

Anti-CD3   Anti-CD20   Anti-CD3(brown)
Anti-CD20(red)

Figure 6.16. Immunohistochemical analysis of human tonsil follicle centers. Human tonsil preparations were stained either with the histochemical stain hematoxylin and eosin (H&E), or were immunostained with antibodies against CD21 (complement receptor 2, expressed on follicular dendritic cells and B-cells), CD68 (expressed on macrophages), CD3 (T-cells), CD20 (B-cells), or a combination of anti-CD3 and anti-CD20, as shown. (Images kindly provided by Dr Andreas Kappeler.)

between a range of standards of known concentration enables the concentration of antigen in the test samples to be calculated.

The nephelometric assay for antigen

If antigen is added to a solution of excess antibody, the amount of complex which can be assessed by forward light scatter in a nephelometer (cf. p. 133) is linearly related to the concentration of antigen. With the ready availability of a wide range of monoclonal antibodies which facilitate the standardization of the method, nephelometry is frequently used for the estimation of immunoglobulins, C3, C4, haptoglobin, ceruloplasmin and C-reactive protein in those favored laboratories which can sport the appropriate equipment. Very small samples down in the range 1–10 μl can be analyzed. Turbidity of the sample can be a problem; blanks lacking antibody can be deducted but a more satisfactory solution is to follow the **rate of formation** of complexes which is proportional to antigen concentration since this obviates the need for a separate blank (figure 6.17). Because soluble complexes begin to be formed in

antigen excess, it is important to ensure that the value for antigen was obtained in antibody excess by running a further control in which additional antigen is included.

Immunoblotting (Western blotting)

This widely adopted technique can be used to determine the **relative molecular mass** of a protein and to explore its behavior within a complex mixture of other proteins. Issues relating to whether the protein of interest is upregulated, downregulated, cleaved, phosphorylated, glycosylated or ubiquitinated in response to a particular stimulus can be addressed by immunoblot analysis. This involves first running a mixture of proteins through a gel matrix that is formed by polymerization of acrylamide and bisacrylamide between a pair of glass plates. **Polyacrylamide gel electrophoresis (PAGE)** of proteins is typically carried out using protein mixtures that have been denatured by heating in the presence of a detergent, sodium dodecyl sulfate (SDS). SDS is a negatively charged molecule that becomes covalently coupled to proteins along their length upon

Milestone 6.1 — Ligand-binding Assays

The appreciation that a ligand could be measured by the fractional occupancy (F) of its specific binding agent heralded a new order of sensitive wide-ranging assays. Ligand-binding assays were first introduced for the measurement of thyroid hormone by thyroxine-binding protein (Ekins) and for the estimation of hormones by antibody (Berson & Yalow). These findings spawned the technology of radioimmunoassay, so called because the antigen had to be trace-labeled in some way and the most convenient candidates for this were radioisotopes.

The relationship between fractional occupancy and analyte concentration [An] is given by the equation:

$$F = 1 - (1/1 + K[An])$$

where K is the association constant of the ligand-binding reaction. F can be measured by noncompetitive or competitive assays (figure M6.1.1) and related to a calibration curve constructed with standard amounts of analyte.

For competitive assays, the maximum theoretical sensitivity is given by the term ε/K where ε is the experimental error (coefficient of variation). Suppose the error is 1% and K is $10^{11}\,\text{M}^{-1}$, the maximum sensitivity will be $0.01 \times 10^{-11}\,\text{M} = 10^{-13}\,\text{M}$ or 6×10^7 molecules/ml. For noncompetitive assays, labels of very high specific activity could give sensitivities down to 10^2–10^3 molecules/ml under ideal conditions. In practice, however, since the sensitivity represents the lowest analyte concentration which can be measured against a background containing zero analyte, the error of the measurement of background poses an ultimate constraint on sensitivity.

Figure M6.1.1. The principle of ligand-binding assays. The ligand-binding agent may be in the soluble phase or bound to a solid support as shown here, the advantage of the latter being the ease of separation of bound from free analyte. After exposure to analyte, the fractional occupancy of the ligand-binding sites can be determined by competitive or noncompetitive assays using labeled reagents (in orange) as shown.

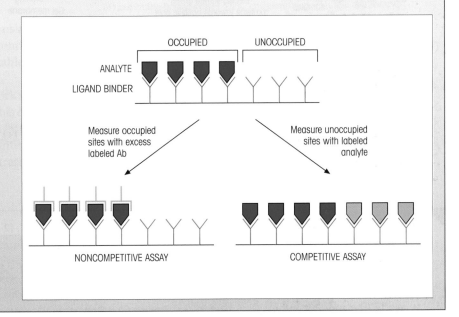

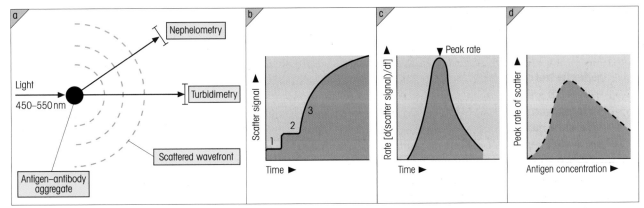

Figure 6.17. Rate nephelometry. (a) On addition of antiserum, small antigen–antibody aggregates form (cf. figure 6.24) which scatter incident light filtered to give a wavelength band of 450–550 nm. For nephelometry, the light scattered at a forward angle of 70° or so is measured. (b) After addition of the sample (1) and then the antibody (2), the rate at which the aggregates form (3) is determined from the scatter signal.

(c) The software in the instrument then computes the maximum rate of light scatter which is related to the antigen concentration as shown in (d). (Copied from the operating manual for the 'Array' rate reaction automated immunonephelometer with permission from Beckman Coulter Ltd.)

With small haptens, equilibrium dialysis can be employed to measure K_a, but usually one is dealing with larger antigens and other techniques must be used. One approach is to add increasing amounts of radiolabeled antigen to a fixed amount of antibody, and then separate the free from bound antibody by precipitating the soluble complex as described above (e.g. by an anti-immunoglobulin). The reciprocal of the bound, i.e. complexed, antibody concentration can be plotted against the reciprocal of the free antigen concentration, so allowing the affinity constant to be calculated (figure 6.26a). For an antiserum this will give an affinity constant representing an average of the heterogeneous antibody components and a measure of the effective number of antigen-binding sites operative at the highest levels of antigen used.

Various types of ELISA have been developed which provide a measure of antibody affinity. In one system the antibody is allowed to first bind to its antigen, and then a chaotropic agent such as thiocyanate is added in increasing concentration in order to disrupt the antibody binding; the higher the affinity of the antibody, the more agent that is required to reduce the binding. Another type of ELISA for measuring affinity is the indirect competitive system devised by Friguet and associates (figure 6.26b). A constant amount of antibody is incubated with a series of antigen concentrations and the free antibody at equilibrium is assessed by

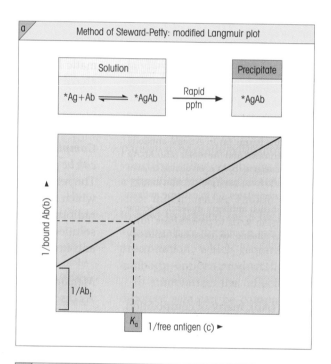

Figure 6.26. Determination of affinity with large antigens. The equilibria between Ab and Ag at different concentrations are determined as follows:
(a) For a polyclonal antiserum one can use the Steward–Petty modification of the Langmuir equation:

$$1/b = 1/(Ab_t.c.K_a) + 1/Ab_t$$

where Ab_t = total Ab combining sites, b = bound Ab concentration, c = free Ag concentration and K_a = average affinity constant. At infinite Ag concentration, all Ab sites are bound and $1/b = 1/Ab_t$. When half the Ab sites are bound, $1/c = K_a$.
(b) The method of Friguet *et al.* for monoclonal antibodies. First, a calibration curve for free antibody is established by estimating the proportion binding to solid-phase antigen, bound antibody being measured by enzyme-labeled anti-Ig (ELISA: see text). Using the calibration curve, the amount of free Ab in equilibrium with Ag in solution is determined by seeing how much of the Ab binds to solid-phase Ag (the amount of solid-phase antigen is insufficient to affect the solution equilibrium materially). Combination of the Klotz and Scatchard equations gives:

$$A_o/A_o - A = 1 + K_d/a_o$$

where A_o = ELISA optical density (OD) for Ab in the absence of Ag, A = OD in the presence of Ag concentration a_o where a_o is approximately $10 \times$ concentration of Ab. The slope of the plot gives K_d. (Labeled molecules are marked with an asterisk.)

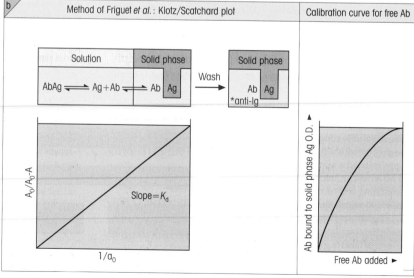

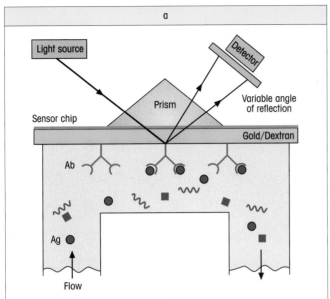

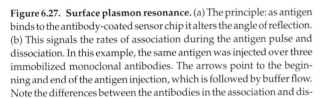

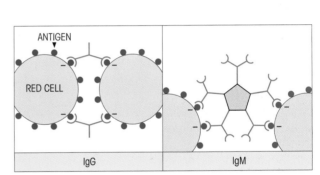

Figure 6.27. Surface plasmon resonance. (a) The principle: as antigen binds to the antibody-coated sensor chip it alters the angle of reflection. (b) This signals the rates of association during the antigen pulse and dissociation. In this example, the same antigen was injected over three immobilized monoclonal antibodies. The arrows point to the beginning and end of the antigen injection, which is followed by buffer flow. Note the differences between the antibodies in the association and dissociation rates. (Data kindly provided by Dr R. Karlsson, Biacore AB, and reproduced from Panayotou G. (1998) Surface plasmon resonance. In Delves P.J. & Roitt I.M. (eds) *Encyclopedia of Immunology*, 2nd edn. Academic Press, with permission.) The system can be used with antigen immobilized on the sensor chip and antibody in the fluid phase, or can be applied to any other single ligand-binding assay.

secondary binding to solid-phase antigen. In this way, values for K_a are not affected by any distortion of antigen by labeling. This again stresses the superiority of determining affinity by studying the **primary reaction** with antigen in the **soluble state** rather than conformationally altered through binding to a solid phase.

Increasingly, affinity measurements are obtained using **surface plasmon resonance**. A sensor chip consisting of a monoclonal antibody coupled to dextran overlying a gold film on a glass prism will totally internally reflect light at a given angle (figure 6.27a). Antigen present in a pulse of fluid will bind to the sensor chip and, by increasing its size, alter the angle of reflection. The system provides data on the kinetics of association and dissociation (and hence K) (figure 6.27b) and permits comparisons between monoclonal antibodies and also assessment of subtle effects of mutations.

Agglutination of antigen-coated particles

Whereas the cross-linking of multivalent protein antigens by antibody leads to precipitation, cross-linking of cells or large particles by antibody directed against surface antigens leads to agglutination. Since most cells are electrically charged, a reasonable number of antibody links between two cells are required before the mutual repulsion is overcome. Thus agglutination of

Figure 6.28. Mechanism of agglutination of antigen-coated particles by antibody cross-linking to form large macroscopic aggregates. If red cells are used, several cross-links are needed to overcome the electrical charge at the cell surface. IgM is superior to IgG as an agglutinator because of its multivalent binding and because the charged cells are further apart.

cells bearing only a small number of determinants may be difficult to achieve unless special methods such as further treatment with an antiglobulin reagent are used. Similarly, the higher avidity of multivalent IgM antibody relative to IgG makes the former more effective as an agglutinating agent, molecule for molecule (figure 6.28).

Agglutination reactions are used to identify bacteria and to type red cells; they have been observed with leukocytes and platelets, and even with spermatozoa in certain cases of male infertility due to sperm agglutinins. Because of its sensitivity and convenience, the test has been extended to the identification of antibodies to soluble antigens which have been artificially coated on to erythrocytes, latex or gelatin particles. Agglutination of IgG-coated latex is used to detect rheumatoid factors. Similar tests using antigen-coated particles can be carried out in U-bottom microtiter plates where the settling pattern on the bottom of the well may be observed (figure 6.29); this provides a more sensitive indicator than macroscopic clumping. Quantification of more subtle degrees of agglutination can be achieved by nephelometry or Coulter counting.

Immunoassay for antibody using solid-phase antigen

The principle

The antibody content of a serum can be assessed by the ability to bind to antigen which has been immobilized by physical adsorption to a plastic tube or microtiter plate with multiple wells; the bound immunoglobulin may then be estimated by addition of a labeled anti-Ig raised in another species (figure 6.30). Consider, for example, the determination of DNA autoantibodies in SLE (cf. p. 414). When a patient's serum is added to a microwell coated with antigen (in this case DNA), the autoantibodies will bind to the antigen and the remaining serum proteins can be readily washed away. Bound antibody can now be estimated by addition of ^{125}I-labeled purified rabbit anti-human IgG; after rinsing out excess unbound reagent, the radioactivity of the tube will clearly be a measure of the autoantibody content of the patient's serum. The distribution of antibody in different classes can be determined by using specific antisera. Take the radioallergosorbent test (RAST) for IgE antibodies in allergic patients. The allergen (e.g. pollen extract) is covalently coupled to an immunoabsorbent,

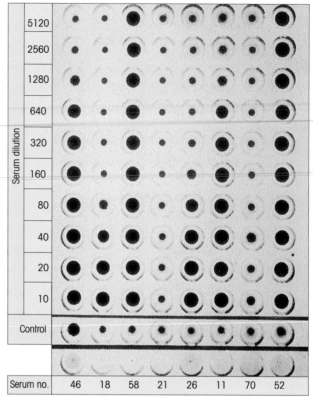

Figure 6.29. Red cell hemagglutination test for thyroglobulin autoantibodies. Thyroglobulin-coated cells were added to dilutions of patients' serums. Uncoated cells were added to a 1:10 dilution of serum as a control. In a positive reaction, the cells settle as a carpet over the bottom of the cup. Because of the 'V'-shaped cross-section of these cups, in negative reactions the cells fall into the base of the 'V', forming a small, easily recognizable button. The reciprocal of the highest serum dilution giving an unequivocally positive reaction is termed the titer. The titers reading from left to right are: 640, 20, >5120, neg, 40, 320, neg, >5120. The control for serum no. 46 was slightly positive and this serum should be tested again after absorption with uncoated cells.

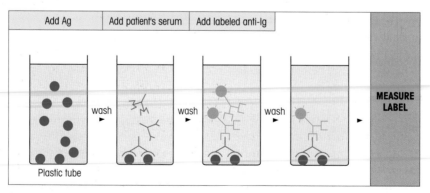

Figure 6.30. Solid-phase immunoassay for antibody. To reduce non-specific binding of IgG to the solid phase after adsorption of the first reagent, it is usual to add an irrelevant protein, such as dried skimmed milk powder or bovine serum albumin, to block any free sites on the plastic. Note that the conformation of a protein often alters on binding to plastic, e.g. a monoclonal antibody which distinguishes between the apo and holo forms of cytochrome c in solution combines equally well with both proteins on the solid phase. Covalent coupling to carboxy-derivatized plastic or capture of the antigen substrate by solid-phase antibody can sometimes lessen this effect.

in this case a paper disk, which is then treated with patient's serum. The amount of specific IgE bound to the paper can now be estimated by the addition of labeled anti-IgE.

A wide variety of labels are available

Whilst providing extremely good sensitivity, radiolabels have a number of disadvantages, including loss of sensitivity during storage due to radioactive decay, the deterioration of the labeled reagent through radiation damage, and the precautions needed to minimize human exposure to radioactivity. Therefore, other types of label are often employed in immunoassays.

ELISA (enzyme-linked immunosorbent assay). Enzymes which give a colored soluble reaction product are currently the most commonly used labels, with horseradish peroxidase (HRP) and calf intestine alkaline phosphatase (AP) being by far the most popular. *Aspergillus niger* glucose oxidase, soy bean urease and *Escherichia coli* β-galactosidase provide further alternatives. One clever ploy for amplifying the phosphatase reaction is to use nicotinamide adenine dinucleotide phosphate (NADP) as a substrate to generate NAD which now acts as a coenzyme for a second enzyme system.

Other labels. Enzyme-labeled streptococcal protein G or staphylococcal protein A will bind to IgG. Conjugation with the vitamin biotin is frequently used since this can readily be detected by its reaction with enzyme-linked avidin or streptavidin (the latter gives lower background binding), both of which bind with ferocious specificity and affinity ($K = 10^{15}\mathrm{M}^{-1}$).

Chemiluminescent systems based on the HRP-catalyzed enhanced luminol reaction, where light from the oxidized luminol substrate is intensified and the signal duration increased by the use of an enhancing reagent, provide increased sensitivity and dynamic range. Special mention should be made of time-resolved fluorescence assays based upon chelates of rare earths such as europium 3^+, although these have a more important role in antigen assays.

DETECTION OF IMMUNE COMPLEX FORMATION

Many techniques for detecting circulating complexes have been described and because of variations in the size, complement-fixing ability and Ig class of different complexes, it is useful to apply more than one method. Two fairly robust methods for general use are:

1 precipitation of complexed IgG from serum at concentrations of polyethylene glycol which do not bring down significant amounts of IgG monomer, followed by estimation of IgG in the precipitate by single radial immunodiffusion (SRID) or laser nephelometry, and

2 binding of C3b-containing complexes to beads coated with bovine conglutinin (cf. p. 17) and estimation of the bound Ig with enzyme-labeled anti-Ig.

Other techniques include: (i) estimation of the binding of ^{125}I-C1q to complexes by coprecipitation with polyethylene glycol, (ii) inhibition by complexes of rheumatoid factor-induced aggregation of IgG-coated particles, and (iii) detection with radiolabeled anti-Ig of serum complexes capable of binding to the C3b (and to a lesser extent the Fc) receptors on the Raji cell line. Sera from patients with immune complex disease often form a cryoprecipitate when allowed to stand at 4°C. Measurement of serum C3 and its conversion product C3c is sometimes useful.

Tissue-bound complexes are usually visualized by the immunofluorescent staining of biopsies with conjugated anti-immunoglobulins and anti-C3 (cf. figure 15.18).

ISOLATION OF LEUKOCYTE SUBPOPULATIONS

Because of the complexity of the interactions between cells of the immune system, it is often well-nigh impossible to sort out who is doing what to whom unless one adopts a reductionist approach by purifying specific cell populations to study in isolation. Clearly, this approach also has its pitfalls as purified cell populations often behave differently *in vitro* to the way they do *in vivo*. However, the combination of *in vitro* and *in vivo* approaches has been very powerful and each has its place in the immunologist's armory. A number of techniques are routinely employed to enrich immune cell populations to varying degrees of purity. Most of these rely upon unique characteristics of particular cell populations ranging from their size, ability to adhere to plastic, or expression of a particular cell surface antigen. Antibodies to particular CD markers are especially useful for isolating specific populations of leukocytes when used in conjunction with a range of clever panning methods as we shall see below.

Bulk techniques

Separation based on physical parameters

Separation of cells on the basis of their differential **sedimentation rate**, which roughly correlates with **cell size**, can be carried out by centrifugation through a density gradient. Cells can be increased in mass by selectively binding particles such as red cells to their surface, the most notable example being the rosettes formed when

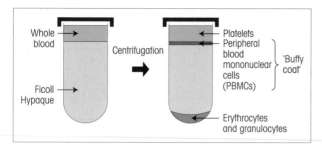

Figure 6.31. Separation of leukocytes by density gradient centrifugation. Whole blood is carefully layered onto Ficoll-Hypaque or similar medium of known density, followed by centrifugation at 800 g for 30 min. This results in the sedimentation of erythrocytes and granulocytes to the bottom of the centrifuge tube. A peripheral blood mononuclear cell 'buffy coat' consisting mainly of T- and B-lymphocytes, NK cells and monocytes is found at the interface between the two layers.

sheep erythrocytes bind to the CD2 marker present on human T-cells.

Buoyant density is another useful parameter. Centrifugation of whole blood over isotonic Ficoll–Hypaque (sodium metrizoate) of density 1.077 g/ml leaves the mononuclear cells (lymphocytes, monocytes and natural killer (NK) cells) floating in a band at the interface, while the erythrocytes and polymorphonuclear leukocytes, being denser, travel right down to the base of the tube (figure 6.31). **Adherence** to plastic surfaces largely removes phagocytic cells, while passage down nylon-wool columns greatly enriches lymphocyte populations for T-cells at the expense of B-cells.

Separation exploiting biological parameters
Actively phagocytic cells which take up small iron particles can be manipulated by a magnet deployed externally. Lymphocytes which divide in response to a polyclonal activator (see p. 178), or specific antigen, can be eliminated by allowing them to incorporate 5-bromodeoxyuridine (BrdU); this renders them susceptible to the lethal effect of UV irradiation.

Selection by antibody
Several methods are available for the selection of cells specifically coated with antibody, some of which are illustrated in figure 6.32. Addition of complement or anti-Ig toxin conjugates will eliminate such populations. Magnetic beads coated with anti-Ig form clusters with antibody-coated cells which can be readily separated from uncoated cells. Another useful bulk selection technique is to pan antibody-coated cells on anti-Ig adsorbed to a surface. One variation on this theme used to isolate bone marrow stem cells with anti-CD34 is to coat the cells with biotinylated antibody and select with an avidin column or avidin magnetic beads. Cocktails of

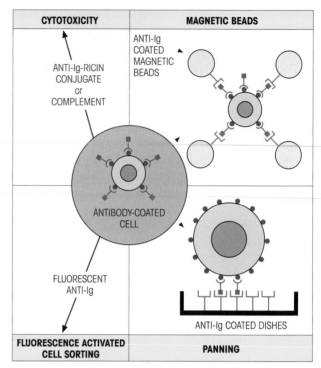

Figure 6.32. Major methods for separating cells coated with a specific antibody.

antibodies coated onto beads are used in cell separation columns for the depletion of specific populations leading to, for example, enriched CD4$^+$ CD45RA$^-$ or CD4$^+$ CD45RO$^-$ lymphocytes.

Cell selection by FACS

Cells coated with fluorescent antibody can be separated by fluorescence-activated cell sorting (FACS) as described in Milestone 6.2 and figure 6.33 (see more in-depth discussion under 'Flow cytometry', p. 123). The technique is relatively simple but the technology required to achieve it is highly sophisticated. Cells are typically stained with antibodies against particular cell surface markers (such as CD4 or CD19) and cells that are positive or negative for this marker are sorted into different collection tubes by the instrument.

Enrichment of antigen-specific populations

Selective expansion of antigen-specific T-cells by repeated stimulation with antigen and presenting cells in culture, usually alternated with interleukin-2 (IL-2) treatment, leads to an enrichment of heterogeneous T-cells specific for different epitopes on the antigen. Such **T-cell lines** can be distributed in microtiter wells at a high enough dilution such that **on average** there is less than one cell per well; pushing the cells to proliferate

Milestone 6.2—The Fluorescence-activated Cell Sorter (FACS)

The FACS was developed by the Herzenbergs and their colleagues to quantify the surface molecules on individual white cells by their reaction with fluorochrome-labeled monoclonal antibodies and to use the signals so generated to separate cells of defined phenotype from a heterogeneous mixture.

In this elegant but complex machine, the fluorescent cells are made to flow obediently in a single stream past a laser beam. Quantitative measurement of the fluorescent signal in a suitably placed photomultiplier tube relays a signal to the cell as it emerges in a single droplet; the cell becomes charged and

can be separated in an electric field (figure M6.2.1). Extra sophistication can be introduced by using additional lasers and fluorochromes, and both 90° and forward light scatter. This is elaborated upon in the section on flow cytofluorimetry describing how this technique can be used for quantitative multiparameter analysis of single-cell populations (cf. figure 6.14). Suffice to state that these latest FACS machines permit the isolation of cells with a complex phenotype from a heterogeneous population with a high degree of discrimination.

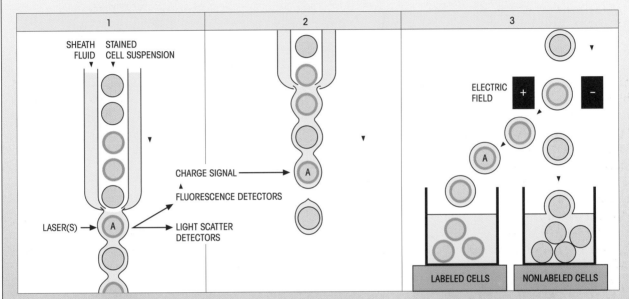

Figure M6.2.1. The principle of the FACS for flow cytofluorimetry of the fluorescence on stained cells (green rimmed circles) and physical separation from unstained cells. The charge signal can be activated to separate cells of high from low fluorescence and, using light scatter, of large from small size and dead from living.

with antigen or anti-CD3 produces single T-cell clones which can be maintained with much obsessional care and attention, but my goodness they can be a pain! Potentially immortal **T-cell hybridomas**, similar in principle to B-cell hybridomas, can be established by fusing cell lines with a T-tumor line and cloning.

Animals populated essentially by a single T-cell specificity can be produced by introducing the T-cell receptor α and β genes from a T-cell clone, as a transgene (see below); since the genes are already rearranged, their presence in every developing T-cell will switch off any other $V\beta$ gene recombinations.

No one has succeeded in cloning primary B-cells as they die rapidly upon introduction to cell culture. It is possible however to culture immortalized B-cell hybridomas or Epstein–Barr virus-transformed cell lines, and, as with T-cells, transgenic animals expressing the same antibody in all of their B-cells have been generated.

GENE EXPRESSION ANALYSIS

The analysis of gene expression patterns can tell us a lot about what a cell or cell population is doing, or about to do, at a particular moment in time. To analyze the cohort of genes that are expressed by a cell population, either at a steady-state level or in response to a particular stimulus, messenger RNA (mRNA) is extracted and is analyzed by a method that enables genes of interest to be detected. mRNA can be analyzed by Northern blot, where a single gene probe is hybridized to the mRNA sample, or by reverse transcriptase (RT)–primed PCR where genes of interest can be amplified by initially making a cDNA copy using RT followed by gene amplification by means of specific primers that are complementary to the sequence of interest. While Northern blotting and RT-PCR can give information concerning more than one transcript, this

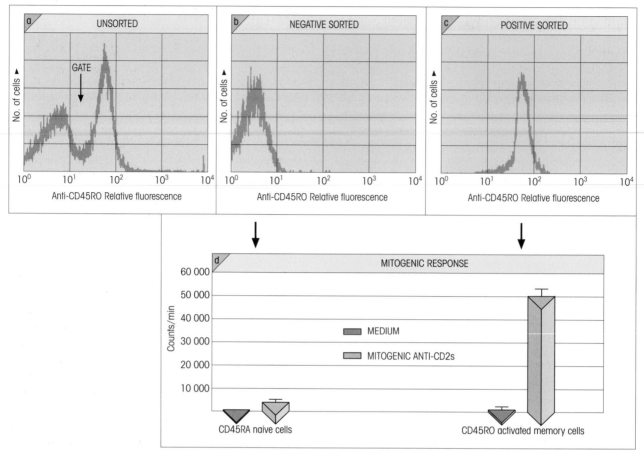

Figure 6.33. Separation of activated peripheral blood memory T-cells (CD45RO positive) from naive T-cells (CD45RO negative; but positive for the CD45RA isoform) in the FACS after staining the surface of the living cells in the cold with a fluorescent monoclonal antibody to the CD45RO (see p. 207). The unsorted cells showed two peaks (a); cells with fluorescence intensity lower than the arbitrary gate were separated from those with higher intensity giving (b) negative (CD45RA) and (c) positive (CD45RO) populations, which were each tested for their proliferative response to a mixture of two anti-CD2 monoclonals (OKT11 and GT2) in the presence of 10% antigen-presenting cells (d). ^{3}H-Thymidine was added after 3 days and the cells counted after 15 h. Clearly the memory cell population proliferated, whereas the naive population did not. (Data kindly provided by D. Wallace and R. Hicks.)

usually requires significant amounts of mRNA and is relatively slow.

The development of microarray technologies now permits the simultaneous measurement of expression of thousands of genes in a single experiment. Oligonucleotides or cDNA fragments are robotically spotted onto a gene chip and cDNA generated from, for example, T-cell mRNA is labeled and hybridized to the genes on the microarray. This provides a quantitative comparison of expression for every gene present on the chip. By accumulating such data it is possible to build up a complete picture of which genes are expressed in which cells (figure 6.34). One area in which this technology is being rapidly deployed is in the analysis of differences in gene expression between a tumor cell and its normal counterpart, thereby illuminating possible targets for therapeutic intervention.

All that glitters is not gold however and it is certainly true to say that DNA microarrays are not a solution to all our problems. Background is a troublesome feature of this type of approach and often threatens to drown out interesting data in a cacophony of experimental noise. Well-controlled experimental set-ups are a must for large-scale microarray approaches, otherwise any gene expression differences observed could well be due to slamming the tissue culture incubator door rather than the intended stimulus. The term 'garbage in, garbage out' comes to mind in these situations.

ASSESSMENT OF FUNCTIONAL ACTIVITY

The activity of phagocytic cells

The major tests employed to assess neutrophil function are summarized in table 6.1.

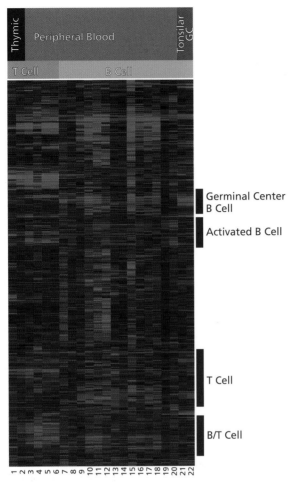

Figure 6.34. Gene expression during lymphocyte development and activation. The data were generated from over 3.8 million measurements of gene expression made on 13 637 genes using 243 microarrays. Each experiment represents a different cell population. For example, experiment 1 utilized polyclonally activated fetal CD4+ thymic cells, whereas experiment 2 shows the same population prior to stimulation. Overexpressed or induced genes are colored red, underexpressed or repressed genes green. Certain gene expression signatures become apparent in the different cell populations, indicated on the right. For example, the T-cell gene expression signature includes CD2, TCR, TCR signaling molecules and many cytokines. (Reproduced with permission of the authors and the publishers from Alizadeh A.A. & Staudt L.M. (2000) *Current Opinion in Immunology* **12**, 219.)

Lymphocyte responsiveness

When lymphocytes are stimulated by antigen or polyclonal activators *in vitro* they usually undergo cell division (cf. figure 2.6b) and release cytokines. Cell division is normally assessed by the incorporation of radiolabeled ^{3}H-thymidine or ^{125}I-UdR (5-iododeoxyuridine) into the DNA of the dividing cells. Cell division can also be measured by incorporation of fluorescent lipophilic dyes, such as CFSE, into the plasma membrane of lymphocytes or other cells. Upon division of cells labeled in this way, the fluorescent dye is equally partitioned to

Table 6.1. Evaluation of neutrophil function.

Function	Test
Phagocytosis	Measure the uptake of particles such as latex or bacteria by counting or by chemiluminescence
Respiratory burst	Measure reduction of nitroblue tetrazolium
Intracellular killing	Microbicidal test using viable *Staphylococcus aureus*
Directional migration	Movement through filters up concentration gradient of chemotactic agent such as formyl.Met.Leu.Phe
Surface LFA-1 and CR3 upregulation	Ascertained with monoclonal antibody staining

each of the daughter cells such that each daughter has only half the dye content of the parent (figure 6.35a). The decrease in membrane dye content can be measured accurately using a flow cytometer and this gives information concerning the number of cell divisions a cell has undergone since it was labeled (figure 6.35b). This method is especially useful when using mixed cell populations where it is important to know which cell type is dividing; by membrane labeling of purified cells, followed by adding these cells into a mixed cell population or even injecting these into an animal, it is possible to track the number of cell divisions the labeled cells subsequently undergo by measuring their dye content.

Cytokines released into the culture medium can be measured by immunoassay or by a bioassay using a cell line dependent on a particular cytokine for its growth and survival. Individual cells synthesizing cytokines can be enumerated in the flow cytometer by permeabilizing and staining intracellularly with labeled antibody; alternatively the ELISPOT technique (see below) can be applied. As usual, molecular biology has a valuable, if more sophisticated, input since T-cells transfected with an IL-2 enhancer–*lacZ* construct will switch on *lacZ* β-galactosidase expression on activation of the IL-2 cytokine response (cf. p. 175) and this can be readily revealed with a fluorescent or chromogenic enzyme substrate.

The ability of cytotoxic T-cells to kill their cell targets extracellularly is usually evaluated by a chromium release assay. Target cells are labeled with ^{51}Cr and the release of radioactive protein into the medium over and above that seen in the controls is the index of cytotoxicity. The test is repeated at different ratios of effector to target cells. A similar technique is used to measure extracellular killing of antibody-coated or uncoated targets by NK cells. Now a word of caution regarding the interpretation of *in vitro* assays. Since one can manipulate the

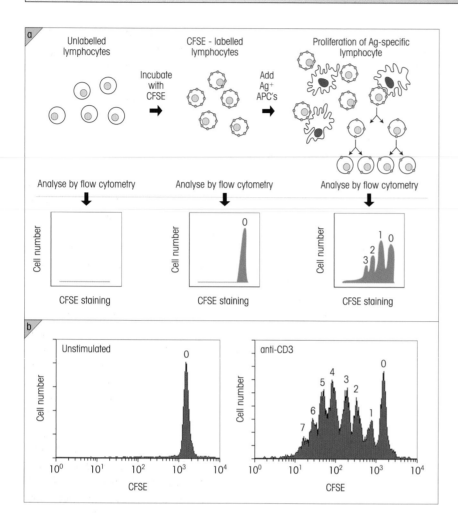

Figure 6.35. Analysis of cell proliferation by CFSE-labeling. Lymphocytes, or other cells with proliferative potential, can be labeled with the fluorescent lipophilic dye, CFSE, and subsequently analyzed for partitioning of fluorescent dye into daughter cells. (a) Schematic depiction of a CFSE-antilabeling experiment and corresponding flow cytometry plots. (b) Human peripheral T-cells were labeled with CFSE and stimulated with plate-coated anti-CD3 monoclonal antibody for 4 days. Left panel: no stimulation; right panel: anti-CD3 stimulation. Numbers and bars on the top of each histogram refer to respective division peaks with the peak of undivided cells to the extreme right in each histogram. (Courtesy of Dr Antione Attinger.)

culture conditions within wide limits, it is possible to achieve a result that might not be attainable *in vivo*. Let us illustrate this point by reference to cytotoxicity for murine cells infected with lymphocytic choriomeningitis virus (LCMV) or vesicular stomatitis virus (VSV). The most sensitive *in vitro* technique proved to be chromium release from target cells after secondary stimulation of the lymphocytes. However, this needs 5 days, during which time a relatively small number of memory CD8 cytotoxic T-cell precursors can replicate and surpass the threshold required to produce a measurable assay. Nonetheless, a weak cytotoxicity assay under these conditions was not reflected by any of the *in vivo* assessments of antiviral function implying that they had no biological relevance.

Apoptosis

Programed cell death occurs frequently in the immune system and is particularly important for the resolution of immune responses. Antigen-driven clonal expansion of T- and B-cells is typically followed by death of many

of these cells within a relatively short period, with the remaining cells making up the memory cell population; interference with this cell elimination process can result in accumulation of lymphocytes that may break tolerance and result in autoimmunity. The Fas (CD95) receptor plays an important role in peripheral tolerance and homeostatic control of lymphocyte cell populations; inactivation of this membrane receptor protein, or its ligand, in the mouse results in severe enlargement of the spleen and lymph nodes due to accumulation of lymphocytes that would normally have been eliminated through Fas-dependent apoptosis (figure 6.36). Engagement of the Fas receptor on activated lymphocytes normally results in rapid induction of apoptosis in these cells (figure 6.7). Cytotoxic T-cells also eliminate target cells by inducing apoptosis through a variety of strategies. Apoptosis is also important in shaping the T- and B-cell repertoires; negative selection of both lymphocyte populations involves triggering apoptosis.

A variety of approaches can be used to measure apoptosis, ranging from morphological assessment (figure 6.7) or by exploiting biochemical alterations to the cell that occurs during this process. One of the most widely used assays for apoptosis takes advantage of the fact that phosphatidylserine (PS), a phospholipid that is normally confined to the inner leaflet of the plasma membrane, becomes exposed on the outer leaflet during apoptosis. This can be readily detected using fluorescently labeled annexin V, a PS-binding protein; apoptotic cells display markedly enhanced binding of annexin V relative to healthy cells (figure 6.37).

Other assays take advantage of the fact that extensive DNA fragmentation is also a common feature of apoptosis and this can be assessed by agarose gel electrophoresis of DNA extracted from apoptotic cells or the TUNEL (*T*dT-mediated d*U*TP (deoxyuridine triphosphate) *n*ick *e*nd *l*abeling) assay; the latter assay utilizes the enzyme terminal deoxynucleotidyl transferase (TdT) to add biotinylated nucleotides to the 3′ ends of DNA frag-

ments and this can then be detected using fluorescently labeled streptavidin. Several members of the caspase family of cysteine proteases become activated during apoptosis and this can be assessed by immunoblot analysis (figure 6.19) or by using labeled synthetic substrate peptides that can be cleaved by active caspases.

Precursor frequency

The magnitude of lymphocyte responses in culture is closely related to the number of antigen-specific lymphocytes capable of responding. Because of the clonality of the responses, it is possible to estimate the frequency of these antigen-specific precursors by **limiting dilution analysis**. In essence, the method depends upon the fact that, if one takes several replicate aliquots of a given cell suspension which would be expected to contain *on average* one precursor per aliquot, then Poisson distribution analysis shows that 37% of the aliquots will contain *no* precursor cells (through the randomness of the sampling). Thus, if aliquots are made from a series of dilutions of a cell suspension and incubated under conditions which allow the precursors to mature and be recognized through some amplification scheme, the dilution at which 37% of the aliquots give negative responses will be known to contain an average of one precursor cell per aliquot, and one can therefore calculate the precursor frequency in the original cell suspension. An example is shown in some detail in figure 6.38.

It has been argued that limiting dilution analysis often underestimates the true precursor frequency. This is likely because cells generally do not survive very well when cultured in isolation (i.e. as a single cell per well) because most cells, with few exceptions, require signals from other cells to survive. Martin Raff showed that in the absence of such signals cells typically undergo apoptosis. An accurate measure of the percentage of lymphocytes bearing a specific antigen receptor can be obtained by flow cytometry of cells stained with labeled antigen.

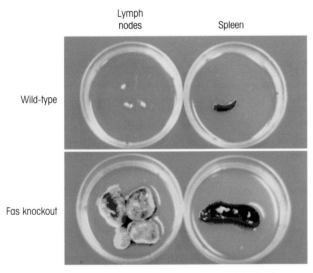

Figure 6.36. Gross enlargement of spleen and lymph nodes from Fas 'knockout' mice. Lymph nodes and spleen from wild type versus Fas knockout mice are compared. Both organs are increased approximately 20-fold in size in the knockout due to accumulation of excess T- and B-cells due to a failure of peripheral deletion in these animals. (Kindly provided by Professor Shigekazu Nagata and adapted from Adachi *et al.*, 1995 *Nature Genetics* **11**, 294, with permission.)

Figure 6.37. Analysis of apoptosis by Annexin V-labeling. Phosphatidylserine (PS) is externalized on the outer leaflet of the plasma membrane during apoptosis and this can be readily detected using the PS-binding protein, Annexin V. (a) Untreated human T-lymphoblastoid cells and (b) apoptotic T-lymphoblastoid cells were stained with FITC-conjugated annexin V. (Data kindly provided by Dr Gabriela Brumatti.)

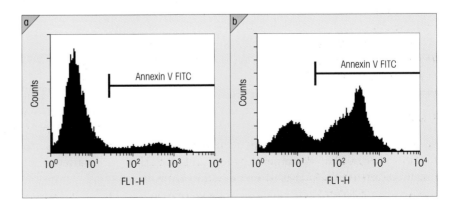

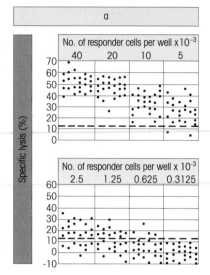

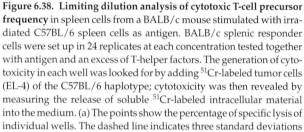

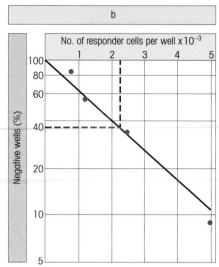

Figure 6.38. Limiting dilution analysis of cytotoxic T-cell precursor frequency in spleen cells from a BALB/c mouse stimulated with irradiated C57BL/6 spleen cells as antigen. BALB/c splenic responder cells were set up in 24 replicates at each concentration tested together with antigen and an excess of T-helper factors. The generation of cytotoxicity in each well was looked for by adding ^{51}Cr-labeled tumor cells (EL-4) of the C57BL/6 haplotype; cytotoxicity was then revealed by measuring the release of soluble ^{51}Cr-labeled intracellular material into the medium. (a) The points show the percentage of specific lysis of individual wells. The dashed line indicates three standard deviations above the medium release control, and each point above that line is counted as positive for cytotoxicity. (b) The data replotted in terms of the percentage of negative wells at each concentration of responder cells over the range in which the data titrated (5×10^{-3}/well to 0.625×10^{-3}/well). The dashed line is drawn at 37% negative wells and this intersects the regression line to give a precursor (T_{cp}) frequency of 1 in 2327 responder cells. The regression line has an r^2 value of 1.00 in this experiment. (Reproduced with permission from Simpson E. & Chandler P. (1986) In Weir D.M. (ed.) *Handbook of Experimental Immunology*, figure 68.2. Blackwell Scientific Publications, Oxford.)

In the case of B-cells this is fairly straightforward given that their antigen receptors recognize native antigen. However, it is only recently that technical finesse, in the form of peptide–MHC tetramers, has brought this technique to T-cells (figure 6.39). This approach overcomes the problem of the relatively weak intrinsic affinity of TCR for peptide–MHC by presenting a tagged peptide–MHC as a multivalent tetramer, thereby exploiting the bonus effect of multivalency (cf. p. 94). Peptide–MHC complexes are produced by permitting recombinant MHC molecules to refold with the appropriate synthetic peptide. The recombinant MHC molecules are biotinylated on a special carboxy-terminal extension, which ensures that the biotin is incorporated at a distance from the site to which the TCR binds, and mixed with fluorescently labeled streptavidin, which not only binds biotin with a very high affinity but also has a valency of four with respect to the biotin—hence the formation of tetramers.

Numerous adaptations of this technology are appearing. For example, incubation of tetramers bound to their cognate TCR leads to internalization at 37°C; by tagging them with a toxin individual T-lymphocytes of a single specificity can be eliminated. Another approach is to use the FACS to directly sort stained cells into an ELISPOT microtiter plate in which cytokine secretion is measured, providing a functional analysis of the cells.

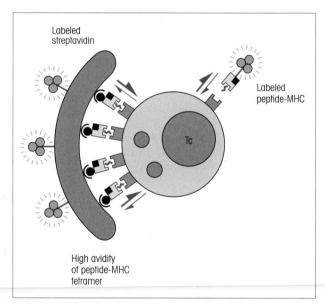

Figure 6.39. Peptide–MHC tetramer. A single fluorochrome-labeled peptide–MHC complex (top right) has only a low affinity for the TCR and therefore provides a very insensitive probe for its cognate receptor. However, by biotinylating (•) the MHC molecules and then mixing them with streptavidin, which has a valency of four with respect to biotin binding, a tetrameric complex is formed which has a much higher functional affinity (avidity) when used as a probe for the specific TCRs on the T-cell surface.

Enumeration of antibody-forming cells

The immunofluorescence sandwich test

This is a double-layer procedure designed to visualize specific intracellular antibody. If, for example, we wished to see how many cells in a preparation of lymphoid tissue were synthesizing antibody to *Pneumococcus* polysaccharide, we would first fix the cells with ethanol to prevent the antibody being washed away during the test, and then treat with a solution of the polysaccharide antigen. After washing, a fluorescein-labeled antibody to the polysaccharide would then be added to locate those cells which had specifically bound the antigen.

The name of the test derives from the fact that antigen is sandwiched between the antibody present in the cell substrate and that added as the second layer (figure 6.8c).

Plaque techniques

Antibody-secreting cells can be counted by diluting them in an environment in which the antibody formed by each individual cell produces a readily observable effect. In one technique, developed from the original method of Jerne and Nordin, the cells from an animal immunized with sheep erythrocytes are suspended together with an excess of sheep red cells and complement within a shallow chamber formed between two microscope slides. On incubation, the antibody-forming cells release their immunoglobulin which coats the surrounding erythrocytes. The complement will then cause lysis of the coated cells and a **plaque**

clear of red cells will be seen around each antibody-forming cell (figure 6.40). Direct plaques obtained in this way largely reveal IgM producers since this antibody has a high hemolytic efficiency. To demonstrate IgG synthesizing cells it is necessary to increase the complement binding of the erythrocyte–IgG antibody complex by adding a rabbit anti-IgG serum; the 'indirect plaques' thus developed can be used to enumerate cells making antibodies in different immunoglobulin subclasses, provided that the appropriate rabbit antisera are available. The method can be extended by coating an antigen such as *Pneumococcus* polysaccharide on to the red cell, or by coupling hapten groups to the erythrocyte surface.

In the **ELISPOT** modification, the antibody-forming cell suspension is incubated in microtiter wells containing filters coated with antigen. The secreted antibody is captured locally and is visualized, after removal of the cells, by treatment with enzyme-labeled anti-Ig and development of the color reaction with the substrate. The macroscopic spots can be readily enumerated (figure 6.41).

Analysis of functional activity by cellular reconstitution

Radiation chimeras

The entire populations of lymphocytes and polymorphs can be inactivated by appropriate doses of X-irradiation. Animals ablated in such a way may be reconstituted by injection of bone marrow hematopoietic stem cells which provide the precursors of all the formed elements of the blood (cf. figure 11.1). These chimeras of host plus

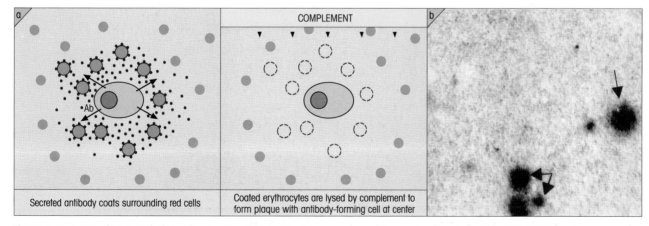

Figure 6.40. Jerne plaque technique for enumerating antibody-forming cells (Cunningham modification). (a) The *direct* technique for cells synthesizing IgM hemolysin is shown. The *indirect* technique for visualizing cells producing IgG hemolysins requires the addition of anti-IgG to the system. The difference between the plaques obtained by direct and indirect methods gives the number of 'IgG' plaques. The *reverse plaque* assay enumerates total Ig-producing cells by capturing secreted Ig on red cells coated with anti-Ig. Multiple plaque assays can be carried out by a modification using microtiter plates. (b) Photograph of plaques which show as circular dark areas (some of which are arrowed) under dark-ground illumination. They vary in size depending upon the antibody affinity and the rate of secretion by the antibody-forming cell. (Courtesy of C. Shapland, P. Hutchings and Professor D. Male.)

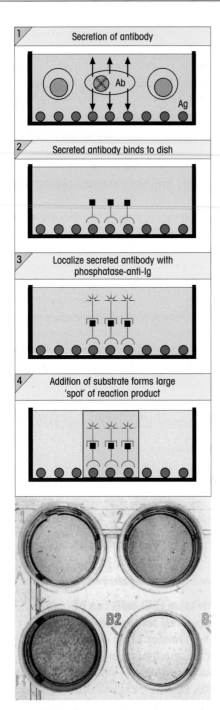

Figure 6.41. ELISPOT (from ELISA spot) system for enumerating antibody-forming cells. The picture shows spots formed by hybridoma cells making autoantibodies to thyroglobulin revealed by alkaline phosphatase-linked anti-Ig (courtesy of P. Hutchings). Increasing numbers of hybridoma cells were added to the top two and bottom left-hand wells which show corresponding increases in the number of 'ELISPOTs'. The bottom right-hand well is a control using a hybridoma of irrelevant specificity.

hematopoietic grafted cells can be manipulated in many ways to analyze cellular function, such as the role of the thymus in the maturation of T-lymphocytes from bone marrow stem cells (figure 6.42).

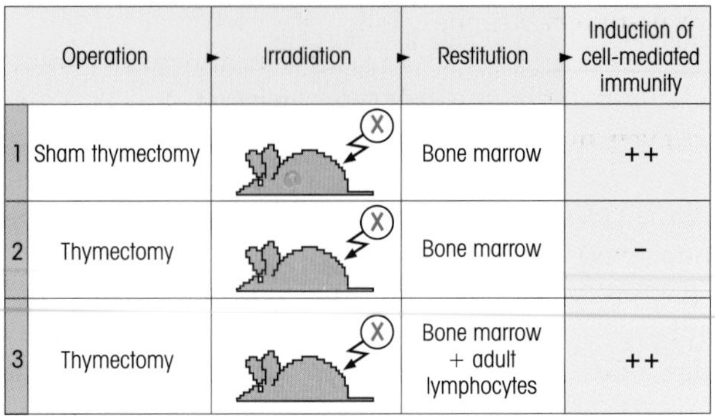

	Operation	Irradiation	Restitution	Induction of cell-mediated immunity
1	Sham thymectomy	(X)	Bone marrow	+ +
2	Thymectomy	(X)	Bone marrow	−
3	Thymectomy	(X)	Bone marrow + adult lymphocytes	+ +

Figure 6.42. Maturation of bone marrow stem cells under the influence of the thymus to become immunocompetent lymphocytes capable of cell-mediated immune reactions. X-irradiation (X) destroys the ability of host lymphocytes to mount a cellular immune response, but the stem cells in injected bone marrow can become immunocompetent and restore the response (1) unless the thymus is removed (2), in which case only already immunocompetent lymphocytes are effective (3). Incidentally, the bone marrow stem cells also restore the levels of other formed elements of the blood (red cells, platelets, neutrophils, monocytes) which otherwise fall dramatically after X-irradiation, and such therapy is crucial in cases where accidental or therapeutic exposure to X-rays or other antimitotic agents seriously damages the hematopoietic cells.

Mice with severe combined immunodeficiency (SCID)

Mice with defects in the genes encoding the IL-2 receptor γ chain, the nucleotide salvage pathway enzymes adenosine deaminase or purine nucleoside phosphorylase, or the RAG enzymes, develop SCID due to a failure of B- and T-cells to differentiate. These special animals can be reconstituted with various human lymphoid tissues and their functions and responses analyzed. Coimplantation of contiguous fragments of human fetal liver (hematopoietic stem cells) and thymus allows T-lymphopoiesis, production of B-cells and maintenance of colony-forming units of myeloid and erythroid lineages for 6–12 months. Adult peripheral blood cells injected into the peritoneal cavity of SCID mice treated with growth hormone can sustain the production of human B-cells and antibodies and can be used to generate human hybridomas making defined monoclonal antibodies. Immunotherapeutic antitumor responses can also be played with in these animals.

Cellular interactions in vitro

It is obvious that the methods outlined earlier for depletion, enrichment and isolation of individual cell populations enable the investigator to study cellular interactions through judicious recombinations. These interactions are usually more effective when the cells are operating within some sort of stromal network resembling the set-up of the tissues where their function is optimally expressed. For example, colonization of murine fetal thymus rudiments in culture with T-cell precursors enables one to follow the pattern of proliferation, maturation, TCR rearrangement and positive and negative selection normally seen *in vivo* (cf. pp. 233–234). An even more refined system involves the addition of selected lymphoid populations to disaggregated stromal cells derived from fetal thymic lobes depleted of endogenous lymphoid cells with deoxyguanosine. The cells can be spun into a pellet and cocultured in hanging drops; on transfer to normal organ culture conditions after a few hours, reaggregation to intact lobes takes place quite magically and the various differentiation and maturation processes then unfold.

GENETIC ENGINEERING OF CELLS

Insertion and modification of genes in mammalian cells

Because gene transfer into primary (i.e. untransformed) mammalian cells is inefficient, it is customary to use immortal cell lines for such **transfections** and to include a selectable marker such as neomycin resistance. Genes can be introduced into cells using bacterial plasmid vectors; however, because cells do not readily take up free DNA, methods to improve the rate of uptake have been developed. Increased uptake can be achieved through precipitating plasmid DNA using calcium phosphate or by electroporation where an electric current is used to open transient pores in the plasma membrane. Another approach is to incorporate the plasmid into liposomes which fuse with the cell membrane. Direct microinjection of DNA is also effective but is labor intensive and requires specialized equipment. Integration of the gene into the genome of a virus such as vaccinia provides an easy ride into the cell, although more stable long-term transfections are obtained with modified retroviral vectors. One of the latest fads is transfection by biolistics, the buzz word for biological ballistics. DNA coated on to gold microparticles is literally fired from a high-pressure helium gun and penetrates the cells; even plant cells with their cellulose coats are easy meat for this technology. Skin and surgically exposed tissues can also be penetrated with ease.

Studying the effect of *adding* a gene, then, does not offer too many technological problems. How does one assess the impact of *removing* a gene? One versatile strategy to delete endogenous gene function is to target the gene's mRNA as distinct from the gene itself. Nucleotide sequences complementary to the mRNA of the target gene are introduced into the cell, usually in a form which allows them to replicate. The **antisense** molecules so produced base pair with the target mRNA and block translation into protein. Although antisense RNA approaches showed early promise, this approach has been largely superseded by a recent innovation called **RNA interference (RNAi)**.

RNAi can be used to 'knock down' expression of particular target genes within a cell by introducing a double-stranded (ds) RNA molecule homologous to the target gene. This method takes advantage of a natural antiviral system that selectively targets mRNA when it is detected in double-stranded form in the cell; normally dsRNA spells trouble, as this form of RNA is rarely present in cells unless they are infected by a virus. The cellular machinery that naturally responds to dsRNA selectively degrades only mRNAs that are homologous to the dsRNA molecule that initiated the response. In theory, this can be mimicked by synthesizing a dsRNA copy of the gene to be silenced and introducing this into the cell; in practice there are problems with this approach when using mammalian cells and so an alternative strategy is widely employed (figure 6.43). Short-interfering RNA (siRNA) molecules of 21–25 nucleotides, homologous to the gene of interest, can be synthesized and these overcome some of the nonspecific effects seen with large dsRNA molecules. Because of the simplicity of the siRNA approach, genome-wide cell-based screens are underway to knockdown essen-

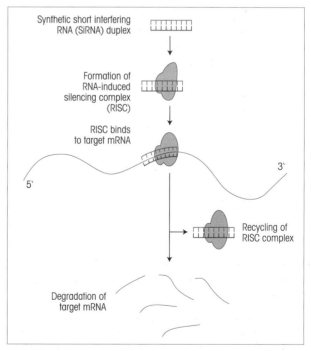

Figure 6.43. Gene silencing via siRNA. Synthetic short-interfering double-stranded RNA molecules (siRNAs), complementary to a gene of interest, are introduced into cells by transfection and, in complex with proteins within the transfected cell, lead to the formation of an RNA-induced silencing complex (RISC) which binds to mRNA molecules complementary to the introduced siRNA. This results in degradation of the target mRNA and recycling of the RISC to target additional mRNA molecules.

tially every gene in the genome and explore the consequences of this. It is important to note however that gene knockdown approaches are rarely, if ever, 100% effective and there is always the uncertainty that any observed effects could also be due to unintentional silencing of other genes along with the gene of interest.

Introducing new genes into animals

Establishing 'designer mice' bearing new genes
Female mice are induced to superovulate and are then mated. The fertilized eggs are microinjected with the gene and surgically implanted in females. Between 5% and 40% of the implanted oocytes develop to term and, of these, 10–25% have copies of the injected gene, stably integrated into their chromosomes, detectable by PCR. These 'founder' transgenic animals are mated with non-transgenic mice and pure transgenic lines are eventually established (figure 6.44).

Expression of the transgene can be directed to particular tissues if the relevant promoter is included in the construct, for example the thyroglobulin promoter will

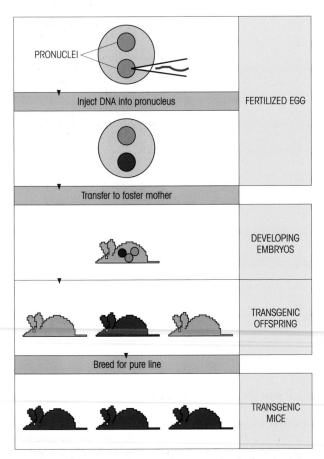

Figure 6.44. Production of pure strain transgenic mice by microinjection of fertilized egg, implantation into a foster mother and subsequent inbreeding.

confine expression to the thyroid. A different approach is to switch a gene on and off at will by incorporating an inducible promoter. Thus, the metallothionine promoter will enable expression of its linked gene only if zinc is added to the drinking water given to the mice. One needs to confirm that only the desired expression is obtained as, in some situations, promoters may misbehave leading to 'leaky' expression of the associated gene.

Transgenes introduced into embryonic stem cells
Embryonic stem (ES) cells can be obtained by culturing the inner cell mass of mouse blastocysts. After transfection with the appropriate gene, the transfected cells can be selected and reimplanted after injection into a new blastocyst. The resulting mice are chimeric, in that some cells carry the transgene and others do not. The same will be true of germ cells and, by breeding for germ-line transmission of the transgene, pure strains can be derived (figure 6.45).

The advantage over microinjection is that the cells can be selected after transfection, and this is especially important if **homologous recombination** is required in order to generate '**knockout mice**' lacking the gene which has been targeted. In this case, a DNA sequence which will disrupt the reading frame of the endogenous gene is inserted into the ES cells. Because homologous recombination is a rare event compared to random integration, selectable markers are incorporated into the construct in order to transfer only those ES cells in which the endogenous gene has been deleted (figure 6.46). This is a truly powerful technology and the whole biological community has been suffused with boxing fever, knocking out genes right, left and center. Just a few examples of knockout mice of interest to immunologists are listed in table 6.2.

It is not a particularly rare finding to observe that knocking out a gene leads to unexpected developmental defects. Whilst this in itself can provide important information concerning the role of the gene in developmental processes, it can frustrate the original aim of the experiment. Indeed, a number of knockouts are nonviable due to embryonic lethality. Never fear, ingenuity once again triumphs, in this case by the harnessing of viral or yeast recombinase systems. Instead of using a nonfunctional gene to create the knockout mouse, the targeting construct contains the normal form of the gene but flanked with recognition sequences (*loxP* sites) for a recombinase enzyme called Cre. These mice are mated with transgenic mice containing the bacteriophage P1-derived *Cre* transgene linked to an inducible or tissue-specific promoter. The endogenous gene of interest will be deleted only when and where Cre is expressed

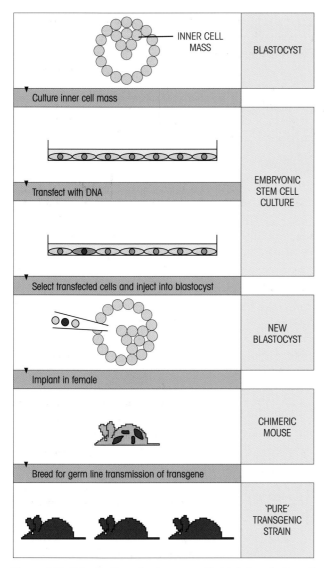

Figure 6.45. Introduction of a transgene through transfection of embryonic stem cells. The transfected cells can be selected, e.g. for homologous recombinant 'knockouts', before reimplantation.

thereby creating a **tissue-specific** or **conditional knock-out** (figure 6.47). The Cre/*loxP* system can also be organized in such a way as to turn on expression of a gene by incorporating a stop sequence flanked by *loxP* sites.

Mice in which an endogenous gene is purposefully replaced by a functional gene, be it a modified version of the original gene or an entirely different gene, are referred to as **'knocked in mice'**. Hence, in the example above, knocking in a *loxP* flanked gene leads eventually to a knocked out gene in a selected cell type.

Table 6.2. Some gene 'knockouts' and their effects.

Knockout target	Phenotype of knockout mice
CD8 α-chain	Absence of cytotoxic T-cells
p59 *fynT*	Defective signaling in thymocytes but not peripheral T-cells
HOX 11	No spleen
FcεRI α-chain	Resistant to cutaneous and systemic anaphylaxis
IgM μ-chain membrane exon	Absence of B-cells
IL-6	No bone loss when ovariectomized (implications for osteoporosis?)
IL-18	Susceptible to *Leishmania major*; shift from Th1 to Th2 response (decreased IFNγ and increased IL-4 production)
MHC class II Aβ	Decreased CD4 T-cells; inflammatory bowel disease
Perforin	Impaired CTL and NK cell function
TAP1	Lack CD8 cells
TNFR-1	Resistant to endotoxic shock; susceptible to *Listeria*

Modified from Brandon (1995) *Current Biology* **5**, 625.

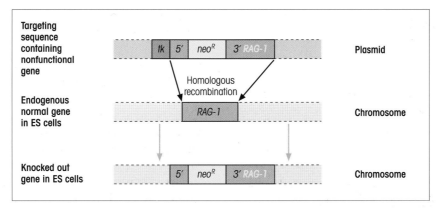

Figure 6.46. Gene disruption by homologous recombination with plasmid DNA containing a copy of the gene of interest (in this example *RAG-1*) into which a sequence specifying neomycin resistance (*neo^R*) has been inserted in such a way as to destroy the *RAG-1* reading frame between the 5′ and 3′ ends of the gene. Embryonic stem (ES) cells in which the targeting sequence has been incorporated into the chromosomal DNA by homologous recombination will be resistant to the neomycin analog G418. Stem cells in which nonhomologous recombination into chromosomal DNA has occurred would additionally incorporate the *thymidine kinase* (*tk*) gene which can be used to destroy such cells by culturing them in the presence of ganciclovir, leaving only ES cells in which homologous recombination has been achieved. These are then used to create a knockout mouse.

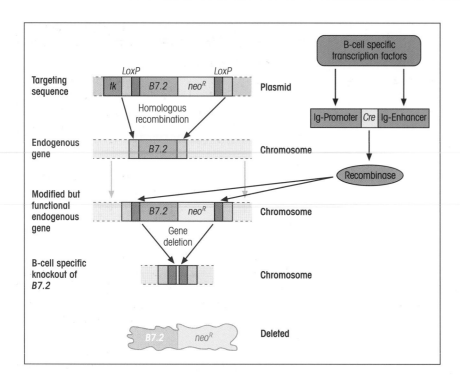

Figure 6.47. Conditional knockout. The endogenous gene that is under study (here *B7.2*) is homologously replaced in ES cells with an identical gene, as in figure 6.46, but here flanked by *loxP* sequences (brown boxes) and with the *neo^R* gene incorporated in a nondisruptive manner purely for selection purposes. Nonhomologous recombinants will contain the *tk* gene and are eliminated using ganciclovir. Transgenic animals are then generated from ES cells which are resistant to G418. If homozygous *B7.2–loxP* transgenics are mated with mice which contain a transgene for the Cre recombinase under the control of specific regulatory elements, only those cells in which the promoter is active will produce the Cre enzyme necessary to delete the sequence flanked by *loxP*. The example given would represent an experiment aimed at investigating the effect of specifically knocking out *B7.2* in B-cells whilst maintaining its expression in, for example, dendritic cells.

Gene therapy in humans

We seem to be catching up with science fiction and are in the early stages of being able to correct genetic misfortune by the introduction of 'good' genes. For example, one form of severe combined immunodeficiency (SCID) is due to a mutation in the γc gene which encodes a subunit of the cytokine receptors for IL-2, -4, -7, -9, -15 and -21. Correction of this defect in children has been achieved by *in vitro* transfer of the normal gene into CD34+ bone marrow stem cells using a vector derived from a Moloney retrovirus, a convincing proof of principle for human gene therapy.

Major problems yet to be overcome concern both the *efficiency* of delivery of replacement genes as well as *targeting* of the gene-delivery vector to the desired cell population. Where it is possible to remove the target cell population and treat *ex vivo* the risk of mis-targeting to other tissues is diminished but not entirely eliminated. In situations where the target tissue cannot be removed for treatment, the efficiency of gene delivery can be poor.

Other risks include insertion of the replacement gene at random chromosomal sites; insertion into a tumor suppressor gene for example would be highly undesirable and may lead to tumor development. Some gene delivery vectors such as adeno-associated virus (AAV) insert at predictable chromosomal locations and seem the way forward in this regard. This still leaves the problem of efficient gene delivery *in vivo*. Viruses represent the most efficient gene delivery vehicles, being perfectly adapted to the task of invading human tissues and inserting their genomes. Thus it is not surprising that the most promising gene delivery vectors are currently assembled around modified forms of adenovirus, AAV, and lentiviruses such as HIV. Ironically, the immune system turns out to be one of the biggest obstacles to efficient gene delivery due to robust immune responses agains these viral vectors. However, some viruses (such as AAV) provoke only modest or ineffective immune responses which can be exploited, in this instance at least, to our benefit.

SUMMARY

Making antibodies to order

• Polyclonal antisera can be generated by repeated immunization with antigen.

• Polyclonal antibodies recognize a mixture of determinants on the antigen.

• Adjuvants are required for efficient immune responses to antigen.

• Immortal hybridoma cell lines making monoclonal antibodies provide powerful immunological reagents and insights into the immune response. Applications include enumeration of lymphocyte subpopulations, cell depletion, immunoassay, cancer diagnosis and imaging, purification of antigen from complex mixtures, and recently the use of monoclonals as artificial enzymes (catalytic antibodies).

• Genetically engineered human antibody fragments can be derived by expanding the V_H and V_L genes from unimmunized, but preferably immunized, donors and expressing them as completely randomized combinatorial libraries on the surface of bacteriophage. Phages bearing the highest affinity antibodies are selected by panning on antigens and the antibody genes can then be cloned from the isolated viruses.

• Single-chain Fv (scFv) fragments encoded by linked V_H and V_L genes and even single heavy chain domains can be created.

• The human anti-mouse antibody (HAMA) response is a significant obstacle to use of mouse monoclonal antibodies for therapeutic purposes.

• The HAMA response against mouse monoclonal antibodies can be reduced by producing chimeric antibodies with mouse variable regions and human constant regions or, better still, using humanized antibodies in which all the mouse sequences except for the CDRs are replaced by human sequences.

• Humanized antibodies are now in clinical use for the treatment of a variety of conditions such as rheumatoid arthritis and B-cell lymphoma.

• Transgenic mice bearing human Ig genes can be immunized. The mice produce high affinity fully human antibodies.

• Recombinant antibodies can be expressed on a large scale in plants.

• Combinatorial libraries of diabodies containing the H1 and H2 V_H CDR may be used to develop new drugs.

Purification of antigen and antibody by affinity chromatography

• Insoluble immunoabsorbents prepared by coupling antibody to Sepharose can be used to affinity-purify antigens from complex mixtures and reciprocally to purify antibodies.

• Affinity chromatography can also be used to co-purify proteins that serve as binding partners of antigens.

Modulation of biological activity

• Antibodies can be detected by inhibition of biological functions such as viral infectivity or bacterial growth.

• Inhibition of biological function by known antibodies helps to define the role of the antigen, be it a hormone or cytokine for example, in complex responses *in vivo* and *in vitro*.

• Activation of biological function by receptor-stimulating or receptor-crosslinking antibodies can substitute for natural ligand and can be used to explore biological function *in vitro* or *in vivo*.

Immunodetection of antigen in cells and tissues

• Antibodies can be used as highly specific probes to detect the presence of antigen in a tissue and to explore the subcellular localization of antigen. Antigens can be localized if stained by fluorescent antibodies and viewed in a fluorescence microscope.

• Fixation and permeabilization of cells permits entry of antibodies and allows intracellular antigens to be detected.

• Confocal microscopy scans a very thin plane at high magnification and provides quantitative data on extremely sharp images of the antigen-containing structures which can also be examined in three dimensions.

• Antibodies can either be labeled directly or visualized by a secondary antibody, a labeled anti-Ig.

• Different fluorescent labels can be conjugated to secondary antibodies enabling simultaneous detection of several different antigens in the same cell.

• Flow cytometry is a highly quantitative means of detecting fluorescence associated with immunolabeled or dye-labeled cells and thousands of cells per minute can be analyzed by such instruments.

• In a flow cytometer single cells in individual droplets are interrogated by one or more lasers and quantitative data using different fluorescent labels can be logged, giving a complex phenotypic analysis of each cell in a heterogeneous mixture. In addition, forward scatter of the laser light defines cell size and 90° scatter, cell granularity.

• Fluorescent antibodies or their fragments can also be used for staining intracellular antigens in permeabilized cells. Intracellular probes for pH, Ca^{2+}, Mg^{2+}, Na^+, thiols and DNA content are also available.

• Antibodies can be enzyme-labeled for histochemical definition of antigens at the light microscope level, or coupled with different-sized colloidal gold particles for ultrastructural visualization in the electron microscope.

Detection and quantitation of antigen by antibody

• Exceedingly low concentrations of antigens can be measured by immunoassay techniques which depend upon the

(Continued p.152)

Storch W.B. (2000) *Immunofluorescence in Clinical Immunology: A Primer and Atlas.* Birkhäuser Verlag AG, Basel.

Vaughan T.J. *et al.* (1996) Human antibodies with subnanomolar affinities isolated from a large nonimmunized phage display library. *Nature Biotechnology* **14**, 309–314.

Weir D.M. *et al.* (eds) (1996) *Handbook of Experimental Immunology*, 5th edn. Blackwell Scientific Publications, Oxford.

Zola H. (1999) *Monoclonal Antibodies.* Bios Scientific Publishers, Oxford.

7 The anatomy of the immune response

INTRODUCTION

Immunologists from the far corners of the world who have produced monoclonal antibodies directed to surface molecules on B- and T-cells, macrophages, neutrophils and natural killer (NK) cells, and so on, get together every so often to compare the specificities of their reagents in international workshops whose spirit of cooperation should be a lesson to most politicians. Where a cluster of monoclonals are found to react with the same polypeptide, they clearly represent a series of reagents defining a given marker and are labeled with a CD (**cluster of differentiation**) number. Currently, there are nearly 340 CD numbers assigned, with some of them having subdivisions, but those in table 7.1 are most relevant to our discussions. It is important to appreciate that the expression level of cell surface molecules often changes as cells differentiate or become activated and that 'subpopulations' of cells exist which differentially express particular molecules. When expressed at a low level the 'presence' or 'absence' of a given CD antigen may be rather subjective, but be aware that low level expression does not necessarily imply biological irrelevance.

THE NEED FOR ORGANIZED LYMPHOID TISSUE

For an effective immune response, an intricate series of cellular events must occur. Antigen must bind and if necessary be processed by antigen-presenting cells, which must then make contact with and activate T- and B-cells; T-helpers must assist B-cells and cytotoxic T-cell precursors, and there have to be mechanisms which amplify the numbers of potential effector cells by proliferation and then bring about differentiation to generate the mediators of humoral and cellular immunity. In addition, memory cells for secondary responses must be formed and the whole response controlled so that it is adequate but not excessive and is appropriate to the type of infection being dealt with. By working hard, we can isolate component cells of the immune system and persuade them to carry out a number of responses to antigen in the test-tube, but compared with the efficacy of the overall development of immunity in the body, our efforts still leave much to be desired. *In vivo* the integration of the complex cellular interactions which form the basis of the immune response takes place within the organized architecture of peripheral, or secondary, lymphoid tissue which includes the lymph nodes, spleen and unencapsulated tissue lining the respiratory, gastrointestinal and genitourinary tracts.

These tissues become populated by cells of reticular origin and by macrophages and lymphocytes derived from bone marrow hematopoietic stem cells, the T-cells first differentiating into immunocompetent cells by a high-pressure training period in the thymus, the B-cells undergoing their education in the bone marrow itself (figure 7.1). In essence, the lymph nodes receive antigen either draining directly from the tissues or carried by MHC class II$^+$ dendritic cells, the spleen monitors the blood and the unencapsulated lymphoid tissue is strategically integrated into mucosal surfaces of the body as a forward defensive system based on IgA secretion.

The anatomical disposition of these lymphoid tissues is illustrated in figure 7.2. The lymphatics and associated lymph nodes form an impressive network, draining the viscera and the more superficial body structures before returning to the blood by way of the thoracic duct (figure 7.3).

Communication between these tissues and the rest of the body is maintained by a pool of recirculating lym-

Table 7.1. Some of the major clusters of differentiation (CD) markers on human cells.

CD	Expression	Functions
CD1	IDC, B subset	Presents glycolipid and other non-peptide antigens to T-cells
CD2	T, NK	Receptor for CD58 (LFA-3) costimulator
CD3	T	Transducing elements of T-cell receptor
CD4	MHC class II restricted T, Mo, Mφ, IDC	Receptor for MHC class II
CD5	T, B subset	Involved in antigen receptor signaling
CD8	MHC class I restricted T	Receptor for MHC class I
CD14	G, Mo, Mφ	Receptor for LPS/LBP complex
CD16	G, NK, B, Mφ, IDC	FcγRIII (medium affinity IgG receptor)
CD19	B, FDC	Part of B-cell antigen receptor complex
CD20	B	Provides signals for B cell activation and proliferation
CD21	B, FDC	CR2. Receptor for C3d and Epstein–Barr virus. Part of B-cell antigen receptor complex
CD23	B, Mo, FDC	FcεRII (low affinity IgE receptor)
CD25	*T, *B, *Mo, *Mφ	IL-2 receptor α chain
CD28	T, *B	Receptor for CD80/CD86 (B7.1 and B7.2) costimulators
CD32	Mo, Mφ, IDC, FDC, G, NK, B	FcγRII (low affinity IgG receptor)
CD34	Progenitors	Adhesion molecule. Stem cell marker
CD40	B, Mφ, IDC, FDC	Receptor for CD154 (CD40L) costimulator
CD45RA	Resting/Naive T-cells, B, G, Mo, NK	Phosphatase, cell activation
CD45RO	Effector T-cell Mo, Mφ, IDC	Phosphatase, cell activation
CD64	Mo, Mφ, DC	FcγRI (high affinity IgG receptor)
CD79a/CD79b	B	Igα/Igβ transducing elements of B-cell receptor
CD80	*B, *T, Mφ, DC	B7.1 receptor for CD28 costimulator and for CTLA4 inhibitory signal
CD86	B, IDC, Mo	B7.2 receptor for CD28 costimulator and for CTLA4 inhibitory signal
CD95	Widespread	Fas receptor for FasL (CD178). Transmits apoptotic signals

*, activated; B, B-lymphocytes; FDC, follicular dendritic cells; G, granulocytes; IDC, interdigitating dendritic cells; Mast, mast cells; Mφ, macrophages; Mo, monocytes; NK, natural killer cells; T, T-lymphocytes.

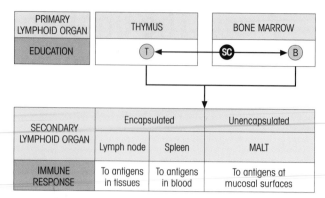

Figure 7.1. The functional organization of lymphoid tissue. Hematopoietic stem cells (SC) arising in the bone marrow differentiate into immunocompetent T- and B-cells in the primary lymphoid organs and then colonize the secondary lymphoid tissues where immune responses are organized. The mucosa-associated lymphoid tissue (MALT) together with diffuse collections of cells in the lamina propria and the lungs produces antibodies for mucosal secretions.

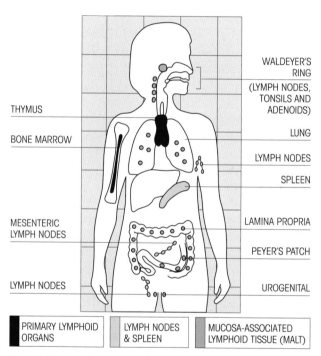

Figure 7.2. The distribution of major lymphoid organs and tissues throughout the body.

LYMPHOCYTES TRAFFIC BETWEEN LYMPHOID TISSUES

This traffic of lymphocytes between the tissues, the bloodstream and the lymph nodes enables antigen-sensitive cells to seek the antigen and to be recruited to sites at which a response is occurring, while the dissemination of memory cells and their progeny enables a more widespread response to be organized throughout the lymphoid system. Thus, antigen-reactive cells are

phocytes which pass from the blood into the lymph nodes, spleen and other tissues and back to the blood by the major lymphatic channels such as the thoracic duct (figures 7.4 and 7.12).

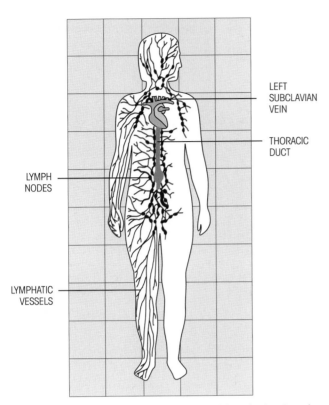

Figure 7.3. The network of lymph nodes and lymphatics. Lymph nodes occur at junctions of the draining lymphatics. The lymph finally collects in the thoracic duct and thence returns to the bloodstream via the left subclavian vein.

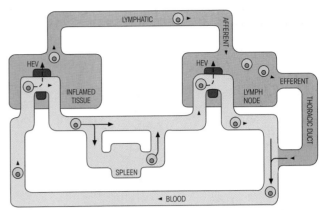

Figure 7.4. Traffic and recirculation of lymphocytes through encapsulated lymphoid tissue and sites of inflammation. Blood-borne lymphocytes enter the tissues and lymph nodes passing through the high-walled endothelium of the postcapillary venules (HEV) and leave via the draining lymphatics. The efferent lymphatics join to form the thoracic duct which returns the lymphocytes to the bloodstream. In the spleen, which lacks HEVs, lymphocytes enter the lymphoid area (white pulp) from the arterioles, pass to the sinusoids of the erythroid area (red pulp) and leave by the splenic vein. Traffic through the mucosal immune system is elaborated in figure 7.12.

depleted from the circulating pool of lymphocytes within 24 hours of antigen first localizing in the lymph nodes or spleen; several days later, after proliferation at the site of antigen localization, a peak of activated cells appears in the thoracic duct. When antigen reaches a lymph node in a primed animal, there is a dramatic fall in the output of cells in the efferent lymphatics, a phenomenon described variously as 'cell shutdown' or 'lymphocyte trapping' and which is thought to result from the antigen-induced release of soluble factors from T-cells (cf. the cytokines, p. 185); this is followed by an output of activated blast cells which peaks at around 80 hours.

Naive lymphocytes home to lymph nodes

Naive lymphocytes enter a lymph node through the afferent lymphatics and by guided passage across the specialized **high-walled endothelium of the postcapillary venules (HEVs)** (figure 7.5). Their destination is determined by a series of **homing receptors** which include members of the **integrin** superfamily (table 7.2), chemokine receptors and selectins. Integrins can bind to extracellular matrix, plasma proteins and to other cell surface molecules, and they are widely involved in

embryogenesis, cell growth, differentiation, adhesion, motility, programed cell death and tissue maintenance. Within the immune system their complementary ligands include cell surface **vascular addressins** such as highly glycosylated and sulfated sialomucins present only on the HEVs of the appropriate blood vessels, in this case peripheral lymph nodes (figure 7.6). Chemokines presented by vascular endothelium play a key role in triggering lymphocyte arrest, the chemokine receptors on the lymphocyte being involved both in binding to their ligand and in the functional activation of integrins. Thus, naive lymphocytes, and also dendritic cells, express CCR7 and are therefore directed into peripheral lymph nodes by virtue of the fact that the HEVs in the nodes have CCL19 and CCL21 (cf. table 9.3) on their luminal surface. Whilst CCL21 is produced by the endothelial cells themselves, CCL19 is secreted by local stromal cells and subsequently transferred to the HEV. The *plt/plt* mouse, which lacks expression of both of these chemokines, not unsurprisingly exhibits defective T-cell migration into peripheral lymph nodes. Chemokine activation of integrins occurs as a result of the chemokine signals facilitating their lateral mobility in the cell membrane and also by inducing structural changes in the integrins which results in a state of increased affinity.

Transmigration occurs in three stages

Step 1: Tethering and rolling
In order for the lymphocyte to become attached to the

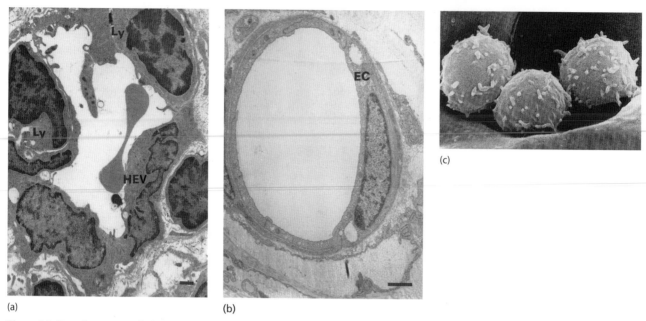

Figure 7.5. Lymphocyte association with postcapillary venules. (a) High-walled endothelial venules (HEV) in rat cervical lymph nodes showing intimate association with lymphocytes (Ly). (b) Flattened capillary endothelial cell (EC) for comparison. (c) Lymphocytes adhering to HEV (scanning electron micrograph). ((a) and (b) Kindly provided by Dr Ann Ager and (c) by Dr W. van Ewijk.)

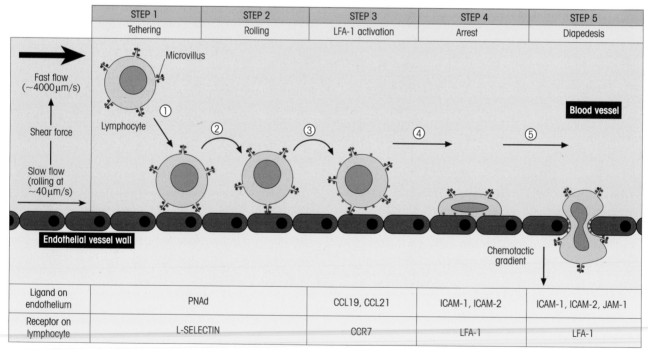

Figure 7.6. Homing and transmigration of lymphocytes into peripheral lymph nodes. Fast-moving lymphocytes are tethered (Step 1) to the vessel walls of the tissue they are being guided to enter through an interaction between specific homing receptors, such as L-selectin (•) located on the microvilli of the lymphocyte, and its peripheral node addressin (PNAd) ligands on the HEV of the vessel wall. PNAd comprises several molecules, including CD34 and GlyCAM-1, which possess fucosylated, sulfated and sialylated Lewis^x structures. Various chemokine receptors (•) are also present on these T- and B-cells. After rolling along the surface of the endothelial cells (Step 2), activation of the lymphocyte LFA-1 integrin (•) (cf. table 7.2) occurs (Step 3) in response to stimulation by chemokines. For T-cells this step is mainly regulated by CCL19 and CCL21 binding to CCR7 as shown, whereas for B-cells CXCL13 binding to CXCR5 provides additional signals. Note that, because LFA-1 is absent from the microvilli, firm binding occurs by the body of the lymphocyte to its ligands, ICAM-1/2, on the endothelium. This process results in cell arrest and flattening (Step 4) followed by migration of the lymphocyte between adjacent endothelial cells, a process referred to as diapedesis which involves LFA-1 binding not only to ICAM-1/2 but additionally to the junctional adhesion molecule-1 (JAM-1) which is present between the endothelial cells (Step 5).

Table 7.2. The integrin superfamily. In general, the integrins are concerned with intercellular adhesion and adhesion to extracellular matrix components. Many of them are also involved in cell signal transduction. They are $\alpha\beta$ heterodimers selected from 18 α chains and 24 β chains which pair to form 24 different combinations. The VLA subfamily took its name from VLA-1 and -2 which appeared as very late antigens (VLA) on T-cells, 2–4 weeks after *in vitro* activation. However, VLA-3, -4 and -5 belong to the same family but are not 'very late' and are found to different extents on lymphocytes, monocytes, platelets and hematopoietic progenitors. A structure called the I (inserted) domain is present in many integrin subunits and contains the metal ion-dependent adhesion site (MIDAS) which, in the presence of Mg^{2+}, is involved in binding the Arg.Gly.Asp. (RGD) motif on many of the ligands essential for cell adhesion.

Integrin	CD designation	Expression	Ligand
$\alpha_1\beta_1$ (VLA-1)	CD49a/CD29	Widespread	LM, CO
$\alpha_2\beta_1$ (VLA-2)	CD49b/CD29	Widespread	LM, CO, CHAD, MMP-1
$\alpha_3\beta_1$ (VLA-3)	CD49c/CD29	Widespread	FN, LM, CO, EN
$\alpha_4\beta_1$ (VLA-4)	CD49d/CD29	Widespread	FN, VCAM-1, OP
$\alpha_5\beta_1$ (VLA-5)	CD49e/CD29	Widespread	FN
$\alpha_6\beta_1$ (VLA-6)	CD49f/CD29	Widespread	LM
$\alpha_7\beta_1$	–/CD29	Widespread	LM
$\alpha_8\beta_1$	–/CD29	Widespread	VN, FN, TN, NN, OP
$\alpha_9\beta_1$	–/CD29	Widespread	TN
$\alpha_{10}\beta_1$	–/CD29	Widespread	CO
$\alpha_{11}\beta_1$	–/CD29	Musculoskeletal	CO
$\alpha_v\beta_1$	CD51/CD29	Most leukocytes	FN, VN
$\alpha_L\beta_2$ (LFA-1)	CD11a/CD18	Most leukocytes	ICAM-1,-2,-3
$\alpha_M\beta_2$ (CR3 [Mac-1])	CD11b/CD18	N, Mo, Mϕ	ICAM-1, C3bi, FG, FX
$\alpha_X\beta_2$ (p150,95)	CD11c/CD18	IDC, IEL, NK, Mo, Mϕ	C3bi, LPS
$\alpha_D\beta_2$	CD11d/CD18	Mϕ	ICAM-3
$\alpha_{IIb}\beta_3$ (GPIIb/IIIa)	CD41/CD61	Megakaryocytes, platelets	FN, VN, FG, VWF, THR
$\alpha_v\beta_3$	CD51/CD61	Widespread	VN, FN, FG, VWF, THR, TN, OP
$\alpha_6\beta_4$	CD49f/CD104	Epithelium, endothelium, Schwann cells, T-cells	LM
$\alpha_v\beta_5$	CD51/–	Widespread	VN
$\alpha_v\beta_6$	CD51/–	Epithelium	FN, TN
$\alpha_4\beta_7$ (LPAM-1)	CD49d/–	T-cells, B-cells	MAdCAM-1, VCAM-1, FN
$\alpha_E\beta_7$	–/–	IEL	E-cadherin
$\alpha_v\beta_8$	CD51/–	Neurons	FN, LM, CO

CHAD, chondroadherin; CO, collagen; CR3, complement receptor 3; EN, entactin; FG, fibrinogen; FN, fibronectin; FX, factor X; GPIIb/IIIa, integrin glycoproteins IIb and IIIa; ICAM, intercellular adhesion molecule; IDC, interdigitating dendritic cell; IEL, intraepithelial lymphocyte; LFA, leukocyte function-associated molecule; LM, laminin; LPAM, lymphocyte Peyer's patch adhesion molecule; Mϕ, macrophage; MAdCAM, mucosal addressin cell adhesion molecule; MMP, matrix metalloproteinase-; Mo, monocyte; N, neutrophil; NK, natural killer cell; NN, nephronectin; OP, osteopontin; THR, thrombospondin; TN, tenascin; VCAM, vascular cell adhesion molecule; VLA, very late antigen (although they are not all expressed late!); VN, vitronectin; VWF, von Willebrand factor. *CD markers are explained on p. 155. –, no CD designation yet assigned.

endothelial cell, it has to overcome the shear forces created by the blood flow. This is effected by a force of attraction between the homing receptors and their ligands on the vessel wall which operates through microvilli on the leukocyte surface (figure 7.6). After this tethering process, the lymphocyte rolls along the endothelial cell, with L-selectin and other adhesion molecules on the lymphocyte binding to their ligands on the endothelium. The selectins generally terminate in a lectin domain (hence 'selectin'), as might be expected given the oligosaccharide nature of the ligands.

Step 2: LFA-1 activation resulting in firm adhesion

This process leads to activation and recruitment of LFA-1 to the nonvillous surface of the lymphocyte. This integrin binds very strongly to ICAM-1 and -2 on the endothelial cell, the intimate contact causing the lymphocyte rolling to be arrested and a flattening of the lymphocyte.

Step 3: Diapedesis

The flattened lymphocyte now uses the LFA-1 to bind to the ICAMs and junctional adhesion molecule-1 (JAM-1) on the endothelial cells to elbow its way between the endothelial cells and into the tissue in response to chemotactic signals.

Lymphocyte homing to other tissues

Homing of activated and memory lymphocytes to other tissues involves a similar process but with different receptors and ligands involved. The codes for skin and gut homing are fairly well established, whilst those for lung and liver are only partially defined (figure 7.7). It appears that dendritic cells from the appropriate tissue play an important role in selectively imprinting the correct address code during their activation of naive T-cells. Cells concerned in mucosal immunity are imprinted to enter Peyer's patches by binding to HEVs in this location. In other cases involving migration into normal and inflamed tissues, the lymphocytes bind to and cross nonspecialized flatter endothelia.

LYMPH NODES

The encapsulated tissue of the lymph node contains a meshwork of reticular cells and their fibers organized into sinuses. These act as a filter for lymph draining the body tissues, and possibly bearing foreign antigens, which enters the subcapsular sinus by the afferent vessels and diffuses past the lymphocytes in the cortex to reach the macrophages of the medullary sinuses

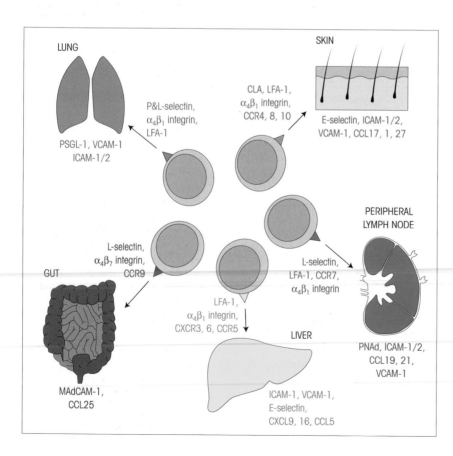

Figure 7.7. Access to tissues require the correct address code. T-cells (and dendritic cells) destined for various locations carry a combination code of cell surface molecules which recognize their respective ligands on the vascular endothelium at their destination. Some ligand–ligand pairs are the same irrespective of the destination tissue, such as LFA-1 binding to ICAM-1 and -2, and $\alpha_4\beta_1$ (VLA-4) integrin binding to VCAM-1. Other interactions utilize adhesion molecules that bind a number of different ligands, each expressed at different locations. Thus, L-selectin recognizes PNAd (peripheral lymph node addressin) on peripheral lymph node endothelium but MAdCAM-1 (mucosal vascular addressin cell adhesion molecule-1), which is also recognized by the $\alpha_4\beta_7$ integrin, on gut endothelium. Both L- and P-selectin bind PSGL-1 (P-selectin glycoprotein ligand-1) on lung endothelium. The recognition of E-selectin by CLA (cutaneous lymphocyte antigen) directs skin bound lymphocytes to the correct location. Chemokine receptors (cf. table 9.3) recognize tissue-specific chemokines.

(figure 7.8a,b) and thence the efferent lymphatics (figures 7.4 and 7.8b). What is so striking about the organization of the lymph node is that the T- and B-lymphocytes are very largely separated into different anatomical compartments, a process directed to a large extent by chemokines. Lymph node stromal cells and

IDCs secrete CCL19 and CCL21 in the T-cell zone which attracts CCR7-bearing T-cells, whilst CXCL13 produced in the B-cell areas attract CXCR5-positive B-cells. T–B interaction occurs when antigen stimulation upregulates CCR7 on B-cells thereby directing them into the T-cell zone.

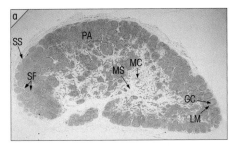

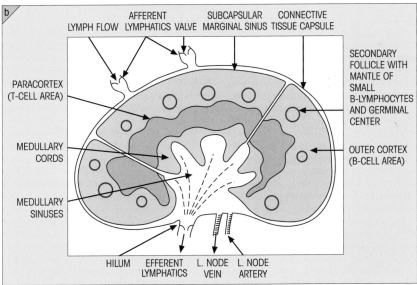

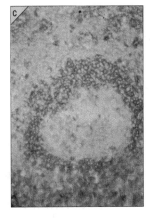

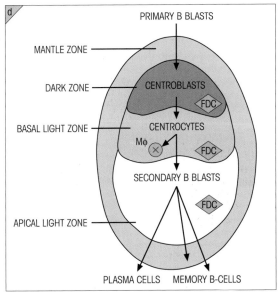

Figure 7.8. Lymph node. (a) Human lymph node, low-power view. (b) Diagrammatic representation of section through a whole node. (c) Secondary lymphoid follicle showing germinal center surrounded by a mantle of small B-lymphocytes stained by anti-human IgD labeled with horseradish peroxidase (brown color). There are few IgD-positive cells in the center but both areas contain IgM-positive B-lymphocytes. (d) Diagram showing differentiation of B-cells during passage through different regions of an active germinal center. FDC, follicular dendritic cell; Mϕ, macrophage; ×, apoptotic B-cell. ((a) Photographed by Professor P.M. Lydyard; (c) by Dr K.A. MacLennan.)

B-cell areas

The follicular aggregations of B-lymphocytes are a prominent feature of the outer cortex. In the unstimulated node they are present as spherical collections of cells termed **primary follicles**, but after antigenic challenge they form **secondary follicles** which consist of a corona or mantle of concentrically packed, resting, small B-lymphocytes possessing both IgM and IgD on their surface surrounding a pale-staining **germinal center** (figure 7.8c,d). This contains large, usually proliferating, B-blasts, a minority of T-cells, scattered conventional reticular macrophages containing 'tingible bodies' of phagocytosed lymphocytes, and a tight network of specialized **follicular dendritic cells** (FDCs). The FDCs are of mesenchymal origin, are nonphagocytic and lack lysosomes but have very elongated processes which make intimate contact with the lymphocytes. The B-cell activating factor BAFF, a TNF family member, is produced by FDCs and promotes B-cell survival in the germinal center by inhibiting apoptosis of proliferating B-cells. Germinal centers are greatly enlarged in secondary antibody responses during which they constitute sites of B-cell maturation and the generation of B-cell memory.

In the absence of antigen drive, the primary follicles are composed of a mesh of FDCs whose spaces are filled with recirculating, but resting, small B-lymphocytes. On priming with a single dose of a T-dependent antigen (i.e. antigen for which the B-cells require cooperation from T-helper cells; cf. p. 178), the FDC network can be colonized by as few as three primary B-blasts which undergo exponential growth, producing around 10^4 so-called centroblasts and displacing the original resting B-cells which now form the follicular mantle. These highly mitotic centroblasts, with no surface IgD (sIgD) and very little sIgM, then differentiate into light zone centrocytes which are noncycling and begin to upregulate their expression of sIg. At this stage there is very extensive apoptotic cell death, giving rise to DNA fragments which are visible as 'tingible bodies' within the macrophages, the final resting place of the dead cells. The survivors undergo their final training in the apical light zone. A proportion of those which are shunted down the **memory** cell pathway take up residence in the mantle zone population, the remainder joining the recirculating B-cell pool. Other cells differentiate into plasmablasts with a well-defined endoplasmic reticulum, prominent Golgi apparatus and cytoplasmic Ig; these migrate to become plasma cells in the medullary cords which project between the medullary sinuses (figure 7.8b). This maturation of antibody-forming cells at a site distant from that at which antigen triggering has occurred is also seen in the spleen, where plasma cells are found predominantly in the marginal zone. One's guess is that this movement of cells acts to prevent the generation of high local concentrations of antibody within the germinal center, so avoiding neutralization of the antigen and premature shutting off of the immune response.

The remainder of the outer cortex is also essentially a B-cell area with scattered T-cells.

T-cell areas

T-cells are mainly confined to a region referred to as the paracortex, or thymus-dependent area (figure 7.8a,b). In nodes taken from children with selective T-cell deficiency (figure 14.6), or from neonatally thymectomized mice, the paracortical region is seen to be virtually devoid of lymphocytes. Techniques such as intravital two photon scanning laser microscopy allow observation of lymphocyte behavior within lymphoid tissue. T-cells are seen to move rapidly and randomly within the paracortex, desperately trying to find an IDC bearing 'their' antigen. Should the TCR on the T-cell recognize the cognate MHC-peptide, a stable binding occurs which is largely cemented by LFA-1 on the T-cell binding to ICAM-1 on the IDC. An immunological synapse is generated and contact maintained for 36–48 hours in order to fully activate the T-cell.

SPLEEN

On a fresh section of spleen, the lymphoid tissue forming the white pulp is seen as circular or elongated gray areas (figure 7.9a) within the erythrocyte-filled red pulp which consists of splenic cords lined with macrophages and venous sinusoids. As in the lymph node, T- and B-cell areas are segregated (figure 7.9b). The spleen is a very effective blood filter removing effete red and white cells and responding actively to blood-borne antigens, the more so if they are particulate. Plasmablasts and mature plasma cells are present in the marginal zone extending into the red pulp (figure 7.9c).

THE SKIN IMMUNE SYSTEM

Pathogens will first be encountered at body surfaces, either the skin or the mucosae (see below). The surfaces of the body are endowed with a variety of external barriers against infection (cf. figure 1.2), and only if these are breached will the cells of the immune system come into play. In a normal, noninflamed, state the epidermis is provided with resident Langerhans cells and T-cells whilst the underlying dermis contains dendritic cells, T-

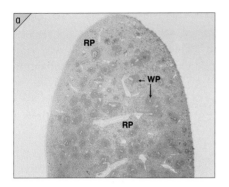

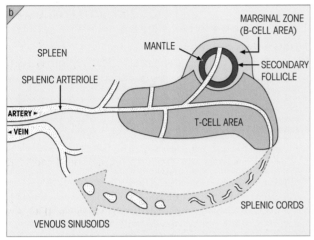

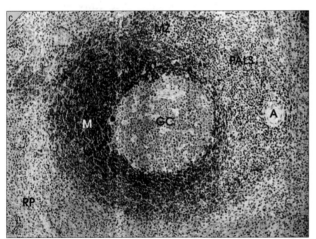

Figure 7.9. Spleen. (a) Low-power view showing lymphoid white pulp (WP) and red pulp (RP). (b) Diagrammatic representation of an area of white pulp surrounded by red pulp. (c) High-power view of germinal center (GC) and lymphocyte mantle (M) surrounded by marginal zone (MZ) and red pulp (RP). Adjacent to the follicle, an arteriole (A) is surrounded by the periarteriolar lymphoid sheath (PALS) predominantly consisting of T-cells. Note that the marginal zone is only present above the secondary follicle. ((a) Photographed by Professor P.M. Lydyard; (c) by Professor I.C.M. MacLennan.)

cells, macrophages and mast cells. There is a continuous migration of leukocytes into the skin from the blood vessels, with these cells looking out for signs of infection and then returning to the circulation via the lymphatic system and lymph nodes. Should a pathogen provoke

an inflammatory reaction in the skin then other cells of the immune system will fairly rapidly appear on the scene, including neutrophils, monocytes, eosinophils and plasma cells. In diseases such as atopic eczema the number of leukocytes in the skin substantially increases. Cutaneous inflammation is directed by several adhesion molecules amongst which LFA-1, $\alpha_1\beta_1$ and $\alpha_4\beta_1$ integrins and cutaneous leukocyte antigen (CLA) have key roles in the recruitment of appropriate cells. The CCR4 chemokine receptor is expressed by most CLA$^+$T-cells, with its ligand CCL17 (TARC, *t*hymus and *a*ctivation *r*egulated *c*hemokine) being presented on blood vessel walls in the skin. Another chemokine, CCL27 (CTACK, *c*utaneous *T*-cell-*a*ttracting *c*hemo*k*ine) is expressed by keratinocytes and its receptor, CCR10, on a subpopulation of CLA$^+$T-cells. Some of the CLA$^+$T-cells present in the skin are CD4$^+$CD25$^+$Foxp3$^+$ regulatory cells.

MUCOSAL IMMUNITY

Many pathogens will first be encountered at mucosal surfaces, for example if ingested, inhaled or sexually transmitted. The gastrointestinal, respiratory and genitourinary tracts are guarded immunologically by subepithelial accumulations of cells and of lymphoid tissues which are not constrained by a connective tissue capsule (figure 7.10). These may occur as diffuse collections of lymphocytes, plasma cells and phagocytes throughout the lung and the lamina propria of the intestinal wall (figure 7.10c), or as organized tissue (mucosa-associated lymphoid tissue, MALT) with well-formed follicles. In humans, the latter includes the lingual, palatine and pharyngeal tonsils, the Peyer's patches of the small intestine (figure 7.10a) and the appendix. Gut lymphoid tissue is separated from the lumen by columnar epithelium with tight junctions and a mucous layer. This epithelium is interspersed with microfold (M)-cells (figures 7.10b and 7.11); specialized antigen-transporting cells with short, irregular microvillae, and strong nonspecific esterase activity. They overlay intraepithelial lymphocytes and macrophages (figure 7.11b,c).

Collectively the cells and tissues involved in mucosal immunity form an interconnected secretory system within which B-cells committed to IgA (and IgE) synthesis may circulate (figure 7.12). It is however noteworthy that, unlike other mucosal tissues, in both the female and male reproductive tract the dominant isotype is IgG.

Peyer's patches form the site for induction of immune responses in the gut

Foreign material, including bacteria, is taken up by M-

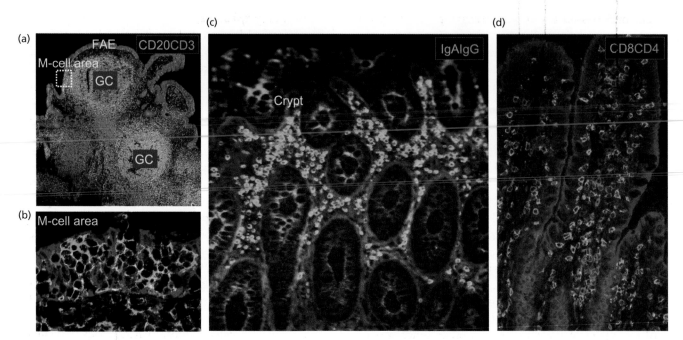

Figure 7.10. Gut-associated immunity. (a) Immunofluorescence staining indicating the B-cells (with anti-CD20, green), T-cells (with anti-CD3, red) and the follicle-associated epithelium (FAE) (with anti-cytokeratin, blue) in Peyer's patch of human small intestine. (b) Details from the antigen-sampling microfold-cell (M-cell) area. (c) Staining for IgA (green) and IgG (red) in a section of human large bowel mucosa. Crypt epithelium shows selective transport of IgA. Only a few scat-tered IgG-producing cells are seen in the lamina propria, together with numerous IgA plasma cells. (d) Staining for CD4 (red) and CD8 (green) T-cells in human duodenal mucosa. The epithelium of the villi is blue (cytokeratin). The weak CD4 expression seen in the background is either macrophages or dendritic cells. (Reproduced from Brandtzaeg P. & Pabst R. (2004) *Trends in Immunology* **25**, 570–577 with permission from the publishers.)

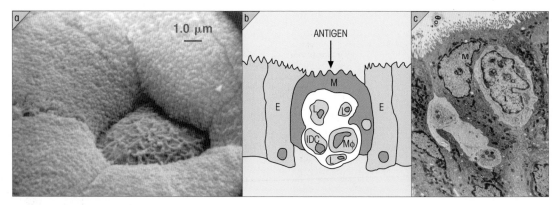

Figure 7.11. M-cell within Peyer's patch epithelium. (a) Scanning electron micrograph of the surface of the Peyer's patch epithelium. The antigen-sampling M-cell in the center is surrounded by absorptive enterocytes covered by closely packed, regular microvilli. Note the irregular and short microfolds of the M-cell. (Reproduced with permission of the authors and publishers from Kato T. & Owen R.L. (1999) In Ogra R. *et al.* (eds) *Mucosal Immunology*, 2nd edn. Academic Press, San Diego.) (b) After uptake and transcellular transport by the M-cell (M), antigen is processed by macrophages and thence by dendritic cells which present antigen to T-cells in Peyer's patches and mesenteric lymph nodes. E, enterocyte; IDC, interdigitating dendritic cell; L, lym-phocyte; Mϕ, macrophage. (c) Electron photomicrograph of an M-cell (M in nucleus) with adjacent lymphocyte (L in nucleus). Note the flank-ing epithelial cells are both absorptive enterocytes with a typical brush border. In some cases, proteases on the surface of the M-cells modify the pathogen so that it can adhere and be taken up. Pathogenic *Salmonella* can invade and destroy M-cells, making a hole through which other bacteria can invade the underlying tissue. (Lead citrate and uranyl acetate, ×1600.) ((b) Based on Sminia T. & Kraal G. (1998) In Delves P.J. & Roitt I.M. (eds) *Encyclopedia of Immunology*, 2nd edn, p. 188. Academic Press, London.)

cells and passed on to the underlying Peyer's patch antigen-presenting cells which then activate the appropriate lymphocytes. Thus, the Peyer's patches constitute the *inductive site* for immune responses in the gut. After their activation is induced the lymphocytes travel via the lymph to the mesenteric lymph nodes where additional activation and proliferation may occur. A feature of dendritic cells from Peyer's patches and mesenteric lymph nodes is that, unlike dendritic cells from peripheral lymph nodes or spleen, they express enzymes which convert vitamin D to retinoic acid. Why is this relevant?—well because it turns out that retinoic acid induces T-cells to upregulate gut homing receptors. These lymphocytes then move via the thoracic duct into the bloodstream and finally on to the lamina propria (figure 7.12). In this **responsive site** they assist IgA-forming B-cells which, because they are now broadly distributed, protect a wide area of the bowel with protective antibody. T- and B-cells also appear in the lymphoid tissue of the lung and in other mucosal sites guided by the interactions of specific homing receptors with appropriate HEV addressins as discussed earlier. Similarly, intranasal immunization is particularly effective at generating antibody production in the genitourinary tract.

Intestinal lymphocytes

The intestinal **lamina propria** is home to a predominantly activated T-cell population rich in the $\alpha_4\beta_7$ (LPAM-1) integrin (table 7.2), the ligand for MAdCAM-1 on the lamina propria postcapillary venules (figure 7.13). These T-cells bear a phenotype roughly comparable to that of peripheral blood lymphocytes: viz. >95% T-cell receptor (TCR) $\alpha\beta$ and a CD4 : CD8 ratio of 7 : 3. Unwarranted immune responses may be dampened down following the secretion of IL-10 and transforming growth factor-β (TGFβ) by inducible regulatory T-cells. Within the lamina propria there is also a generous sprinkling of activated B-blasts and plasma cells secreting IgA for transport by the poly-Ig receptor to the intestinal lumen (cf. p. 51).

Intestinal **intraepithelial lymphocytes** (IELs) are quite a different 'kettle of fish'. They are also mostly T-cells, in humans about 10% of which have a $\gamma\delta$ TCR although in other species $\gamma\delta$ T-cells may represent up to 40% of the IEL T-cells. Of those bearing an $\alpha\beta$ TCR, most are CD8+ positive and can be divided into two populations. One-third of them possess the conventional form of CD8, which is a heterodimer composed of a CD8 α chain and a CD8 β chain. However, two-thirds of them instead express a CD8 $\alpha\alpha$ homodimer which is almost

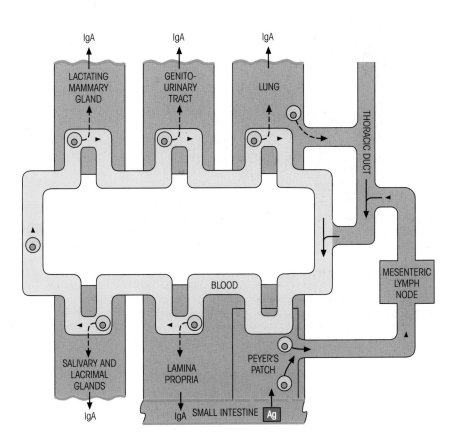

Figure 7.12. Circulation of lymphocytes within the mucosa-associated lymphoid system. Antigen-stimulated cells move from Peyer's patches to colonize the lamina propria and the other mucosal surfaces (〜〜〜), forming what has been described as a common mucosal immune system.

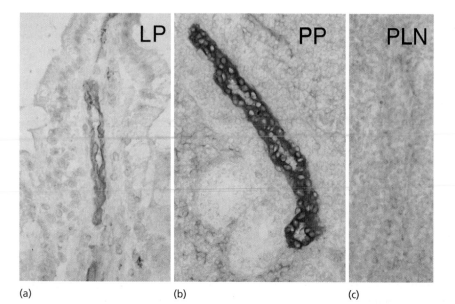

(a)   (b)   (c)

Figure 7.13. Selective expression of the mucosal vascular addressin MAdCAM-1 on endothelium involved in lymphocyte homing to gastrointestinal sites. Immunohistologic staining reveals the presence of MAdCAM-1 (a) on postcapillary venules in the small intestinal lamina propria and (b) on HEV in Peyer's patches, but its absence from (c) HEV in peripheral lymph nodes. (Reproduced with permission from Butcher E.C. *et al.* (1999) *Advances in Immunology* **72**, 209.) At least some component of intestinal trafficking appears to operate as a subcomponent of a common mucosal immune system (cf. figure 7.12), MAdCAM-1 being largely absent from the genitourinary tract, lung, salivary and lacrimal gland, although it is present on vascular endothelium in the mammary gland.

exclusively found only on IELs. Whilst the CD8 αβ TCR αβ IELs are conventional T-cells restricted by classical MHC class I molecules for the recognition of foreign peptides, CD8 αα TCR αβ IELs are efficiently generated in class I knockout mice. Whether or not they are restricted by nonclassical MHC molecules (cf. p. 83) such as TL and Qa1 remains somewhat unclear. Intraepithelial lymphocytes and intraepithelial dendritic cells express high levels of the $\alpha_E\beta_7$ integrin which binds E-cadherin on intestinal epithelial cells.

There is a relatively high proportion of TCR γδ intestinal T-cells in many species, and most of these cells also express the CD8 αα characteristic of IELs. It has been postulated that they act as a relatively primitive first line of defense at the outer surfaces of the body. Reflect for a moment on the fact that roughly 10^{14} bacteria reside in the intestinal lumen of the normal adult human. That is a pretty impressive number of 'noughts' to swallow. Yet combined with the barrier of mucins produced by goblet cells and the protective zone of secreted IgA antibodies, these collections of intestinal lymphocytes represent a crucial line of defense. Indeed, the number of IEL in the small intestine of the mouse accounts for nearly 50% of the total number of T-cells in all lymphoid organs.

It is not only the intestine that has a localized immune system composed mostly of resident T-lymphocytes; we have already mentioned the resident T-cells in skin and a similar set-up appears to apply to the liver which in the human contains 10^{10} lymphocytes, mostly long lived memory T-cells but also a relatively high proportion of NK and NKT cells. Nonclassical MHC antigens seem to play an important role in these specialized locales, with the MHC class I chain-related (MIC) family members MICA and MICB (cf. p. 84) involved in the activation of

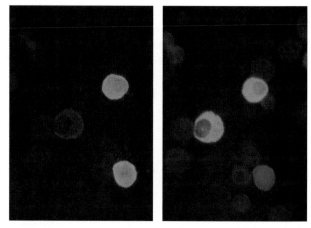

Figure 7.14. Plasma cells in human bone marrow. Cytospin preparation stained with rhodamine (orange) for IgA heavy chain and fluorescein (green) for lambda light chain. One cell is IgA.λ, another IgA.non-λ and the third is non-IgA.λ positive. (Photograph kindly supplied by Drs Benner, Hijmans and Haaijman.)

human γδ TCR IELs, and CD1d in the presentation of glycolipids to liver NKT cells (cf. p. 105).

BONE MARROW CAN BE A MAJOR SITE OF ANTIBODY SYNTHESIS

A few days after a secondary response, activated memory B-cells migrate to the bone marrow where they mature into plasma cells (figure 7.14). The bone marrow is a major source of serum Ig, contributing up to 80% of the total Ig-secreting cells in the 100-week-old mouse. The peripheral lymphoid tissue responds rapidly to antigen, but only for a relatively short time, whereas bone marrow starts slowly and gives a long-lasting massive production of antibody to antigens which repeatedly challenge the host.

THE ENJOYMENT OF PRIVILEGED SITES

Certain locations in the body, for example brain, anterior chamber of the eye and testis, are referred to as **immunologically privileged sites** because antigens located within them do not provoke reactions against themselves. It has long been known, for example, that foreign corneal grafts can take up long-term residence, and a number of viruses have been expanded by repeated passage through animal brain.

Generally, privileged sites are protected by rather strong blood–tissue barriers and low permeability to hydrophilic compounds and carrier-mediated transport systems. Functionally insignificant levels of complement reduce the threat of acute inflammatory reactions and unusually high concentrations of immunomodulators, such as IL-10 and TGFβ (cf. p. 187), endow macrophages with an immunosuppressive capacity. Immune privilege may also be maintained by Fas (CD95)-induced apoptosis of autoaggressive cells. Lesley Brent put it rather well: 'It may be supposed that it is beneficial to the organism not to turn the anterior chamber or the cornea of the eye, or the brain, into an inflammatory battle-field, for the immunological response is sometimes more damaging than the antigen insult that provoked it.'

THE HANDLING OF ANTIGEN

Where does antigen go when it enters the body? If it penetrates the tissues, it will tend to finish up in the draining lymph nodes. Antigens which are encountered in the upper respiratory tract or intestine are trapped by local MALT, whereas antigens in the blood provoke a reaction in the spleen. Macrophages in the liver will filter blood-borne antigens and degrade them without producing an immune response since they are not strategically placed with respect to lymphoid tissue.

Macrophages are general antigen-presenting cells

'Classically', it has always been recognized that antigens draining into lymphoid tissue are taken up by macrophages. The antigens are then partially, if not completely, broken down in the phagolysosomes; some may escape from the cell in a soluble form to be taken up by other antigen-presenting cells and a fraction may reappear at the surface, either as a large fragment or as a processed peptide associated with class II major histocompatibility molecules. Although resting, resident macrophages do not express MHC class II, antigens are usually encountered in the context of a microbial infectious agent which can induce the expression of class II by

its adjuvant-like properties involving molecules such as bacterial lipopolysaccharide (LPS) which activates the macrophage through TLR4.

Interdigitating dendritic cells present antigen to T-lymphocytes

Notwithstanding the impressive ability of the mighty macrophage to present antigen, there is one function where it is deficient, namely the priming of naive lymphocytes. Animals which have been depleted of macrophages, by selective uptake of liposomes containing the drug dichloromethylene diphosphonate, are as good as their controls with intact macrophages in responding to T-dependent antigens. We must conclude that cells other than macrophages prime T-helper cells, and it is now generally accepted that these are the interdigitating dendritic cells (IDCs). These cells, which are of bone marrow origin, have the awesome capacity to process four times their own volume of extracellular fluid in 1 hour, thereby facilitating antigen capture and processing in their abundant intracellular MHC class II-rich compartments (MIIC; cf. p. 97).

The IDCs are the *crème de la crème* of the antigen-presenting cells and, if pulsed with antigen before injection into animals, usually produce stunning immune responses. In this connection, it is relevant to note that large numbers of these dendritic cells can be generated from peripheral blood by cultivation with granulocyte–macrophage colony-stimulating factor (GM-CSF) (cf. p. 187) to promote proliferation and IL-4 to suppress macrophage overgrowth. Their use in immunotherapy is beginning to be explored, e.g. by pulsing autologous dendritic cells with the patient's tumor antigens and then reinjecting them to evoke an immune response.

Precursor dendritic cells in the blood that are destined to become skin Langerhans' cells express cutaneous leukocyte antigen (CLA), directing their homing to skin via interaction with E-selectin on the relevant vascular endothelial cells just as occurs for cutaneous T-cells. The Langerhans' cells, and dendritic cells in other tissues, act as antigen sampling agents. They are only moderately phagocytic but display extremely active endocytosis. Receptors involved in antigen capture, including the mannose receptor and Fc receptors for both IgG and IgE, are present on dendritic cells. The expression of cell surface MHC class II, and of adhesion and costimulatory molecules, is low at this early stage of the dendritic cells' life. However, as they differentiate into fully fledged antigen-presenting cells, they decrease their phagocytic and endocytic activity, show reduced levels of molecules involved in antigen capture, but dramati-

unencapsulated and somewhat structured (tonsils, Peyer's patches, appendix). There are also diffuse cellular collections in the lamina propria. Intraepithelial lymphocytes are mostly T-cells and include some novel subsets, e.g. CD8 $\alpha\alpha$-bearing cells which use nonclassical MHC molecules as restriction elements for antigen presentation.

• Together with the subepithelial accumulations of cells lining the mucosal surfaces of the respiratory and genitourinary tracts, these cells and lymphoid tissues form the 'secretory immune system' which bathes the surface with protective antibodies.

Other sites

• T-cells in the skin characteristically bear cutaneous lymphocyte antigen (CLA) and the chemokine receptor CCR4.
• Bone marrow is a major site of antibody production.
• The respiratory tract and the liver contain substantial numbers of lymphocytes and phagocytic cells.
• The brain, anterior chamber of the eye and testis are privileged sites in which antigens can be safely sequestered.

Lymphocyte traffic

• Lymphocyte recirculation between the blood and tissues is guided by specialized homing receptors on the surface of the high-walled endothelium of the postcapillary venules.

• Lymphocytes are tethered and then roll along the surface of the selected endothelial cells through interactions between selectins, integrins and chemokine receptors, and their respective ligands. Arrest of the lymphocyte following LFA-1 activation results in cell flattening and subsequent transmigration across the endothelial cell.

The handling of antigen

• Macrophages are general antigen-presenting cells for primed lymphocytes but cannot stimulate naive T-cells.
• This is effected by dendritic cells of hematopoietic origin which process antigen, migrate to the draining lymph node and settle down as interdigitating dendritic cells. They can present antigen-derived peptides to naive T-cells, thereby powerfully initiating primary T-cell responses.
• Follicular dendritic cells in germinal centers bind immune complexes to their surface through Ig and C3b receptors. The complexes are long-lived and can provide a sustained source of antigenic stimulation for B-cells.

See the accompanying website (**www.roitt.com**) for multiple choice questions.

FURTHER READING

Barclay A.N. *et al.* (1997) *The Leucocyte Antigen Factsbook*, 2nd edn. Academic Press, London.

Bos J.D. (ed) (2004) *Skin Immune System (SIS): cutaneous immunology and clinical immmunodermatology*, 3rd edn. Boca Raton. CRC Press.

Brandtzaeg P. & Pabst R. (2004) Let's go mucosal: communication on slippery ground. *Trends in Immunology* **25**, 570–577.

Caligaris-Cappio F. (1998) Germinal centers. In Delves P.J. & Roitt I.M. (eds) *Encyclopedia of Immunology*, 2nd edn, pp. 992–995. Academic Press, London.

Cheroutre H. (2004) Starting at the beginning: new perspectives on the biology of mucosal T cells. *Annual Reviews of Immunology* **22**, 217–246.

Iwata M., Hirakiyama A., Eshima Y. *et al.* (2004) Retinoic acid imprints gut-homing specificity on T cells. *Immunity* **21**, 527–538.

Kraehenbuhl J.P. & Neutra M.R. (2000) Epithelial M cells: differentiation and function. *Annual Reviews of Cell and Developmental Biology* **16**, 301–332.

Lefrançois L. & Puddington L. (2006) Intestinal and pulmonary mucosal T-cells: Local heroes fight to maintain the status quo. *Annual Review of Immunology* **24**, 681–704.

McHeyzer-Williams L.J., Driver D.J. & McHeyzer-Williams M.G. (2001) Germinal center reaction. *Current Opinion in Hematology* **8**, 52–59.

Pribila J.T., Quale A.C., Mueller K.L & Shimizu Y. (2004) Integrins and T cell-mediated immunity. *Annual Reviews of Immunology* **22**, 157–180.

Wardlaw, A.J., Guillen C. & Morgan A. (2005) Mechanisms of T cell migration to the lung. *Clinical and Experimental Allergy* **35**, 4–7.

8 Lymphocyte activation

INTRODUCTION

The adaptive immune response begins as a result of an encounter between a B- or T-lymphocyte and its specific antigen which typically results in 'activation' of the lymphocyte and a radical shift in cell behavior—from a quiescent nondividing state, to a more active proliferative one. This simultaneously achieves two goals: the number of cells that are capable of responding to a particular antigen are multiplied (clonal expansion), and these new recruits are equipped with the ability to produce large quantities of cytokines or antibodies to help repel the intruder. Because of the potential dangers associated with inappropriate lymphocyte activation (to 'self' or innocuous substances), signals that promote T- or B-cell activation usually require costimulation by other cells of the immune system. The requirement for costimulation raises the threshold for lymphocyte activation and provides a safeguard against autoimmunity (see Chapter 18).

In previous chapters we learned that B- or T-cells use related, but nonetheless distinct, antigen receptors to 'see' antigen. Stimulation of T- or B-cells through their respective antigen receptors initiates a cascade of signal transduction events that rely heavily upon protein kinases; proteins that can add phosphate groups to other proteins. While there are differences in the nature of the specific kinases that relay signals from the B- and T-cell receptors, there are also many similarities. In both cases, these signal transduction events result in the activation of many of the same transcription factors, entry into the cell division cycle, and the expression of an array of new proteins by the activated lymphocyte.

CLUSTERING OF MEMBRANE RECEPTORS LEADS TO THEIR ACTIVATION

All cells use plasma membrane-borne receptors to extract information from their environment. This information is propagated within the cell by signaling molecules and enables the cell to make the appropriate response; whether this is reorganization of the cell cytoskeleton (to facilitate movement), expression of new gene products, increased cellular adhesiveness, or all of the above. In many instances, occupation of the receptor with its specific ligand (whether this is a growth factor, a hormone or an antigen) results in aggregation of the receptor and creates the conditions under which the receptors, or proteins associated with the receptor cytoplasmic tails, can mutually interact. Because many plasma membrane receptors are protein kinases, or can recruit protein kinases upon engagement with their specific ligands, aggregation of the receptors typically results in phosphorylation of the receptor, or of associated proteins. In the case of the B- and T-cell receptors, the receptors themselves do not have any intrinsic enzymatic activity but are associated with invariant accessory molecules (the CD3 $\gamma\delta\epsilon$ and ζ chains in the case of the T-cell receptor, and the Ig-α/β complex in the case of the B-cell receptor) that can attract the attentions of a particular class of kinases. Central to this attraction is the presence of special motifs called **ITAMs (Immunoreceptor tyrosine-based activation motifs)** within the cytoplasmic tails of these accessory molecules (see also p. 63, Chapter 4). Phosphorylation of ITAMs at tyrosine residues—in response to TCR or BCR stimulation—enables these motifs to interact with adaptor proteins that have an affinity for phosphorylated tyrosine motifs, thereby initiating signal transduction. We will deal, in turn, with the signaling events that take place upon encounter of a T-cell or a B-cell with antigen.

T-LYMPHOCYTES AND ANTIGEN-PRESENTING CELLS INTERACT THROUGH SEVERAL PAIRS OF ACCESSORY MOLECULES

Before we delve into the nuts and bolts of TCR-driven signaling events, it is important to recall that T-cells can only recognize antigen when presented within the peptide-binding groove of major histocompatibility complex (MHC) molecules. Furthermore, while the TCR is the primary means by which T-cells interact with the MHC–peptide complex, T-cells also express coreceptors for MHC (either CD4 or CD8) that define functional T-cell subsets. Recall that CD4 molecules act as coreceptors for MHC class II and are found on T-helper cell populations which provide 'help' for activation and maturation of B-cells and cytotoxic T-cells (figure 8.1). CD8 molecules act as coreceptors for MHC class I molecules and are a feature of cytotoxic T-cells that can kill virally infected or precancerous cells (figure 8.1). Note, however, that the affinity of an individual TCR for its specific MHC–antigen peptide complex is relatively low (figure 8.2). Thus, a sufficiently stable association with an antigen-presenting cell (APC) can only be achieved by the interaction of several complementary pairs of accessory molecules such as LFA-1/ICAM-1, CD2/LFA-3 and so on (figure 8.3). However, these

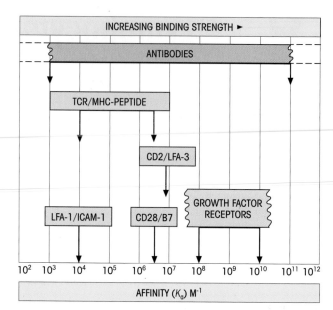

Figure 8.2. The relative affinities of molecular pairs involved in interactions between T-lymphocytes and cells presenting antigen. The ranges of affinities for growth factors and their receptors, and of antibodies, are shown for comparison. (Based on Davies M.M. & Chien Y.-H. (1993) *Current Opinion in Immunology* **5**, 45.)

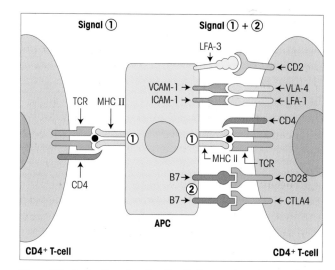

Figure 8.3. Activation of resting T-cells. Interaction of costimulatory molecules leads to activation of resting T-lymphocyte by antigen-presenting cell (APC) on engagement of the T-cell receptor (TCR) with its antigen–MHC complex. Engagement of the TCR signal 1 without accompanying costimulatory signal 2 leads to anergy. Note, a cytotoxic rather than a helper T-cell would, of course, involve coupling of CD8 to MHC class I. Signal 2 is delivered to a resting T-cell primarily through engagement of CD28 on the T-cell by B7.1 or B7.2 on the APC. CTLA-4 competes with CD28 for B7 ligands and has a much higher affinity than CD28 for these molecules. Engagement of CTLA-4 with B7 down-regulates signal 1. ICAM-1/2, *i*ntercellular *a*dhesion *m*olecule-1/2; LFA-1/2, *l*ymphocyte *f*unction-*a*ssociated molecule-1/2; VCAM-1, *v*ascular *c*ell *a*dhesion *m*olecule-1; VLA-4, *v*ery *l*ate *a*ntigen-4.

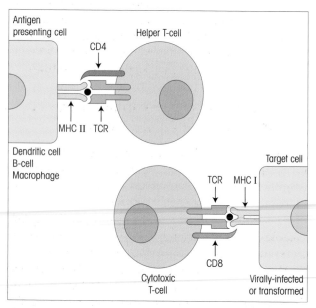

Figure 8.1. Helper and cytotoxic T-cell subsets are restricted by MHC class. CD4 on helper T-cells acts as a coreceptor for MHC class II and helps to stabilize the interaction between the TCR and peptide–MHC complex; CD8 on cytotoxic T-cells performs a similar function by associating with MHC class I.

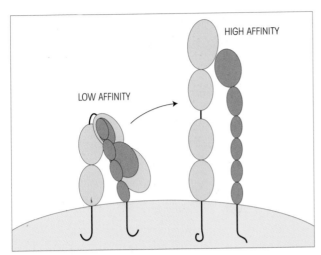

Figure 8.4. Integrin activation. Integrins such as LFA-1 can assume different conformations that are associated with different affinities. The bent head-piece conformation has a low affinity for ligand but can be rapidly transformed into the extended high-affinity conformation by activation signals that act on the cytoplasmic tails of the integrin α and β subunits; a process known as 'inside-out' signaling.

molecular couplings are not necessarily concerned with intercellular adhesion alone; some of these interactions also provide the necessary costimulation that is essential for proper lymphocyte activation.

Unstimulated lymphocytes are typically nonadherent but rapidly adhere to extracellular matrix components or other cells (such as APCs) within seconds of encountering chemokines or antigen. Integrins such as LFA-1 and VLA-4 appear to be particularly important for lymphocyte adhesion. The ease with which lymphocytes can alter their adhesiveness seems to be related to the ability of integrins to change conformation; from a closed, low-affinity state, to a more open, high-affinity, one (figure 8.4). Thus, upon encounter of a T-cell with an APC displaying an appropriate MHC–peptide complex, the affinity of LFA-1 for ICAM-1 is rapidly increased and this helps to stabilize the interaction between the T-cell and the APC. This complex has come to be known, in fashionable terms, as the **immunological synapse**. Activation of the small GTPase **Rap1** by TCR stimulation appears to contribute to the rapid change in integrin adhesiveness. How Rap1 achieves this remains somewhat hazy, but it is likely that modification of the integrin cytoplasmic tail serves to trigger a conformational change in the integrin extracellular domains; a process that has been termed 'inside-out' signaling.

THE ACTIVATION OF T-CELLS REQUIRES TWO SIGNALS

Stimulation of the TCR by MHC–peptide (which can be mimicked by antibodies directed against the TCR or CD3 complex) is not sufficient to fully activate resting helper T-cells on their own. Upon addition of interleukin-1 (IL-1), however, RNA and protein synthesis is induced, the cell enlarges to a blast-like appearance, interleukin-2 (IL-2) synthesis begins and the cell moves from G0 into the G1 phase of the cell division cycle. Thus, two signals are required for the activation of a resting helper T-cell (figure 8.3).

Antigen in association with MHC class II on the surface of APCs is clearly capable of fulfilling these requirements. Complex formation between the TCR and MHC–peptide provides signal 1, through the receptor–CD3 complex, and this is greatly enhanced by coupling of CD4 with the MHC. The T-cell is now exposed to a costimulatory signal (signal 2) from the APC. Although this could be IL-1, it would appear that the most potent costimulator is B7 on the APC which interacts with CD28 on the T-cell. Thus activation of resting T-cells can be blocked by anti-B7; surprisingly, this renders the T-cell **anergic**, i.e. unresponsive to any further stimulation by antigen. As we shall see in later chapters, the principle that two signals activate, but one may induce anergy in, an antigen-specific cell provides a potential for targeted immunosuppressive therapy. However, unlike resting T-lymphocytes, **activated T-cells proliferate in response to a** *single* **signal**.

Adhesion molecules such as ICAM-1, VCAM-1 and LFA-3 are not intrinsically costimulatory but augment the effect of other signals (figure 8.3); an important distinction. Early signaling events also involve the aggregation of **lipid rafts** composed of membrane subdomains enriched in cholesterol and glycosphingolipids. The cell membrane molecules involved in activation become concentrated within these structures.

PROTEIN TYROSINE PHOSPHORYLATION IS AN EARLY EVENT IN T-CELL SIGNALING

As we shall see shortly, the signaling cascades that result from TCR stimulation can become quite complex (figure 8.5); but take it one step at a time and a sense of order can be extracted from the apparent chaos.

Interaction between the TCR and MHC–peptide complex is greatly enhanced by recruitment of either coreceptor for MHC, CD4 or CD8, into the complex. Furthermore, because the cytoplasmic tails of CD4 and CD8 are constitutively associated with **Lck**, a protein tyrosine kinase (PTK) that can phosphorylate the three tandemly arranged ITAMs within the TCR ζ **chains**, recruitment of CD4 or CD8 to the complex results in stable association between Lck and its ζ chain substrate (figure 8.6).

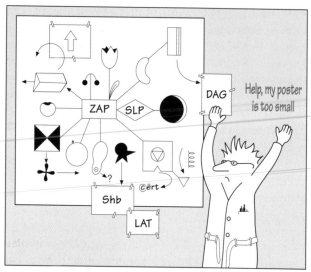

Figure 8.5. Signaling pathways can become quite complex. (Reproduced with permission from Zolnierowicz S. & Bollen M. (2000) *EMBO Journal* **19**, 483.)

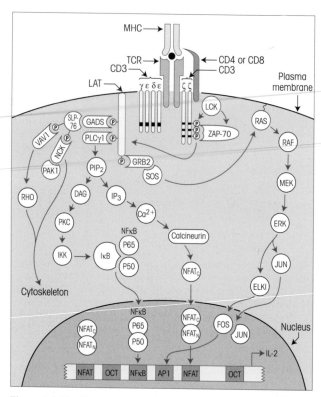

Figure 8.6. T-cell signaling leads to activation. Signals through the MHC–antigen complex (signal 1) and costimulator B7 (signal 2) initiate a cascade of protein kinase activation events and a rise in intracellular calcium, thereby activating transcription factors which control entry in the cell cycle from G0 and regulate the expression of IL-2 and many other cytokines. Stable recruitment of CD4 or CD8 to the TCR complex initiates the signal transduction cascade through phosphorylation of the tandemly arranged ITAM motifs within the CD3 ζ chains which creates binding sites for the ZAP-70 kinase. Subsequent events are marshaled through ZAP-70-mediated phosphorylation of LAT; recruitment of several signaling complexes to LAT result in triggering of the Ras/MAPK and PLCγ1 signaling pathways. The latter pathways culminate in activation of a range of transcription factors including NFκB, NFAT and Fos/Jun heterodimers. Note that other molecules can also contribute to this pathway but have been omitted for clarity. See main body of text for further details. Abbreviations: DAG, diacylglycerol; ERK, *e*xtracellular signal *r*egulated *k*inase; IP$_3$, inositol triphosphate; LAT, *l*inker for *a*ctivated *T*-cells; NFκB, *n*uclear *f*actor κβ; NFAT, *n*uclear *f*actor of *a*ctivated *T*-cells; OCT-1, octamer-binding factor; Pak1, *p*21-*a*ctivated *k*inase; PIP$_2$, phosphatidylinositol diphosphate; PKC, protein kinase C; PLC, phospholipase C; SH2, *S*rc-*h*omology domain 2; SLAP, *SL*P-76-*a*ssociated *p*hosphoprotein; SLP-76, *SH*2-domain containing *l*eukocyte-specific 76 kDa *p*hosphoprotein; ZAP-70, ζ chain-*a*ssociated *p*rotein kinase. ⟶, Positive signal transduction.

Phosphorylation of ζ chain by Lck creates binding sites for the recruitment of another PTK, **ZAP-70 (zeta chain associated protein of 70 kDa)**, into the TCR signaling complex. Recruitment of ZAP-70 into the receptor complex results in activation of this PTK by Lck-mediated phosphorylation. ZAP-70, in turn, phosphorylates two adaptor proteins, **LAT (linker for activation of T-cells)** and **SLP76 (SH2-domain containing leukocyte protein of 76 kDa)** that can instigate divergent signaling cascades downstream (figure 8.6).

LAT plays an especially significant role in subsequent events by serving as a platform for the recruitment of several additional players to the TCR complex. LAT contains many tyrosine residues that, upon phosphorylation by ZAP-70, can bind to other adaptor proteins through motifs (called SH2 domains) that bind phosphotyrosine residues. Thus, phosphorylation of LAT results in recruitment of **GADS (GRB2-related adapter protein)** which is constitutively associated with SLP76. SLP76 has been implicated in cytoskeletal rearrangements due to its ability to associate with Vav1 and NCK (figure 8.6). Thus, TCR-stimulation induced cell shape changes are most likely due to recruitment of SLP76 into the TCR signaling complex.

Phosphorylated LAT also attracts the attentions of two additional phosphotyrosine-binding proteins; the γ1 isoform of **phospholipase C (PLCγ1)**, and the adaptor protein **GRB2 (growth factor receptor-binding protein 2)**. From this point on, at least two distinct signaling cascades can ensue; the **Ras/MAPK pathway** and the **phosphatidylinositol pathway**.

DOWNSTREAM EVENTS FOLLOWING TCR SIGNALING

The Ras/MAPK pathway

Ras is a small G-protein that is constitutively associated with the plasma membrane and is frequently activated

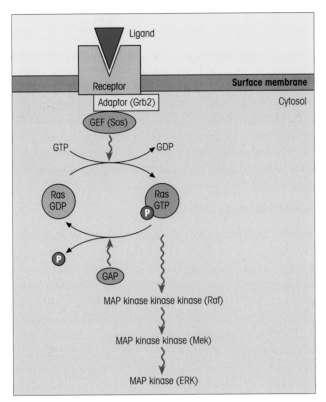

Figure 8.7. Regulation of Ras activity controls kinase amplification cascades. A number of cell surface receptors signal through Ras-regulated pathways. Ras cycles between inactive Ras–GDP and active Ras–GTP, regulated by guanine nucleotide exchange factors (GEFs) which promote the conversion of Ras–GDP to Ras–GTP, and by GTPase-activating proteins (GAPs) which increase the intrinsic GTPase activity of Ras. Upon ligand binding to receptor, receptor tyrosine kinases recruit adaptor proteins, e.g. Grb2, and GEF proteins, such as Sos ('son of sevenless'), to the plasma membrane. These events generate Ras–GTP which activates Raf. (Modified with permission from Olson M.F. & Marais R. (2000) *Seminars in Immunology* **12**, 63.)

in response to diverse stimuli that promote cell division (figure 8.7). Ras can exist in two states, GTP-bound (active) and GDP-bound (inactive). Thus, exchange of GDP for GTP stimulates Ras activation and enables this protein to recruit one of its downstream effectors, Raf. So how does TCR stimulation result in activation of Ras? One of the ways in which Ras activation can be achieved is through the activity of **GEFs (guanine-nucleotide exchange factors)** that promote exchange of GDP for GTP on Ras. One such GEF, SOS (son of sevenless), is recruited to phosphorylated LAT via the phosphotyrosine-binding protein GRB2 (figure 8.6). Thus, phosphorylation of LAT by ZAP-70 leads directly to the recruitment of the GRB2/SOS complex to the plasma membrane where it can stimulate activation of Ras through promoting exchange of GDP for GTP.

In its GTP-bound state, Ras can recruit a kinase, **Raf (also called MAPKKK, mitogen-associated protein kinase kinase kinase!),** to the plasma membrane which

then sets in motion a series of further kinase activation events culminating in phosphorylation of the transcription factor Elk1. Elk1 phosphorylation permits translocation of this protein to the nucleus and results in the expression of Fos, yet another transcription factor. The appearance of Fos results in the formation of heterodimers with Jun to form the AP-1 complex which has binding sites on the IL-2 promoter as well as on many other genes (figure 8.6). Deletion of AP-1 binding sites from the IL-2 promoter abrogates 90% of IL-2 enhancer activity.

The phosphatidylinositol pathway

Phosphorylation of LAT by ZAP-70 not only promotes docking of the GRB2/SOS complex on LAT, but also stimulates recruitment of the $\gamma 1$ isoform of **phospholipase C** (PLC$\gamma 1$; figure 8.6). PLC$\gamma 1$ plays a crucial role in propagating the cascade further. Phosphorylation of PLC$\gamma 1$ activates this lipase which enables it to hydrolyze the membrane phospholipid, **phosphatidylinositol biphosphate (PIP$_2$),** into diacylglycerol (DAG) and inositol triphosphate (IP$_3$) (figure 8.6). Interaction of IP$_3$ with specific receptors in the endoplasmic reticulum triggers the release of Ca^{2+} into the cytosol which also triggers an influx of extracellular calcium. The **raised Ca^{2+}** concentration within the T-cell has at least two consequences. First, it synergizes with DAG to activate **protein kinase C** (PKC); second, it acts together with **calmodulin** to increase the activity of **calcineurin**, a protein phosphatase that can promote activation of an important transcription factor (NFAT) required for IL-2 production.

The **Ca^{2+}**-dependent activation of PKC by DAG is instrumental in the activation of yet another transcription factor, NFκB. NFκB is actually a family of related transcription factors that are involved in the regulation of transcription of many genes, including cytokines (such as IL-2), as well as genes that can promote cell survival by blocking signals that promote apoptosis.

Control of IL-2 gene transcription

Transcription of IL-2 is one of the key elements in preventing the signaled T-cell from lapsing into anergy and is controlled by multiple binding sites for transcriptional factors in the promoter region (figure 8.6).

Under the influence of calcineurin, the cytoplasmic component of the *n*uclear *f*actor of *a*ctivated *T*-cells (**NFAT$_c$**) becomes dephosphorylated and this permits its translocation to the nucleus where it forms a binary complex with NFAT$_n$, its partner which is constitutively expressed in the nucleus. The NFAT complex binds to two different IL-2 regulatory sites (figure 8.6). Note here that the calcineurin effect is blocked by the anti-T-cell drugs cyclosporine and tracolimus (see Chapter 16). PKC- and calcineurin-dependent pathways synergize in activating the multisubunit IκB kinase (IKK), which phosphorylates the inhibitor IκB thereby targeting it for ubiquitination and subsequent degradation by the proteasome. Loss of IκB from the IκB–NFκB complex exposes the nuclear localization signal on the NFκB transcription factor which then swiftly enters the nucleus. In addition, the ubiquitous transcription factor **Oct-1** interacts with specific octamer-binding sequence motifs.

We have concentrated on IL-2 transcription as an early and central consequence of T-cell activation, but more than 70 genes are newly expressed within 4 hours of T-cell activation, leading to proliferation and the synthesis of several cytokines and their receptors (see Chapter 9).

CD28 costimulation amplifies TCR signals

As discussed earlier, naive T-cells typically require two signals for proper activation; one derived from TCR ligation (signal 1), and the other most likely provided by simultaneous engagement of CD28 on the T-cell (signal 2) by B7.1 or B7.2 on the APC (figure 8.3). Indeed, T-cells derived from CD28-deficient mice, or cells treated with anti-CD28 blocking antibodies, display severely reduced capacity to proliferate in response to TCR stimulation *in vitro* and *in vivo*. Moreover, CD28 deficiency also impairs T-cell differentiation and the production of cytokines required for B-cell help. Similar effects are also seen when B7.1 or B7.2 expression is interfered with. So what does tickling the CD28 receptor do that is so special?

While early studies suggested that CD28 stimulation may result in *qualitatively* different signals to those that are generated through the TCR, recent studies suggest that this might not be the case. Instead, these studies suggest that while CD28 engagement undoubtedly activates pathways within the T-cell that TCR stimulation alone does not (such as the phosphatidylinositol 3-kinase [PI3K] pathway), the primary purpose of costimulation through CD28 may be to *quantitatively* amplify signals through the TCR by converging on similar transcription factors such as NFκB and NFAT. In support of this view, microarray analyses of genes upregulated in response to TCR ligation alone, versus TCR ligation in the presence of CD28 costimulation, found, rather surprisingly, that essentially the same cohorts of genes were expressed in both cases. While signals through CD28 enhanced the expression of many of the genes switched

on in response to TCR ligation, no new genes were expressed. This indicates that CD28 costimulation may be required in order to cross signaling thresholds that are not achievable via TCR ligation alone. One is reminded here of the choke that earlier generations of cars were supplied with to provide a slightly more fuel-rich mixture to help start a cold engine! CD28 costimulation of naive T-cells may serve a similar purpose, with the CD28 'choke' no longer needed when these cells have warmed up as a result of previous stimulation.

Further thoughts on T-cell triggering

A serial TCR engagement model for T-cell activation
We have already commented that the major docking forces which conjugate the APC and its T-lymphocyte counterpart must come from the complementary accessory molecules such as ICAM-1/LFA-1 and LFA-3/CD2, rather than through the relatively low affinity TCR–MHC plus peptide links (figure 8.3). Nonetheless, cognate antigen recognition by the TCR remains a *sine qua non* for T-cell activation. Fine, but how can as few as 100 MHC–peptide complexes on an APC, through their low affinity complexing with TCRs, effect the Herculean task of sustaining a raised intracellular calcium flux for the 60 minutes required for full cell activation? Any fall in calcium flux, as may be occasioned by adding an antibody to the MHC, and NFAT$_c$ dutifully returns from the nucleus to its cytoplasmic location, so aborting the activation process.

Surprisingly, Valitutti and Lanzavecchia have shown that as few as 100 MHC–peptide complexes on an APC can downregulate 18 000 TCRs on its cognate T-lymphocyte partner. They suggest that each MHC–peptide complex can *serially* engage up to 200 TCRs. In their model, conjugation of an MHC–peptide dimer with two TCRs activates signal transduction, phosphorylation of the CD3-associated ζ chains with subsequent downstream events, and then downregulation of those TCRs. Intermediate affinity binding favors dissociation of the MHC–peptide, freeing it to engage and trigger another TCR, so sustaining the required intracellular activation events. The model for **agonist** action would also explain why peptides giving interactions of lower or higher affinity than the optimum could behave as **antagonists** (figure 8.8). The important phenomenon of modified peptides behaving as **partial agonists**, with differential effects on the outcome of T-cell activation, is addressed in the legend to figure 8.8.

The immunological synapse
Experiments using peptide–MHC and ICAM-1 molecules labeled with different fluorochromes and inserted

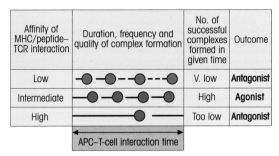

Affinity of MHC/peptide–TCR interaction	Duration, frequency and quality of complex formation	No. of successful complexes formed in given time	Outcome
Low		V. low	**Antagonist**
Intermediate		High	**Agonist**
High		Too low	**Antagonist**

APC–T-cell interaction time

Figure 8.8. Serial triggering model of TCR activation (Valitutti S. & Lanzavecchia A. (1995) *The Immunologist* **3**, 122). Intermediate affinity complexes between MHC–peptide and TCR survive long enough for a successful activation signal to be transduced by the TCR, and the MHC–peptide dissociates and fruitfully engages another TCR. A sustained high rate of formation of successful complexes is required for full T-cell activation. Low affinity complexes have a short half-life which either has no effect on the TCR or produces inactivation, perhaps through partial phosphorylation of ζ chains (●, successful TCR activation; ●, TCR inactivation; —, no effect: the length of the horizontal bar indicates the lifetime of that complex). Being of low affinity, they recycle rapidly and engage and inactivate a large number of TCRs. High affinity complexes have such a long lifetime before dissociation that insufficient numbers of successful triggering events occur. Thus modified peptide ligands of either low or high affinity can act as antagonists by denying the agonist access to adequate numbers of vacant TCRs. Some modified peptides act as partial agonists in that they produce differential effects on the outcomes of T-cell activation. For example, a single residue change in a hemoglobin peptide reduced IL-4 secretion 10-fold but completely knocked out T-cell proliferation. The mechanism presumably involves incomplete or inadequately transduced phosphorylation events occurring through a truncated half-life of TCR engagement, allosteric effects on the MHC–TCR partners, or orientational misalignment of the peptide within the complex. (Reproduced with permission of Hogrefe & Huber Publishers.)

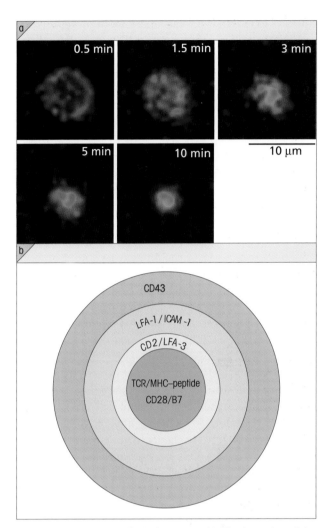

Figure 8.9. The immunological synapse. (a) The formation of the immunological synapse. T-cells were brought into contact with planar lipid bilayers and the positions of engaged MHC–peptide (green) and engaged ICAM-1 (red) at the indicated times after initial contact are shown. (Reproduced with permission from Grakoui A., Dustin M.L. *et al.* (1999) *Science* **285**, 221. © American Association for the Advancement of Science.). (b) Diagrammatic representation of the resolved synapse in which the adhesion molecule pairs CD2/LFA-3 and LFA-1/ICAM-1, which were originally in the center, have moved to the outside and now encircle the antigen recognition and signaling interaction between TCR and MHC–peptide and the costimulatory interaction between CD28 and B7. The CD43 molecule has been reported to bind to ICAM-1 and E-selectin, and upon ligation is able to induce IL-2 mRNA, CD69 and CD154 (CD40L) expression and activate the DNA-binding activity of the AP-1, NFκB and NFAT transcription factors.

into a planar lipid bilayer on a glass support have provided evidence for the idea that T-cell activation occurs in the context of an **immunological synapse**. A clustered area of integrins acts as an anchor to permit optimal interaction between the opposing cell surfaces. Initially unstable TCR–MHC interactions occur in a broad outer ring surrounding the integrins. The peptide–MHC molecules then move towards the center of the synapse, changing places with the adhesion molecules which now form the outer ring (figure 8.9). It has been suggested that the generation of the immunological synapse only occurs after a certain initial threshold level of TCR triggering has been achieved, its formation being dependent upon cytoskeletal reorganization and leading to potentiation of the signal.

Damping T-cell enthusiasm

We have frequently reiterated the premise that no self-respecting organism would permit the operation of an expanding enterprise such as a proliferating T-cell population without some sensible controlling mechanisms.

Whereas CD28 is constitutively expressed on T-cells, CTLA-4 is not found on the resting cell but is rapidly upregulated following activation. It has a 10- to 20-fold higher affinity for both B7.1 and B7.2 and, in contrast to costimulatory signals generated through CD28, B7 engagement of CTLA-4 downregulates T-cell activation. The mechanism by which CTLA-4 suppresses T-cell activation remains enigmatic, as this receptor appears to recruit a similar repertoire of proteins (such as PI3K) to its intracellular tail as CD28 does. It has been proposed, however, that CTLA-4 may antagonize the recruitment of the TCR complex to lipid rafts, which is where many of the signaling proteins that propagate TCR signals reside.

A number of adaptor molecules have been identified which may be involved in reigning in T-cell activation. These include SLAP, SIT and members of the Cbl family. Cbl-b appears to influence the CD28 dependence of IL-2 production during T-cell activation, perhaps via an effect on the guanine nucleotide exchange factor Vav. Another member of the Cbl family, Cbl-c, is a negative regulator of Syk and ZAP-70, and may thereby alter the triggering threshold of the antigen receptors on both T- and B-cells.

Tempting though it might be, phosphatases should not automatically be equated with downregulation of a phosphorylation cascade. The observation that T-cell mutants lacking CD45 do not possess signal transduction capacity was at first sight deemed to be strange because CD45 has phosphatase activity and was thought thereby to downregulate signaling. However, the Lck kinase in the CD45-deficient T-cells is phosphorylated on tyrosine-505 which is a negative regulatory site for kinase activity; hence dephosphorylation by CD45 activates the Lck enzyme and the paradox is resolved.

B-CELLS RESPOND TO THREE DIFFERENT TYPES OF ANTIGEN

1 Type 1 thymus-independent antigens

Certain antigens, such as bacterial lipopolysaccharides, at a high enough concentration, have the ability to activate a substantial proportion of the B-cell pool polyclonally, i.e. without reference to the antigen specificity of the surface receptor hypervariable regions. They do this through binding to a surface molecule which bypasses the early part of the biochemical pathway mediated by the specific antigen receptor. At concentrations which are too low to cause polyclonal activation through unaided binding to these mitogenic bypass molecules, the B-cell population with Ig receptors specific for these antigens will selectively and passively focus them on their surface, where the resulting high local concentration will suffice to drive the activation process (figure 8.10a).

2 Type 2 thymus-independent antigens

Certain linear antigens which are not readily degraded in the body and which have an appropriately spaced, highly repeating determinant—*Pneumococcus* polysaccharide, ficoll, D-amino acid polymers and polyvinylpyrrolidone, for example—are also thymus-independent in their ability to stimulate B-cells directly without the need for T-cell involvement. They persist for long periods on the surface of specialized macrophages located at the subcapsular sinus of the lymph nodes and the splenic marginal zone, and can bind to antigen-specific B-cells with great avidity through their multivalent attachment to the complementary Ig receptors which they cross-link (figure 8.10b).

In general, the thymus-independent antigens give rise to predominantly low affinity IgM responses, some IgG3 in the mouse, and relatively poor, if any, memory. Neonatal B-cells do not respond well to type 2 antigens and this has important consequences for the efficacy of carbohydrate vaccines in young children.

3 Thymus-dependent antigens

The need for collaboration with T-helper cells
Many antigens are thymus-dependent in that they

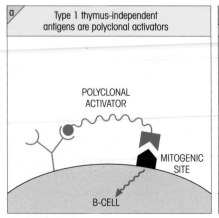
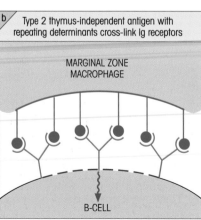

Figure 8.10. B-cell recognition of (a) type 1 and (b) type 2 thymus-independent antigens. The complex gives a sustained signal to the B-cell because of the long half-life of this type of molecule. ⤳, activation signal; ⌇, surface Ig receptor; – – –, cross-linking of receptors.

provoke little or no antibody response in animals which have been thymectomized at birth and have few T-cells (Milestone 8.1). Such antigens cannot fulfil the molecular requirements for direct stimulation; they may be univalent with respect to the specificity of each determinant; they may be readily degraded by phagocytic cells; and they may lack mitogenicity. If they bind to B-cell receptors, they will sit on the surface just like a hapten and do nothing to trigger the B-cell (figure 8.11). Cast your mind back to the definition of a hapten—a small molecule like dinitrophenyl (DNP) which binds to preformed antibody (e.g. the surface receptor of a spe-

cific B-cell) but fails to stimulate antibody production (i.e. stimulate the B-cell). Remember also that haptens become immunogenic when coupled to an appropriate carrier protein (see p. 89). Building on the knowledge that both T- and B-cells are necessary for antibody responses to thymus-dependent antigens (Milestone 8.1), we now know that the carrier functions to stimulate T-helper cells which cooperate with B-cells to enable them to respond to the hapten by providing accessory signals (figure 8.11). It should also be evident from figure 8.11 that, while one determinant on a typical protein antigen is behaving as a hapten in binding to the

Milestone 8.1 — T–B Collaboration for Antibody Production

In the 1960s, as the mysteries of the thymus were slowly unraveled, our erstwhile colleagues pushing back the frontiers of knowledge discovered that neonatal thymectomy in the mouse abrogated not only the cellular rejection of skin grafts, but also the antibody response to some but not all antigens (figure M8.1.1). Subsequent investigations showed that both thymocytes and bone marrow cells were needed for optimal antibody responses to such **thymus-dependent antigens** (figure M8.1.2). By carrying out these transfers with cells from animals bearing a recognizable chromosome marker (T6), it became evident that the antibody-forming cells were derived from the bone marrow inoculum, hence the nomenclature 'T' for Thymus-derived lymphocytes and 'B' for antibody-forming cell precursors originating in the Bone marrow. This convenient nomenclature has stuck even though bone marrow contains embryonic T-cell precursors since the immunocompetent T- and B-cells differentiate in the thymus and bone marrow respectively (see Chapter 11).

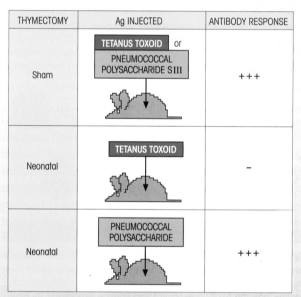

Figure M8.1.1. The antibody response to some antigens is thymus-dependent and, to others, thymus-independent. The response to tetanus toxoid in neonatally thymectomized animals could be restored by the injection of thymocytes.

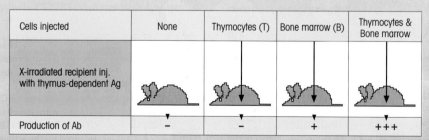

Cells injected	None	Thymocytes (T)	Bone marrow (B)	Thymocytes & Bone marrow
X-irradiated recipient inj. with thymus-dependent Ag				
Production of Ab	–	–	+	+++

Figure M8.1.2. The antibody response to a thymus-dependent antigen requires two different T-cell populations. Different populations of cells from a normal mouse histocompatible with the recipient (i.e. of the same H-2 haplotype) were injected into recipients which had been X-irradiated to destroy their own lymphocyte responses. They were then primed with a thymus-dependent antigen such as sheep red blood cells (i.e. an antigen which fails to give a response in neonatally thymectomized mice; figure M8.1.1) and examined for the production of antibody after 2 weeks. The small amount of antibody synthesized by animals receiving bone marrow alone is due to the presence of thymocyte precursors in the cell inoculum which differentiate in the intact thymus gland of the recipient.

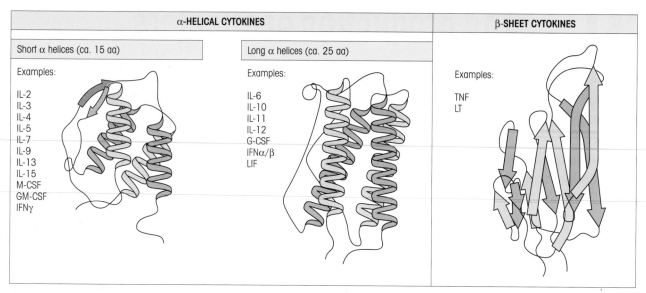

Figure 9.1. Cytokine structures. Cytokines can be divided into a number of different structural groups. Illustrated here are three of the main types of structure and some named examples of each type: (a) four short (~15 amino acids) α-helices, (b) four long (~25 amino acids) α-helices and (c) a β-sheet structure. (Reproduced with permission from Michal G. (ed.) (1999) *Biochemical Pathways: An Atlas of Biochemistry and Molecular Biology.* John Wiley & Sons, New York.)

viral replication (interferons). It is important to note, however, that cytokines often do much more than their somewhat descriptive (and often misleading) names would suggest. Indeed, the response that these molecules elicit depends, to a large extent, on the context in which the cytokine signal is delivered. Thus, factors such as the differentiation stage of the cell, its position within the cell cycle (whether quiescent or proliferating) and the presence of other cytokines, can all influence the response made to a particular cytokine.

Cytokine action is transient and usually short range

Cytokines are typically low molecular weight (15–25 kDa) secreted proteins that mediate cell division, inflammation, immunity, differentiation, migration and repair. Because they regulate the amplitude and duration of the immune–inflammatory responses, cytokines must be produced in a transient manner tightly coupled to the presence of foreign material. Cytokine production can also occur in response to the release of endogenous 'danger signals' that betray the presence of cells dying by necrosis, a mode of cell death that is typically seen in pathological situations and is typically provoked by infectious agents or tissue injury. It is relevant that the AU-rich sequences in the 3′ untranslated regions of the mRNA of many cytokines prime these mRNAs for rapid degradation thereby ensuring that cytokine production rapidly declines in the absence of appropriate stimulation. Unlike endocrine hormones, the majority of cytokines normally act locally in a paracrine or even

autocrine fashion. Thus cytokines derived from lymphocytes rarely persist in the circulation, but nonlymphoid cells can be triggered by bacterial products to release cytokines which may be detected in the bloodstream, often to the detriment of the host. Septic shock, for example, is a life-threatening condition that largely results from massive overproduction of cytokines such as TNF and IL-1 in response to bacterial infection and highlights the necessity to keep a tight rein on cytokine production. Certain cytokines, including IL-1 and tumor necrosis factor (TNF), also exist as membrane-anchored forms and can exert their stimulatory effects without becoming soluble.

Cytokines act through cell surface receptors

Cytokines are highly potent, often acting at femtomolar (10^{-15} M) concentrations, combining with small numbers of high affinity cell surface receptors to produce changes in the pattern of RNA and protein synthesis in the cells they act upon. Cytokine receptors typically possess specific protein–protein interaction domains or phosphorylation motifs within their cytoplasmic tails to facilitate recruitment of appropriate adaptor proteins upon receptor stimulation. A recurring theme in cytokine receptor activation pathways is the ligand-induced dimer- or trimerization of receptor subunits; this facilitates signal propagation into the cell through the interplay of the transiently associated receptor cytoplasmic tails. There are six major cytokine receptor structural families (figure 9.2).

Table 9.1. Cytokines: their origin and function.

CYTOKINE	SOURCE	EFFECTOR FUNCTION
INTERLEUKINS		
IL-1α, IL-1β	Mono, Mφ, DC, NK, B, Endo	Costimulates T activation by enhancing production of cytokines including IL-2 and its receptor; enhances B proliferation and maturation; NK cytotoxicity; induces IL-1,-6,-8, TNF, GM-CSF and PGE$_2$ by Mφ; proinflammatory by inducing chemokines and ICAM-1 and VCAM-1 on endothelium; induces fever, APP, bone resorption by osteoclasts
IL-2	Th1	Induces proliferation of activated T- and B-cells; enhances NK cytotoxicity and killing of tumor cells and bacteria by monocytes and Mφ
IL-3	T, NK, MC	Growth and differentiation of hematopoietic precursors; MC growth
IL-4	Th2, Tc2, NK, NKT, γδ T, MC	Induces Th2 cells; stimulates proliferation of activated B, T, MC; upregulates MHC class II on B and Mφ, and CD23 on B; downregulates IL-12 production and thereby inhibits Th1 differentiation; increases Mφ phagocytosis; induces switch to IgG1 and IgE
IL-5	Th2, MC	Induces proliferation of eosino and activated B; induces switch to IgA
IL-6	Th2, Mono, Mφ, DC, BM stroma	Differentiation of myeloid stem cells and of B into plasma cells; induces APP; enhances T proliferation
IL-7	BM and thymic stroma	Induces differentiation of lymphoid stem cells into progenitor T and B; activates mature T
IL-8	Mono, Mφ, Endo	Mediates chemotaxis and activation of neutrophils
IL-9	Th	Induces proliferation of thymocytes; enhances MC growth; synergizes with IL-4 in switch to IgG1 and IgE
IL-10	Th (Th2 in mouse), Tc, B, Mono, Mφ	Inhibits IFNγ secretion by mouse, and IL-2 by human, Th1 cells; downregulates MHC class II and cytokine (including IL-12) production by mono, Mφ and DC, thereby inhibiting Th1 differentiation; inhibits T proliferation; enhances B differentiation
IL-11	BM stroma	Promotes differentiation of pro-B and megakaryocytes; induces APP
IL-12	Mono, Mφ, DC, B	Critical cytokine for Th1 differentiation; induces proliferation and IFNγ production by Th1, CD8$^+$ and γδ T and NK; enhances NK and CD8$^+$ T cytotoxicity
IL-13	Th2, MC	Inhibits activation and cytokine secretion by Mφ; co-activates B proliferation; upregulates MHC class II and CD23 on B and mono; induces switch to IgG1 and IgE; induces VCAM-1 on endo
IL-15	T, NK, Mono, Mφ, DC, B	Induces proliferation of T-, NK and activated B and cytokine production and cytotoxicity in NK and CD8$^+$ T; chemotactic for T; stimulates growth of intestinal epithelium
IL-16	Th, Tc	Chemoattractant for CD4 T, mono and eosino; induces MHC class II
IL-17	T	Proinflammatory; stimulates production of cytokines including TNF,IL-1β,-6,-8, G-CSF
IL-18	Mφ, DC	Induces IFNγ production by T; enhances NK cytotoxicity
IL-19	Mono	Modulation of Th1 activity
IL-20	Mono, Keratinocytes	Regulation of inflammatory responses to skin
IL-21	Th	Regulation of hematopoiesis; NK differentiation; B activation; T costimulation
IL-22	T	Inhibits IL-4 production by Th2
IL-23	DC	Induces proliferation and IFNγ production by Th1; induces proliferation of memory cells
IL-24	Th2, Mono, Mφ	Induction of TNF, IL-1, IL-6, anti-tumor activity
IL-25	Th1, Mφ, Mast	Induction of IL-4, IL-5, IL-13 and Th2-associated pathologies
IL-26	T, NK	Enhanced production of IL-8 and IL-10 by epithelium
IL-27	DC, Mono	Induction of TH1 responses, enhanced IFN-γ production
IL-28	Mono, DC	Type 1 IFN-like activity, inhibition of viral replication
IL-29	Mono, DC	Type 1 IFN-like activity, inhibition of viral replication
IL-31	T	Promotes inflammatory responses in skin
IL-32	NK, T	Promotes inflammation. Role in activation-induced T-cell apoptosis.
IL-33	DC, Mφ	Induction of IL-4, IL-5, IL-13
COLONY STIMULATING FACTORS		
GM-CSF	Th, Mφ, Fibro, MC, Endo	Stimulates growth of progenitors of mono, neutro, eosino and baso; activates Mφ
G-CSF	Fibro, Endo	Stimulates growth of neutro progenitors
M-CSF	Fibro, Endo, Epith	Stimulates growth of mono progenitors
SLF	BM stroma	Stimulates stem cell division (c-kit ligand)
TUMOR NECROSIS FACTORS		
TNF (TNFα)	Th, Mono, Mφ, DC, MC, NK, B	Tumor cytotoxicity; cachexia (weight loss); induces cytokine secretion; induces E-selectin on endo; activates Mφ; antiviral
Lymphotoxin (TNFβ)	Th1, Tc	Tumor cytotoxicity; enhances phagocytosis by neutro and Mφ; involved in lymphoid organ development; antiviral
INTERFERONS		
IFNα	Leukocytes	Inhibits viral replication; enhances MHC class I
IFNβ	Fibroblasts	Inhibits viral replication; enhances MHC class I
IFNγ	Th1, Tc1, NK	Inhibits viral replication; enhances MHC class I and II; activates Mφ; induces switch to IgG2a; antagonizes several IL-4 actions; inhibits proliferation of Th2
OTHERS		
TGFβ	Th3, B, Mφ, MC	Proinflammatory by, e.g. chemoattraction of mono and Mφ but also anti-inflammatory by, e.g. inhibiting lymphocyte proliferation; induces switch to IgA; promotes tissue repair
LIF	Thymic epith, BM stroma	Induces APP
Eta-1	T	Stimulates IL-12 production and inhibits IL-10 production by Mφ
Oncostatin M	T, Mφ	Induces APP

APP, acute phase proteins; B, B-cell; baso, basophil; BM, bone marrow; Endo, endothelium; eosino, eosinophil; Epith, epithelium; Fibro, fibroblast; GM-CSF, granulocyte–macrophage colony-stimulating factor; IL, interleukin; LIF, leukemia inhibitory factor; Mφ, macrophage; MC, mast cell; Mono, monocyte; neutro, neutrophil; NK, natural killer; SLF, steel locus factor; T, T-cell; TGFβ, transforming growth factor-β. Note that there is not an interleukin-14. This designation was given to an activity that, upon further investigation, could not be unambiguously assigned to a single cytokine. IL-30 also awaits assignment. IL-8 is a member of the chemokine family. These cytokines are listed separately in table 9.3.

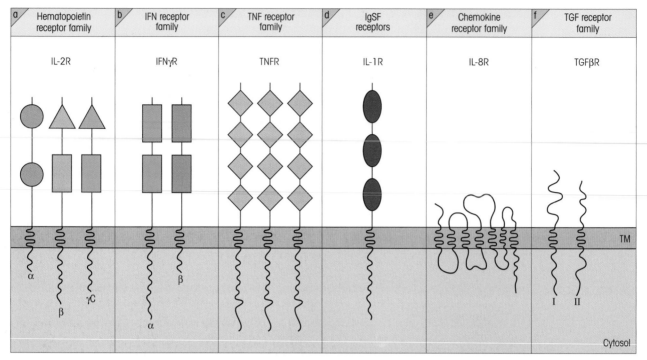

Figure 9.2. Cytokine receptor families. One example is shown for each family. (a) The **hematopoietin receptors** operate through a common subunit (γc, βc or gp130, depending on the subfamily) which transduces the signal to the interior of the cell. In essence, binding of the cytokine to its receptor must initiate the signaling process by mediating hetero- or homodimer formation involving the common subunit. In some cases the cytokine is active when bound to the receptor either in soluble or membrane-bound form (e.g. IL-6). The IL-2 receptor is interesting with respect to its ligand binding. The α chain (CD25, reacting with the Tac monoclonal) of the receptor possesses two complement control protein structural domains and binds IL-2 with a low affinity; the β chain (CD122) has a membrane proximal fibronectin type III structural domain and a membrane distal cytokine receptor structural domain, and associates with the common γ chain (CD132) which has a similar structural organization. The β chain binds IL-2 with intermediate affinity. IL-2 binds to and dissociates from the α chain very rapidly but the same processes involving the β chain occur at two or three orders of magnitude more slowly. When the α, β and γ chains form a single receptor, the α chain binds the IL-2 rapidly and facilitates its binding to a separate site on the β chain from which it can only dissociate slowly. Since the final affinity (K_d) is based on the ratio of dissociation to association rate constants, then $K_d = 10^{-4} s^{-1}/10^7 M^{-1} s^{-1} = 10^{-11} M$, which is a very high affinity. The γ chain does not itself bind IL-2 but contributes towards signal transduction. (b) The **interferon receptor** family consists of heterodimeric molecules each of which bears two fibronectin type III domains. (c) The receptors for **TNF** and related molecules consist of a single polypeptide with four TNFR domains. The receptor trimerizes upon ligand binding and, in common with a number of other receptors, is also found in a soluble form which, when released from a cell following activation, can act as an antagonist. (d) Another group of receptors contains varying numbers of **Ig superfamily domains**, whereas (e) **chemokine receptors** are members of the G-protein-coupled receptor superfamily and have seven hydrophobic transmembrane domains. (f) The final family illustrated are the **TGF receptors** which require association between two molecules, referred to as TGFR type I and TGFR type II, for signaling to occur.

Hematopoietin receptors

These are the largest family, sometimes referred to simply as the cytokine receptor superfamily, and are named after the first member of this family to be defined—the hematopoietin receptor. These receptors generally consist of one or two polypeptide chains responsible for cytokine binding and an additional shared (common or 'c') chain involved in signal transduction. The γc (CD132) chain is used by the IL-2 receptor (figure 9.2a) and IL-4, IL-7, IL-9, IL-15 and IL-21 receptors, a βc (CDw131) chain by IL-3, IL-5 and granulocyte–macrophage colony-stimulating factor (GM-CSF) receptors, and gp130 (CD130) shared chain by the IL-6, IL-11, IL-12, oncostatin M, ciliary neurotrophic factor and leukemia inhibitory factor (LIF) receptors.

Interferon receptors

These also consist of two polypeptide chains and, in addition to the IFNα, IFNβ and IFNγ receptors (figure 9.2b), this family includes the IL-10 receptor.

TNF receptors

Members of the TNF receptor superfamily possess cysteine-rich extracellular domains and most likely exist as preformed trimers that undergo a conformational change in their intracellular domains upon ligand binding. They include the tumor necrosis factor (TNF) receptor (figure 9.2c) and the related Fas (CD95/APO-1) and TRAIL receptors. This family also contains the lymphotoxin (LT) and nerve growth factor (NGF) receptors, as well as the CD40 receptor, which plays an important role in costimulation of B-cells and dendritic cells by activated T-cells.

IgSF cytokine receptors

Immunoglobulin superfamily members are broadly utilized in many aspects of cell biology (cf. p. 252) and include the IL-1 receptor (figure 9.2d), and the macrophage colony-stimulating factor (M-CSF) and stem cell factor (SCF/c-kit) receptors.

Chemokine receptors

Chemokines share a common functional property of promoting chemotaxis and their receptors comprise a family of approximately 20 different G-protein-coupled, seven transmembrane segment polypeptides (figure 9.2e). Each receptor subtype is capable of binding multiple chemokines within the same family. For example, CXC receptor 2 (CXCR2) is capable of binding seven different ligands within the CXC ligand (CXCL) family.

TGF receptors

Receptors for transforming growth factors such as the TGFβ receptor (figure 9.2f) possess cytoplasmic signaling domains with serine/threonine kinase activity.

Signal transduction through cytokine receptors

The ligand-induced homo- or heterodimerization of cytokine receptor subunits represents a common theme for signaling by cytokines. The two major routes that are utilized are the Janus kinase (JAK)–STAT and the Ras–MAP kinase pathways. Members of the cytokine receptor superfamily (hematopoietin receptors) lack catalytic domains but are constitutively associated with one or more JAKs (figure 9.3). There are four members of the mammalian JAK family: JAK1, JAK2, JAK3 and Tyk2 (tyrosine kinase 2) and all phosphorylate their downstream substrates at tyrosine residues. Genetic knockout studies have shown that the various JAKS have highly specific functions and produce lethal or severe phenotypes relating to defects in lymphoid development, failure of erythropoiesis and hypersensitivity to pathogens.

Upon cytokine-induced receptor dimerization, JAKs reciprocally phosphorylate, and thereby activate, each other. Active JAKs then phosphorylate specific tyrosine residues on the receptor cytoplasmic tails to create docking sites for members of the **STAT** (signal *t*ransducers and *a*ctivators of *t*ranscription) family of SH2 domain-containing transcription factors. STATs reside in the cytoplasm in an inactive state but, upon recruitment to cytokine receptors (via their SH2 domains),

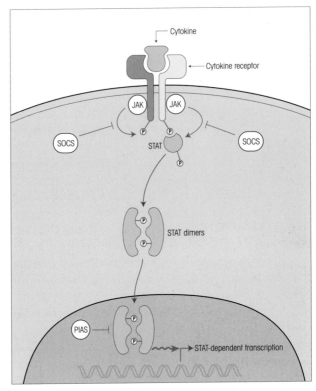

Figure 9.3. Cytokine receptor-mediated pathways for gene transcription. Cytokine-induced receptor oligomerization activates JAK kinases that are constitutively associated with the receptor cytoplasmic tails. Upon activation, JAK kinases phosphorylate tyrosine residues within the receptor tails, thereby creating binding sites for STAT transcription factors which then become recruited to the receptor complex and are, in turn, phosphorylated by JAKs. Phosphorylation of STATs triggers their dissociation from the receptor and promotes the formation of STAT dimers which translocate to the nucleus to direct transcription of genes that have the appropriate binding motifs within their promoter regions. Members of the SOCS family of inhibitors can suppress cytokine signaling at several points, either through inhibition of JAK kinase activity directly or by promoting polyubiquitination and proteasome-mediated degradation of JAKs. The PIAS family of STAT inhibitors can form complexes with STAT proteins that either result in decreased STAT-binding to DNA or recruitment of transcriptional corepressors that can block STAT-mediated transcription. Cytokine receptors can also recruit additional adaptor proteins such as Shc, Grb2 and Sos, that can activate the MAP kinase (see figure 8.7) and PI3 kinase signaling cascades, but these have been omitted for clarity.

become phosphorylated by JAKs and undergo dimerization and dissociation from the receptor. The dimerized STATs then translocate to the nucleus where they play an important role in pushing the cell through the mitotic cycle by activating transcription of various genes (figure 9.3). Seven mammalian STATs have been described and each plays a relatively nonredundant role in distinct cytokine signaling pathways. Individual cytokines usually employ more than one type of STAT to exert their biological effects; this is because the hematopoietin receptors are composed of two different receptor chains that are capable of recruiting distinct

STAT proteins. Further complexity is achieved due to the ability of STATs to form heterodimers with each other, with the result that a single cytokine may exert its transcriptional effects via a battery of STAT combinations. JAKs may also act through src family kinases to generate other transcription factors via the Ras–MAP kinase route (see figure 8.7). Some cytokines also activate phosphatidylinositol 3-kinase (PI3K) and phospholipase C (PLCγ).

Downregulation of JAK-STAT signaling is achieved by proteins that belong to the SOCS (suppressor of cytokine signaling) and PIAS (protein inhibitor of activated STAT) families (figure 9.3). SOCS proteins are induced in a STAT-dependent manner and therefore represent a classical feedback inhibition mechanism where cytokine signals induce expression of proteins that dampen down their own signaling cascades. The SOCS family contains eight members (namely CIS and SOCS1–SOCS7), and these proteins utilize two distinct mechanisms to downregulate cytokine signals. On the one hand, SOCS proteins can interact with JAKs, as well as other signaling proteins such as Vav, and target these proteins for degradation by the ubiquitin-proteasome pathway (cf. p. 98). Alternatively, SOCS family proteins can interact with SH2-domain binding sites found within the activation loop of the JAK kinase domains, thereby blocking access of JAKs to their downstream substrates (figure 9.3). Some SOCS family members, such as CIS (cytokine-inducible src homology domain 2 [SH2]-containing), can also directly interact with the STAT-binding SH2 domains found on cytokine receptors and by doing so can block recruitment of STAT molecules to the receptor complex. Targeted deletion of SOCS genes in the mouse has revealed the importance of these proteins for normal cytokine signaling. *SOCS-1*-deficient mice display marked growth retardation and lymphocytopenia and die from inflammation-associated multi-organ failure within 3 weeks of birth. Consistent with the role of SOCS proteins as negative regulators of cytokine signaling, lymphocytes derived from *SOCS-1*-deficient mice undergo spontaneous activation even in pathogen-free conditions. *SOCS-1*-deficient mice generated on a *RAG2*-deficient background do not display any of the phenotypes observed on a normal genetic background, confirming that SOCS-1 exerts its effects primarily within the lymphocyte compartment.

The PIAS family consists of four members (PIAS1, PIAS3, PIASX and PIASY) and can act to repress STAT-induced transcriptional activity by interacting with these proteins to either restrict their ability to interact with the DNA promoter elements they associate with, or alternatively, by recruiting transcriptional corepressor proteins such as histone deacetylase to the STAT transcriptional complexes (figure 9.3).

JAK-STAT pathways can also be regulated by other mechanisms such as protein tyrosine phosphatase-mediated antagonism of JAK activity, for example.

Cytokines often have multiple effects

In general, cytokines are **pleiotropic**, i.e. exhibit multiple effects on a variety of cell types (table 9.1), and there is considerable overlap and *redundancy* between them with respect to individual functions, partially accounted for by the sharing of receptor components and the utilization of common transcription factors. For example, many of the biological activities of IL-4 overlap with those of IL-13. However, it should be pointed out that virtually all cytokines have at least some unique properties.

Their roles in the generation of T- and B-cell effectors, and in the regulation of chronic inflammatory reactions (figure 9.4a,b), will be discussed at length later in this chapter. We should note here the important role of cytokines in the control of hematopoiesis (figure 9.4c). The differentiation of stem cells to become the formed elements of blood within the environment of the bone marrow is carefully nurtured through the production of cytokines by the stromal cells. These include GM-CSF, G-CSF (granulocyte colony-stimulating factor), M-CSF, IL-6 and -7 and LIF (table 9.1), and many of them are also derived from T-cells and macrophages. It is not surprising therefore that, during a period of chronic inflammation, the cytokines that are produced recruit new precursors into the hematopoietic differentiation pathway—a useful exercise in the circumstances. One of the cytokines, IL-3, should be highlighted for its exceptional ability to support the early cells in this pathway, particularly in synergy with IL-6 and G-CSF.

Network interactions

The complex and integrated relationships between the different cytokines are mediated through cellular events. The genes for IL-3, -4 and -5 and GM-CSF are all tightly linked on chromosome 5 in a region containing genes for M-CSF and its receptor and several other growth factors and receptors. Interaction may occur through a cascade in which one cytokine induces the production of another, through transmodulation of the receptor for another cytokine and through synergism or antagonism of two cytokines acting on the same cell (figure 9.5). Because of the number of combinations that are possible and the almost yearly discovery of new cytokines, the means by which target cells integrate

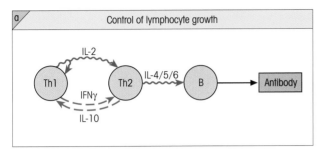

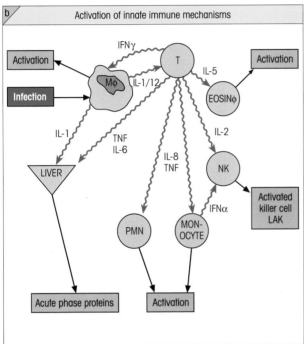

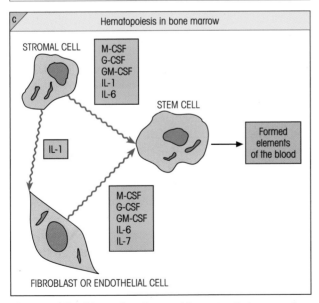

Figure 9.4. Cytokine action. A general but not entirely comprehensive guide to indicate the scope of cytokine interactions (e.g. for reasons of simplicity we have omitted the inhibitory effects of IL-10 on monocytes and the activation of NK cells by IL-12). EOSINϕ, eosinophil; LAK, lymphokine-activated killer; Mϕ, macrophage; NK, natural killer cell; PMN, polymorphonuclear neutrophil.

and interpret the complex patterns of stimuli induced by these multiple soluble factors is only slowly unfolding.

DIFFERENT T-CELL SUBSETS CAN MAKE DIFFERENT CYTOKINE PATTERNS

The bipolar Th1/Th2 concept

Helper T-cell clones can be divided into two main phenotypes, Th1 and Th2, with each displaying distinct cytokine secretion profiles (table 9.2). This makes biological sense in that Th1 cells producing cytokines such as IFNγ would be especially effective against **intracellular infections** with viruses and organisms which grow in macrophages, whereas Th2 cells are very good helpers for B-cells and would seem to be adapted for defense against parasites and other **extracellular pathogens** which are vulnerable to IL-4-switched IgE, IL-5-induced eosinophilia and IL-3/4-stimulated mast cell proliferation. Thus, studies on the infection of mice with the pathogenic protozoan *Leishmania major* demonstrated that intravenous or intraperitoneal injection of killed promastigotes leads to protection against challenge with live parasites associated with high expression of IFNγ mRNA and low levels of IL-4 mRNA; the reciprocal finding of low IFNγ and high IL-4 expression was made after subcutaneous immunization which failed to provide protection. Furthermore, nonvaccinated mice infected with live organisms could be saved by injection of IFNγ and anti-IL-4. These results are consistent with the preferential expansion of a population of protective IFNγ-secreting Th1 cells by intraperitoneal or intravenous immunization, and of nonprotective Th2 cells producing IL-4 in the subcutaneously injected animals. The ability of IFNγ, the characteristic Th1 cytokine, to inhibit the proliferation of Th2 clones, and of Th2-derived IL-4 and -10 to block both proliferation and cytokine release by Th1 cells, would seem to put the issue beyond reasonable doubt (figure 9.6).

The original Mosmann–Coffman classification into Th1 and Th2 subsets was predicated on data obtained with clones which had been maintained in culture for long periods and might have been artifacts of conditions *in vitro*. The use of cytokine-specific monoclonal antibodies for intracellular fluorescent staining, and of ELISPOT assays (cf. p. 145) for the detection of the secreted molecules, has demonstrated that the Th1/Th2 dichotomy is also apparent in freshly sampled cells and thus also applies *in vivo*. Nonetheless, it is perhaps best not to be too rigidly constrained in one's thinking by the Th1/Th2 paradigm, but rather to look upon activated T-cells as potentially producing a whole spectrum of

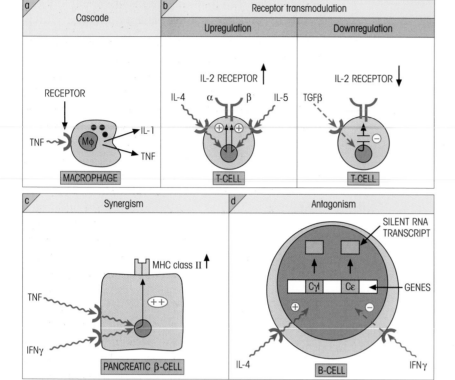

Figure 9.5. Network interactions of cytokines. (a) Cascade: in this example TNF induces secretion of IL-1 and of itself (autocrine) in the macrophage. (Note that all diagrams in this figure are simplified in that the effects on the nucleus are due to messengers resulting from the combination of cytokine with its surface receptor.) (b) Receptor transmodulation showing upregulation of each chain forming the high affinity IL-2 receptor in an activated T-cell by individual cytokines and downregulation by TGFβ. (c) Synergy of TNF and IFNγ in upregulation of surface MHC class II molecules on cultured pancreatic insulin-secreting cells. (d) Antagonism of IL-4 and IFNγ on transcription of silent ('sterile') mRNA relating to isotype switch (cf. figure 9.17).

Table 9.2. Cytokine patterns of helper T-cell clones. Interleukin-10 is not listed in the table. Although classed as a Th2 cytokine in the mouse, it is produced by both Th1 and Th2 cells in the human.

CYTOKINE PATTERNS OF T-CELL CLONES		
	Th1	Th2
IFNγ	++	
IL-2	++	
Lymphotoxin (TNFβ)	++	
TNF (TNFα)	++	++
GM-CSF	++	++
IL-3	++	++
IL-4		++
IL-5		++
IL-6		++
IL-13		++

++   +   Negative

Th1/2, T-helper 1/2.

cytokine profiles (Th0, figure 9.6), with possible skewing of the responses towards the extreme Th1 and Th2 patterns depending on the nature of the antigen stimulus. Thus, other subsets may also exist, in particular the transforming growth factor-β (TGFβ) and IL-10-producing Th3/Tr1 (T-regulatory 1) cells, which are of interest because these cytokines can mediate immuno-suppressive effects and may be involved in the induction of mucosally induced tolerance (cf. p. 451).

Interactions with cells of the innate immune system biases the Th1/Th2 response

The cytokine milieu that becomes established by cells of the innate immune system during the early stages of infection has a major influence on the adaptive immune response. Typically, innate immune responses dominate initially as T-lymphocytes require priming by DCs or other APCs to initiate clonal expansion and maturation to effectors. Upon migration of antigen-specific T-cells to lymph nodes where they come in contact with mature DCs fresh from their encounters with microbial pathogens, the pathogen products encountered by the DC will have polarized the latter in favor of secreting particular cytokines. This in turn can polarize T-cell responses in favor of differentiating towards a Th1 or Th2 phenotype. The reader will be well aware by now that efficient T-cell activation requires two signals from the APC; signal 1 is provided by stimulation through the TCR and signal 2 is provided by costimulation through CD28. Polarization of T-cells towards a Th1, Th2 or other fate is achieved via signal 3 and the nature of this signal is strongly influenced by the conditions under which the APC is primed (figure 9.6).

IL-12 and its recently discovered relatives, IL-23 and

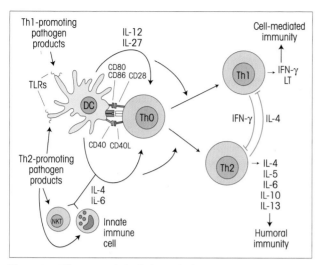

Figure 9.6. The generation of Th1 and Th2 CD4 subsets. Following initial stimulation of T-cells, a range of cells producing a spectrum of cytokine patterns emerges. Depending on the nature of the pathogen and the response of cells of the innate immune system during the initial stages of infection, the resulting T-helper cell population can be biased towards two extremes. Th1-promoting pathogen products (such as LPS) engage Toll-like receptors (TLRs) on dendritic cells (DC) or macrophages and induce the secretion of Th1-polarizing cytokines such as IL-12 and IL-27. The latter cytokines promote the development of Th1 cells which produce the cytokines characteristic of *cell-mediated immunity*. IL-4, possibly produced by interaction of microorganisms with the lectin-like NK1.1$^+$ receptor on NKT-cells or through interaction of Th2-promoting pathogen products with TLRs on DCs, skews the development to the production of Th2 cells whose cytokines assist the progression of B-cells to antibody secretion and the provision of *humoral immunity*. Cytokines produced by polarized Th1 and Th2 subpopulations are mutually inhibitory. LT, lymphotoxin (TNFβ); Th0, early helper cell producing a spectrum of cytokines; other abbreviations as in table 9.1.

IL-27, are instrumental in polarizing towards a Th1 cell phenotype while IL-4 is pivotal for the production of a Th2 cell phenotype. Polarization of T-cells towards an *inducible* regulatory phenotype (Th3/Tr1) can also occur during this phase, with IL-10 and TGFβ being influential in this situation. Invasion of phagocytic cells by intracellular pathogens induces copious secretion of IL-12, which in turn stimulates IFNγ production by NK cells. Engagement of many of the known Toll-like receptors (TLRs) on DCs by microbial products (such as LPS, dsRNA and bacterial DNA) triggers DC maturation and induces IL-12 production, thereby favoring Th1 responses. Bacterial priming also induces CD40 receptor expression on DCs and induces responsiveness to CD40L, expressed by activated T-cells, for optimal IL-12 synthesis. IL-12 is also particularly effective at inducing IFNγ by activated T-cells and secretion of the latter by the T-cell further enhances IL-12 production and secretion by DCs; this acts as a classical positive feedback loop for enhancement of IL-12 production and further skews the response towards Th1.

While IL-12 and IFNγ promote a Th1 response, these cytokines also inhibit Th2 responses (figure 9.6). However, IL-4 effects appear to be dominant over IL-12 and therefore the amounts of IL-4 relative to the amounts of IL-12 and IFNγ will be of paramount importance in determining the differentiation of Th0 cells into Th1 or Th2. IL-4 downregulates the expression of the IL-12R β$_2$ subunit necessary for responsiveness to IL-12, further polarizing the Th2 dominance. It is still unclear whether signals from the innate immune system drive T-cells in the direction of a Th2 response or whether this is a default differentiation pathway for Th cells unless suppressed by Th1-polarizing signals such as IL-12 or IFNγ. A special cell population, the NKT-cells bearing the NK1.1$^+$ marker, rapidly releases an IL-4-dominated pattern of cytokines on stimulation. These cells have many unusual features. They may be CD4$^-$8$^-$ or CD4$^+$8$^-$ and express low levels of T-cell αβ receptors with an invariant α chain and very restricted β, many of these receptors recognizing the nonclassical MHC-like CD1 molecule. Their morphology and granule content are intermediate between T-cells and NK cells. Although they express TCRαβ, there is an inclination to classify them on the fringe of the 'innate' immune system with regard to their primitive characteristics and possession of the lectin-like NK1.1 receptor which may be involved in the recognition of microbial carbohydrates.

Whilst there is a certain amount of evidence indicating the existence of subpopulations of dendritic cells specialized for the stimulation of either Th1 or Th2 populations, it seems that DCs are relatively plastic and can adopt a Th1- or Th2-polarizing phenotype depending on the priming signals they encounter from microbial and tissue-derived sources. However, it should be obvious from the above discussion that the cytokines produced in the immediate vicinity of the T-cell will be important. To give one recent example, Cantor and colleagues homologously deleted the gene for the cytokine Eta-1 (osteopontin) in mice and found that these animals had severely impaired immunity to infection with herpes simplex virus and to the intracellular bacterium *Listeria monocytogenes*. This was due to a deficient Th1 immunity caused by reduced IL-12 and IFNγ and enhanced IL-10 production. It appears that Eta-1 production by activated T-cells stimulates IL-12 production by macrophage lineage cells and downregulates IL-10 production. Interestingly, both serine phosphorylated and nonphosphorylated forms of Eta-1 are secreted by T-cells, and the IL-12 effect is phosphorylation-dependent whereas the IL-10 effect is not, indicating that phosphorylation can regulate the activity of secreted proteins.

Regulatory T-cells dampen immune responses and protect against autoimmunity

Another subset of T-cells, the **naturally-occurring regulatory T-cells (Tregs)**, has been the subject of much attention in recent years. These cells are a population of CD25$^+$ CD4$^+$ T-cells that can suppress immune responses of autoreactive T-cells by mechanisms that are still poorly understood but do not seem to involve cytokines. These Tregs are a *natural*, as opposed to an *inducible*, population of regulatory T-cells distinct from TGFβ-secreting Th3 cells and IL10-secreting Tr1 cells (cf. figure 10.10). The current view is that these self-antigen-reactive T-cells develop in the thymus and are released as functionally mature cells that can act to suppress the activation of other self-reactive T-cells that escape negative selection in the thymus, possibly through competition for self-antigens presented by APCs or through CTLA4-mediated signals from the Treg to the APC. IL-2 is crucial for the maintenance of natural Tregs as these T-cells are incapable of making their own IL-2, unlike activated T-cells, and rely fully on paracrine IL-2 for their survival. Consequently, the number of such cells is drastically reduced in *IL-2* and *IL-2R* knockout mice, with the result that these mice develop lymphoproliferation followed by lethal autoimmunity. The source of IL-2 for the maintenance of Tregs is unresolved but could come from autoreactive or antigen-activated T-cells that are interacting on the same DC as the Treg.

In contrast to natural regulatory T-cells, Th3/Tr1 cells are generated from naive T-cells in the periphery after encounter with antigen presented by DCs. The conditions under which DCs polarize towards Th3/Tr1cells remain uncertain but there is some evidence that such DCs have a semi-mature phenotype with low levels of CD40 and ICAM1. Pathogen molecules that induce IL-10 and suppress IL-12 production by DCs may be instrumental in evoking a Th3/Tr1 response.

Cytotoxic T-cells can also be subdivided into Tc1/Tc2

Clones of human cytotoxic T-cells obtained by limiting dilution also characteristically secrete particular cytokines. Thus, Tc1 cells secrete IFNγ but not IL-4, whilst Tc2 cells secrete IL-4 but not IFNγ. These clones show no differences in their cytolytic function but, when cocultured with CD4$^+$ T-cells, Tc1 clones induce Th1 cells, whilst Tc2 clones induce Th2 cells.

ACTIVATED T-CELLS PROLIFERATE IN RESPONSE TO CYTOKINES

In so far as T-cells are concerned, amplification follow-

ing activation is critically dependent upon IL-2 (figure 9.7). This cytokine is a single peptide of molecular weight 15.5 kDa which acts only on cells which express high affinity IL-2 receptors (figure 9.2). These receptors are not present on resting cells, but are synthesized within a few hours after activation.

Separation of an activated T-cell population into those with high and low affinity IL-2 receptors showed clearly that an adequate number of high affinity receptors were mandatory for the mitogenic action of IL-2. The numbers of these receptors on the cell increase under the action of antigen and of IL-2 and, as antigen is cleared, so the receptor numbers decline and, with that, the responsiveness to IL-2. It should be appreciated that, although IL-2 is an immunologically nonspecific T-cell growth factor, it only functions appropriately in specific responses because unstimulated T-cells do not express IL-2 receptors.

The T-cell blasts also produce an impressive array of

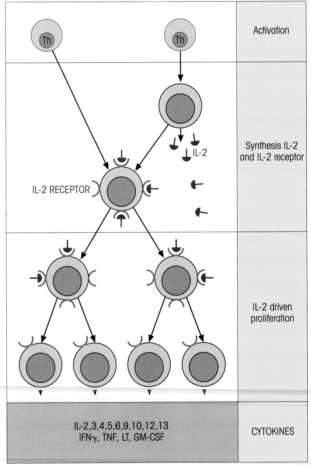

Figure 9.7. Activated T-blasts expressing surface receptors for IL-2 proliferate in response to IL-2 produced by itself or by another T-cell subset. Expansion is controlled through downregulation of the IL-2 receptor by IL-2 itself. The expanded population secretes a wide variety of biologically active cytokines of which IL-4 also enhances T-cell proliferation.

other cytokines, and the proliferative effect of IL-2 is reinforced by the action of IL-4 and, to some extent, IL-6, which react with corresponding receptors on the dividing T-cells. We must not lose sight of the importance of control mechanisms, and obvious candidates to subsume this role are TGFβ, which blocks IL-2-induced proliferation (figure 9.5b) and the production of TNF (TNFα) and lymphotoxin (TNFβ), and the cytokines IFNγ, IL-4 and IL-12, which mediate the mutual antagonism of Th1 and Th2 subsets.

T-CELL EFFECTORS IN CELL-MEDIATED IMMUNITY

Cytokines mediate chronic inflammatory responses

In addition to their role in the adaptive response, T-cell cytokines are responsible for generating antigen-specific chronic inflammatory reactions which deal with intracellular parasites (figures 9.4b and 9.8), although there is a different emphasis on the pattern of factors involved (cf. p. 282).

Early events

The initiating event is probably a local inflammatory response to tissue injury caused by the infectious agent which provokes the synthesis of adhesion molecules such as VCAM-1 (vascular cell adhesion molecule) and ICAM-1 on adjacent vascular endothelial cells. These adhesion molecules permit entry of memory T-cells to the infected site through their VLA-4 and LFA-1 homing receptors (cf. p. 159). Contact with processed antigen derived from the intracellular parasite will activate the specific T-cell and induce the release of secreted cytokines. TNF will further enhance the expression of endothelial accessory molecules and increase the chances of other memory cells in the circulation homing in to meet the antigen provoking inflammation.

Chemotaxis

The recruitment of T-cells and macrophages to the inflammatory site (figure 9.8) is greatly enhanced by the action of chemotactic cytokines termed **chemokines** (*chemo*attractant cyto*kine*). These can be produced by a variety of cell types and are divided into four families

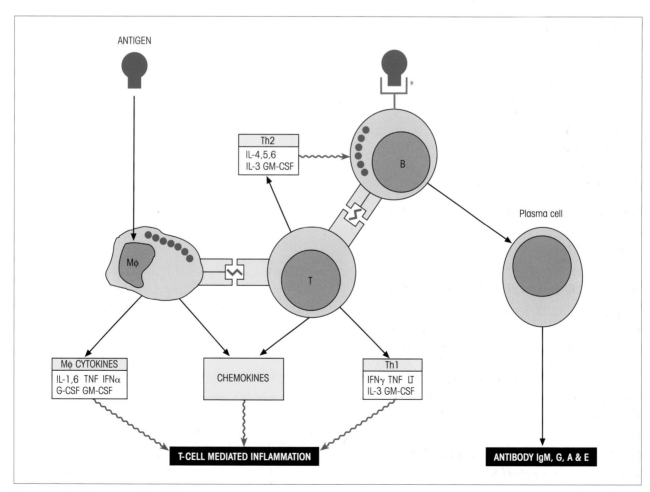

Figure 9.8. Cytokines controlling the antibody and T-cell-mediated inflammatory responses. Abbreviations as in table 9.1.

based on the disposition of the first (N-terminal) two of the four canonical cysteine residues (table 9.3). CXC chemokines have one amino acid and CX3C have three amino acids between the two cysteines. CC chemokines have adjacent cysteines at this location, whereas C chemokines lack cysteines 1 and 3 found in other chemokines. Chemokines bind to G-protein-coupled seven transmembrane receptors (figure 9.2). Despite the fact that a single chemokine can sometimes bind to more than one receptor, and a single receptor can bind several chemokines, many chemokines exhibit a strong tissue and receptor specificity. They play important roles in inflammation, lymphoid organ development, cell trafficking, cellular compartmentalization within lym-

Table 9.3. Chemokines and their receptors. The chemokines are grouped according to the arrangement of their cysteines (see text). The letter L designates ligand (i.e. the individual chemokine), whereas the letter R designates receptors. Names in parentheses refer to the murine homologs of the human chemokine where the names of these differ, or the murine chemokine alone if no human equivalent has been described.

FAMILY	CHEMOKINE	ALTERNATIVE NAMES	CHEMOTAXIS	RECEPTORS
CXC	CXCL1	GROα/MGSAα	Neutro	CXCR2>CXCR1
	CXCL2	GROβ/MGSAβ	Neutro	CXCR2
	CXCL3	GROγ/MGSAγ	Neutro	CXCR2
	CXCL4	PF4	Eosino, Baso, T	CXCR3-B
	CXCL5	ENA-78	Neutro	CXCR2
	CXCL6	GCP-2/(CKα-3)	Neutro	CXCR1, CXCR2
	CXCL7	NAP-2	Neutro	CXCR2
	CXCL8	IL-8	Neutro	CXCR1, CXCR2
	CXCL9	Mig	T, NK	CXCR3-A, CXCR3-B
	CXCL10	IP-10	T, NK	CXCR3-A, CXCR3-B
	CXCL11	I-TAC	T, NK	CXCR3-A, CXCR3-B
	CXCL12	SDF-1α/β	T, B, DC, Mono	CXCR4
	CXCL13	BLC/BCA-1	B	CXCR5
	CXCL14	BRAC/Bolekine	?	DC, Mono
	CXCL15	Lungkine	Neutro	?
	CXCL16	None	T, NKT	CXCR6
C	XCL1	Lymphotactin/SCM-1α/ATAC	T	XCR1
	XCL2	SCM-1β	T	XCR1
CX3C	CX3CL1	Fractalkine/Neurotactin	T, NK, Mono	CX3CR1
CC	CCL1	I-309/(TCA-3/P500)	Mono	CCR8
	CCL2	MCP-1/MCAF	T, NK, DC, Mono, Baso	CCR2
	CCL3	MIP-1α/LD78α	T, NK, DC, Mono, Eosino	CCR1, CCR5
	CCL4	MIP-1β	T, NK, DC, Mono	CCR5
	CCL5	RANTES	T, NK, DC, Mono, Eosino, Baso	CCR1, CCR3, CCR5
	(CCL6)	(C10/MRP-1)	Mono, Mφ, T, Eosino	CCR1
	CCL7	MCP-3	T, NK, DC, Mono, Eosino, Baso	CCR1,CCR2, CCR3
	CCL8	MCP-2	T, NK, DC, Mono, Baso	CCR3
	(CCL9/10)	(MRP-2/CCF18/MIP-1γ)	T, Mono	CCR1
	CCL11	Eotaxin-1	T, DC, Eosino, Baso	CCR3
	(CCL12)	(MCP-5)	T, NK, DC, Mono, Baso	CCR2
	CCL13	MCP-4	T, NK, DC, Mono, Eosino, Baso	CCR2, CCR3
	CCL14	HCC-1/HCC-3	T, Mono, Eosino	CCR1
	CCL15	HCC-2/Leukotactin-1/MIP-1δ	T	CCR1, CCR3
	CCL16	HCC-4/LEC/(LCC-1)	T	CCR1
	CCL17	TARC	T, DC, Mono	CCR4
	CCL18	DCCK1/PARC/AMAC-1	T, DC	?
	CCL19	MIP-3β/ELC/Exodus-3	T, B, DC	CCR7
	CCL20	MIP-3α/LARC/Exodus-1	DC	CCR6
	CCL21	6Ckine/SLC/Exodus-2/(TCA-4)	T, DC	CCR7
	CCL22	MDC/STCP-1/ABCD-1	T, DC, Mono	CCR4
	CCL23	MPIF-1	T	CCR1
	CCL24	MPIF-2/Eotaxin-2	T, DC, Eosino, Baso	CCR3
	CCL25	TECK	T, DC, Mono	CCR9
	CCL26	SCYA26/Eotaxin-3	T	CCR3
	CCL27	CTACK/ALP/ESkine	T	CCR10
	CCL28	MEC	T, B, Eosino	CCR3/CCR10

B, B-cell; Baso, basophil; DC, dendritic cell; Eosino, eosinophil; MEC, mucosal epithelial chemokine; Mono, monocyte; Neutro, neutrophil; NK, natural killer; T, T-cell.

phoid tissues, Th1/Th2 development, angiogenesis and wound healing.

Macrophage activation

Macrophages with intracellular organisms are activated by agents such as IFNγ, GM-CSF, IL-2 and TNF and should become endowed with microbicidal powers. During this process, some macrophages may die (probably helped along by cytotoxic T-cells) and release living parasites, but these will be dealt with by fresh macrophages brought to the site by chemotaxis and newly activated by local cytokines so that they have passed the stage of differentiation at which the intracellular parasites can subvert their killing mechanisms (cf. p. 269).

Combating viral infection

Virally infected cells require a different strategy and one strand of that strategy exploits the innate interferon mechanism to deny the virus access to the cell's replicative machinery. IFNγ, TNF and lymphotoxin all induce 2′–5′ (A) synthetase, a protein which is involved in viral protection. TNF has another string to its bow in terms of its ability to kill certain cells, since death of an infected cell before viral replication has occurred is obviously beneficial to the host. The cytotoxic potential of TNF was first recognized using tumor cells as targets (hence the name), and IFNγ and lymphotoxin can act synergistically, with IFNγ setting up the cell for destruction by inducing the formation of TNF receptors. It is worth pointing out, however, that TNF kills by inducing apoptosis rather than necrosis in the majority of cases.

Killer T-cells

The generation of cytotoxic T-cells

Cytotoxic T-cells (Tc), also referred to as cytotoxic T-lymphocytes (CTLs), represent the other major arm of the cell-mediated immune response and are of strategic importance in the killing of virally infected cells and possibly in contributing to the postulated surveillance mechanisms against cancer cells (see p. 388).

CTL precursors recognize antigen on the surface of cells in association with class I major histocompatibility complex (MHC) molecules and, like B-cells, they usually require help from T-cells. The mechanism by which help is proffered may, however, be quite different. As explained earlier (see p. 180), effective T–B collaboration is usually 'cognate' in that the collaborating cells recognize two epitopes that are physically linked (usually on the same molecule). If we may remind the reader without causing offense, the reason for this is that the surface Ig receptors on the B-cell capture native antigen, process it internally and present it to the Th as a peptide in association with MHC class II. Although it has been shown that linked epitopes on the antigen are also necessary for cooperation between Th and the cytotoxic T-cell precursor (Tcp), the nature of T-cell recognition prevents native antigen being focused onto the Tcp by its receptor for subsequent processing, even if that cell were to express MHC II, which in its resting state it does not. It seems most likely that Th and Tcp bind to the same APC, for example a dendritic cell, which has processed viral antigen and displays processed viral peptides in association with both class II (for the Th cell) and class I (for the Tcp) on its surface; one cannot exclude the possibility that the APC could be the virally infected cell itself. Cytokines from the triggered Th will be released in close proximity to the Tcp which is engaging the antigen–MHC signal and will be stimulated to proliferate and differentiate into a Tc under the influence of IL-2 and -6 (figure 9.9a). However, interaction of the APC with the Th and the Tc cell can be temporally separated and, in this case, it appears that the helper T-cell 'licenses' the dendritic cell for future interaction with the cytotoxic T-cell. It does this by activating the dendritic cell through CD40, thereby upregulating costimulatory molecules and cytokine production, in particular IL-12, by the dendritic cell (figure 9.9b). An entirely Th-independent mechanism of Tc activation is also thought to occur. This has been demonstrated in, for example, the response to protein antigens given with potent adjuvants such as immunostimulatory DNA sequences (ISSs), in this case possibly involving adjuvant-induced production of proinflammatory cytokines and cell surface costimulatory molecules.

The lethal process

Cytotoxic T-cells (Tc) are generally of the CD8 subset, and their binding to the target cell through TCR-mediated recognition of peptide presented on class I MHC is assisted by interactions between CD8, the co-receptor for class I, and by other accessory molecules such as LFA-1 and CD2 which increase the affinity of the interaction between the CTL and the target cell (see figure 8.3).

Tc are **unusual secretory cells** which contain modified lysosomes equipped with a battery of cytotoxic proteins. Following activation of the Tc, the **cytotoxic granules** are driven at a rare old speed (up to 1.2 μm/sec) along the microtubule system and delivered to the point of contact between the Tc and its target (figure 9.10). This ensures the specificity of killing dictated by TCR recognition of the target and limits collateral damage to surrounding cells, as well as to the killer cell itself. As with NK cells, which have comparable

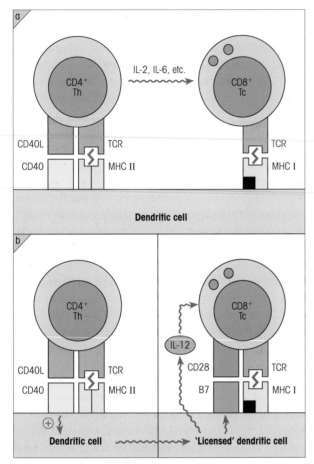

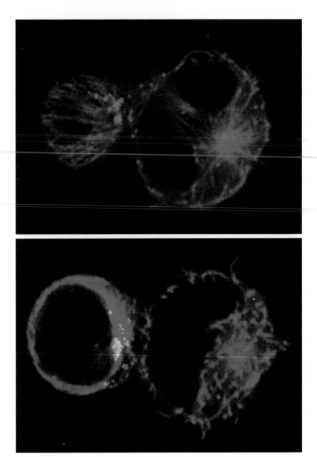

Figure 9.9. T-helper cell activation of cytotoxic T-cells. Activation of the CD4+ helper T-cells (Th) by the dendritic cell involves a CD40–CD40 ligand (CD154) costimulatory signal and recognition of an MHC class II peptide presented by the T-cell receptor. (a) If both the Th and the cytotoxic T-lymphocyte (Tc) are present at the same time, the release of cytokines from the activated Th cells stimulates the differentiation of the CD8+ precursor into an activated, MHC class I-restricted Tc. However, as shown in (b), the Th and the Tc do not need to interact with the APC at the same time. In this case, the Th cell 'licenses' the dendritic cell for future interaction with a Tc cell. Thus the Th cell, by engaging CD40, drives the dendritic cell from a resting state into an activated state with upregulation of costimulatory molecules such as B7.1 and B7.2 (CD80 and CD86, respectively) and increased cytokine production, particularly of IL-12.

Figure 9.10. Conjugation of a cytotoxic T-cell (on left) to its target, here a mouse mastocytoma, showing polarization of the granules towards the target at the point of contact. The cytoskeletons of both cells are revealed by immunofluorescent staining with an antibody to tubulin (green) and the lytic granules with an antibody to granzyme A (red). Twenty minutes after conjugation the target cell cytoskeleton may still be intact (above), but this rapidly becomes disrupted (below). (Photographs kindly provided by Dr Gillian Griffiths.)

granules (cf. p. 18), exocytosis of the cytotoxic granules delivers a range of cytotoxic proteins into the target cell cytosol that cooperate to promote apoptosis of the target. Videomicroscopy shows that Tc are serial killers. After the 'kiss of death', the T-cell can disengage and seek a further victim, there being rapid synthesis of new granules.

Cytotoxic T-cell granules contain perforin, a pore-forming protein similar to the C9 component of complement, and a battery of cathepsin-like proteases that are collectively referred to as **granzymes**. Perforin facilitates the entry of the other granule constituents into the target cell in a manner that is still much debated, but all

are agreed that perforin plays an essential role in the killing process; mice deficient in perforin are severely impaired in clearing several viral pathogens. It is not clear how all of the granzymes contribute to target cell death upon delivery into the cell cytoplasm but granzyme A and B are known to play particularly significant roles in this process. Granzyme A can promote the activation of a nuclease through proteolysis of its inhibitor and this results in the formation of numerous single-stranded DNA breaks within the target cell (figure 9.11). Granzyme B can directly process and activate several members of the **caspase** family of cysteine proteases that can rapidly initiate apoptosis through restricted proteolysis of hundreds of proteins within the target cell. Granzyme B can also promote caspase activation indirectly, through activation of Bid, a protein that promotes permeabilization of mitochondria and release of mitochondrial cytochrome *c* into the cytosol; the latter

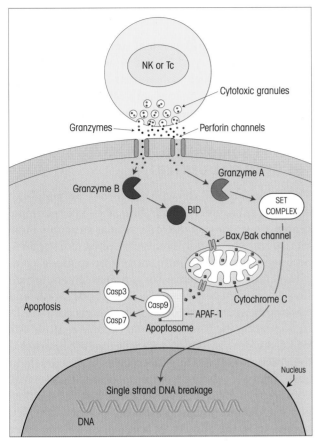

Figure 9.11. Cytotoxic granule-dependent killing of target cells by cytotoxic T-cells and NK cells. In response to an appropriate stimulus, Tc and NK cells deliver the contents of their cytotoxic granule onto the surface of target cells. The cytotoxic granule protein perforin is thought to polymerize within the target cell membrane forming pores that permit passage of other granule constituents, which includes several serine proteases (granzymes), into the target cell. Upon entry into the target, granzyme B orchestrates apoptosis by cleaving and activating BID, which translocates to mitochondria and triggers the opening of a pore or channel within the mitochondrial outer membrane composed of Bax and/or Bak; the latter channel permits the release of cytochrome *c* from the mitochondrial intermembrane space into the cytoplasm where it acts as a co-factor for the assembly of a caspase-9-activating complex (the apoptosome). The apoptosome promotes activation of downstream caspases, such as caspase-3 and caspase-7, and the latter proteases coordinate apoptosis through restricted proteolysis of hundreds of substrate proteins. Granzyme B can also proteolytically process and activate caspases-3 and -7 directly, providing a more direct route to caspase activation. Another granule protein, granzyme A, can cleave a protein within the SET complex (an endoplasmic reticulum-associated protein complex). This permits the translocation of a nuclease (NM23-H1) to the nuclear compartment that can catalyze single-strand DNA breaks. Cytotoxic granules also contain other granzymes that contribute to target cell killing but substrates for these proteases have yet to be identified.

event arms a caspase-activating complex that has been termed 'the apoptosome' and this complex promotes the activation of several downstream caspases (figure 9.11). Several additional granzymes have also been found within cytotoxic granules but their precise func-

tional role in Tc killing remains the subject of ongoing investigation. Collectively, entry of the full spectrum of granzymes into the target cells results in very swift cell killing (within 60 minutes or so) and several parallel pathways to apoptosis are most likely engaged during this process. Tc also express protease inhibitors, such as PI-9, that may protect them from the lethal effects of their own granule contents.

The induction of apoptosis, as opposed to necrosis, by the Tc is likely to have several benefits. Apoptotic cells, by virtue of specific alterations to their plasma membranes, are swiftly recognized by macrophages and other phagocytic cells and undergo phagocytosis before their intracellular contents can leak; this has the desirable effect of minimizing collateral damage to neighboring cells and may also prevent escape of viral particles from an infected cell. Moreover, nucleases and caspase proteases that become activated within the target cell during apoptosis are also likely to degrade viral nucleic acids and structural proteins and may also contribute to ensuring that infectious viral particle release is kept to a minimum.

Tc are also endowed with a second killing mechanism involving Fas and its ligand (cf. p. 19). In this situation, engagement of the trimeric Fas receptor by membrane-borne Fas ligand on the Tc initiates a signaling pathway within the target cell that results in the recruitment and activation of caspase-8 at the receptor complex. Upon activation, caspase-8 can further propagate the death signal through restricted proteolysis of Bid, similar to the granzyme B pathway discussed above, or can directly process and activate downstream caspases such as caspase-3. However, the inability of perforin knockout mice to clear viruses effectively suggests that the secretory granules provide the dominant means of killing virally infected cells. One should also not lose sight of the fact that CD8 cells synthesize other cytokines such as IFNγ which also have potent antiviral effects.

Inflammation must be regulated

Once the inflammatory process has cleared the inciting agent, the body needs to switch it off. IL-10 has profound anti-inflammatory and immunoregulatory effects, acting on macrophages and Th1 cells to inhibit release of factors such as IL-1 and TNF. It induces the release of soluble TNF receptors which are endogenous inhibitors of TNF, and downregulates surface TNF receptor. Soluble IL-1 receptors released during inflammation can act to 'decoy' IL-1 itself. IL-4 not only acts to constrain Th1 cells but also upregulates production of the natural inhibitor of IL-1, the IL-1 receptor antagonist

(IL-1Ra). The role of TGFβ is more difficult to tease out because it has some pro- and other anti-inflammatory effects, although it undoubtedly promotes tissue repair after resolution of the inflammation.

PROLIFERATION AND MATURATION OF B-CELL RESPONSES ARE MEDIATED BY CYTOKINES

The activation of B-cells by Th cells, through the TCR recognition of MHC-linked antigenic peptide plus the costimulatory **CD40L–CD40 interaction**, leads to upregulation of the surface receptor for IL-4. Copious local release of this cytokine from the Th then drives powerful clonal proliferation and expansion of the activated B-cell population. IL-2 and IL-13 also contribute to this process (figure 9.12).

Under the influence of IL-4 and IL-13, the expanded clones can differentiate and mature into IgE synthesizing cells. TGFβ and IL-5 encourage cells to switch their Ig class to IgA. IgM plasma cells emerge under the tutelage of IL-4 plus -5, and IgG producers result from the combined influence of IL-4, -5, -6, -13 and IFNγ (figure 9.12).

Type 2 thymus-independent antigens can activate B-cells directly (cf. p. 178) but nonetheless still need cytokines for efficient proliferation and Ig production. These may come from accessory cells such as NK and NKT-cells which bear lectin-like receptors.

WHAT IS GOING ON IN THE GERMINAL CENTER?

The secondary follicle with its corona or mantle of small lymphocytes surrounding the pale germinal center is a striking and unique cellular structure. First, let us recall the overall events described in Chapter 8. Secondary challenge with antigen or immune complexes induces enlargement of germinal centers, formation of new ones, appearance of memory B-cells and development of Ig-producing cells of higher affinity. B-cells entering the germinal center become **centroblasts** which divide with a very short cycle time of 6 hours, and then become nondividing **centrocytes** in the basal light zone, many of which die from apoptosis (figure 9.13). As the surviving centrocytes mature, they differentiate either into **immunoblast plasma cell precursors**, which secrete Ig in the absence of antigen, or into **memory B-cells**.

What then is the underlying scenario? Following secondary antigen challenge, primed B-cells may be activated by paracortical Th cells in association with interdigitating dendritic cells or macrophages, and migrate to the germinal center. There they divide in response to powerful stimuli from complexes on follicular dendritic cells (cf. p. 169) and from cytokines released by T-cells in response to antigen-presenting B-cells. During this particularly frenetic bout of cell division, **somatic hypermutation** of B-cell Ig genes occurs. The cells also undergo **Ig class switching**. Thereafter, as they transform to centrocytes, they are vulnerable and die readily, whence they are taken up as the 'tingible bodies' by macrophages, unless rescued by association with antigen on a follicular dendritic cell. This could result from cross-linking of surface Ig receptors and is accompanied by expression of Bcl-x and Bcl-2 which protect against apoptosis. Interactions between BAFF (*B-cell-activating factor* of the tumor necrosis factor *family*; also called BLyS) on the T-helper cell and TACI (*transmembrane activator* and *calcium modulator* and cyclophilin ligand [CAML] *interactor*), its receptor on the B-cell, may also be important for the maintenance of germinal center B-cells. Signaling through CD40 and TACI, during presentation of antigen to Th cells, would also prolong the life of the centrocyte. In either case, the

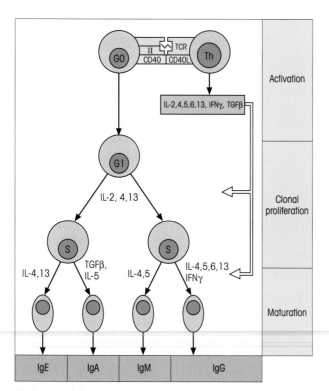

Figure 9.12. B-cell response to thymus-dependent (TD) antigen: clonal expansion and maturation of activated B-cells under the influence of T-cell-derived soluble factors. Costimulation through the CD40L–CD40 interaction is essential for primary and secondary immune responses to TD antigens and for the formation of germinal centers and memory. c-*myc* expression, which is maximal 2 hours after antigen or anti-μ stimulation, parallels sensitivity to growth factors; transfection with c-*myc* substitutes for anti-μ.

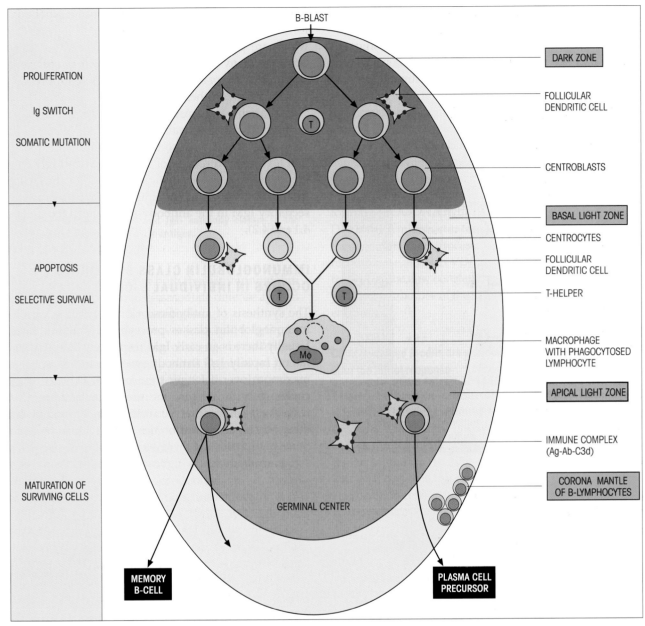

Figure 9.13. The events occurring in lymphoid germinal centers. Germinal center B-cells can be enriched through their affinity for the peanut agglutinin lectin. They show numerous mutations in the antibody genes. Expression of LFA-1 and ICAM-1 on B-cells and follicular dendritic cells (FDCs) in the germinal center makes them 'sticky'. Centroblasts at the base of the follicle are strongly CD77 positive. The Th cells bear the unusual CD57 marker. The FDCs all express CD21 and CD54; those in the apical light zone are strongly CD23 positive, those in the basal light zone express little CD23. Through their surface recep-

tors, FDCs bind immune complexes containing antigen and C3 which, in turn, are very effective B-cell stimulators since coligation of the surface receptors for antigen and C3 (CR2) lowers their threshold for activation. The costimulatory molecules CD40 and B7 play pivotal roles. Antibodies to CD40 prevent formation of germinal centers and anti-CD40L can disrupt established germinal centers within 12 hours. Anti-B7.2, given early in the immune response, prevents germinal center formation and, when given at the onset of hypermutation, suppresses that process.

interactions will only occur if the mutated surface Ig receptor still binds antigen and, as the concentration of antigen gradually falls, only if the receptor is of high affinity. In other words, the system can deliver high affinity antibody by a Darwinian process of high frequency mutation of the Ig genes and selection by antigen of the cells bearing the antibody which binds

most strongly (figure 9.14). This increase of affinity as the antibody level falls late in the response is of obvious benefit, since a small amount of high affinity antibody can do the job of a large amount of low affinity (as in boxing, a small 'goodun' will generally be a match for a mediocre 'bigun').

Further differentiation now occurs. The cells either

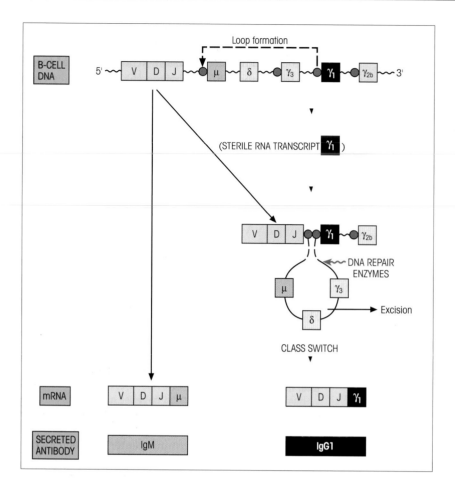

Figure 9.17. Class switching to produce antibodies of identical specificity but different immunoglobulin isotype (in this example from IgM to IgG1) is achieved by a recombination process which utilizes the specialized switch sequences (●) and leads to a loss of the intervening DNA loop (μ, δ and γ3). Each switch sequence is 1–10 kilobases in length and comprises guanosine-rich repeats of 20–100 base pairs. Because the switch sequence associated with each C_H gene has a unique nucleotide sequence, recombination cannot occur homologously and therefore probably depends upon nonhomologous end joining. DNA repair proteins including Ku70, Ku80 and the catalytic subunit of the DNA-dependent protein kinase (DNA-PK$_{CS}$) are involved in this process.

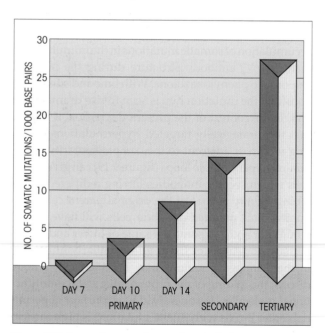

Figure 9.18. Increasing somatic mutations in the immunodominant germ-line antibody observed in hybridomas isolated following repeated immunization with phenyloxazolone. (Data from Berek C. & Apel M. (1989) In Melchers F. *et al.* (eds) *Progress in Immunology* **7**, 99. Springer-Verlag, Berlin.)

FACTORS AFFECTING ANTIBODY AFFINITY IN THE IMMUNE RESPONSE

The effect of antigen dose

Other things being equal, the binding strength of an antigen for the surface receptor of a B-cell will be determined by the affinity constant of the reaction:

$$Ag+(surface)Ab \rightleftharpoons AgAb$$

and the reactants will behave according to the laws of thermodynamics (cf. p. 91).

It may be supposed that, when a sufficient number of antigen molecules are bound to the receptors on the cell surface and processed for presentation to T-cells, the lymphocyte will be stimulated to develop into an antibody-producing clone. When only small amounts of antigen are present, only those lymphocytes with high affinity receptors will be able to bind sufficient antigen for stimulation to occur and their daughter cells will, of course, also produce high affinity antibody. Consideration of the antigen–antibody equilibrium equation will show that, as the concentration of antigen is increased, even antibodies with relatively low affinity will bind

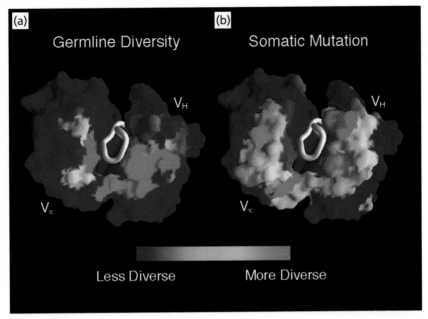

Figure 9.19. An 'antigen's eye view' of sequence diversity in human antibodies. The sequence diversity has been plotted on a scale of blue (more conserved) to red (more diverse). The V_H domain is on the right and the V_κ domain on the left in both pictures. (a) Germ-line diversity prior to somatic hypermutation is focused at the center of the antigen-binding site. (b) Somatic hypermutation spreads diversity to regions at the periphery of the binding site that are highly conserved in the germ-line V gene repertoire. Somatic hypermutation is therefore complementary to germ-line diversity. The V_H CDR3, which lies at the center of the antigen-binding site, was not included in this analysis and therefore is shown in gray as a loop structure. The end of the V_κ CDR3 (also excluded) lies at the center of the binding site and is not visible in this representation. (Reproduced with kind permission from Tomlinson I.M. *et al.* (1996) *Journal of Molecular Biology* **256**, 813.)

more antigen; therefore, at high doses of antigen, the lymphocytes with lower affinity receptors will also be stimulated and, as may be seen from figure 9.20, these are more abundant than those with receptors of high affinity. Furthermore, there is a strong possibility that cells with the highest affinity will bind so much antigen as to become tolerized (cf. p. 247). Thus, in summary, low amounts of antigen produce high affinity antibodies, whereas high antigen concentrations give rise to an antiserum with low to moderate affinity.

Maturation of affinity

In addition to being brisker and fatter, secondary responses tend to be of higher affinity. There are probably two main reasons for this maturation of affinity after primary stimulation. First, once the primary response gets under way and the antigen concentration declines to low levels, only successively higher affinity cells will bind sufficient antigen to maintain proliferation. Second, at this stage the cells are mutating madly in the germinal centers, and any mutants with an adventitiously higher affinity will bind well to antigen on follicular dendritic cells and be positively selected for by its persistent clonal expansion. Modification of antibody specificity by somatic point mutations allows gradual

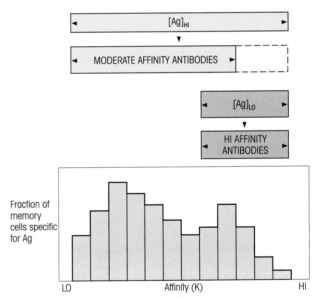

Figure 9.20. Relationship of antigen concentration to affinity of antibodies produced. Low concentrations of antigen ($[Ag]_{LO}$) bind to and permit stimulation of a range of high affinity memory cells and the resulting antibodies are of high affinity. High doses of antigen ($[Ag]_{HI}$) are able to bind sufficiently to the low affinity cells and thereby allow their stimulation, whilst the highest affinity cells may bind an excess of antigen and be tolerized (dashed line); the resulting antiserum will have a population of low to moderate affinity antibodies.

diversification on which positive selection for affinity can act during clonal expansion.

It is worth noting that responses to thymus-independent antigens, which have poorly developed memory with very rare mutations, do not show this phenomenon of affinity maturation. Overall, the ability of Th to facilitate responses to nonpolymeric, nonpolyclonally activating antigens, to induce expansive clonal proliferation, to effect class switching and, lastly, to fine-tune responses to higher affinity has provided us with bigger, better and more flexible immune responses.

MEMORY CELLS

As the immune response subsides, the majority of recently expanded effector cells are culled by large-scale induction of apoptosis in this population. However, a subpopulation of cells escape the culling process and these form the **memory compartment** that live to mount a more rapid and efficient secondary immune response upon re-exposure to the same antigen. It is possible that the memory cell population represents a subpopulation of cells that bypass the effector cell stage entirely, but this concept remains controversial. The process of memory cell generation is central to the concept of vaccination and memory cells have been the subjects of much investigation as a consequence.

Antibodies encoded by unmutated germ-line genes represent a form of evolutionary memory, in the sense that they tend to include specificities for commonly encountered pathogens and are found in the so-called 'natural antibody' fraction of serum. Memory acquired during the adaptive immune response requires contact with antigen and expansion of antigen-specific memory cells, as seen for example in the 20-fold increase in cytotoxic T-cell precursors after immunization of females with the male H-Y antigen.

Memory of early infections such as measles is long-lived and the question arises as to whether the memory cells are long-lived or are subject to repeated antigen stimulation from persisting antigen or subclinical reinfection. Fanum in 1847 described a measles epidemic on the Faroe Islands in the previous year in which almost the entire population suffered from infection except for a few old people who had been infected 65 years earlier. While this evidence favors the long half-life hypothesis, memory function of B-cells transferred to an irradiated syngeneic recipient is lost within a month unless antigen is given or the donor is transgenic for the *bcl-2* gene (remember that signals in the germinal center which prevent apoptosis of centrocytic B-cells also upregulate *bcl-2* expression). It is envisaged that B-cell memory is a dynamic state in which survival of the memory cells is maintained by recurrent signals from follicular dendritic cells in the germinal centers, the only long-term repository of antigen.

Evidence from mouse models strongly suggests that memory T-cells can, at least in principle, persist in the absence of antigen. T-cells isolated from mice several months after they were immunized with lymphocytic choriomeningitis virus (LCMV) were transferred into two groups of genetically modified mice which lacked endogenous T-cells, one of the groups additionally lacking MHC class I expression. T-cells were parked in these mice for 10 months and then analysed *in vitro*. Functional virus-specific CD8$^+$ CTLs were still present in both groups of mice, and in similar numbers, even though those from the class I$^-$ mice could not have had antigen presented to their TCR. Indeed, these memory T-cells undergo antigen- and MHC-independent proliferation *in vivo*, their numbers controlled, at least in part, by a balance between proliferation-inducing signals from IL-15 and cell death-inducing signals from IL-2 released in the local environment, both cytokines binding to the IL-2R β chain (cf. figure 9.2). Other recent findings indicate that helper T-cell memory also does not require the continued presence of antigen or MHC and, at least in some cases, Th memory is maintained in the absence of cell division.

However, we should not lose sight of the fact that, while these experiments in transgenic and knockout animals clearly demonstrate that immunological memory *can* be maintained in the absence of antigen, usually antigen persists as complexes on follicular dendritic cells. Therefore, there is the potential for antigen-presenting cells within the germinal center to capture and process this complexed antigen and then present it to memory T-cells. Some evidence, again recent, suggests that it is a type of dendritic cell, and not the germinal center B-cells, that may subserve this function. To add complexity, there is also accumulating evidence that the mechanisms used to maintain memory T-cells in the mouse, a relatively short-lived animal, may differ significantly from those employed by the human immune system. Specific antigen may play a much more important role in maintaining T-lymphocyte memory in man, not least because ongoing entry of new memory cells specific for diverse antigens to the memory compartment will generate competition between memory cells. Because the naive and memory cell pools are maintained at a relatively constant size, it is likely that memory cells which receive periodic re-stimulation with antigen are likely to persist for longer than those that fail to re-encounter antigen. Competition may be absent or diminished in mouse models where animals are typically maintained in artificially clean environments; such cosseting is likely to reduce the rate of entry of new T-cell specificities to the memory compartment and therefore reduce competition between memory cell populations. In support of this view, while there is evidence that T-cell memory in humans can persist for decades after exposure to particular antigens, immunity does indeed decline over time and estimates of the half-life of T-cell responses have put this between 8 and 15 years. In addition, because the lifespan of the laboratory mouse is far shorter than the average human, the problems associated with retention of memory cells in the human are likely to be greater than those faced by laboratory mice. Ongoing attrition of memory T-cells, in the absence of antigenic re-stimulation, may contribute to the increased rate and severity of infectious diseases in the elderly and may also explain why latent viruses, such as varicella zoster (human herpesvirus 3), may reactivate many years after initial infection.

The memory population is not simply an expansion of corresponding naive cells

In general, memory cells are more readily stimulated by a given dose of antigen because they have a higher affinity. In the case of B-cells, we are satisfied by the evidence that links mutation and antigen-driven selection, occurring within the germinal centers of secondary lymph node follicles, to the creation of high affinity memory cells. The receptors for antigen on memory T-cells also have higher affinity but, since they do not undergo significant somatic mutation during the priming response, it would seem that cells with **pre-existing receptors of relatively higher affinity in the population of naive cells proliferate selectively through preferential binding to the antigen**.

Intuitively one would not expect to improve on affinity to the same extent that somatic hypermutation can achieve for the B-cells, but nonetheless memory T-cells augment their binding avidity for the antigen-presenting cell through increased expression of accessory adhesion molecules, CD2, LFA-1, LFA-3 and ICAM-1. Since several of these molecules also function to enhance signal transduction, the memory T-cell is more readily triggered than its naive counterpart. Indeed, memory cells enter cell division and secrete cytokines more rapidly than naive cells, and there is some evidence that they may secrete a broader range of cytokines than do naive cells.

A phenotypic change in the isoform of the leukocyte common antigen CD45R, derived by differential splicing, allows some distinction to be made between naive

and memory cells. Expression of CD45RA has been used as a marker of naive T-cells and of CD45RO as a marker of memory cells capable of responding to recall antigens. However, most of the features associated with the CD45RO subset are in fact manifestations of **activated cells** and CD45RO cells can revert to the CD45RA phenotype. Memory cells, perhaps in the absence of antigenic stimulation, may therefore lose their activated status and join a resting pool. Another marker used for differentiating naive from memory cells takes one step back on the CD ladder and utilizes differences in the relative expression of the adhesion molecule CD44; naive T-cells seem to express low levels of CD44 whilst memory T-cells express high levels.

Lanzavecchia and colleagues have proposed that the CCR7 chemokine receptor allows a distinction to be made between CCR7$^+$ 'central memory' T-cells, which differentiate from naive T-cells, and CCR7$^-$ 'effector memory' T-cells, which subsequently arise from the central memory T-cells (figure 9.21). Both populations are long-lived. The central memory cells provide a clonally expanded pool of antigen-primed cells which can travel to secondary lymphoid organs under the influence of the CCL21 (SLC) chemokine (cf. table 9.3) and, following re-encounter with antigen, can stimulate dendritic cells, help B-cells and generate effector cells. In contrast, effector memory T-cells possess CCR1, CCR3 and CCR5 receptors for proinflammatory chemokines and constitute tissue-homing cells which mediate inflammatory reactions or cytotoxicity.

Recently, IL-7 has emerged as a key regulator of peripheral T-cell survival and homeostatic turnover. Unlike most other cytokines that use receptors containing the common γ-(CD132), IL-7 is produced constitutively at low levels, is detectable in human serum, and may contribute to the antigen-independent maintenance of CD4 and CD8 memory T-cells by stimulating homeostatic division of these cells. Whereas studies using MHC-deficient mice have shown that peptide–MHC interactions are not essential for the persistence of memory T-cells, CD4 T-cells decline rapidly in the absence of IL-7. The expression of IL-7R is highest on resting cells, ensuring that these cells compete more effectively for available IL-7 than activated effector T-cells. Indeed, stimulation via the TCR induces downregulation of the receptor for IL-7 as effector T-cells come under the influence of cytokines produced during immune responses (such as IL-2, IL-4, IL-7, IL-15 and IL-21). As the response subsides, T-cells become dependent on IL-7 for their continued survival once more. Thus, the current view is that IL-7 contributes to the antigen-independent maintenance of T-cells by permitting homeostatic division of these cells in the absence of

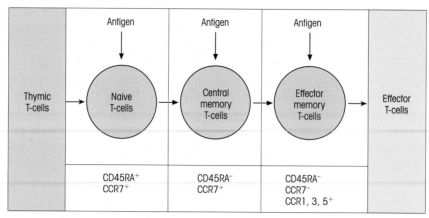

Figure 9.21. Central and effector memory T-cells. Naive T-cells bear the CD45RA splice variant of the CD45 molecule and are attracted from the thymus into secondary lymphoid tissue under the influence of CCR7-binding chemokines such as CCL19 (MIP-3β) and CCL21 (6Ckine/SLC). Upon encounter with antigen, some of these cells become effectors of the primary immune response, whilst others differentiate into central memory T-cells which retain the CCR7 chemokine receptor but lose expression of CD45RA. Subsequent re-encounter with antigen will push these cells into the effector memory compartment with replacement of CCR7 by other chemokine receptors such as CCR1, CCR3 and CCR5. This changes the homing characteristics of these cells which can now relocate as cytokine-secreting or cytotoxic T-cells to inflammatory sites under the influence of a number of chemokines including CCL3 (MIP-1α), CCL4 (MIP-1β) and CCL5 (RANTES) (see table 9.3). Note that whilst the activation and subsequent differentiation of these cells is dependent on antigen, both central memory and effector memory T-cells are thought to be long-lived in the absence of antigen.

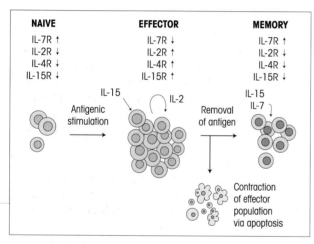

Figure 9.22. Cytokine receptor expression and cytokine availability control T-cell proliferation and survival. Naive CD4 and CD8 T-cells express high levels of IL-7R and low levels of receptors for other cytokines, such as IL-2, IL-4 and IL-15, which can influence T-cell proliferation and survival. Antigenic stimulation induces downregulation of IL-7R and upregulation of receptors for IL-2, IL-4 and IL-15 as these cytokines sustain T-cell clonal expansion and survival during the effector phase of the immune response. During resolution of the immune response, massive apoptosis occurs within the effector cell compartment leaving only the 'fittest' cells to become memory cells. The memory cell compartment appears to rely upon IL-7 for long-term survival with IL-15 also thought to be required, particularly for the maintenance of memory CD8 T-cells.

antigenic stimulation (figure 9.22). IL-15 also appears to be more important for the maintenance of CD8 memory T-cells as mice deficient in either IL-15 or IL-15Rα chain display reduced CD8 T-cell memory which can be rescued by transfer of these cells to normal mice. Thus, IL-7 and IL-15 appear to act in concert to maintain the memory T-cell pool, the latter being particularly important for the maintenance of CD8 memory T-cells (figure 9.22).

The persistence of memory cells may also be influenced by physical factors, such as the length of **chromosomal telomeres**, that impose limits on the number of divisions that most mammalian cells can undergo; the so-called **Hayflick limit**. The progressive erosion of chromosomal telomeres during each cell division can result in cells entering a state of senescence from which they cannot exit. In this situation, cells are unable to divide further and are likely to be functionally compromised and therefore of little further use to the immune system. For many cell types, the Hayflick limit is typically reached within 40–50 cell divisions, but lymphocytes may be permitted somewhat more cell divisions than this due to the upregulation of the telomere-lengthening enzyme, **telomerase**, within activated lymphocytes. It has been reported that CD8 T-cells fail to upregulate telomerase after four restimulations with antigen while CD4 T-cells may retain this ability for longer.

Virgin B-cells lose their surface IgM and IgD and switch receptor isotype on becoming memory cells, and the differential expression of these surface markers has greatly facilitated the separation of B- and T-cells into naive and memory populations for further study. The costimulatory molecules B7.1 (CD80) and B7.2 (CD86) are rapidly upregulated on memory B-cells, and the potent ability of these cells to present antigen to T-cells could well account for the brisk and robust nature of secondary responses. A scheme similar to that outlined in figure 9.21 for T-cells may also exist for the B-lymphocyte compartment, with an initial population of memory cells possessing the B220 marker developing into B220⁻ memory B-cells which then go on to generate antibody-secreting effector cells.

SUMMARY

A succession of genes are upregulated by T-cell activation

- Within 15–30 minutes, genes for transcription factors concerned in the progression G0 to G1 and in the control of IL-2 are expressed.
- Up to 14 hours, cytokines and their receptors are expressed.
- Later, a variety of genes related to cell division and adhesion are upregulated.

Cytokines act as intercellular messengers

- Cytokines act transiently and usually at short range, although circulating IL-1 and IL-6 can mediate release of acute phase proteins from the liver.
- Cytokines are mostly small proteins that act through surface receptors belonging to six structural families.
- Cytokine-induced dimerization of individual subunits of the main (hematopoietin) receptor family activates protein tyrosine kinases, including JAKs, and leads to phosphorylation and activation of STAT transcription factors.
- Cytokine signaling can be downregulated by members of the SOCS and PIAS family of inhibitors that act to suppress JAK activity or STAT-dependent transcription, respectively.
- Cytokines are pleiotropic, i.e. have multiple effects in the general areas of: (i) control of lymphocyte growth, (ii) activation of innate immune mechanisms (including inflammation), and (iii) control of bone marrow hematopoiesis (cf. figure 9.4).
- Cytokines may act sequentially, through one cytokine inducing production of another or by transmodulation of the receptor for another cytokine; they can also act synergistically or antagonistically.
- The roles of cytokines *in vivo* can be assessed by gene 'knockout', transfection or inhibition by specific antibodies.

Different T-cell subsets can make different cytokines

- The cytokine milieu that is established within the initial stages of infection has a significant influence on the pattern of cytokines secreted by Th cell populations.
- As immunization proceeds, Th tend to develop into two subsets: Th1 cells concerned in inflammatory processes, macrophage activation and delayed sensitivity make IL-2 and -3, IFNγ, TNF, lymphotoxin and GM-CSF; Th2 cells help B-cells to synthesize antibody and secrete IL-3, -4, -5, -6 and -13, TNF and GM-CSF. IL-10 is secreted by Th2 cells in mice but by both Th1 and Th2 subsets in humans.

- Interaction of antigen with macrophages or dendritic cells, via their Toll-like receptors (TLRs) and other pattern recognition receptors, leads to production of IL-12 and IL-27 which skews T-cell responses to the Th1 type, or IL-4 which will skew the responses to the Th2 pole.
- Other subsets may exist, including natural Tregs and inducible TGFβ-secreting Th3 (Tr1) regulatory cells.
- Tc1 (IFNγ) and Tc2 (IL-4) populations can also be distinguished.

Activated T-cells proliferate in response to cytokines

- IL-2 acts as an autocrine growth factor for Th1 and paracrine for Th2 cells which have upregulated their IL-2 receptors.
- Cytokines act on cells which express the appropriate cytokine receptor.

T-cell effectors in cell-mediated immunity

- Cytokines mediate chronic inflammatory responses and induce the expression of MHC class II on endothelial cells, a variety of epithelial cells and many tumor cell lines, so facilitating interactions between T-cells and nonlymphoid cells.
- Differential expression of chemokine receptors permits selective recruitment of neutrophils, macrophages, dendritic cells and T- and B-cells.
- TNF synergizes with IFNγ in killing cells.
- Cytotoxic T-cells are generated against cells (e.g. virally infected) which have intracellularly derived peptide associated with surface MHC class I. They kill using lytic granules containing perforin, granzymes and TNF.
- The cytotoxic granule-dependent pathway to apoptosis is orchestrated by granzyme B, a serine protease that can process and activate the mitochondrial-permeabilizing protein, Bid, as well as members of the caspase family of cell death proteases. Granzyme A also plays an important role in granule-dependent killing.
- T-cell-mediated inflammation is strongly downregulated by IL-4 and IL-10.

Proliferation of B-cell responses is mediated by cytokines

- Early proliferation is mediated by IL-4 which also aids IgE synthesis.
- IgA producers are driven by TGFβ and IL-5.
- IL-4 plus IL-5 promote IgM and IL-4, -5, -6 and -13 plus IFNγ stimulate IgG synthesis.

(Continued p.210)

Events in the germinal center

- There is clonal expansion, isotype switch and mutation in the dark zone centroblasts.
- The B-cell centroblasts die through apoptosis unless rescued by certain signals which upregulate *bcl-2*. These include cross-linking of surface Ig by complexes on follicular dendritic cells and engagement of the CD40 receptor which drives the cell to the memory compartment.
- The selection of mutants by antigen guides the development of high affinity B-cells.

The synthesis of antibody

- RNA for variable and constant regions is spliced together before leaving the nucleus.
- Differential splicing allows coexpression of IgM and IgD with identical V regions on a single cell and the switch from membrane-bound to secreted IgM.

Ig class switching occurs in individual B-cells

- IgM produced early in the response switches to IgG, particularly with thymus-dependent antigens. The switch is largely under T-cell control.
- IgG, but not IgM, responses improve on secondary challenge.

Antibody affinity during the immune response

- Low doses of antigen tend to select high affinity B-cells and hence antibodies since only these can be rescued in the germinal center.
- For the same reasons, affinity matures as antigen concentration falls during an immune response.

Memory cells

- Upon disappearance of the source of antigen that initiated their production, the vast majority of effector lymphocytes are eliminated via apoptosis. A fraction of antigen-responsive cells are retained, possibly those with the highest affinity for antigen, and these form the memory compartment.
- Murine memory T-cells can be maintained in the absence of antigen but human T-cell memory may require periodic restimulation with antigen.
- Immune complexes on the surface of follicular dendritic cells in the germinal centers provide a long-term source of antigen.
- Memory cells have higher affinity than naive cells, in the case of B-cells through somatic mutation, and in the case of T-cells through selective proliferation of cells with higher affinity receptors and through upregulated expression of associated molecules such as CD2 and LFA-1, which increase the avidity (functional affinity) for the antigen-presenting cell.
- Activated memory and naive T-cells are distinguished by the expression of CD45 isoforms, the former having the CD45RO phenotype, the latter CD45RA. It seems likely that a proportion of the CD45RO population reverts to a CD45RA pool of resting memory cells. CD45RA⁻ memory cells can be divided into $CCR7^+$ central memory and $CCR7^-$ effector memory cells.
- High levels of CD44 expression are also characteristic of memory T-cells, low level expression being associated with naive T-cells.
- IL-7 appears to be critical for the long-term survival of CD4 T-cell populations and is preferentially bound by resting T-cells. Memory CD8 T-cells require IL-15 for their long-term survival.

FURTHER READING

Beverly P.C.L. (2004) Kinetics and clonality of immunological memory in humans. *Seminars in Immunology* **16**, 315–321.

Bradley L.M., Haynes L. & Swain S.L. (2005) IL-7: maintaining T-cell memory and achieving homeostasis. *Trends in Immunology* **26**, 172–176.

Camacho S.A., Kosco-Vilbois M.H. & Berek C. (1998) The dynamic structure of the germinal center. *Immunology Today* **19**, 511–514.

Fujimoto M. & Naka T. (2003) Regulation of cytokine signaling by SOCS family molecules. *Trends in Immunology* **24**, 659–666.

Kapsenberg M.L. (2003) Dendritic cell control of pathogen-driven T-cell polarization. *Nature Reviews Immunology* **3**, 984–993.

Kinoshita K. & Honjo T. (2000) Unique and unprecedented recombination mechanisms in class switching. *Current Opinion in Immunology* **12**, 195–198.

Lanzavecchia A. & Sallusto F. (2002) Progressive differentiation and selection of the fittest in the immune response. *Nature Reviews Immunology* **2**, 982–987.

Mills K.H.G. (2004) Regulatory T-cells: friend or foe in immunity to infection? *Nature Reviews Immunology* **4**, 841–855.

Moser B. & Loetscher P. (2001) Lymphocyte traffic control by chemokines. *Nature Immunology* **2**, 123–128.

Sallusto F., Mackay C.R. & Lanzavecchia A. (2000) The role of chemokine receptors in primary, effector, and memory immune responses. *Annual Review of Immunology* **18**, 593–620.

Schluns K.S. & Lefrançois L. (2003) Cytokine control of memory T-cell development and survival. *Nature Reviews Immunology* **3**, 269–279.

Shuai K. & Liu B. (2003) Regulation of JAK-STAT signaling in the immune system. *Nature Reviews Immunology* **3**, 900–911.

Sprent J. & Surh C.D. (2001) Generation and maintenance of memory T-cells. *Current Opinion in Immunology* **13**, 248–254.

Tough D.F., Sun S., Zhang X. & Sprent J. (1999) Stimulation of naive and memory T-cells by cytokines. *Immunological Reviews* **170**, 39–47.

Trinchieri G. (2003) Interleukin-12 and the regulation of innate resistance and adaptive immunity. *Nature Reviews Immunology* **3**, 133–146.

Zlotnik A. & Yoshie O. (2000) Chemokines: a new classification system and their role in immunity. *Immunity* **12**, 121–127.

10 Control mechanisms

INTRODUCTION

The acquired immune response evolved so that it would come into play upon contact with an infectious agent. The appropriate antigen-specific cells expand, often to form a sizable proportion of the lymphocytes in the local lymphoid tissues, the effectors eliminate the antigen and then the response quietens down and leaves room for reaction to other infections. Feedback mechanisms must operate to limit the response; otherwise, after antigenic stimulation, we would become overwhelmed by the responding clones of T-cells and antibody-forming cells and their products—obviously an unwelcome state of affairs, as may be clearly seen in multiple myeloma, where control over lymphocyte proliferation is lost. It makes sense for **antigen to be a major regulatory factor** and for lymphocyte responses to be driven by the presence of antigen, falling off in intensity as the antigen concentration drops (figure 10.1). There is abundant evidence to support this view. Antigens can stimulate the proliferation of specific lymphocytes *in vitro*. Clearance of antigen *in vivo* by injection of excess antibody during the course of an immune response leads to a dramatic drop in antibody synthesis and the number of antibody-secreting cells.

ANTIGENS CAN INTERFERE WITH EACH OTHER

The presence of one antigen in a mixture of antigens can drastically diminish the immune response to the others. This is true even for epitopes within a given molecule; for example, the response to epitopes on the Fab fragment of IgG is far greater when the Fab rather than whole IgG is used for immunization due to the inhibitory nature of the Fc region. Factors which determine immunodominance include the precursor frequency of the B-cells bearing antigen receptors for different epitopes on the antigen, the relative affinity of these antigen receptors for their respective epitopes, the degree to which the surface membrane antibody protects the epitope from proteolysis following internalization of the antibody–antigen complex, and the level of competition of processed antigenic peptides for the *m*ajor *h*istocompatibility *c*omplex (MHC) groove. There is a clear hierarchy of epitopes with respect to this competitive binding based on differential accessibility to proteases as the molecule unfolds, and the presence or absence of particular amino acid sequences which facilitate breakdown to yield peptides in high abundance and with relatively high affinity for the MHC (figure 10.2). Thus, Sercarz envisages **dominant epitopes**, which bag the lion's share of the available MHC grooves, **subdominant epitopes**, which are less successful, and **cryptic epitopes**, which generate miserably low concentrations of peptide–MHC that are ignored by potentially reactive naive T-cells.

Clearly, the possibility that certain antigens in a mixture, or particular epitopes in a given antigen, may block a desired protective immune response has obvious implications for vaccine design. Contrariwise, the identification of inhibitory peptides with a predatory affinity for the MHC groove(s) should provide therapeutic agents to quash unwanted hypersensitivity reactions.

COMPLEMENT AND ANTIBODY ALSO PLAY A ROLE

Innate immune mechanisms are usually first on the scene and activation of the alternative pathway of complement will lead to C3d deposition on the microbe. When C3d-coated antigens are recognized by the B-cell, cross-linking of the BCR and the CD21 complement receptor, with its associated signal-transducing molecule CD19, enhances B-cell activation (figure 10.3a). By contrast, cross-linking of the BCR with FcγRIIB1 (cf. p. 46) delivers a negative signal by suppressing tyrosine phosphorylation of CD19 (figure 10.3b). Thus, removal of circulating antibody by plasmapheresis during an ongoing response leads to an increase in synthesis, whereas injection of preformed IgG antibody markedly

hastens the fall in the number of antibody-forming cells (figure 10.4) consistent with feedback control on overall synthesis.

In complete contrast, injection of IgM antibodies enhances the response (figure 10.4), presumably by cross-linking antigen bound to the sIgM receptors without activating the Fcγ inhibitory receptor, and

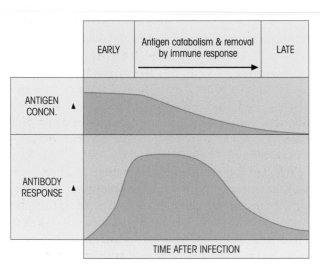

Figure 10.1. Antigen drives the immune response. As antigen concentration falls due to catabolism and elimination by antibody, the intensity of the immune response declines, but is maintained for some time at a lower level by antigen trapped on germinal center follicular dendritic cells.

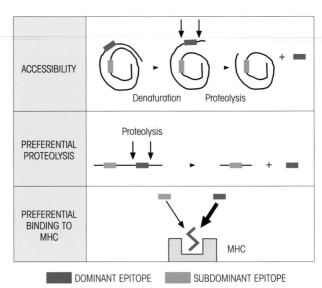

Figure 10.2. Mechanisms of epitope dominance at the MHC level. The other factor which can influence dominance is the availability of reactive T-cells; if these have been eliminated, e.g. through tolerization by cross-reacting self-antigens, a peptide which may have dominated the MHC groove would be unable to provoke an immune response.

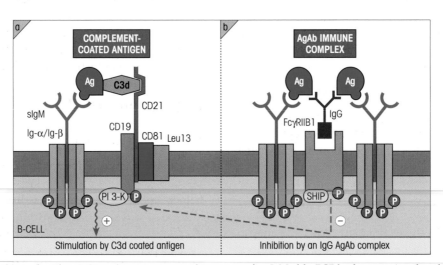

Figure 10.3. Cross-linking of surface IgM antigen receptor to the CD21 complement receptor stimulates, and to the Fcγ receptor FcγRIIB1 inhibits, B-cells. (a) Following activation of complement, C3d becomes covalently bound to the microbial surface. The CD21 complement receptor binds C3d and signals through its associated CD19 molecule. The CD21 and CD81 (TAPA-1) Leu13 molecules form the B-cell coreceptor (cf. p. 181) and cross-linking of this complex to the surface IgM of the BCR leads to tyrosine phosphorylation of CD19 and subsequent binding of phosphatidylinositol 3-kinase (PI 3-K), leading to B-cell activation. (b) The FcγRIIB1 molecule possesses a cytoplasmic immunoreceptor tyrosine-based inhibitory motif (ITIM) and, upon cross-linking to membrane Ig, becomes phosphorylated and binds the inositol polyphosphate 5'-phosphatase SHIP. This suppresses phosphorylation of CD19 and thus inhibits B-cell activation.

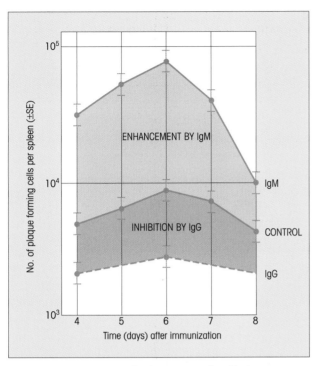

Figure 10.4. Time-course of enhancement of antibody response to sheep red blood cells (SRBC) due to injection of preformed IgM, and of suppression by preformed IgG antibodies. Mice received monoclonal IgM anti-SRBC, IgG anti-SRBC or medium alone intravenously 2 hours prior to immunization with 10^5 SRBC. (Data provided by J. Reiter, P. Hutchings, P. Lydyard and A. Cooke.)

perhaps also via the generation of C3d by the classical pathway of complement activation. Since antibodies of this isotype are either already present amongst the broadly reactive natural antibodies, or if not will certainly appear at an early stage after antigen challenge, they would be useful in boosting the initial response.

ACTIVATION-INDUCED CELL DEATH

Although clearance of antigen from the body by the immune system will clearly lead to a downregulation of lymphocyte proliferation due to the absence of a signal through the antigen receptor, even in the presence of antigen the signals provided do not lead to the continuous proliferation of cells, but rather set off a train of events that, unless the cells are protected in some way, leads to activation-induced cell death (AICD) by apoptosis. Subsequent to activation, T-cells upregulate death receptors and their ligands. If the ligands remain associated with the cell surface they can activate apoptosis in adjacent cells. However, they are often released from the cell surface by proteases, producing soluble forms which in some cases retain activity, for example the soluble version of the *TNF-related apoptosis-inducing*

ligand (TRAIL/Apo2L) retains the ability to signal through the receptor TRAIL-R1. Such soluble ligands can potentially mediate either paracrine or autocrine cell death *in vivo*, and show promise as tumor therapeutics. The death receptors are members of the tumor necrosis factor receptor (TNF-R) family and include TNFRI, CD95 (Fas), TRAMP (TNF receptor apoptosis-mediating protein), the aforementioned TRAIL-R1 (*death receptor* DR4), TRAIL-R2 (DR5), DR3 and DR6. Apoptosis induction through these receptors initially involves cleavage of the inactive cysteine protease pro-caspase 8 to yield active caspase 8. Ultimately, this activation pathway converges with the apoptosis pathway induced by cellular stress, both leading to the activation of downstream effector caspases (figure 10.5). There are also a number of *decoy receptors*, including the membrane bound TRAIL-R3 (DcR1) and TRAIL-R4 (DcR2) and the soluble TRAIL-R5 (osteoprotegerin), which bind the potentially apoptosis-inducing ligands but do not signal.

When initially activated by peptide–MHC, T-cells are resistant to apoptosis but become progressively sensitive. A number of molecules are known to be protective against apoptosis; for example, bcl-2 and bcl-X_L, which appear to act as watchdogs preventing the release of pro-apoptotic proteins from the mitochondria. Of particular relevance to death receptor-mediated AICD, however, is the molecule FLIP (*FLICE inhibitory protein*, FLICE being an older name for caspase 8). FLIP bears structural similarity to caspase 8, and therefore by competitive inhibition prevents recruitment of this caspase into the *death-inducing signaling complex* (DISC) (figure 10.5). Thus, FLIP levels can determine the fate of the cell when the death receptor is engaged by its ligand but does not affect apoptosis induced by the stress-activated mitochondrial pathway (figure 10.6).

T-CELL REGULATION

Helper T-cell specialization

There is abundant evidence to suggest that different populations of Th cells are specialized for different helper functions. With respect to help for antibody production, T-cell lines derived from Peyer's patches are much better at helping IgA-producing B-cells from Peyer's patch precursors than are splenic T-cell lines. The help is for IgA-precommitted B-cells rather than for induction of the class switch to IgA, since Peyer's patch T-cells do not markedly enhance IgA production by splenic B-cells. It should also be evident from the previous discussion of AICD that Th cells will not be around to expand B-cell and Tc clone sizes indefinitely.

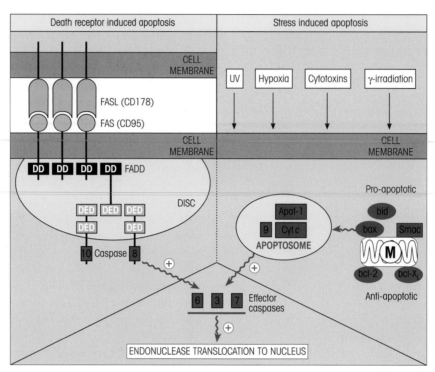

Figure 10.5. Activation-induced cell death. Receptor-based induction of apoptosis involves the trimerization of TNF-R family members (e.g. Fas) by trimerized ligands (e.g. Fas-ligand). This brings together cytoplasmic death domains (DD) which can recruit a number of death effector domain (DED)-containing adaptor molecules to form the death-inducing signaling complex (DISC). The different receptors use different combinations of DED-containing adaptors; Fas uses FADD (*F*as-*a*ssociated protein with *d*eath *d*omain). The DISC, which also includes caspase 10, induces the cleavage of inactive procaspase 8 into active caspase 8 with subsequent activation of downstream effector caspases. This process eventually leads to the release of the endonuclease known as caspase-activated DNase (CAD) from a restraining protein (inhibitor of CAD; ICAD) in the cytoplasm, with subsequent translocation of the endonuclease to the nucleus. A second pathway of apoptosis induction, often triggered by cellular stress, involves a number of mitochondria-associated proteins including cytochrome *c*, Smac/DIABLO and the bcl-2 family member bax. Caspase 9 activation is the key event in this pathway and requires association of the caspase with a number of other proteins including the cofactor Apaf-1; the complex formed incorporates cytochrome *c* and is referred to as the apoptosome. The activated caspase 9 then cleaves procaspase 3. Although the death receptor and mitochondrial pathways are shown as initially separate in the figure, there is cross-talk between them. Thus, caspase 8 can cleave the bcl-2 family member bid, a process which promotes cytochrome *c* release from mitochondria. Other members of the bcl-2 family, such as bcl-2 itself and bcl-X$_L$, inhibit apoptosis, perhaps by preventing the release of pro-apoptotic molecules from the mitochondria. M, mitochondrion.

T-cell suppression

It is perhaps inevitable that nature, having evolved a functional set of T-cells which promote immune responses, should also develop a regulatory set whose job would be to modulate the helpers. T-cell mediated suppression was first brought to the serious attention of the immunological fraternity by a phenomenon colorfully named by its discoverer, Dick Gershon, as 'infectious tolerance'. Quite surprisingly it was shown that, if mice were made unresponsive by injection of a high dose of sheep red blood cells (SRBC), their T-cells would suppress specific antibody formation in normal recipients to which they had been transferred (figure 10.7). It may not be apparent to the reader why this result was at all surprising, but at that time antigen-induced tolerance was regarded essentially as a negative phenomenon involving the depletion or silencing of clones rather than a state of active suppression. Over the years, T-cell mediated suppression has been shown to modulate a variety of humoral and cellular responses, the latter including delayed-type hypersensitivity, cytotoxic T-cells and antigen-specific T-cell proliferation. However, the existence of dedicated professional T-suppressor cells is a question which has generated a great deal of heat.

Suppressor and helper epitopes can be discrete

Detailed analysis of murine responses to antigens such as hen egg-white lysozyme tells us that certain determinants can evoke very strong suppression rather than help depending on the mouse strain, and also that T-cell mediated suppression directed to one determinant can switch off helper and antibody responses to other deter-

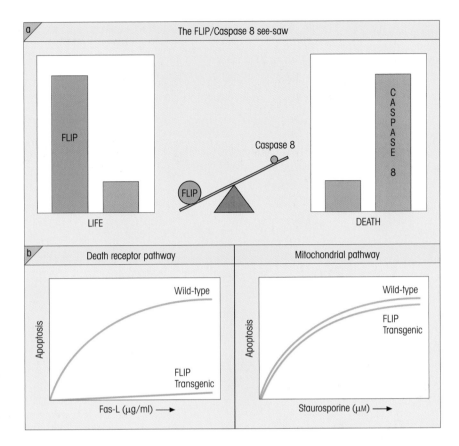

Figure 10.6. Life and death decisions. (a) The relative amounts of anti-apoptotic FLIP and pro-apoptotic caspase 8 can determine the fate of the cell. (b) Experiments involving overexpression of FLIP in transgenic mice indicate that this protein protects T-cells from AICD stimulated through the death receptor pathway by Fas-ligand, but not from cell death triggered via the mitochondrial pathway using the drug staurosporine. (Based on data obtained by J. Tschopp and colleagues.)

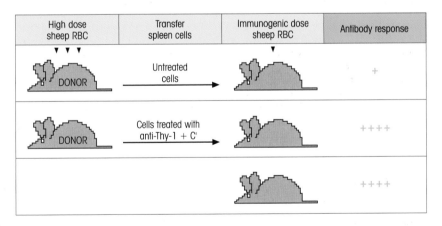

Figure 10.7. Demonstration of T-suppressor cells. A mouse of an appropriate strain immunized with an immunogenic dose of sheep erythrocytes makes a strong antibody response. However, if spleen cells from a donor of the same strain previously injected with a high dose of antigen are first transferred to the syngeneic animal, they depress the antibody response to a normally immunogenic dose of the antigen. The effect is lost if the spleen cells are first treated with a T-cell-specific antiserum (anti-Thy-1) plus complement, showing that the suppressors are T-cells. (After Gershon R.K. & Kondo K. (1971) *Immunology* **21**, 903–914.)

minants on the same molecule. Thus mice of *H-2^b* haplotype respond poorly to lysozyme because they develop dominant suppression; however, if the three N-terminal amino acids are removed from the antigen, these mice now make a splendid response, showing that the T-regulation directed against the determinant associated with the N-terminal region has switched off the response to the remaining determinants on the antigen. Similar results have been obtained in several other systems. This must imply that the antigen itself acts as a form of bridge to allow communication between regulatory T-cells and cells reacting to the other determinants,

as might occur through these cells binding to an antigen-presenting cell expressing several different processed determinants of the same antigen on its surface (figure 10.8).

Characteristics of suppression

Originally, suppressor T-cells in mice were found to possess Ly2 (now called CD8α) and Ly3 (CD8β) on their surface. As researchers began to characterize these CD8+ T-suppressor cells they were described as expressing a molecule called I-J encoded within the MHC region and able to produce soluble suppressor factors that were

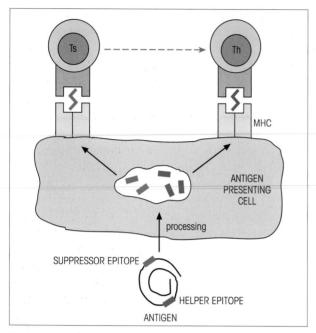

Figure 10.8. Possible mechanism to explain the need for a physical linkage between suppressor and helper epitopes. The helper and suppressor cells can interact by binding close together on the surface of an antigen-presenting cell, which processes the antigen and displays the different epitopes on separate MHC molecules on its surface.

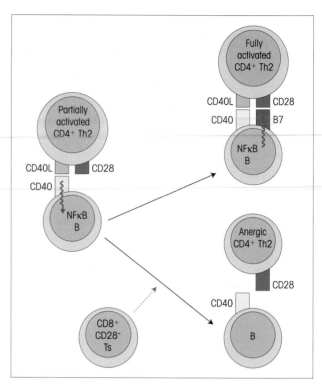

Figure 10.9. CD8+ suppressor T-cells can inhibit T-cell activation by B-cells. Upon stimulation by peptide–MHC through the T-cell receptor, the CD40 ligand (CD40L, CD154) is upregulated on the partially activated Th2 cell. Interaction with CD40 on B-cells leads to NFκB-mediated upregulation of B7.1 and B7.2 (CD80 and CD86, respectively) on the B-cell leading to mutual stimulation of the helper T-cell and the B-cell through B7–CD28 interactions. In the presence of CD8+CD28− suppressor T-cells there is a failure to upregulate B7 and the lack of costimulation results in the Th2 cells becoming anergic. Unlike T-cells in various stages of activation, resting anergic T-cells do not express CD40L.

frequently antigen-specific. These suppressor factors proved impossible to define biochemically, and when the entire MHC was cloned it was found that I-J didn't exist! There then, perhaps not unsurprisingly under the circumstances, followed a period of extreme skepticism regarding the very existence of suppressor T-cells. However, during the last decade they have made a dramatic comeback, although it is now appreciated that the majority of these cells belong to the CD4 rather than the CD8 T-cell lineage, and the current vogue is to refer to them as regulatory T-cells (Tregs). The characterization of these cells has itself, however, not been without its problems and there seem to be several different types of Tregs. Whilst some require cell–cell contact in order to be suppressive, others depend upon soluble cytokines to mediate their effect.

Let us first look at CD8+ T suppressors. One experimental example that relates to the B10.A (2R) mouse strain which has a low immune response to lactate dehydrogenase β (LDHβ) associated with the possession of the H-2Eβ gene of k rather than b haplotype. Lymphoid cells taken from these animals after immunization with LDHβ proliferate poorly *in vitro* in the presence of antigen, but if CD8+ cells are depleted, the remaining CD4+ cells give a much higher response. Adding back the CD8+ cells reimposes the active suppression. Human suppressor T-cells can also belong to the CD8

subset. Thus, CD8+ CD28− cells can prevent antigen-presenting B-cells from upregulating costimulatory B7 molecules in response to CD40-mediated signals from the CD40 ligand on Th cells (figure 10.9). Following interaction with the CD8 T-cells, the APCs are then capable of inducing anergy in Th cells. This effect on B7 is mediated by inhibition of NFκB activation in the APC, an event necessary for transcription of both the B7.1 (CD80) and B7.2 (CD86) genes.

Although it is clear from such experiments that CD8+ T-cells can mediate suppression, the current view is that regulatory CD4+ cells are perhaps the major effectors of suppression. If anti-CD25 and complement are used to deplete the CD25+ cells from the lymph nodes or spleen of BALB/c mice and then the remaining CD25− cells transferred into athymic (nude) BALB/c mice, the recipients develop multiple autoimmune diseases. However, if CD4+CD25+ cells are subsequently given shortly after the CD25− cells the mice do not develop autoimmune disease, suggesting that the CD4+CD25+ population contains Tregs. Many similar experiments have established that CD4$^+$CD25$^+$ T-cells do indeed include a population of Tregs able to mediate suppression of autoimmunity, allograft rejection and allergic responses. However, because CD25 (the α-chain of the IL-2 receptor) is a general marker of cell activation, it is not possible to use this as a defining molecule for the regulatory subset. These naturally occurring Tregs also express CTLA-4, OX40, GITR (*glucocorticoid-induced TNF receptor family related molecule*), cell surface TGFβ and the forkhead transcription factor Foxp3. Whilst the presence of each of these molecules is helpful in defining the regulatory population, it is their expression of Foxp3 which is currently thought to uniquely define these cells as regulatory T-cells. Indeed, if the *Foxp3* gene is introduced into naive CD4$^+$CD25$^-$ T-cells they are converted into cells capable of suppressing the development of autoimmune disease in a number of animal models.

The activation of CD4$^+$CD25$^+$Foxp3$^+$ naturally occurring Tregs is usually antigen-specific but they can subsequently suppress the responses to other antigens, a situation referred to as linked suppression. The precise

mechanism they use to suppress immune responses to either the initiating antigen or to other antigens is still being established, but usually requires cell–cell contact between the regulator and the regulated. Several other types of Tregs have also been described, many of which do not require cell–cell contact (figure 10.10). Human CD4 cells stimulated with antigen in the presence of IL-10 can develop into Tr1 cells which themselves secrete IL-10, a cytokine that can mediate immunosuppressive functions. Although these cells constitutively express Foxp3, they only express CD25 upon activation. Th3 cells are defined by the fact that they secrete TGFβ, another cytokine with the capacity to be immunosuppressive. Immunoregulatory $\gamma\delta$ T-cells may recognize activation-induced nonclassical MHC molecules, as appears to be the case with the recognition of the class Ib molecules T22 and T10 in the mouse, although the precise role of such cells is still being elucidated. It is, however, known that some $\gamma\delta$ T-cells secrete IL-10 and TGFβ and such cells would clearly have the potential for immunosuppression. Ongoing research will hopefully help clarify the roles of these different types of regulatory cell.

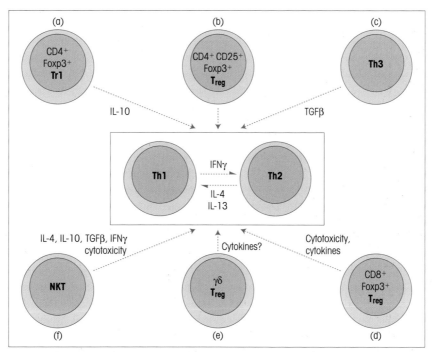

Figure 10.10. T-cell mediated control of immune responses. Th1 and Th2 cells tend to show a mutual antagonism based upon the fact that some of the cytokines they produce downregulate the opposing population. Superimposed on this are a number of different types of suppressor/regulatory T-cell populations. These may include: (a) IL-10 secreting Tr1 cells which acquires CD25 expression upon activation; (b) the naturally occurring Tregs which arise in the thymus and constitutively express CD25 and Foxp3. Their mode of suppression usually requires cell–cell contact, perhaps utilizing a membrane-bound version of TGFβ; (c) Th3 cells which function via their ability to secrete TGFβ; (d) CD8 cells which may suppress using cytotoxicity or cytokines; (e) immunosuppressive T-cells bearing a $\gamma\delta$ TCR; and (f) NKT cells for which cytokine and cytotoxicity mediated modes of operation have been proposed. Whilst it is thought that these various types of T-cell can act directly on effector T-cells, they (and perhaps other) populations of suppressor/regulatory T-cells may also function via effects on dendritic cells.

Suppression is a regulated phenomenon

We have already entertained the idea that antigen-linked T–T interactions can occur on the surface of an antigen-presenting cell (figure 10.8) and the concept of Tc1 and Tc2 CD8 subsets paralleling the Th1/Th2 dichotomy. Furthermore, there is mutual antagonism (suppression) between Th1 and Th2 cells. One could postulate downregulation of Th1 cells by type 2 IL-4-producing **CD8** cells, and suppression of Th2 cells by type 1 IFNγ-producing **CD8** cells, interacting on the surface of an antigen-presenting cell (figure 10.11). In this model, when the immune response has locked onto a particular mode, e.g. Th1-mediated cellular immunity, other types of response, such as T–B collaboration, are restricted through a cytokine inhibitory effect. Although these cells mediate T-suppression, they would not be called dedicated professional suppressors since, in a sense, their suppressive powers are a by-product of their main defensive function. Perhaps we need these cytokine-secreting Tc cells to prevent Th cells getting out of hand by excessive proliferation, just as IgG holds back the B-cells by feedback control.

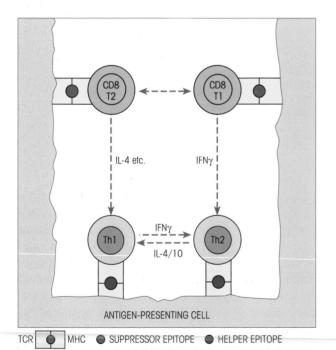

TCR ▢●▢ MHC ● SUPPRESSOR EPITOPE ● HELPER EPITOPE

Figure 10.11. Mutual antagonisms between T-cell subsets linked indirectly by processed antigen on an antigen-presenting cell lead to functionally distinct modes of suppression. (Leaning heavily on Bloom B.R., Salgame P. & Diamond B. (1992) *Immunology Today* **13**, 131–136.) Yet another mechanism may prove to be important. Unlike the mouse, many other mammalian species can express MHC class II on a proportion of their activated T-cells; presentation of processed peptide by these cells can induce CD4+ cytotoxic cells with suppressor potential. We also need to know more about the circumstances leading to the production of TGFβ by suppressors since this cytokine inhibits T-cell proliferation.

The activities of Tregs are to some extent controlled by dendritic cells, with resting dendritic cells favoring the development of a regulatory phenotype. The activation of dendritic cells which occurs through microbial engagement of pattern recognition receptors will lead to the production of IL-6 and other soluble mediators which can curb the Tregs when an anti-pathogen response is required.

IDIOTYPE NETWORKS

Jerne's network hypothesis

In 1974 the Nobel laureate Neils Jerne published a paper entitled 'Towards a network theory of the immune system' in which he proposed that structures formed by the variable regions of antibodies (i.e. the antibody idiotype) could recognize other antibody variable regions in such a way that they would form a network based upon mutual idiotype–anti-idiotype interactions. Because B-cells use the antibody molecule as their antigen receptor this would provide a connectivity between different clones of B-cells, and therefore the potential for regulation of the individual clones that are members of the network (figure 10.12). This concept was later extended to include the idiotypes present on the T-cell receptors of both CD4+ and CD8+ T-cells. There is no doubt that the elements which can form an idiotypic network are present in the body, and autoanti-idiotypes occur during the course of antigen-induced responses. For example, certain strains of mice injected with pneumococcal vaccines make an antibody response to the phosphorylcholine groups in which the germ-line-encoded idiotype T15 dominates. Waves of T15+ and of anti-T15 (i.e. autoanti-idiotype) cells are demonstrable. Anti-idiotypic reactivity has also been demonstrated in T-cell populations using various experimental systems. Indeed, anti-idiotypic T-cells recognizing peptide derived from the CDR2, CDR3 and framework regions of other TCRs appear to form a part of the normal human T-cell repertoire.

A network is evident in early life

If the spleens of fetal mice which are just beginning to secrete immunoglobulin are used to produce hybridomas, an unusually high proportion are interrelated as idiotype–anti-idiotype pairs. This high level of idiotype connectivity is not seen in later life and suggests that these early cells, largely the CD5+ **B-1 subset** (cf. p. 244), are programed to synthesize germ-line gene specificities which have network relationships.

Private and public idiotypes

Whilst certain idiotypes (private idiotypes) are present

Ab$_{2\beta}$	Ab$_1$	Ab$_{2\alpha}$	Ab$_3$
ANTI-IDIOTYPE (internal image)	IDIOTYPE	ANTI-IDIOTYPE	ANTI-ANTI-IDIOTYPE

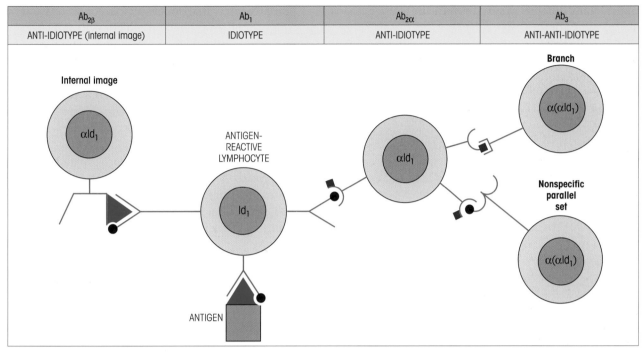

Figure 10.12. Elements in an idiotypic network in which the antigen receptors on one lymphocyte reciprocally recognize an idiotype on the receptors of another. T-helper, T-suppressor and B-lymphocytes interact through idiotype–anti-idiotype reactions producing either stimulation or suppression. T–T interactions could occur through direct recognition of one T-cell receptor (TCR) by the other, or more usually by recognition of a processed TCR peptide associated with MHC. One of the anti-idiotype sets, Ab$_{2\beta}$, may bear an idiotype of similar shape to (i.e. provides an **internal image** of) the antigen. The same idiotype (?) may be shared by receptors of different specificity, the nonspecific parallel set (since the several hypervariable regions provide a number of potential idiotypic determinants and a given idiotype does not always form part of the epitope-binding site, i.e. the paratope), so that the anti-(anti-Id$_1$) does not necessarily bind the original antigen. (The following abbreviations are often employed: α as a prefix = anti; Id = idiotype; Ab$_1$ = Id; Ab$_2\alpha$ = αId not involving the paratope; Ab$_2\beta$ = internal image αId involving the paratope; Ab$_3$ = $\alpha(\alpha$Id).)

only on antibodies of a defined single specificity, cross-reacting idiotypes (public idiotypes) are present on a variety of antibodies (and thus B-cell receptors) of different specificities. Such frequently occurring and usually germ-line-encoded public idiotypes seem to be provoked fairly readily with anti-Id and are therefore candidates for **regulatory Id** which can be under some degree of control by a limited idiotypic network. The phenomenon of '**original antigenic sin**' occurs when the immune response becomes 'locked in' to particular epitopes originally encountered on a microorganism, such that it largely ignores even normally immunodominant epitopes during a subsequent encounter with an antigenically related but nonidentical microorganism. Although competition for antigen by the expanded population which forms the memory B-cells plays a major role, idiotype-specific memory Th cells could also contribute to this phenomenon.

Idiotype networks may also, by a mutual low-level stimulation of lymphocytes within a network, allow the immune response to 'tick over' for extended periods and maintain the memory cell population.

Manipulation of the immune response through idiotypes

Quite low doses of anti-idiotype, of the order of nanograms, can greatly enhance the expression of the idiotype in the response to a given antigen, whereas doses in the microgram range lead to a suppression (figure 10.13). Thus the idiotypic network provides interesting opportunities to manipulate the immune response, particularly in hypersensitivity states such as autoimmune disease, allergy and graft rejection. However, the B-cell response is normally so diverse, suppression by anti-Id is likely to prove difficult; even when the response is dominated by a public Id and that Id is suppressed, compensatory expansion of clones bearing other idiotypes ensures that the fall in the total antibody titer is relatively undramatic (cf. figure 10.13). Conceivably, Th cells may express a narrower spectrum of idiotypes, thereby being more susceptible to suppression by Id autoimmunization. Reports that 'vaccination' with irradiated lines of Th cells specific for brain or thyroid antigens prevents the induction of experimental autoimmunity against the relevant organ are encouraging. A totally different approach would be to use monoclonal anti-Id of the 'antigen internal image' set (figure 10.12) to stimulate antigen-specific regulatory T-cells capable of turning off B-cells directed to other epitopes on the antigen through bridging by the antigen itself (cf. figure 10.8).

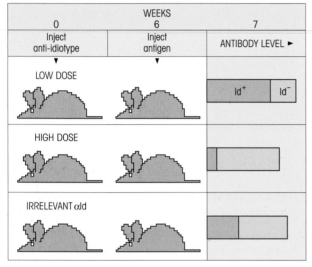

Figure 10.13. Modulation of a major idiotype in the antibody response to antigen by anti-idiotype. In the example chosen, the idiotype is present in a substantial proportion of the antibodies produced in controls injected with irrelevant anti-Id plus antigen (i.e. this is a public or cross-reacting Id; see p. 52). Pretreatment with 10 ng of a monoclonal anti-Id greatly expands the Id$^+$ antibody population, whereas prior injection of 10 µg of anti-Id almost completely suppresses expression of the idiotype without having any substantial effect on total antibody production due to a compensatory increase in Id$^-$ antibody clones.

Since we know that under suitable conditions anti-Id can also stimulate antibody production, it might be possible to use 'internal image' monoclonal anti-Ids as 'surrogate' antigens for immunization in cases where the antigen is difficult to obtain in bulk — for example, antigens from parasites such as filaria or the weak embryonic antigens associated with some cancers. Another example is where protein antigens obtained by chemical synthesis or gene cloning fail to fold into the configuration of the native molecule; this is not a problem with the anti-Id which by definition has been selected to have the shape of the antigenic epitope.

The main factors currently thought to modulate the immune response are summarized in figure 10.14.

THE INFLUENCE OF GENETIC FACTORS

Some genes affect general responsiveness

Mice can be selectively bred for high or low antibody responses through several generations to yield two lines, one of which consistently produces high-titer antibodies to a variety of antigens, and the other, antibodies of relatively low titer (figure 10.15; Biozzi and colleagues). Out of the ten or so different genetic loci involved, some give rise to a higher rate of B-cell proliferation and differentiation, while one or more affect macrophage behavior.

Antigen receptor genes are linked to the immune response

Clearly, the Ig and TCR *V*, *D* and *J* genes encoding the specific recognition sites of the lymphocyte antigen

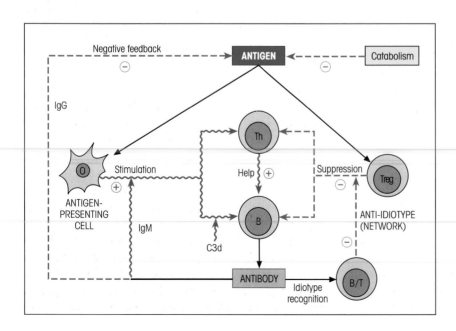

Figure 10.14. Regulation of the immune response. T-help for cell-mediated immunity will be subject to similar regulation. Some of these mechanisms may be interdependent; for example, one could envisage regulatory T-cells with specificity for the idiotype on Th or B-cells. To avoid too many confusing arrows, we have omitted the recruitment of B-cells by anti-idiotypic Th cells. Th, T-helper cell; Treg, regulatory T-cell.

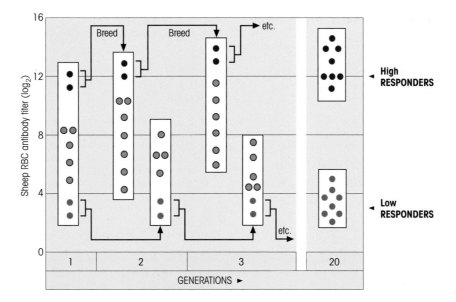

Figure 10.15. Selective breeding of high and low antibody responders (after Biozzi and colleagues). A foundation population of wild mice (with crazy mixed-up genes and great variability in antibody response) is immunized with sheep red blood cells (SRBC), a multi-determinant antigen. The antibody titer of each individual mouse is shown by a circle. The male and female giving the highest titer antibodies (●) were bred and their litter challenged with antigen. Again, the best responders were bred together and so on for 20 generations when all mice were high responders to SRBC and a variety of other antigens. The same was done for the poorest responders (●), yielding a strain of low responder animals. The two lines are comparable in their ability to clear carbon particles or sheep erythrocytes from the blood by phagocytosis, but macrophages from the high responders present antigen more efficiently (cf. p. 167). On the other hand, the low responders survive infection by *Salmonella typhimurium* better and their macrophages support much slower replication of *Listeria* (cf. p. 268), indicative of an inherently more aggressive microbicidal ability.

receptors are of fundamental importance to the acquired immune response. However, since the mechanisms for generating receptor diversity from the available genes are so powerful (cf. p. 68), immunodeficiency is unlikely to occur as a consequence of a poor Ig or TCR variable region gene repertoire. Nevertheless, just occasionally, we see holes in the repertoire due to the absence of a gene; failure to respond to the sugar polymer α1–6 dextran is a feature of animals without a particular immunoglobulin *V* gene, and mice lacking the $V\alpha_2$ TCR gene cannot mount a cytotoxic T-cell response to the male H-Y antigen.

Immune response can be influenced by the MHC

There was much excitement when it was first discovered that the antibody responses to a number of thymus-dependent antigenically simple substances are determined by genes mapping to the MHC. For example, mice of the *H-2^b* haplotype respond well to the synthetic branched polypeptide (T,G)-A–L, whereas *H-2^k* mice respond poorly (table 10.1).

It was said that mice of the *H-2^b* haplotype (i.e. a particular set of *H-2* genes) are **high responders** to (T,G)-A–L because they possess the appropriate immune

Table 10.1. H-2 haplotype linked to high, low and intermediate immune responses to synthetic peptides. (T,G)-A–L, polylysine with polyalanine side-chains randomly tipped with tyrosine and glutamine; (H,G)-A–L, the same with histidine in place of tyrosine.

ANTIGEN	H-2 HAPLOTYPE				
	b	k	d	a	s
(T,G)-A–L	Hi	Lo	Int	Lo	Lo
(H,G)-A–L	Lo	Hi	Int	Hi	Lo

response (*Ir*) gene. With another synthetic antigen, (H,G)-A–L, having histidine in place of tyrosine, the position is reversed, the 'poor (T,G)-A–L responders' now giving a good antibody response and the 'good (T,G)-A–L responders' a weak one, showing that the capacity of a particular strain to give a high or low response varies with the individual antigen (table 10.1). These relationships are only apparent when antigens of highly restricted structure are studied because the response to each single determinant is controlled by an *Ir* gene and it is less likely that the different determinants on a complex antigen will all be associated with consistently high or consistently low responder *Ir* genes; however, although one would expect an average of randomly high and low responder genes, since the various determinants on most thymus-dependent complex antigens are structurally unrelated, the outcome will be biased by the dominance of one or more epitopes (cf. p. 211). Thus H-2-linked immune responses have been observed not only with relatively simple polypeptides, but also with transplantation antigens from another strain and autoantigens where merely one or two determinants are recognized as foreign by the host. With complex antigens, in most but not all cases, H-2 linkage is usually only seen when the dose administered is so low that just one immunodominant determinant is recognized by the immune system. In this way, reactions controlled by *Ir* genes are distinct from the overall responsiveness to a variety of complex antigens which is a feature of the Biozzi mice (above).

The Ir genes map to the H-2I region and control T–B cooperation

Table 10.2 gives some idea of the type of analysis used to map the *Ir* genes. The three high responder strains have individual *H-2* genes derived from prototypic pure strains which have been interbred to produce recombinations within the H-2 region. The only genes they have in common are A^k and D^b; since the B.10 strain bearing the D^b gene is a low responder, high response must be linked in this case to possession of A^k. The I region molecules must represent the *Ir* gene product since a point mutation in the H-2A subregion in one strain led to a change in the class II molecule at a site affecting its polymorphic specificity and changed the mice from high to low responder status with respect to their thymus-dependent antibody response to antigen *in vivo*. The mutation also greatly reduced the proliferation of T-cells from immunized animals when challenged *in vitro* with antigen plus appropriate presenting cells, and there is a good correlation between antigen-specific T-cell proliferation and the responder status of the host. The implication that **responder status may be linked to the generation of Th cells** is amply borne out by adop-

tive transfer studies showing that irradiated (H-2^b×H-2^k) F1 mice make good antibody responses to (T,G)-A–L when reconstituted with antigen-primed B-cells from another F1 plus T-cells from a primed H-2^b (high responder); T-cells from the low responder H-2^k mice only gave poor help for antibody responses. This also explains why these *H-2* gene effects are seen with thymus-dependent but not T-independent antigens.

Three mechanisms can account for class II-linked high and low responsiveness.

1 *Defective presentation.* In a high responder, processing of antigen and its recognition by a corresponding T-cell lead to lymphocyte triggering and clonal expansion (figure 10.16a). Although there is (and has to be) considerable degeneracy in the specificity of the class II groove for peptide binding, variation in certain key residues can alter the strength of binding to a particular peptide (cf. p. 101) and convert a high to a low responder because the MHC fails to present antigen to the reactive T-cell (figure 10.16b). Sometimes the natural processing of an antigen in a given individual does not produce a peptide which fits well into their MHC molecules. One study showed that a cytotoxic T-cell clone restricted to HLA-A2, which recognized residues 58–68 of influenza A virus matrix protein, could cross-react with cells from an HLA-A69 subject pulsed with the same peptide; nonetheless, the clone failed to recognize HLA-A69 cells *infected* with influenza A virus. Interestingly, individuals with the HLA-A69 class I MHC develop immunity to a different epitope on the same protein.

2 *Defective T-cell repertoire.* T-cells with moderate to high affinity for self-MHC molecules and their complexes with processed self-antigens are tolerized (cf. p. 237), so creating a 'hole' in the T-cell repertoire. If there is a cross-reaction, i.e. similarity in shape at the T-cell recognition level between a foreign antigen and a self-molecule which has already induced unresponsiveness, the host will lack T-cells specific for the foreign antigen and therefore be a low responder (figure 10.16c). To take a concrete example, mice of DBA/2 strain respond well to the synthetic peptide polyglutamyl, polytyrosine (GT), whereas BALB/c mice do not, although both have identical class II genes. BALB/c B-cell blasts express a structure which mimics GT and the presumption would be that self-tolerance makes these mice unresponsive to GT. This was confirmed by showing that DBA/2 mice made tolerant by a small number of BALB/c hematopoietic cells were changed from high to low responder status. To round off the story in a very satisfying way, DBA/2 mice injected with BALB/c B-blasts, induced by the polyclonal activator lipopolysaccharide, were found to be primed for GT.

Table 10.2. Mapping of the *Ir* gene for (H,G)-A–L responses by analysis of different recombinant strains.

Strain	H-2 region				(H,G)-A–L Response
	K	A	E	D	
A	k	k	k	b	Hi
A.TL	s	k	k	b	Hi
B.IO.A (4R)	k	k	b	b	Hi
B.IO	b	b	b	b	Lo
A.SW	s	s	s	s	Lo

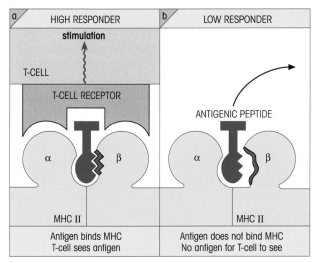

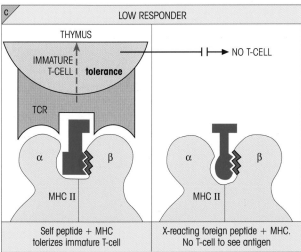

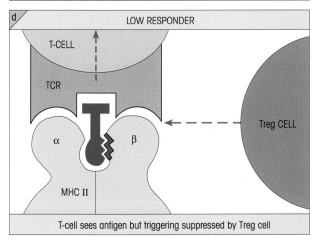

Figure 10.16. Different mechanisms can account for low T-cell response to antigen in association with MHC class II.

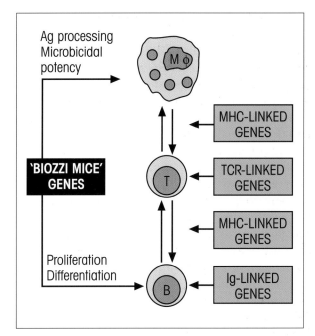

Figure 10.17. Genetic control of the immune response.

result of regulatory cell activity (figure 10.16d). Low response can be dominant in class II heterozygotes, indicating that suppression can act against Th restricted to any other class II molecule. In this it differs from models 1 and 2 above where high response is dominant in a heterozygote because the factors associated with the low responder gene cannot influence the activity of the high responder.

Factors influencing the genetic control of the immune response are summarized in figure 10.17.

REGULATORY IMMUNONEUROENDOCRINE NETWORKS

There is a danger, as one focuses more and more on the antics of the immune system, of looking at the body as a collection of myeloid and lymphoid cells roaming around in a big sack and of having no regard to the integrated physiology of the organism. Within the wider physiological context, attention has been drawn increasingly to interactions between immunological and neuroendocrine systems.

Immunological cells have the receptors which enable them to receive signals from a whole range of hormones: corticosteroids, insulin, growth hormone, estradiol, testosterone, prolactin, β-adrenergic agents, acetylcholine, endorphins and enkephalins. By and large, glucocorticoids and androgens depress immune responses, whereas estrogens, growth hormone, thyroxine and insulin do the opposite.

3 *T-suppression.* We would like to refer again to the MHC-restricted low responsiveness which can occur to relatively complex antigens (see p. 214), since it illustrates the notion that low responder status can arise as a

A neuroendocrine feedback loop affecting immune responses

The secretion of **glucocorticoids** is a major response to stresses induced by a wide range of stimuli, such as extreme changes of temperature, fear, hunger and physical injury. They are also released as a consequence of immune responses and limit those responses in a neuroendocrine feedback loop. Thus, IL-1 (figure 10.18), IL-6 and TNF are capable of stimulating glucocorticoid synthesis and do so through the hypothalamic–pituitary–adrenal axis. This, in turn, leads to the downregulation of Th1 and macrophage activity, so completing the negative feedback circuit (figure 10.19). However, the glucocorticoid dexamethasone can prevent *a*ctivation-*i*nduced *c*ell *d*eath (AICD) in T-cells by inducing expression of GILZ (*g*lucocorticoid-*i*nduced *l*eucine *z*ipper). The situation is therefore somewhat complex because glucocorticoids can themselves trigger apoptosis in T-cells, yet counteract apoptosis activated by peptide–MHC interaction with the TCR. In the absence of glucocorticoid, the activation of T-cells by peptide–MHC leads to a progressive loss of GILZ and eventual cell death by apoptosis. By contrast, if activation through the TCR occurs in the presence of glucocorticoids, then expression of GILZ is increased and this directly inhibits activation and nuclear translocation of NFκB, thereby protecting the cells from AICD.

It has been shown that adrenalectomy prevents spontaneous recovery from *e*xperimental *a*llergic *e*ncephalomyelitis (EAE). This demyelinating disease is associated with progressive paralysis and is produced by immunization with myelin basic protein in complete Freund's adjuvant. Induction of the disease can be blocked by implants of corticosterone. Spontaneous recovery from EAE in intact animals is associated with a dominance of Th2 autoantigen-specific clones, indicative of the view that glucocorticoids suppress Th1 and may augment Th2 cells. Individuals with a genetic predisposition to high levels of stress-induced glucocorticoids might therefore be expected to have increased susceptibility to infections with intracellular pathogens

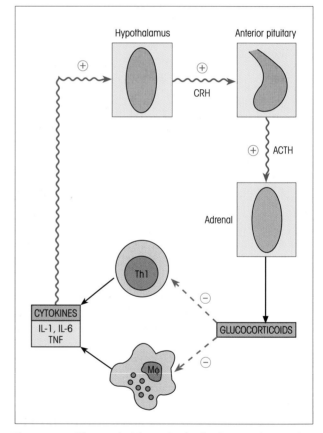

Figure 10.19. Glucocorticoid negative feedback on cytokine production. Additional regulatory circuits based on neuroendocrine interactions with the immune system are almost certain to exist given that lymphoid and myeloid cells in both primary and secondary lymphoid organs can produce hormones and neuropeptides, and classical endocrine glands as well as neurons and glial cells can synthesize cytokines and appropriate receptors. Production of prolactin and its receptors by peripheral lymphoid cells and thymocytes is worthy of attention. Lymphocyte expression of the prolactin receptor is upregulated following activation and, in autoimmune disease, witness the beneficial effects of bromocriptine, an inhibitor of prolactin synthesis, in the NZB × W model of murine systemic lupus erythematosus (cf. p. 82). CRH, corticotropin-releasing hormone; ACTH, adrenocorticotropic hormone.

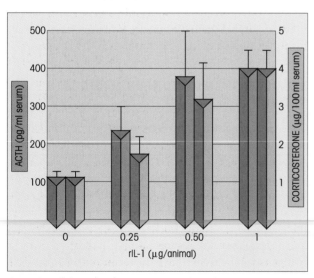

Figure 10.18. Enhancement of ACTH and corticosterone blood levels in C3H/HeJ mice 2 hours after injection of recombinant IL-1 (values are means ± SEM for groups of seven or eight mice). The significance of the mouse strain used is that it lacks receptors for bacterial lipopolysaccharide (LPS), and so the effects cannot be attributed to LPS contamination of the IL-1 preparation. (Reprinted from Besedovsky H., del Rey A., Sorkin E. & Dinarello C.A. (1986) *Science* **233**, 652–654, with permission. Copyright © 1986 by the AAAS.)

such as *Mycobacterium leprae* which require effective Th1 cell-mediated immunity for their eradication.

Neonatal exposure to bacterial endotoxin (LPS) not only exerts a long-term influence on endocrine and central nervous system development, but substantially affects predisposition to inflammatory disease and therefore appears to program or 'reset' the functional development of both the endocrine and immune systems. Thus, in adult life, rats which had been exposed to endotoxin during the first week of life had higher basal levels of corticosterone compared with control animals, and showed a greater increase in corticosterone levels in response to noise stress and a more rapid rise in corticosterone levels following challenge with LPS.

Sex hormones come into the picture

Females are far more susceptible to autoimmune disease, an issue that will be discussed in greater depth in Chapter 18, but here let us note that estrogen receptors are present on various cell types in the immune system, including lymphocytes and macrophages. Although investigations into the role of estrogen in immune responses have often led to apparently contradictory data, some of its more clearly established effects on different populations of lymphocytes are highlighted in figure 10.20. It has often been found to enhance T-cell proliferation, B-cell survival, and humoral responses. Conversely, androgen deprivation induced by castration of postpubertal male mice increases the levels of T-cells in secondary lymphoid tissues and enhances T-cell proliferation.

Estrogen also has effects on regulatory cells, expanding CD4+CD25+ T-cells and upregulating Foxp3 expression. Another type of regulatory cell is the NKT cell that

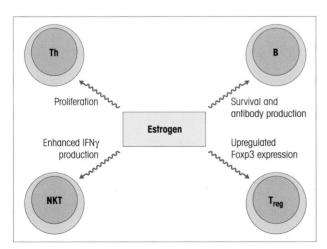

Figure 10.20. Some effects of estrogen on lymphocyte function.

bears an invariant TCR, responds to the synthetic glycolipid α-galactosylceramide presented by CD1d (cf. p. 83), and is able to produce both the Th1 cytokine interferon-γ (IFNγ) and the Th2 cytokine IL-4. Substantially enhanced levels of IFNγ are produced by these cells when stimulated with antigen in the presence of physiological concentrations of estrogen, providing a possible explanation for the observation that female mice produce higher levels of this cytokine in response to antigen challenge.

'Psychoimmunology'

The thymus, spleen and lymph nodes are richly innervated by the sympathetic nervous system. The enzyme dopamine β-hydroxylase catalyses the conversion of dopamine to the catecholamine neurotransmitter norepinephrine which is released from sympathetic neurons in these tissues. Mice in which the gene for this enzyme has been deleted by homologous recombination exhibited enhanced susceptibility to infection with the intracellular pathogen *Mycobacterium tuberculosis* and impaired production of the Th1 cytokines IFNγ and TNF in response to the infection. Although these animals showed no obvious developmental defects in their immune system, impaired Th1 responses were also found following immunization of these mice with the hapten TNP coupled to KLH. These observations suggest that norepinephrine can play a role in determining the potency of the immune response.

Denervated skin shows greatly reduced leukocyte infiltration in response to local damage, implicating cutaneous neurons in the recruitment of leukocytes. Sympathetic nerves which innervate lymphatic vessels and lymph nodes are involved in regulating the flow of lymph and may participate in controlling the migration of β-adrenergic receptor-bearing dendritic cells from inflammatory sites to the local lymph nodes. Mast cells and nerves often have an intimate anatomical relationship and nerve growth factor causes mast cell degranulation. The gastrointestinal tract also has extensive innervation and a high number of immune effector cells. In this context, the ability of substance P to stimulate, and of somatostatin to inhibit, proliferation of Peyer's patch lymphocytes may prove to have more than a trivial significance. The pituitary hormone prolactin has also been brought to our attention by the experimental observation that inhibition of prolactin secretion by bromocriptine suppresses Th activity.

There seems to be an interaction between inflammation and nerve growth in regions of wound healing and repair. Mast cells are often abundant, IL-6 induces neurite growth and IL-1 enhances production of nerve growth factor in sciatic nerve explants. IL-1 also increases slow-wave sleep when introduced into the lateral ventricle of the brain, and both IL-1 and interferon produce pyrogenic effects through their action on the temperature-controlling center.

Although it is not clear just how these diverse neuroendocrine effects fit into the regulation of immune responses, at a more physiological level, stress and circadian rhythms modify the functioning of the immune system. Factors such as restraint, noise and exam anxiety have been observed to influence a number of immune functions including phagocytosis, lymphocyte proliferation, NK activity and IgA secretion. Amazingly, it has been reported that the delayed-type hypersensitivity Mantoux reaction in the skin can be modified by hypnosis. An elegant demonstration of nervous system control is provided by studies showing suppression of conventional immune responses and enhancement of NK cell activity by Pavlovian conditioning. In the classic Pavlovian paradigm, a stimulus such as food that unconditionally elicits a particular response, in this case salivation, is repeatedly paired with a neutral stimulus that does not elicit the same response. Eventually, the neutral stimulus becomes a conditional stimulus and will elicit salivation in the absence of food. Rats were given cyclophosphamide as a unconditional and saccharin as a conditional stimulus repeatedly; subsequently, there was a depressed antibody response when the animals were challenged with antigen together with just the conditional stimulus, saccharin. As more and more data accumulate, it is becoming clearer how immunoneuroendocrine networks could play a role in allergy and in autoimmune diseases such as rheumatoid arthritis, type I diabetes and multiple sclerosis.

EFFECTS OF DIET, EXERCISE, TRAUMA AND AGE ON IMMUNITY

Malnutrition diminishes the effectiveness of the immune response

The greatly increased susceptibility of undernourished individuals to infection can be attributed to many factors: poor sanitation and personal hygiene, overcrowding and inadequate health education. But, in addition, there are gross effects of **protein-calorie malnutrition** on immunocompetence. The widespread atrophy of lymphoid tissues and the 50% reduction in circulating CD4 T-cells underlie **serious impairment of cell-mediated immunity**. Antibody responses may be intact but they are of lower affinity; phagocytosis of bacteria is relatively normal but the subsequent intracellular destruction is defective.

Deficiencies in pyridoxine, folic acid and vitamins A, C and E result in generally impaired immune responses. **Vitamin D is an important regulator**. It is produced not only by the UV-irradiated dermis, but also by activated macrophages, the hypercalcemia associated with sarcoidosis being attributable to production of the vitamin by macrophages in the active granulomas. The vitamin is a potent inhibitor of T-cell proliferation and of Th1 cytokine production. This generates a neat feedback loop at sites of inflammation where macrophages activated by IFNγ produce vitamin D which suppresses the T-cells making the interferon. It also downregulates antigen presentation by macrophages and promotes multinucleated giant cell formation in chronic granulomatous lesions. Nonetheless, as a further emphasis of the potential duality of the CD4 helper subsets, it promotes Th2 activity, especially at mucosal surfaces: quite a busy little vitamin. Zinc deficiency is rather interesting; this greatly affects the biological activity of thymus hormones and has a major effect on cell-mediated immunity, perhaps as a result. Iron deficiency impairs the oxidative burst in neutrophils since the flavocytochrome NADP oxidase is an iron-containing enzyme.

Of course there is another side to all this in that moderate restriction of total calorie intake and/or marked reduction in fat intake ameliorates age-related diseases such as autoimmunity. Oils with an n-3 double bond, such as fish oils, are also protective, perhaps due to increased synthesis of immunosuppressive prostaglandins.

Given the overdue sensitivity to the importance of environmental contamination, it is important to monitor the nature and levels of pollution that may influence immunity. Here is just one example: polyhalogenated organic compounds (such as polychlorinated biphenyls) steadily pervade the environment and, being stable and lipophilic, accumulate readily in the aquatic food chain where they largely resist metabolic breakdown. It was shown that Baltic herrings with relatively high levels of these pollutants, as compared with uncontaminated Atlantic herrings, were immunotoxic when fed to captive harbor seals, suggesting one reason why seals along the coasts of northwestern Europe succumbed so alarmingly to infection with the otherwise nonvirulent phocine distemper virus in 1988.

Other factors

Exercise, particularly severe exercise, induces stress and raises plasma levels of cortisol, catecholamines, IFNα, IL-1, β-endorphin and metenkephalin. It can lead to reduced IgA levels, immune deficiency and increased susceptibility to infection. Maniacal joggers and other such like masochists—you have been warned!

Multiple traumatic injury, surgery and major burns are also immunosuppressive and so contribute to the

increased risk of sepsis. Corticosteroids produced by stressful conditions, the immunosuppressive prostaglandin E$_2$ released from damaged tissues and bacterial endotoxin derived from the disturbance of gut flora are all factors which influence the outcome after trauma.

Accepting that the problem of understanding the mechanisms of **aging** is a tough nut to crack, it is a trifle disappointing that the easier task of establishing the influence of age on immunological phenomena is still not satisfactorily accomplished. Perhaps the elderly population is skewed towards individuals with effective immune systems which give a survival advantage. Be that as it may, IL-2 production by peripheral blood lymphocytes (figure 10.21) and T-cell-mediated functions such as delayed-type hypersensitivity reactions to common skin test antigens decline with age and so, it is thought, does T-cell mediated suppression, although this is a notoriously elusive function to measure.

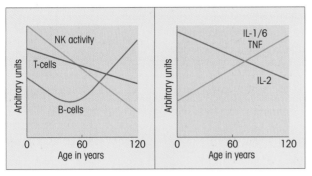

Figure 10.21. Age trends in some immunological parameters. (Based on Franceschi C., Monti D., Sansoni P. & Cossarizza A. (1995) *Immunology Today* **16**, 12–16.)

SUMMARY

Control by antigen

• Immune responses are largely antigen driven. As the level of antigen falls, so does the intensity of the response.

• Antigens can compete with each other: a result of competition between processed peptides for the available MHC grooves.

Feedback control by complement and antibody

• Early IgM antibodies and C3d boost antibody responses, whereas IgG inhibits responses via the Fcγ receptor on B-cells.

T-cell regulation

• Activated T-cells express members of the TNF receptor family, including Fas, which act as death receptors and restrain unlimited clonal expansion by a process referred to as activation-induced cell death (AICD).

• Regulatory T-cells (Tregs) can suppress the activity of helper T-cells, presumably as feedback control of excessive Th expansion.

• Suppressor and helper epitopes on the same molecule can be discrete.

• Effectors of suppression include naturally occurring CD4$^+$CD25$^+$Foxp3$^+$ cell-contact dependent Tregs, IL-10 secreting Tr1 cells, TGFβ-secreting Th3 cells, immunoregulatory γδ T-cells and CD8$^+$ suppressors.

• Resting dendritic cells can preferentially promote the development of regulatory cells.

• Suppression can occur due to T–T interaction on the

surface of antigen-presenting cells. Just as Th1 and Th2 cells mutually inhibit each other through production of their respective cytokines IFNγ and IL-4/10, so there may be two types of CD8 cells with suppressor activity: one of Tc2 type making IL-4 and suppressing Th1 cells, and the other Tc1 cells making IFNγ capable of suppressing Th2 cells.

Idiotype networks

• Antigen-specific receptors on lymphocytes can interact with the idiotypes on the receptors of other lymphocytes to form a network (Jerne).

• Anti-idiotypes can be induced by autologous idiotypes.

• An idiotype network involving mostly CD5 B-1 cells is evident in early life.

• T-cell idiotypic interactions can also be demonstrated.

• Idiotypes which occur frequently and are shared by a multiplicity of antibodies (public or cross-reacting Id) are targets for regulation by anti-idiotypes in the network, thus providing a further mechanism for control of the immune response.

• The network offers the potential for therapeutic intervention to manipulate immunity.

Genetic factors influence the immune response

• Multiple genes control the overall antibody response to complex antigens: some affect macrophage antigen processing and microbicidal activity and some the rate of proliferation of differentiating B-cells.

(Continued p.228)

- Immunoglobulin and TCR genes are very adaptable because they rearrange to create the antigen receptors, but 'holes' in the repertoire can occur.
- Immune response genes are located in the MHC class II locus and control the interactions required for T–B collaboration.
- Class II-linked high and low responsiveness may be due to defective presentation by MHC, a defective T-cell repertoire caused by tolerance to MHC+self-peptides and T-suppression.

Immunoneuroendocrine networks

- Immunological, neurological and endocrinological systems interact, forming regulatory circuits.
- Feedback by cytokines augments the production of corticosteroids and is important because this shuts down Th1 and macrophage activity.

- Estrogens can enhance both T- and B-cell responses, but can also promote the activity of regulatory cells.

Effects of diet and other factors on immunity

- Protein-calorie malnutrition grossly impairs cell-mediated immunity and phagocyte microbicidal potency.
- Exercise, trauma, age and environmental pollution can all act to impair immune mechanisms. The pattern of cytokines produced by peripheral blood cells changes with age, IL-2 decreasing and TNF, IL-1 and IL-6 increasing; the latter is associated with a lowered DHEA level.

Factors influencing the bias between Th1 and Th2 subsets

- These have figured with some prominence in this chapter and a summary of some of the major influences on the balance between Th1 and Th2 responses is presented in figure 10.22.

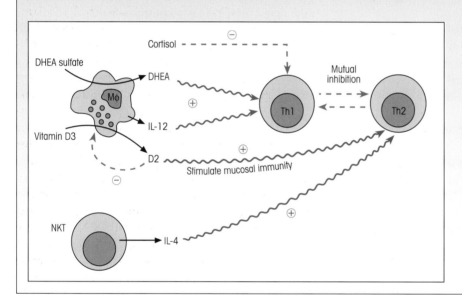

Figure 10.22. Summary of major factors affecting Th1/Th2 balance. Preferential stimulation of mucosal antibody synthesis by vitamin D involves the promotion of dendritic cell migration to the Peyer's patches. By downregulating macrophage activity, Th1 effectiveness is decreased. Cortisol and dehydroepiandrosterone (DHEA) are products of the adrenal and have opposing effects on the Th1 subset. A relative deficiency of DHEA will lead to poor Th1 performance. NKT cells bear an αβ TCR, the natural killer cell marker NK1.1, and secrete cytokines including IL-4 which stimulate Th2 cells.

FURTHER READING

Bevan M.J. (2004) Helping the CD8+ T-cell response. *Nature Reviews Immunology* **4**, 595–602.

Chandra R.K. (1998) Nutrition and the immune system. In Delves P.J. & Roitt I.M. (eds) *Encyclopedia of Immunology*, 2nd edn, pp. 1869–1871. Academic Press, London. (See also other relevant articles in the *Encyclopedia*: 'Aging and the immune system', pp.59–61; 'Behavioral regulation of immunity', pp. 336–340; 'Neuroendocrine regulation of immunity', p. 1824; 'Sex hormones and immunity', pp. 2175–2178; 'Stress and the immune system', pp. 2220–2228; 'Vitamin D', pp. 2494–2499.)

Cohen I.R. (2000) *Tending Adam's Garden*. Academic Press, London.

Crowley M.P. *et al.* (2000) A population of murine γδ T cells that recognize an inducible MHC class Ib molecule. *Science* **287**, 314–316.

Fearon D.T. & Carroll M.C. (2000) Regulation of B lymphocyte responses to foreign and self-antigens by the CD19/CD21 complex. *Annual Reviews of Immunology* **18**, 393–422.

Jiang H. & Chess L. (2006) Regulation of immune responses by T cells. *The New England Journal of Medicine* **354**, 1166–1176.

Krammer P.H. (2000) CD95's deadly mission in the immune system. *Nature* **407**, 789–795.

O'Garra A. & Vieira P. (2004) Regulatory T-cells and mechanisms of immune system control. *Nature Medicine* **10**, 801–805.

Randolph D.A. & Garrison Fathman C. (2006) CD4+ CD25+ regulatory T-cells and their therapeutic potential. *Annual Review of Medicine* **57**, 381–402.

Reiche E.M.V., Nunes S.O.V. & Morimoto H.K. (2004) Stress, depression, the immune system, and cancer. *Lancet Oncology* **5**, 617–625.

Shanks N. *et al.* (2000) Early life exposure to endotoxin alters hypothalamic–pituitary–adrenal function and predisposition to inflammation. *Proceedings of the National Academy of Sciences of the United States of America* **97**, 5645–5650.

Steinman L. (2004) Elaborate interactions between the immune and nervous systems. *Nature Immunology* **5**, 575–581.

11 Ontogeny and phylogeny

INTRODUCTION

Hematopoiesis originates in the early yolk sac but, as embryogenesis proceeds, this function is taken over by the fetal liver and finally by the bone marrow where it continues throughout life. The **hematopoietic stem cell (HSC) which gives rise to the formed elements of the blood** (figure 11.1) can be shown to be multipotent, to seed other organs and, under the influence of the cytokine leukemia inhibitory factor (LIF), to have a relatively unlimited capacity to renew itself through the creation of further stem cells. Thus an animal can be completely protected against the lethal effects of high doses of irradiation by injection of bone marrow cells which will repopulate its lymphoid and myeloid systems. The capacity for self-renewal is not absolute and declines with age in parallel with a shortening of the telomeres and a reduction in telomerase, the enzyme which repairs the shortening of the ends of chromosomes which would otherwise occur at every round of cell division.

HEMATOPOIETIC STEM CELLS

The bone marrow contains at least two types of stem cell, the HSC mentioned above and the mesenchymal stem cell (MSC) which constitute the bone marrow stroma and under appropriate signals can differentiate into adipocytes, osteocytes, chondrocytes and myocytes. The HSC in the mouse is CD34$^{low/-}$, Sca-1$^+$, Thy-1$^{+/low}$, CD38$^+$, c-kit (CD117)$^+$ and lin$^-$, whereas the surface phenotype of the equivalent cell in human is CD34$^{+,}$ CD59$^+$, Thy-1$^+$, CD38$^{low/-}$, c-kit$^{-/low}$ and lin$^-$. Impressively, less than 100 HSCs can prevent death in a lethally irradiated animal.

The hematopoietic stem cells differentiate within the microenvironment of the sessile stromal cells which produce various growth factors including IL-3, -4, -6 and -7, G-CSF, GM-CSF, stem cell factor (SCF), flt-3 (flk-2 ligand), erythropoietin (EPO), thrombopoietin (TPO) and so on. SCF remains associated with the extracellular matrix and acts on primitive stem cells through the tyrosine kinase membrane receptor c-kit. The importance of this interaction between undifferentiated stem cells and the microenvironment which guides their differentiation is clearly shown by studies on mice homozygous for mutations at the *w* or the *sl* loci which, amongst other defects, have severe macrocytic anemia. *sl/sl* mutants have normal stem cells but defective stromal production of SCF which can be corrected by transplantation of a normal spleen fragment; *w/w* mutant myeloid progenitors lack the c-kit surface receptor for SCF, and so can be restored by injection of normal bone marrow cells (figure 11.2). Hematopoiesis needs to be kept under tight control, for example by transforming growth factor β (TGFβ) which exerts a cytostatic effect on HSCs via induction of the cyclin-dependent kinase inhibitor p57KIP2.

Mice with *s*evere *c*ombined *i*mmuno*d*eficiency (SCID) provide a happy environment for fragments of human fetal liver and thymus which, if implanted contiguously, will produce formed elements of the blood for 6–12 months.

THE THYMUS PROVIDES THE ENVIRONMENT FOR T-CELL DIFFERENTIATION

The thymus is organized into a series of lobules based upon meshworks of epithelial cells derived embryologically from an outpushing of the gut endoderm of the third pharyngeal pouch and which form well-defined cortical and medullary zones (figure 11.3). This framework of epithelial cells provides the microenvironment

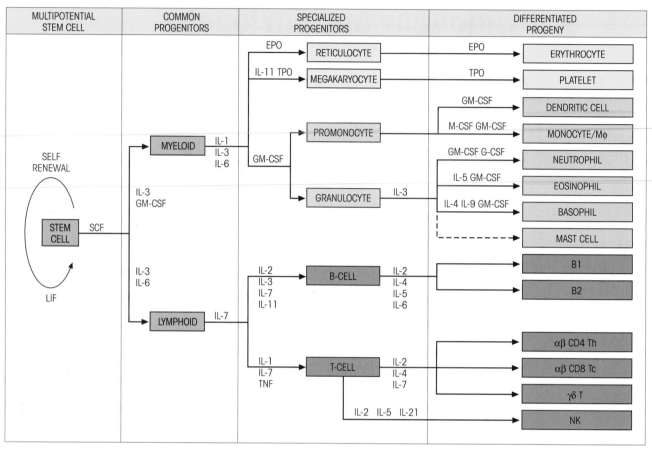

Figure 11.1. The multipotential hematopoietic stem cell and its progeny which differentiate under the influence of a series of soluble growth factors within the microenvironment of the bone marrow. The expression of various nuclear transcription factors directs the differentiation process. For example, the *Ikaros* gene encodes a zinc-fingered transcription factor critical for driving the development of a common myeloid/lymphoid precursor into a lymphoid-restricted progenitor giving rise to T-, B- and NK cells. SCF, stem cell factor; LIF, leukemia inhibitory factor; IL-3, interleukin-3, often termed the multi-CSF because it stimulates progenitors of platelets, erythrocytes, all the types of myeloid cells, and also the progenitors of B-, but not T-, cells; GM-CSF, granulocyte–macrophage colony-stimulating factor, so-called because it promotes the formation of mixed colonies of these two cell types from bone marrow progenitors either in tissue culture or on transfer to an irradiated recipient where they appear in the spleen; G-CSF, granulocyte colony-stimulating factor; M-CSF, monocyte colony-stimulating factor; EPO, erythropoietin; TPO, thrombopoietin; TNF, tumor necrosis factor; TGFβ, transforming growth factor β.

for T-cell differentiation. In both neonatal and adult mice c-kit⁺ CD44⁺ T-cell progenitors arrive from the bone marrow in waves of immigration that appear to be regulated by the accessibility of putative niches in the thymus. There are subtle interactions between the extracellular matrix proteins and a variety of adhesion/homing molecules which, in addition to CD44, include the α_6 integrin. Several chemokines also play an essential role, with CXCL12 (stromal-derived factor-1, SDF-1) being a particularly potent chemoattractant for the CXCR4⁺ progenitor cells in man. In addition, the epithelial cells produce a series of peptide hormones which mostly seem capable of promoting the appearance of T-cell differentiation markers and a variety of T-cell functions on culture with bone marrow cells *in vitro*. The circulating levels of these hormones *in vivo* begin to decline from puberty onwards, reaching vanishingly

small amounts by the age of 60 years. Several have been well characterized and sequenced, including thymulin, thymosin α_1, *t*hymic *h*umoral *f*actor (THF) and thymopoietin (and its active pentapeptide thymopontin, TP-5). Of these, only thymulin is of exclusively thymic origin. This zinc-dependent nonapeptide tends to normalize the balance of immune responses: it restores antibody avidity and antibody production in aged mice and yet stimulates suppressor activity in animals with autoimmune hemolytic anemia induced by cross-reactive rat red cells (cf. p. 428). Thymulin may be looked upon as a true hormone, secreted by the thymus in a regulated fashion and acting at a distance from the thymus as a fine physiological immunoregulator contributing to the maintenance of T-cell subset homeostasis.

Specialized large epithelial cells in the outer cortex, known as 'nurse' cells, are associated with large

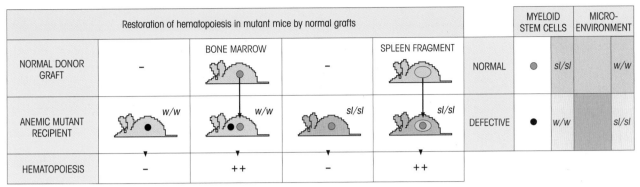

Restoration of hematopoiesis in mutant mice by normal grafts						MYELOID STEM CELLS		MICRO-ENVIRONMENT	
NORMAL DONOR GRAFT	–	BONE MARROW	–	SPLEEN FRAGMENT	NORMAL	●	sl/sl		w/w
ANEMIC MUTANT RECIPIENT	w/w	w/w	sl/sl	sl/sl	DEFECTIVE	●	w/w		sl/sl
HEMATOPOIESIS	–	++	–	++					

Figure 11.2. Hematopoiesis requires normal bone marrow stem cells differentiating in a normal microenvironment. The *w* locus codes for c-kit, a stem cell tyrosine kinase membrane receptor for the stem cell factor (SCF) encoded by the *sl* locus. Mice which are homozygous for mutant alleles at these loci develop severe macrocytic anemia which can be corrected by transplantation of appropriate normal cells. The experiments show that the *w/w* mutant lacks normal stem cells and the *sl/sl* mutant lacks the environmental factor needed for their development.

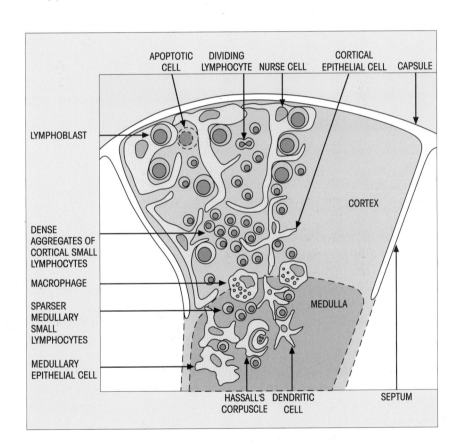

Figure 11.3. Cellular features of a thymus lobule. See text for description. (Adapted from Hood L.E., Weissman I.L., Wood W.B. & Wilson J.H. (1984) *Immunology*, 2nd edn, p. 261. Benjamin Cummings, California.)

numbers of lymphocytes which lie within pockets produced by the long membrane extensions of these epithelial cells. The epithelial cells of the deep cortex have branched processes, rich in class II MHC, and connect through desmosome cell junctions to form a network through which cortical lymphocytes must pass on their way to the medulla (figure 11.3). The cortical lymphocytes are densely packed compared with those in the medulla, many are in division and large numbers of them are undergoing apoptosis. On their way to the medulla, the lymphocytes pass a cordon of 'sentinel' macrophages at the corticomedullary junction. A number of bone marrow-derived dendritic cells are present in the medulla and the epithelial cells have broader processes than their cortical counterparts and express high levels of both class I and class II MHC. Whorled keratinized epithelial cells in the medulla form the highly characteristic Hassall's corpuscles beloved of histopathology examiners. These structures serve as a disposal system for dying thymocytes, perhaps follow-

Milestone 11.1—The Immunological Function of the Thymus

Ludwig Gross had found that a form of mouse leukemia could be induced in low-leukemia strains by inoculating filtered leukemic tissue from high-leukemia strains provided that this was done in the immediate neonatal period. Since the thymus was known to be involved in the leukemic process, Jacques Miller decided to test the hypothesis that the Gross virus could only multiply in the neonatal thymus by infecting neonatally thymectomized mice of low-leukemia strains. The results were consistent with this hypothesis but, strangely, animals of one strain died of a wasting disease which Miller deduced could have been due to susceptibility to infection, since fewer mice died when they were moved from the converted horse stables which served as an animal house to 'cleaner' quarters.

Autopsy showed the animals to have atrophied lymphoid tissue and low blood lymphocyte levels, and Miller therefore decided to test their immunocompetence before the onset of wasting disease. To his astonishment, skin grafts, even from rats (figure M11.1.1) as well as from other mouse strains, were fully accepted. These phenomena were not induced by thymectomy later in life and, in writing up his preliminary

results in 1961 (Miller J.F.A.P., *Lancet* **ii**, 748–479), Miller opined that 'during embryogenesis the thymus would produce the originators of immunologically competent cells, many of which would have migrated to other sites at about the time of birth'. All in all a superb example of the scientific method and its application by a top-flight scientist.

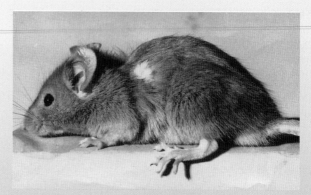

Figure M11.1.1. Acceptance of a rat skin graft by a mouse which had been neonatally thymectomized.

---

ing their phagocytosis by dendritic cells, and are the only location where apoptotic cells are found in the medulla.

A fairly complex relationship with the nervous system awaits discovery; the thymus is richly innervated with both adrenergic and cholinergic fibers. Both thymocytes and thymic stromal cells express receptors for a number of neurotransmitters and neuropeptides. Somatostatin is expressed by both cortical and medullary thymic epithelial cells and is able to induce the migration of thymocytes which express the SSTR2 receptor for this neuropeptide. The *g*lial cell line-*d*erived *n*eurotrophic *f*actor (GDNF) and the GFRα1 component of the GDNF receptor are expressed in CD4⁻CD8⁻ ('double negative', DN) thymocytes. Furthermore, fetal thymocyte precursors fail to grow in a serum-free medium culture system unless recombinant GDNF is added. Thus, GDNF may be involved in the survival of the DN immature thymocytes. Glucocorticoid hormones, such as hydrocortisone (cortisol) and cortisone, are classically associated with the adrenal gland but are also produced by thymic epithelial cells. During stress the output of these hormones increases and directly provokes thymic involution and apoptosis of thymocytes. The sex hormones testosterone, estrogen and progesterone can also promote thymic involution.

In the human, thymic involution naturally commences within the first 12 months of life, reducing by

around 3% a year to middle age and by 1% thereafter. The size of the organ gives no clue to these changes because there is replacement by adipose tissue. In a sense, the thymus is progressively disposable because, as we shall see, it establishes a long-lasting peripheral T-cell pool which enables the host to withstand loss of the gland without catastrophic failure of immunological function—witness the minimal effects of thymectomy in the adult compared with the **dramatic influence in the neonate** (Milestone 11.1). Nevertheless, the adult thymus retains a residue of corticomedullary tissue containing a normal range of thymocyte subsets with a broad spectrum of TCR gene rearrangements. Adult patients receiving either T-cell-depleted bone marrow or peripheral blood hematopoietic stem cells following ablative therapy are able to generate new naive T-cells at a rate that is inversely related to the age of the individual. These observations establish that new T-cells can be generated in adult life, either in the thymus or in the still rather mysterious 'extrathymic' sites that have been proposed as additional locations for T-cell differentiation and which might include the intestinal cryptopatches of the gut-associated lymphoid tissues.

Bone marrow stem cells become immunocompetent T-cells in the thymus

The evidence for this comes from experiments on the

reconstitution of irradiated hosts. An irradiated animal is restored by bone marrow grafts through the immediate restitution of granulocyte precursors; in the longer term, also through reconstitution of the T- and B-cells destroyed by irradiation. However, if the animal is thymectomized before irradiation, bone marrow cells will not reconstitute the T-lymphocyte population (cf. figure 6.42).

By day 11–12 in the mouse embryo, lymphoblastoid stem cells from the bone marrow begin to colonize the periphery of the epithelial thymus rudiment. If the thymus is removed at this stage and incubated in organ culture, a whole variety of mature T-lymphocytes will be generated. This is not seen if 10-day thymuses are cultured and shows that the lymphoblastoid colonizers give rise to the immunocompetent small lymphocyte progeny.

T-CELL ONTOGENY

Differentiation is accompanied by changes in surface markers

T-cell progenitors arriving from the bone marrow enter the thymus through venules at the cortico-medullary junction. These early thymocytes lack both the CD4 and CD8 coreceptors and are therefore referred to as **double negative** (DN) cells. They do, however, express the chemokine receptor CCR7 and, under the influence of chemokines such as CCL19 and CCL21, they migrate through the thymic cortex towards the outer subcapsular zone (figure 11.4). The earliest of these progenitors, the DN1 cells, retain pluripotentiality, still express the stem cell marker CD34, and also express high levels of the adhesion molecule CD44 and the stem cell factor (SCF) receptor (c-kit, CD117) (p. 229). As they mature into DN2 cells they lose CD34 expression and begin to express the IL-2 receptor α chain (CD25). These cells are restricted to producing T-cells and lymphoid dendritic cells. T-cell development is severely impaired in Notch-1[−/−] knockout mice, Notch-1 signaling being necessary for T-cell lineage commitment of the DN1 and DN2 cells. Indeed, the Notch-1 ligands with the rather exotic names of Jagged-1, Jagged-2 and δ-like-1 are expressed on thymic epithelial cells in a highly regulated way. Further differentiation into DN3 cells and a downregulation of CCR7 expression accompanies their arrival in the subcapsular zone. Transient expression of the recombinase-activating genes RAG-1 and RAG-2, together with an increase in chromatin accessibility around one allele of the TCR β-chain genes, results in β-chain rearrangement and commitment to the T-cell lineage. Expression of CD3, the invariant signal trans-

ducing complex of the TCR, occurs at this stage, whilst CD44 and c-kit are lost. The later loss of CD25 signifies passage into the DN4 population, which subsequently differentiate into the CD4+ (the marker for MHC class II recognition) **and** CD8+ (class I recognition) **double positive (DP)** thymocytes. TCR α-chain gene rearrangement occurs when RAG-1 and RAG-2 are again transiently expressed in either the DN4 cells or immediately following expression of CD4 and CD8. The DP thymocytes then begin to re-express high amounts of CCR7 causing them to migrate back through the cortex, eventually crossing the cortico-medullary junction into the medulla. The CD4 and CD8 markers segregate in parallel with differentiation into separate immunocompetent populations of **single positive (SP) CD4+** (mostly **T-helpers)** and **CD8+** (mostly **cytotoxic) T-cell precursors**.

In addition to the factors mentioned above, thymocyte development is critically dependent on IL-7 which is necessary for the transition to the DN3 stage. This cytokine is produced by the thymic epithelial cells and is thought to be retained locally by binding to glycoaminoglycans in the extracellular matrix. Signaling through the IL-7 receptor and c-kit also help drive the early extensive proliferation that occurs in thymocytes prior to the rearrangement of the TCR genes, with thymic stromal lymphopoietin (TSLP) acting as an additional ligand for the IL-7 receptor α-chain. SCF, IL-7 and TSLP are aided and abetted in this task by activation through the Wnt/β-catenin/nuclear T-cell factor (TCF) pathway, which also causes the upregulation of adhesion molecules required for the ordered migration of the chemokine-responsive thymocytes through the thymus. Stimulation of this pathway occurs through binding of Wnt family members to cell surface Frizzled (Fz) receptors on the thymocytes, Wnt-4, -7a, -7b, -10a and -10b being expressed by thymic epithelium. The γδ cells remain double negative, i.e. CD4−8−, except for a small subset which express CD8.

The factors which determine whether the double-positive cells become single-positive CD4+ class II-restricted cells or CD8+ class I-restricted cells in the thymus are still not fully established. Two major scenarios have been put forward. The **stochastic/selection** hypothesis suggests that expression of either the CD4 or CD8 coreceptor is randomly switched off and then cells that have a TCR–coreceptor combination capable of recognizing an appropriate peptide–MHC are selected for survival. By contrast, the **instructive** hypothesis declares that interaction of the TCR with MHC–peptide results in signals which instruct the T-cells to switch off expression of the 'useless' coreceptor incapable of recognizing that particular class of MHC. In order to reconcile the fact that there is supporting data for both

Milestone 11.2—The Discovery of Immunological Tolerance

Over 60 years ago, Owen made the intriguing observation that nonidentical (dizygotic) twin cattle, which shared the same placental circulation and whose circulations were thereby linked, grew up with appreciable numbers of red cells from the other twin in their blood; if they had not shared the same circulation at birth, red cells from the twin injected in adult life would have been rapidly eliminated by an immunological response. From this finding, Burnet and Fenner conceived the notion that potential antigens which reach the lymphoid cells during their developing immunologically immature phase can in some way specifically suppress any future response to that antigen when the animal reaches immunological maturity. This, they considered, would provide a means whereby unresponsiveness to the body's own constituents could be established and thereby enable the lymphoid cells to make the important distinction between 'self' and 'nonself'. On this basis, any foreign cells introduced into the body during immunological development should trick the animal into treating them as 'self'-components in later life, and the studies of Medawar and his colleagues have shown that **immunological tolerance**, or unresponsiveness, can be artificially induced in this way. Thus neonatal injection of CBA mouse cells into newborn A strain animals suppresses their ability to reject a CBA graft immunologically in adult life (figure M11.2.1). Tolerance can also be induced with soluble antigens; for example, rabbits injected with bovine serum albumin without adjuvant at birth fail to make antibodies on later challenge with this protein.

Persistence of antigen is required to maintain tolerance. In Medawar's experiments, the tolerant state was long lived because the injected CBA cells survived and the animals continued to be chimeric (i.e. they possessed both A and CBA cells). With nonliving antigens, such as soluble bovine serum albumin, tolerance is gradually lost; the most likely explanation is that, in the absence of antigen, newly recruited immunocompetent cells which are being generated throughout life are not being rendered tolerant. Since recruitment of newly competent T-lymphocytes is drastically curtailed by

removal of the thymus, it is of interest to note that the tolerant state persists for much longer in thymectomized animals.

The vital importance of the experiments by Medawar and his team was their demonstration that a state of immunological tolerance can result from exposure to an antigen. As will be discussed in the text, there is a window of susceptibility to clonal deletion of self-reacting T-lymphocytes at an immature phase in their ontogenic development within the thymus (and in the case of B-cells within the bone marrow). The concept of a neonatal window for tolerance induction is more apparent than real and stems from the relatively low number of peripheralized immunocompetent T-cells, which do not differ in behavior from resting T-cells in the adult in their tolerizability or capacity for an immune response. Note that resting T-cells are generally more readily tolerizable than memory cells.

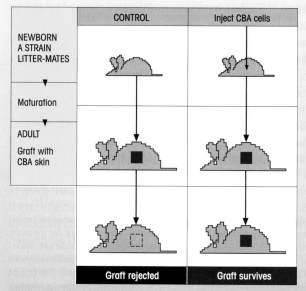

Figure M11.2.1. Induction of tolerance to foreign CBA skin graft in A strain mice by neonatal injection of antigen. The effect is antigen specific since the tolerant mice can reject third-party grafts normally. (After Billingham R., Brent L. & Medawar P.B. (1953) *Nature* **172**, 603–606.)

Self-tolerance can be induced in the thymus

Since developing T-cells are to be found in the thymus, one might expect this to be the milieu in which exposure to self-antigens on the surrounding cells would induce tolerance. The expectation is reasonable. If stem cells in bone marrow of $H-2^k$ haplotype are cultured with fetal thymus of H-2^d origin, the maturing cells become tolerant to H-2^d, as shown by their inability to give a mixed lymphocyte proliferative response when cultured with stimulators of H-2^d phenotype; third-

party responsiveness is not affected. Further experiments with deoxyguanosine-treated thymuses showed that the cells responsible for tolerance induction were deoxyguanosine-sensitive, bone marrow-derived macrophages or dendritic cells which are abundant at the corticomedullary junction (table 11.2).

Intrathymic clonal deletion leads to self-tolerance

There seems little doubt that strongly self-reactive T-cells can be physically deleted within the thymus. If we look at the experiment in table 11.1b, we can see that SCID males bearing the rearranged transgenes coding for the αβ receptor reacting with the male H-Y antigen do not possess any immunocompetent thymic cells expressing this receptor, whereas the females which lack H-Y do. Thus, when the developing T-cells react with self-antigen in the thymus, they are deleted. In other words, self-reactive cells undergo a **negative selection** process in the thymus, a process which constitutes **central tolerance** of the T-cells. Expression of the *AIRE* (*au*toimmune *re*gulator) gene in medullary thymic epithelial cells acts as a master switch directing the transcriptional activation of the genes for a number of organ-specific self antigens. The ectopic expression of these antigens provokes the elimination of the corresponding self-reactive thymocytes. Confirmation of the importance of AIRE expression for such clonal deletion has come from experiments using a double transgenic model developed by Goodnow and colleagues. In these mice a membrane-bound version of hen egg lysozyme (HEL) is transgenically expressed as a 'neo-self' antigen (because it is always present it becomes essentially a self antigen), and high numbers of thymocytes specific for this antigen are also generated by introduction of the relevant TCR as the other transgene. When the HEL transgene is linked to the tissue-specific *r*at *i*nsulin *p*romoter (RIP), expression of the 'self' antigen occurs in both the β-cells in the islets of Langerhans of the pancreas *and* in the thymus. In the absence of AIRE the RIP-driven expression of HEL fails to occur in thymic epithelium, but still occurs in the pancreatic islets. The developing transgenic T-cells which are normally deleted in the thymus escape deletion in the AIRE deficient mice (figure 11.7).

Table 11.2. Induction of tolerance in bone marrow stem cells by incubation with deoxyguanosine (dGuo)-sensitive macrophages or dendritic cells in the thymus. Clearly, the bone marrow cells induce tolerance to their own haplotype. Thus the thymic tolerance-inducing cells can be replaced by progenitors in the bone marrow inoculum (Jenkinson E.J., Jhittay P., Kingston R. & Owen J.J. (1985) *Transplantation* **39**, 331) or by adult dendritic cells from spleen, showing that it is the stage of differentiation of the immature T-cell rather than any special nature of the thymic antigen-presenting cell which leads to tolerance (Matzinger P. & Guerder S. (1989) *Nature* **338**, 74).

Bone marrow cells	Incubate with H-2^d thymus	Tolerance induction to *H-2* haplotype		
		k	d	b
k	Untreated	+	+	−
k	dGuo-treated	+	−	−
k + d	dGuo-treated	+	+	−

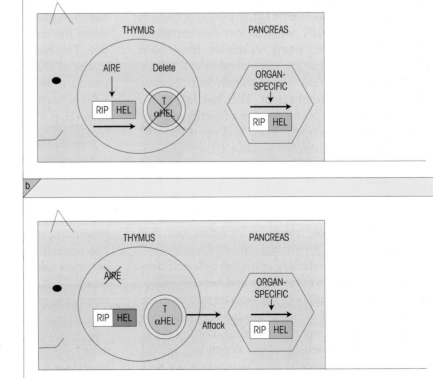

Figure 11.7. AIRE directs the ectopic expression of organ-specific self antigens in the thymus. Double transgenic mice were generated by crossing transgenic mice expressing hen egg lysozyme (HEL) under the control of the rat insulin promoter (RIP) with mice expressing the transgenic 3A9 αβ TCR specific for the amino acid 46–61 peptide from HEL presented by the I-A^k MHC class II molecule. These mice normally tolerize the transgenic T-cells in the thymus (a), but this did not occur if the mice were backcrossed to mice in which the AIRE gene had been knocked out (b). The incidence of type I diabetes was dramatically increased in the absence of AIRE expression. (Based on data from Liston A. *et al.* (2004) *Journal of Experimental Medicine* **200**, 1015–1026.)

cells might also be capable of inducing apoptosis in dendritic cells via CD95-CD95L interactions, or cause the dendritic cells to induce apoptosis in responder T-cells, again by the CD95 pathway. We shall see later in Chapter 16 that the induction of transplantation immunosuppression with a nondepleting anti-CD4 can be long-lasting because the production of anergic regulatory T-cells prevents the priming of newly immunocompetent T-lymphocytes by the transplantation antigen(s).

Lack of communication can cause unresponsiveness

It takes two to tango: if the self-molecule cannot engage the TCR, there can be no response. The anatomical isolation of molecules, like the lens protein of the eye and myelin basic protein in the brain, virtually precludes them from contact with lymphocytes, except perhaps for minute amounts of breakdown metabolic products which leak out and may be taken up by antigen-presenting cells, but at concentrations way below that required to trigger the corresponding naive T-cell.

Even when a tissue is exposed to circulating lymphocytes, the concentration of processed peptide on the cell surface may be insufficient to attract attention from a potentially autoreactive cell in the absence of costimulatory B7. This was demonstrated rather elegantly in animals bearing two transgenes: one for the TCR of a CD8 cytotoxic T-cell specific for LCM virus glycoprotein, and the other for the glycoprotein itself expressed on pancreatic β-cells through the insulin promoter. The result? A deafening silence: the T-cells were not deleted or tolerized, nor were the β-cells attacked. If these mice were then infected with LCM virus, the naive transgenic T-cells were presented with adequate concentrations of the processed glycoprotein within the adjuvant context of a true infection and were now stimulated. Their *primed* progeny, having an increased avidity (cf. p. 424) and thereby being able to recognize the low concentrations of processed glycoprotein on the β-cells, attacked their targets even in the absence of B7 and caused diabetes (figure 11.10). This may sound a trifle tortuous, but the principle could have important implications for the induction of autoimmunity by cross-reacting T-cell epitopes.

Molecules that are specifically restricted to particular organs which do not normally express MHC class II represent another special case, since they would not have the opportunity to interact with organ-specific CD4 T-helper cells.

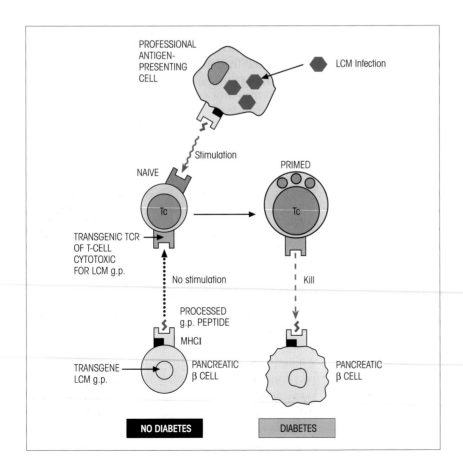

Figure 11.10. Mutual unawareness of a naive cytotoxic precursor T-cell and its B7-negative cellular target bearing epitopes present at low concentrations. Priming of the naive cell by a natural infection and subsequent attack by the higher avidity primed cells on the target tissue. LCM, lymphocytic choriomeningitis virus; g.p., glycoprotein. (From Ohashi P.S. *et al.* (1991) *Cell* **65**, 305–317.)

Immunological silence would also result if an individual has no genes coding for lymphocyte receptors directed against particular self-determinants; analysis of the experimentally induced autoantibody response to cytochrome c suggests that only those parts of the molecule which show species variation are autoantigenic, whereas the highly conserved regions where the genes have not altered for a much longer time appear to be silent, supposedly because the autoreactive specificities have had time to disappear.

B-CELLS DIFFERENTIATE IN THE FETAL LIVER AND THEN IN BONE MARROW

The B-lymphocyte precursors, pro-B-cells, are present among the islands of hematopoietic cells in fetal liver by 8–9 weeks of gestation in humans and 14 days in the mouse. Production of B-cells by the liver wanes and is mostly taken over by the bone marrow for the remainder of life. Stromal reticular cells, which express adhesion molecules and secrete IL-7, extend long dendritic processes making intimate contact with IL-7 receptor-positive B-cell progenitors. Although early B-cells comprise only a minor subpopulation of the cells in those cultures, it is possible to analyze the different stages in their development by *in vitro* rescue with the Abelson murine leukemia virus (A-MuLV), a replication-defective retrovirus capable of transforming pre-B-cells at various points in their development into clones. A series of differentiation markers associated with B-cell maturation have now been established (figure 11.11).

Pax5 is a major determining factor in B-cell differentiation

Development of hematopoietic cells along the B-cell lineage requires expression of E2A and of early B-cell factor (EBF); the absence of either of these prevents pro-B-cells progressing to the pre-B-cell stage (figure 11.12). Also required is expression of the *Pax5* gene which encodes the BSAP (*B-cell-specific activator protein*) transcription factor. Thus, in $Pax5^{-/-}$ knockout mice, early pre-B-cells (containing partially rearranged immunoglobulin heavy chain genes) fail to differentiate into mature, surface Ig+, B-cells (figure 11.12). However, if the pre-B-cells from $Pax5^{-/-}$ knockout mice are provided with the appropriate cytokines *in vitro*, they can be driven to produce T-cells, NK cells, macrophages, dendritic cells, granulocytes and even osteoclasts! These unexpected findings clearly show that the early pre-B-cell has the potential to be diverted from its chosen path and instead provide a source of cells for many other hematopoietic lineages. However, these pre-B-cells are not pluripotent as, unlike bone marrow hematopoietic

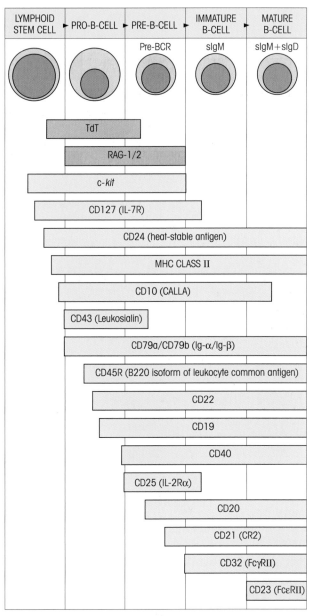

Figure 11.11. Some of the differentiation markers of developing B-cells. The time of appearance of enzymes involved in Ig gene rearrangement and diversification (blue boxes) and of surface markers defined by monoclonal antibodies (orange boxes, see table 7.1 for list of CD members) is shown.

stem cells, they are unable to rescue lethally irradiated mice. It is clear that *Pax5* acts as a critical master gene by directing B-cell development along the correct pathway, and does this by repressing expression of genes such as those encoding Notch-1, myeloperoxidase and monocyte/macrophage colony-stimulating factor receptor which are associated with other lineages, whilst activating B-cell specific genes including Ig-α, CD19 and the adaptor protein BLNK.

MEDIATOR ACTION					
	DILATATION	CONSTRICTION	INCREASE PERMEABILITY	UPREGULATE ADHESION MOL.		NEUTROPHIL CHEMOTAXIS
				ENDOTHELIUM	NEUTROPHIL	
HISTAMINE	+		+	+ +		
BRADYKININ	+		+ +			
PGE$_2$/I$_2$	+ + +		Potentiate other mediators			
VIP	+ + +					
NITRIC OXIDE	+ + +		+ + +			
LEUKOTRIENE-D4		+				
LEUKOTRIENE-C4		+ +	+			
C5a			+ +	+	+ +	+ + +
LEUKOTRIENE-B4			+ +		+ +	+ + +
f.Met.Leu.Phe			+ +		+	+
PLATELET ACTIVATING FACTOR	+		+ +		+ +	
IL-8					+ + +	+ + +
NAP-2 (CXCL7)					+ +	+ +
IL-1				+ +	+ +	
TNF				+ +	+ +	

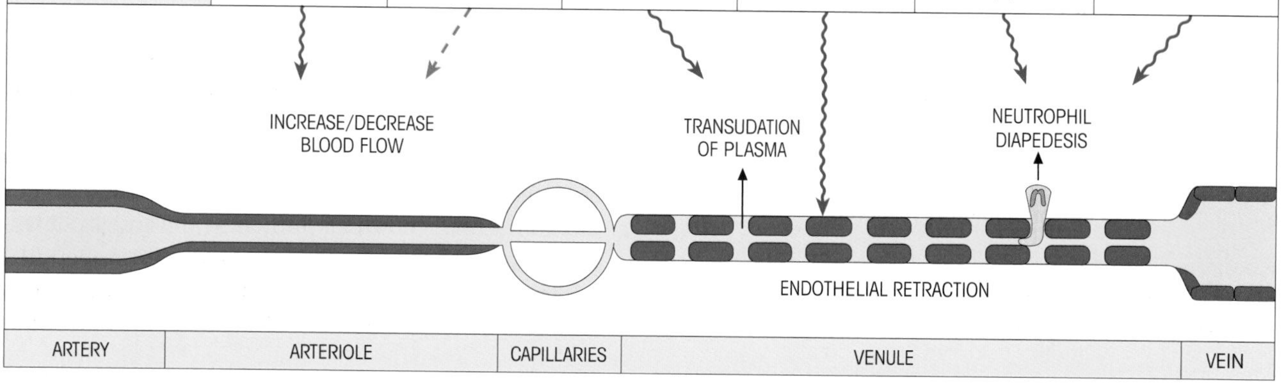

INCREASE/DECREASE BLOOD FLOW · TRANSUDATION OF PLASMA · NEUTROPHIL DIAPEDESIS · ENDOTHELIAL RETRACTION

ARTERY · ARTERIOLE · CAPILLARIES · VENULE · VEIN

Figure 12.2. The principal mediators of acute inflammation. The reader should refer back to figure 1.15 to recall the range of products generated by the mast cell. The later acting cytokines such as IL-1 are largely macrophage-derived and these cells also secrete prostaglandin E$_2$ (PGE$_2$), leukotriene B$_4$ and the neutrophil activating chemokine NAP-2 (CXCL7). VIP, vasoactive intestinal peptide.

another chemokine, MCP-1 (CCL2), which attracts mononuclear phagocytes to the inflammatory site to strengthen and maintain the defensive reaction to infection.

Perhaps this is a good time to remind ourselves of the important role of chemokines (table 9.3) in selectively attracting multiple types of leukocytes to inflammatory foci. Inflammatory chemokines are typically induced by microbial products such as lipopolysaccharide (LPS) and by proinflammatory cytokines including IL-1, TNF and IFNγ. As a very broad generalization, chemokines of the CXC subfamily, such as IL-8, are specific for neutrophils and, to varying extents, lymphocytes, whereas chemokines with the CC motif are chemotactic for T-cells, monocytes, dendritic cells, and variably for natural killer (NK) cells, basophils and eosinophils.

Eotaxin (CCL11) is chemotactic for eosinophils, and the presence of significant concentrations of this mediator together with RANTES (regulated upon activation normal T-cell expressed and secreted, CCL5) in mucosal surfaces contribute towards the enhanced population of eosinophils in those tissues. The different chemokines bind to particular heparin and heparan sulfate glycosaminoglycans so that, after secretion, the chemotactic gradient can be maintained by attachment to the extracellular matrix as a form of scaffolding.

Clearly, this whole operation serves to focus the immune defenses around the invading microorganisms. These become coated with antibody, C3b and certain acute phase proteins and are ripe for phagocytosis by the neutrophils and macrophages; under the influence of the inflammatory mediators these have

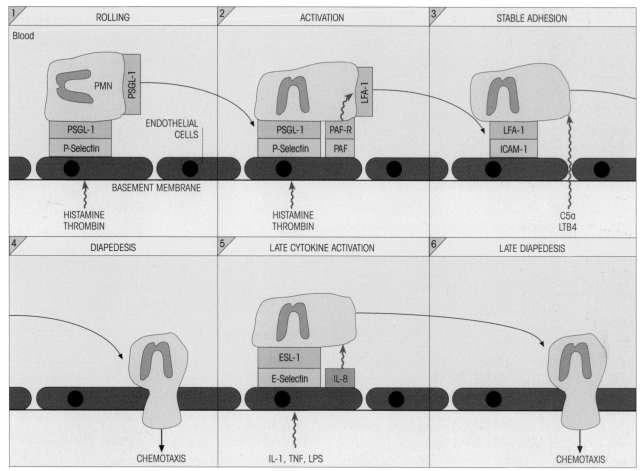

Figure 12.3. Early events in inflammation affecting neutrophil margination and diapedesis. Induced upregulation of P-selectin on the vessel walls plays the major role in the initial leukocyte–endothelial interaction (rolling) by interaction with ligands on the neutrophil such as P-selectin glycoprotein ligand-1 (PSGL-1, CD162). Recognition of extracellular gradients of the chemotactic mediators by receptors on the polymorphonuclear neutrophil (PMN) surface triggers intracellular signals which generate motion. Neutrophil migration along the extracellular matrix vitronectin is dependent upon very rapid cycles of integrin-dependent adhesion and detachment regulated by calcineurin. The cytokine-induced expression of E-selectin, which is recognized by the glycoprotein E-selectin ligand-1 (ESL-1) on the neutrophil, occurs as a later event. Chemotactic factors such as IL-8, which is secreted by a number of cell types including the endothelium itself, are important mediators of the inflammatory process. (Compare events involved in homing and transmigration of lymphocytes, figure 7.6.)

Figure 12.4. Neutrophil extracellular traps. Release of granule proteins and chromatin from neutrophils leads to the formation of neutrophil extracellular traps (NETs) which prevent bacterial spreading and ensure that microbicidal substances released from the neutrophils are kept in the immediate vicinity of the bacteria for optimal killing of the microbe and minimal collateral damage to host tissues. Scanning electron micrograph of NETs from IL-8 activated neutrophils trapping: (A) *Staphylococcus aureus*; (B) *S. typhimurium*; (C) *S. flexneri*. The bar indicates 500 nm. (Reproduced from Brinkman *et al.* (2004) *Science* **303**, 1532, with permission from the Publishers.)

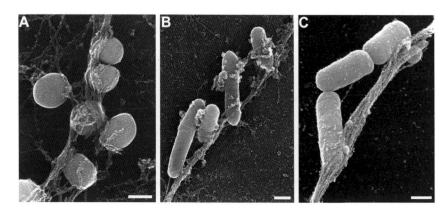

upregulated complement and Fc receptors, enhanced phagocytic responses and hyped-up killing powers, all adding up to bad news for the bugs.

Of course it is beneficial to recruit lymphocytes to sites of infection and we should remember that endothelial cells in these areas express VCAM-1 (cf. p. 160) which acts as a homing receptor for VLA-4-positive activated memory T-cells, while many chemokines (cf. table 9.3) are chemotactic for lymphocytes.

Regulation and resolution of inflammation

With its customary prudence, evolution has established regulatory mechanisms to prevent inflammation from getting out of hand. At the humoral level we have a series of complement regulatory proteins: C1 inhibitor, C4b-binding protein, the C3 control proteins factors H and I, complement receptor CR1 (CD35), *decay accelerating factor* (DAF, CD55), *membrane cofactor protein* (MCP, CD46), immunoconglutinin and homologous restriction factor 20 (HRF20, CD59) (cf. p. 314). Some of the acute phase proteins derived from the plasma transudate, including α-1 antichymotrypsinogen, α-1 antitrypsin, heparin cofactor-2 and plasminogen-activator inhibitor-1, are protease inhibitors.

At the cellular level, PGE_2, transforming growth factor-β (TGFβ) and glucocorticoids are powerful regulators. PGE_2 is a potent inhibitor of lymphocyte proliferation and cytokine production by T-cells and macrophages. TGFβ deactivates macrophages by inhibiting the production of reactive oxygen intermediates, inhibiting the class II MHC transactivator (CIITA) and thus downregulating class II expression, and quelling the cytotoxic enthusiasm of both macrophages and NK cells. Endogenous glucocorticoids produced via the hypothalamic–pituitary–adrenal axis exert their anti-inflammatory effects both through the repression of a number of genes for proinflammatory cytokines and adhesion molecules, and the induction of the inflammation inhibitors lipocortin-1, secretory leukocyte proteinase inhibitor (SLPI, an inhibitor of neutrophil elastase) and IL-1 receptor antagonist. IL-10 inhibits antigen presentation, cytokine production and nitric oxide killing by macrophages, the latter inhibition being greatly enhanced by synergistic action with IL-4 and TGFβ.

Once the agent that has provoked the inflammatory reaction has been cleared, these regulatory processes will normalize the site. When the inflammation traumatizes tissues through its intensity and extent, TGFβ plays a major role in the subsequent wound healing by stimulating fibroblast division and the laying down of new extracellular matrix elements.

Chronic inflammation

If an inflammatory agent persists, either because of its resistance to metabolic breakdown or through the inability of a deficient immune system to clear an infectious microbe, the character of the cellular response changes. The site becomes dominated by macrophages with varying morphology: many have an activated appearance, some form what are termed 'epithelioid' cells and others fuse to form giant cells. Lymphocytes in various guises are also often present. This characteristic **granuloma** walls off the persisting agent from the remainder of the body (see type IV hypersensitivity in Chapter 15, p. 356).

EXTRACELLULAR BACTERIA SUSCEPTIBLE TO KILLING BY PHAGOCYTOSIS AND COMPLEMENT

Bacterial survival strategies

As with virtually all infectious agents, if you can think of a possible avoidance strategy, some microbe will already have used it (table 12.1).

Evading phagocytosis
The cell walls of bacteria are multifarious (figure 12.5) and in some cases are inherently resistant to microbicidal agents; but many other strategies are used to evade the immune response (figure 12.6). A common mechanism by which virulent forms escape phagocytosis is by synthesis of an outer **capsule**, which does not adhere readily to phagocytic cells and covers carbohydrate molecules on the bacterial surface which could otherwise be recognized by phagocyte receptors. For example, as few as 10 encapsulated pneumococci can kill a mouse but, if the capsule is removed by treatment with hyaluronidase, 10 000 bacteria are required for the job. Many pathogens evolve capsules which physically prevent access of phagocytes to C3b deposited on the bacterial cell wall.

Other organisms have actively **antiphagocytic** cell surface molecules and some go so far as to secrete **exotoxins**, which actually poison the leukocytes. Yet another ruse is to gain entry into a nonphagocytic cell and thereby hide from the professional phagocyte. Presumably, some organisms try to avoid undue provocation of phagocytic cells by adhering to and *colonizing the external mucosal surfaces* of the intestine.

Challenging the complement system
Poor activation of complement. Normal mammalian cells are protected from complement destruction by regula-

Table 12.1. Examples of mechanisms used by bacteria to avoid the host immune response. (Partly based on Merrell D.S. and Falkow S. (2004) *Nature* **430**, 250.)

Immune process	Example	Mechanism
Phagocytosis	*Yersinia*	Inhibition of actin skeleton in phagocytes by YopT cleavage of RhoA (see figure 12.7)
	Legionella	Dot/icm intracellular multiplication genes inhibit phagolysosome fusion
Complement	*Streptococcus pyogenes*	M protein binding of C4b-binding protein reduces C3 convertase activity
Apoptosis	*Shigella flexneri*	IpaB-mediated activation of Caspase-1 induces apoptosis (see figure 12.7)
	Mycobacterium tuberculosis	Increased expression of *bcl2* and Rb inhibits apoptosis
Cytokine production	*Vibrio cholerae*	Cholera toxin inhibition of IL-12 secretion
	Bordetella pertussis	Pertussis toxin induction of IL-1 and IL-4
Antibody	*Staphylococcus aureus*	IgG opsonization for phagocytosis blocked by Protein A binding the antibody the 'wrong way' round
	Neisseria gonorrhoeae	Antigenic variation by recombination within *pilE* gene
T-cell activation	*Helicobacter pylori*	VacA vacuolating cytotoxin inhibits calcineurin signaling pathways

tory proteins such as MCP and DAF, which cause C3 convertase breakdown (see p. 314 for further discussion). Microorganisms lack these regulatory proteins so that, even in the absence of antibody, most of them would activate the alternative complement pathway by stabilization of the C$\overline{3bBb}$ convertase on their surfaces. However, bacterial capsules in general tend to be poor activators of complement and selective pressures have favored the synthesis of capsules whose surface components do not permit stable binding of the convertase.

Acceleration of complement breakdown. Members of the regulators of complement activation (RCA) family which diminish C3 convertase activity include C4b-binding protein (C4BP), factor H and factor H-like protein 1 (FHL-1). Certain bacterial surface molecules, notably those rich in sialic acid, bind factor H (figure 12.6), which then acts as a focus for the degradation of C3b by the serine protease factor I (cf. p. 10). This is seen, for example, with *Neisseria gonorrhoeae*. Similarly, the hypervariable regions of the M-proteins of certain *Streptococcus pyogenes* (group A streptococcus) strains are able to bind FHL-1, whilst other strains downregulate complement activation by interacting with C4BP, this time acting as a cofactor for factor I-mediated degradation of the C4b component of the classical pathway C3 convertase C$\overline{4b2a}$. All group A streptococci, and group B, C and G streptococci of human origin, produce a C5a peptidase which acts as a virulence factor by proteolytically cleaving and thereby inactivating C5a.

Complement deviation. Some species manage to avoid lysis by deviating the complement activation site either to a secreted decoy protein or to a position on the bacterial surface distant from the cell membrane.

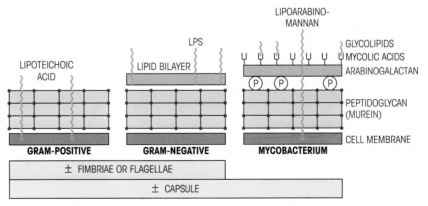

Figure 12.5. The structure of bacterial cell walls. All types have an inner cell membrane and a peptidoglycan wall which can be cleaved by lysozyme and lysosomal enzymes. The outer lipid bilayer of Gram-negative bacteria, which is susceptible to the action of complement or cationic proteins, sometimes contains lipopolysaccharide (LPS; also known as endotoxin; composed of a membrane-distal hydrophilic polysaccharide (which forms the highly polymorphic O-specific antigens) attached to a basal core polysaccharide, itself linked to the hydrophobic membrane-anchoring lipid A. 179 O antigen variants of *Escherichia coli* are known). The mycobacterial cell wall is highly resistant to breakdown. When present, outer capsules may protect the bacteria from phagocytosis.

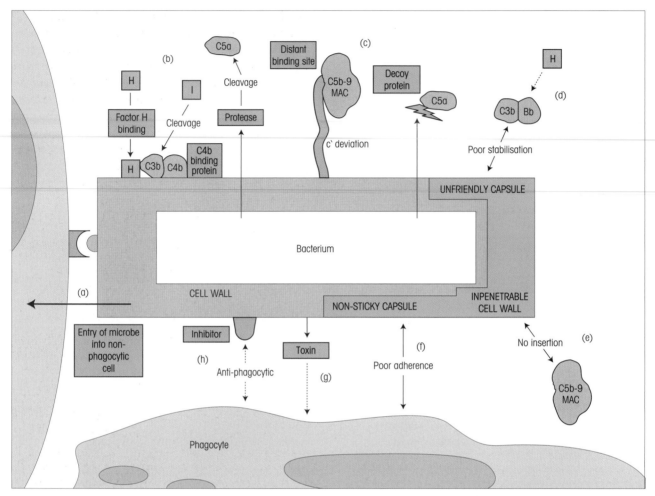

Figure 12.6. Avoidance strategies by extracellular bacteria. Clockwise from left: (a) microbe attaches to surface component to enter non-phagocytic cell; (b) accelerating breakdown of complement by action of microbial products; (c) complement effectors are deviated from the microbial cell wall; (d) capsule provides nonstabilizing surface for alternative pathway convertase; (e) cell wall impervious to complement membrane attack complex (MAC); (f) capsule gives poor phagocyte adherence; (g) exotoxin poisons phagocyte; (h) surface inhibitor of phagocytosis.

Resistance to insertion of terminal complement components. Gram-positive organisms (cf. figure 12.5) have evolved thick peptidoglycan layers which prevent the insertion of the lytic C5b–9 membrane attack complex into the bacterial cell membrane (figure 12.6). Many capsules do the same.

Interfering with internal events in the macrophage

Enteric Gram-negative bacteria in the gut have developed a number of ways of influencing macrophage activity, including inducing apoptosis, enhancing the production of IL-1, preventing phagosome–lysosome fusion and affecting the actin cytoskeleton (figure 12.7).

Antigenic variation

Individual antigens can be altered in the face of a determined host antibody response. Examples include variation of surface lipoproteins in the lyme disease spirochete *Borrelia burgdorferi*, of enzymes involved in synthesizing surface structures in *Campylobacter jejuni*, and of the pili in *Neisseria meningitidis*. In addition, new strains can arise, as has occurred with the life-threatening *E. coli* O157:H7 which can cause hemolytic uremic syndrome and appears to have emerged about 50 years ago by incorporation of *Shigella* toxin genes into the *E. coli* 055 genome.

The host counter-attack

Antibodies can defeat these devious attempts to avoid engulfment by neutralizing the antiphagocytic molecules and by binding to the surface of the organisms to focus the site for fixation of complement, so 'opsonizing' them for ingestion by neutrophils and macrophages or preparing them for the terminal membrane attack complex (Milestone 12.1). However, antibody produc-

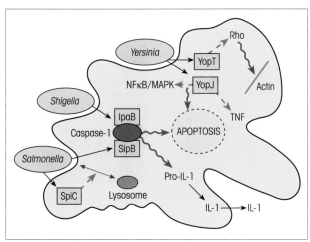

Figure 12.7. Evasion of macrophage defenses by enteric bacteria. The IpaB (*invasion plasmid antigen B*) and SipB (*Salmonella invasion protein B*) molecules secreted by *Shigella* and *Salmonella*, respectively, can activate caspase 1 and thereby set off a train of events that will lead to the death of the macrophage by apoptosis. Activated caspase 1 also triggers a protease which cleaves pro-IL-1, thereby causing the release of large amounts of this proinflammatory cytokine from the macrophage. Paradoxically, this may be advantageous to the bacteria because the subsequent migration of neutrophils to the intestinal lumen results in a loosening of intercellular junctions between the enterocytes, permitting cellular invasion of the basolateral surface by organisms from the lumen. The SpiC (*Salmonella pathogenicity island C*) protein from *Salmonella* inhibits the trafficking of cellular vesicles, and therefore is able to prevent lysosomes fusing with phagocytic vesicles. *Yersinia* produces a number of Yop molecules (*Yersinia outer proteins*) able to interfere with the normal functioning of the phagocyte. For example, YopJ inhibits TNF production and downregulates NFκB and MAP kinases, thereby facilitating apoptosis by inhibiting anti-apoptotic pathways. YopT prevents phagocytosis by modifying the GTPase RhoA involved in regulating the actin cytoskeleton. (Based on Donnenberg M.S. (2000) *Nature* **406**, 768.)

tion by B-cells usually requires T-cell help, and the T-cells need to be activated by antigen-presenting cells.

As already discussed in Chapter 1, but so important that it is worth repeating, *pathogen-associated molecular patterns* (PAMPs), such as the all-important lipopolysaccharide (LPS) endotoxin of Gram-negative bacteria, peptidoglycan, lipoteichoic acids, mannans, bacterial DNA, double-stranded RNA and glucans, are molecules which are broadly expressed by microbial pathogens but not present on host tissues. Thus these molecules serve as an alerting service for the immune system, which detects their presence using pattern recognition receptors (PRRs) expressed on the surface of antigen-presenting cells. It will be recalled that such receptors include the mannose receptor (CD206) which facilitates phagocytosis of microorganisms by macrophages and the scavenger receptor (CD204) which mediates clearance of bacteria from the circulation. LPS-binding protein (LBP) transfers LPS to the CD14 PRR on monocytes, macrophages, dendritic cells and B-cells. This leads to the recruitment of the toll-like receptor 4 (TLR4) molecule which triggers expression of proinflammatory genes, including those for IL-1, IL-6, IL-12 and TNF, and the upregulation of the CD80 (B7.1) and CD86 (B7.2) costimulatory molecules. Other TLRs, e.g. TLR2, recognize Gram-positive bacterial cell wall components. Although each of the 11 or so toll-like receptors so far characterized recognize broadly expressed microbial structures, it has been suggested that collectively they are able to some extent to discriminate between different pathogens by detection of partic-

Milestone 12.1 — The Protective Effects of Antibody

The pioneering research which led to the recognition of the antibacterial protection afforded by antibody clustered in the last years of the 19th century. A good place to start the story is the discovery by Roux and Yersin in 1888, at the Pasteur Institute in Paris, that the exotoxin of diphtheria bacillus could be isolated from a bacterium-free filtrate of the medium used to culture the organism. von Behring and Kitasato at Koch's Institute in Berlin in 1890 then went on to show that animals could develop an immunity to such toxins which was due to the development of specific neutralizing antidotes referred to generally as **antibodies**. They further succeeded in passively transferring immunity to another animal with serum containing the antitoxin. The dawning of an era of serotherapy came in 1894 with Roux's successful treatment of patients with diphtheria by injection of immune horse serum.

Sir Almroth Wright in London in 1903 proposed that the main action of the increased antibody produced after infec-

tion was to reinforce killing by the phagocytes. He called the antibodies **opsonins** (Gk. *opson*, a dressing or relish), because they prepared the bacteria as food for the phagocytic cells, and amply verified his predictions by showing that antibodies dramatically increased the phagocytosis of bacteria *in vitro*, thereby cleverly linking *innate* to *adaptive* immunity.

George Bernard Shaw even referred to Almroth Wright's proposal in his play *The Doctor's Dilemma*. In the preface he gave an evocative description of the function of opsonins: 'the white corpuscles or phagocytes which attack and devour disease germs for us do their work only when we butter the disease germs appetizingly for them with a natural sauce which Sir Almroth named opsonins. . . .' (A more extended account of immunology at the turn of the 19th century may be found in Silverstein A.M. (1989) *A History of Immunology.* Academic Press, San Diego.)

(Continued p.264)

antigen-specific and nonantigen-specific mechanisms. Among the nonspecific mechanisms, antimicrobial peptides are produced not only by neutrophils and macrophages but also by mucosal epithelium. As described in Chapter 1, the group of antimicrobial peptides called defensins lyse bacteria via disruption of their surface membranes. Specific immunity is provided by secretory IgA and IgM, with IgA1 predominating in the upper areas and IgA2 in the large bowel. Most other mucosal surfaces are also protected predominantly by IgA with the exception of the reproductive tract tissues of both male and female, where the dominant antibody isotype is IgG. The size of the task is highlighted by the fact that 80% of the Ig-producing B-cells in the body are present in the secretory mucosae and exocrine glands. IgA antibodies afford protection in the external body fluids, tears, saliva, nasal secretions and those bathing the surfaces of the intestine and lung by coating bacteria and viruses and preventing their adherence to the epithelial cells of the mucous membranes, which is essential for viral infection and bacterial colonization. Secretory IgA molecules themselves have very little innate adhesiveness for epithelial cells, but high affinity Fc receptors for this Ig class are present on macrophages and neutrophils and can mediate phagocytosis (figure 12.10a).

If an infectious agent succeeds in penetrating the IgA barrier, it comes up against the next line of defense of the secretory system (see p. 163) which is manned by IgE. Indeed, most serum IgE arises from plasma cells in mucosal tissues and their local draining lymph nodes. Although present in low concentration, IgE is firmly bound to the Fc receptors of the mast cell (see p. 48) and contact with antigen leads to the release of mediators which effectively recruit agents of the immune response and generate a local acute inflammatory reaction. Thus histamine, by increasing vascular permeability, causes the transudation of IgG and complement into the area, while chemotactic factors for neutrophils and eosinophils attract the effector cells needed to dispose of the infectious organism coated with specific IgG and C3b (figure 12.10b). Engagement of the Fcγ and C3b receptors on local macrophages by such complexes will lead to secretion of factors which further reinforce these vascular permeability and chemotactic events. Broadly, one would say that immune exclusion in the gut is noninflammatory, but immune elimination of organisms which penetrate the mucosa is proinflammatory.

Where the opsonized organism is too large to be engulfed, phagocytes can employ *antibody-dependent cellular cytotoxicity* (ADCC, p. 32) and there is evidence for its involvement in parasitic infections (see p. 279).

The mucosal tissues contain various T-cell populations, but their role and that of the mucosal epithelial cells, other than in a helper function for local antibody production, is of less relevance for the defense against extracellular bacteria.

Some specific bacterial infections

First let us see how these considerations apply to defense against infection by common organisms such as streptococci and staphylococci. The β-hemolytic **streptococci** were classified by Lancefield according to their carbohydrate antigen, the most important for human disease belonging to group A. *Streptococcus pyogenes* most commonly causes acute pharyngitis (strep sore

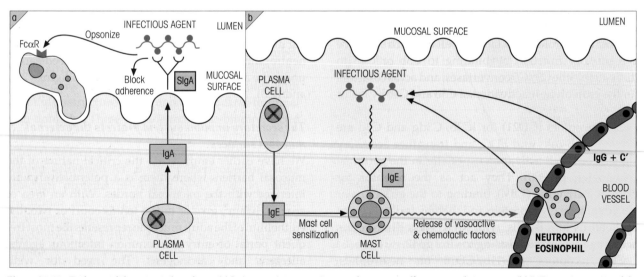

Figure 12.10. Defense of the mucosal surfaces. (a) IgA opsonizes organisms and prevents adherence to the mucosa. (b) IgE recruits agents of the immune response by firing the release of mediators from mast cells.

throat) and the skin condition impetigo, but is also responsible for scarlet fever and has emerged as a cause of the much rarer but often fatal toxic shock syndrome and of the always alarming necrotizing faciitis (flesh-eating disease). Rheumatic fever and glomerular nephritis sometimes occur as serious postinfection sequelae.

The most important virulence factor is the surface M-protein (variants of which form the basis of the Griffith typing). This protein is an acceptor for factor H which facilitates C3b breakdown, and binds fibrinogen and its fragments which cover sites that may act as complement activators. It thereby inhibits opsonization and the protection afforded by antibodies to the M-component is attributable to the striking increase in phagocytosis which they induce. The ability of group A streptococci to elicit cross-reactive autoantibodies which bind to cardiac myosin is implicated in poststreptococcal autoimmune disease. High titer antibodies to the streptolysin O exotoxin (ASO), which damages membranes, indicate recent streptococcal infection. The streptococcal pyrogenic exotoxins SPE-A, -C and -H, and the streptococcal mitogenic exotoxin SMEZ-2, are superantigens associated with scarlet fever and toxic shock syndrome. The toxins are neutralized by antibody and the erythematous intradermal reaction to injected toxin (the Dick reaction) is only seen in individuals lacking antibody. Antibody can also neutralize bacterial enzymes like hyaluronidase which act to spread the infection.

The mutans streptococci (*Streptococcus mutans* and *S. sobrinus*) are an important cause of dental caries. The organisms possess a glucosyltransferase enzyme which converts sucrose to glucose polymers (glucans) that aid adhesion to the tooth surface. Small scale clinical trials with vaccines based upon the glucosyltransferase, usually together with components of the surface antigen I/II fibrillar adhesins, have shown that salivary IgA against mutans streptococci can be increased and, in some cases, interfere with colonization.

Virulent forms of **staphylococci**, of which *Staphylococcus aureus* is perhaps the most common, resist phagocytosis. Both staphylococci and streptococci express surface proteins which act as FcγRs (Protein A and Protein G, respectively) and might serve to limit antibody-mediated effector functions by binding the antibodies the 'wrong way' round. Virulence factors encoded by *S. aureus* genes also include adhesins and cell wall teichoic acid on the surface of the bacterium, toxic shock syndrome toxin-1, enterotoxins and enzymes. The penicillin-binding protein 2a is able to synthesize peptidoglycan even in the presence of β-lactam antibiotics. Other virulence factors are acquired from lysogenic bacteriophages, including Panton-Valentine leucocidin and chemotaxis inhibitory protein (CHIP). Although *S. aureus* is readily phagocytosed in the presence of *adequate* amounts of antibody, a small proportion of the ingested bacteria survives and they are difficult organisms to eliminate completely. Where the infection is inadequately controlled, severe lesions may occur in the immunized host as a consequence of type IV delayed hypersensitivity reactions. Thus, staphylococci were found to be avirulent when injected into mice passively immunized with antibody, but caused extensive tissue damage in animals previously given sensitized T-cells. The *methicillin-resistant S. aureus* (MRSA) 'superbug', which was already also resistant to all the β-lactam antibiotics, has now become vancomycin resistant following transfer of drug-resistance from *Enterococcus*. New drugs such as linezolid and synercid can be used to treat MRSA infections but there is no guarantee that the organism won't become resistant to these as well—pretty scary stuff.

Other examples where antibodies are required to overcome the inherently antiphagocytic properties of **bacterial capsules** are seen in immunity to pneumococci, meningococci and *Haemophilus influenzae*. *Bacillus anthrax* possesses an antiphagocytic capsule composed of a γ-polypeptide of D-glutamic acid but, although anticapsular antibodies effectively promote uptake by neutrophils, the exotoxin is so potent that vaccines are inadequate unless they also stimulate antitoxin immunity. In addition to releasing such lethal exotoxins, *Pseudomonas aeruginosa* also produces an elastase that inactivates C3a and C5a; as a result, only minimal inflammatory responses are made in the absence of neutralizing antibodies.

The ploy of **diverting complement activation** to insensitive sites is seen rather well with different strains of Gram-negative *Salmonella* and *Escherichia coli* organisms which vary in the number of O-specific oligosaccharide side-chains attached to the lipid-A-linked core polysaccharide of the endotoxin (cf. figure 12.5). Variants with long side-chains are relatively insensitive to killing by serum through the alternative complement pathway (see p. 10); as the side-chains become shorter and shorter, the serum sensitivity increases. Although all variants activate the alternative pathway, only those with short or no side-chains allow the cytotoxic membrane attack complex to be inserted near to the outer lipid bilayer (figure 12.6c). On the other hand, antibodies focus the complex to a more vulnerable site.

The destruction of gonococci by serum containing antibody is dependent upon the formation of the membrane attack complex, and rare individuals lacking C8 or C9 are susceptible to *Neisseria* infection. *N. gonor-*

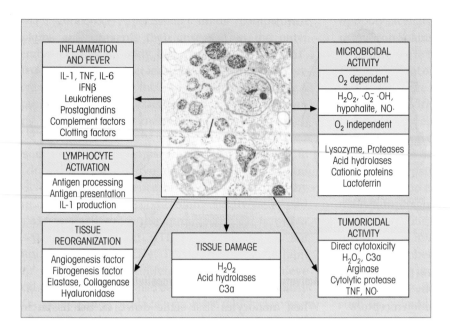

Figure 12.14. The role of the activated macrophage in the initiation and mediation of chronic inflammation with concomitant tissue repair, and in the killing of microbes and tumor cells. It is possible that macrophages differentiate along distinct pathways to subserve these different functions. The electron micrograph shows a highly activated macrophage with many lysozomal structures which have been highlighted by the uptake of thorotrast; one (arrowed) is seen fusing with a phagosome containing the protozoan *Toxoplasma gondii*. (Courtesy of Professor C. Jones.)

most amongst the killing mechanisms which are up-regulated are those mediated by reactive oxygen intermediates and NO·. The activated macrophage is undeniably a formidable cell, capable of secreting the 60 or so substances which are concerned in chronic inflammatory reactions (figure 12.14)—not the sort to meet in an alley on a dark night!

The mechanism of T-cell-mediated immunity in the Mackaness experiments now becomes clear. Specifically primed T-cells react with processed antigen derived from the intracellular bacteria present on the surface of the infected macrophage in association with MHC II; the subsequent release of cytokines activates the macrophage and endows it with the ability to kill the organisms it has phagocytosed (figure 12.15).

Examples of intracellular bacterial infections

Listeria

The organism *Listeria monocytogenes*, usually acquired by humans following the ingestion of contaminated foods such as unpasteurized dairy products, poses a particular risk to pregnant women due to its association with septic abortion. Following interaction of the bacterial cell surface molecule internalin A with E-cadherin on the epithelial cells, the organism passes through the epithelium and enters the bloodstream. Dissemination occurs to the spleen and liver where phagocytic internalization into macrophages occurs, and into hepatocytes via binding of another microbial surface molecule, internalin B, to the hepatocyte growth factor receptor. The actin-assembly-inducing protein ActA produced by the *Listeria* facilitates its intercellular transmission. IFNγ secreted by NK and Th1 cells drives the macrophage

activation required for the ultimate elimination of intracellular *Listeria* (figure 12.16) The bactericidal action of neutrophils and the central role of IL-12 also warrant our attention, as does the recruitment by the chemokine CCL2 (MCP-1) of dendritic cells producing TNF and nitric oxide. These or other populations of dendritic cells are thought to cross-prime CD8+ T-cells with *Listeria* antigens derived from infected macrophages. During primary infection, CD8 T-cells that are restricted to the nonclassical MHC molecule H2-M3 seem to play a particularly important role, whereas the classical class I restricted CD8 T-cells make a more profound contribution during secondary infection. Mutant mice lacking αβ and/or γδ T-cells reveal that these two cell types make comparable contributions to resistance against primary *Listeria* infection, but that the αβ TCR set bears the major responsibility for conferring protective immunity. γδ T-cells control the local tissue response at the site of microbial replication and γδ knockout mutants develop huge abscesses when infected with *Listeria*.

Tuberculosis

Tuberculosis (TB) is on the rampage, aided by the emergence of multidrug-resistant strains of *Mycobacterium tuberculosis*. It is estimated that two million deaths resulted from TB in 2002. The problem is not helped by the fact that human immunodeficiency virus (HIV)-infected individuals with low CD4 counts have increased susceptibility to *M. tuberculosis* infection, with about 20% of patients with AIDS dying of tuberculosis.

With respect to host defense mechanisms, as seen with *Listeria* infection, murine macrophages activated by IFNγ can destroy intracellular mycobacteria, largely

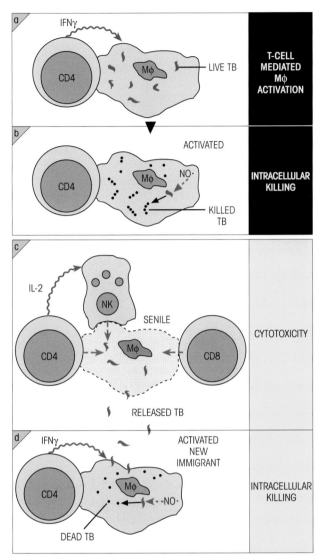

Figure 12.15. The 'cytokine connection': nonspecific murine macrophage killing of intracellular bacteria triggered by a specific T-cell-mediated immunity reaction. (a) Specific CD4 Th1 cell recognizes mycobacterial peptide associated with MHC class II and releases Mφ activating IFNγ. (b) The activated Mφ kills the intracellular TB, mainly through generation of toxic NO·. (c) A 'senile' Mφ, unable to destroy the intracellular bacteria, is killed by CD8 and CD4 cytotoxic cells and possibly by IL-2-activated NK cells. The Mφ then releases live tubercle bacilli which are taken up and killed by newly recruited Mφ susceptible to IFNγ activation (d). Human monocytes require activation by both IFNγ and IL-4 plus a CD23-mediated signal for induction of iNO synthase and production of NO·.

through the generation of toxic NO·. Some parasitized macrophages reach a stage at which they are too incapacitated to be stirred into action by T-cell messages, and here a somewhat ruthless strategy has evolved in which the host deploys cytotoxic CD8, and possibly CD4 and NK cells, to execute the helpless macrophage and release the live mycobacteria; these should now be taken up by newly immigrant phagocytic cells susceptible to activation by IFNγ and summarily disposed of

(figure 12.15). A vital role for both αβ and γδ T-cells in murine TB is indicated by an inability to control the infection in both TCR β-chain knockout mice (which lack an αβ TCR) and TCR δ-chain knockout mice (which lack a γδ TCR).

The position is more complicated in the human because IFNγ-stimulated human macrophages are unable to eliminate intracellular TB. Detection by TLR2 of the 19 kDa lipoprotein PAMP of *M. tuberculosis* stimulates macrophage production of proinflammatory cytokines, inducible NO synthase and expression of costimulatory molecules. However, interference with the phagosome and a resistance to macrophage killing ensure the initial survival of the mycobacteria. Although at first immunostimulatory, prolonged exposure of the macrophage TLR2 to the mycobacterial 19 kDa lipoprotein seems to block IFNγ-mediated activation and inhibit MHC class II expression. Thus, during the persistent phase of the infection CD4⁺ helper T cells are less able to detect the presence of the intracellular mycobacteria.

On the positive side, the mycobacterial products Ag85B (a mycolyl transferase) and ESAT-6 (*e*arly *s*ecreted *a*ntigenic *t*arget-6) are potent inducers of IFNγ from CD4 cells. Human T-cells bearing αβ TCR proliferate in response to mycobacterial lipid-bearing antigens such as didehydroxymycobactins presented by host CD1a molecules and mycolic acid presented by CD1b, while human Vγ$_2$Vδ$_2$ T-cells recognize protein antigens, isopentenyl pyrophosphates and prenyl pyrophosphates from *M. tuberculosis*.

Inbred strains of mice differ dramatically in their susceptibility to infection by *Salmonella typhimurium*, *Leishmania donovani* and various mycobacteria. Resistance is associated with a T-cell-independent enhanced state of macrophage priming for bactericidal activity involving oxygen and nitrogen radicals. Moreover, macrophages from resistant strains have increased MHC class II expression and a higher respiratory burst, are more readily activated by IFNγ, and induce better stimulation of T-cells. By contrast, macrophages from susceptible strains tend to have suppressor effects on T-cell proliferation to mycobacterial antigens. The *M. tuberculosis*-infected macrophages secrete IL-6 which has the property of inhibiting IFNγ signaling in the surrounding macrophages. Susceptibility and resistance to *M. tuberculosis* in murine models depend upon a number of genes, including *SLC11A1* (solute carrier family 11 member 1, a proton-coupled divalent metal ion transporter previously called Nramp1) and genes in the *sst1* gene locus (susceptibility to tuberculosis 1, also involved in immunity to *Listeria monocytogenes* infection). A number of polymorphisms have been identified in the human *SLC11A1* gene and studies

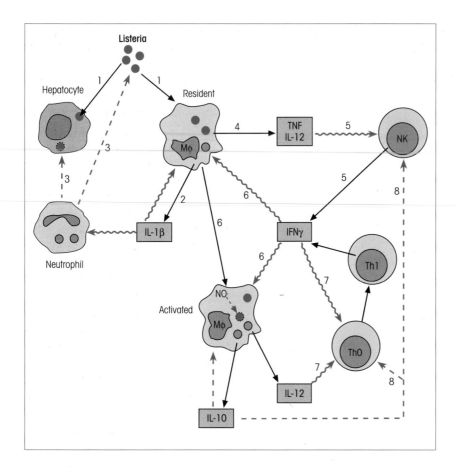

Figure 12.16. Macrophage activation in response to *Listeria* infection. (1) *Listeria* infects resident macrophages and hepatocytes; (2) the Mφ release IL-1β which activates neutrophils; (3) the activated neutrophils destroy *Listeria* bacilli by direct contact and are cytotoxic for infected hepatocytes; (4) the infected Mφ release TNF and IL-12 which stimulate NK cells; (5) NK cells secrete IFNγ, which (6) activates the macrophage to produce NO· and kill intracellular *Listeria*; (7) IFNγ plus Mφ-derived IL-12 recruit Th1 cells which reinforce Mφ activation through the production of IFNγ. (8) Eventual synthesis of IL-10, encouraged by the action of immune complexes, downregulates Mφ, NK and Th1 activity. (Based on an article by Rogers H.W., Tripps C.S. & Unanue E.R. (1995) *The Immunologist* **3**, 152.)

are ongoing to link individual polymorphisms to susceptibility.

Where the host has difficulty in effectively eliminating these organisms, the chronic CMI response to local antigen leads to the accumulation of densely packed macrophages which release angiogenic and fibrogenic factors and stimulate the formation of granulation tissue and ultimately fibrosis. The activated macrophages, probably under the stimulus of IL-4, transform to epithelioid cells and fuse to become giant cells. As suggested earlier, the resulting granuloma represents an attempt by the body to isolate a site of persistent infection.

Leprosy

Human leprosy presents as a spectrum ranging from the tuberculoid form, with lesions containing small numbers of viable organisms, to the lepromatous form, characterized by an abundance of *Mycobacterium leprae* within the macrophages. CMI rather than humoral immunity is important for the control of the leprosy bacillus. Although the tuberculoid state is associated with good cell-mediated dermal hypersensitivity reactions and a bias towards Th1-type responses, these are still not good enough to eradicate the bacilli completely.

In the lepromatous form, there is poor T-cell reactivity to whole bacilli and poor lepromin dermal responses, although there are numerous plasma cells which contribute to a high level of circulating antibody and indicate a more prominent Th2 activity. Leukocyte Ig-like receptor-7 (LIR-7) expression is increased in lesions of lepromatous patients, causing a block in TLR-directed antimicrobial activity and a reduced production of proinflammatory IL-12, but enhanced secretion of immunosuppressive IL-10, by monocytes.

IMMUNITY TO VIRAL INFECTION

Viruses constitute a formidable enemy. HIV and influenza virus, amongst others, can quickly change their antigens by genetic mutation. Other viruses seem to come at us out of nowhere. Take the severe acute respiratory syndrome (SARS) caused by the SARS-associated coronavirus (SARS-CoV). This emerged as a human infection in Guangdong province in China in November 2002, almost certainly arising from one of the related coronaviruses found in a number of animal species. It spread rapidly to Hong Kong, and then on to Beijing, Hanoi and Singapore. Shortly afterwards it was brought into Toronto by an infected traveler. Fortunately the infection was swiftly brought under control by isolating infected individuals and tracing their contacts, and the chain of transmission was broken by July 2003. According to WHO figures, 8098 people became ill in 26 countries and 774 of these died. Hardly worth mentioning compared to the 7000 deaths per day from HIV infection, but nevertheless the brief SARS epidemic had a substantial economic effect, particularly in the Far East, and it is impossible to predict if and when there will be a future SARS outbreak.

Genetically controlled constitutional factors which render a host's cells nonpermissive (i.e. resistant to takeover of their replicative machinery by virus) play a dominant role in influencing the vulnerability of a given individual to infection. A group of proteins referred to as restriction factors have recently been shown to provide a form of innate resistance to retroviruses via their ability to block the replication of some types of virus. Thus, the TRIM5α (*tri*partite *i*nteraction *m*otif 5α) protein targets the retroviral capsid in monkey cells and is responsible for the inability of HIV-1 to infect cells from most nonhuman primates. The APOBEC3 cytidine deaminases also act as restriction factors, in this case by hypermutating the retroviral genome.

Macrophages may readily take up viruses nonspecifically and kill them. However, in some instances, the macrophages allow replication and, if the virus is capable of producing cytopathic effects in various organs, the infection may be lethal; with noncytopathic agents, such as lymphocytic choriomeningitis, Aleutian mink disease and equine infectious anemia viruses, a persistent infection may result. Viruses can avoid recognition by the host's immune system by latency or by sheltering in privileged sites, but they have also evolved a maliciously cunning series of evasive strategies.

Immunity can be evaded by antigen changes

Changing antigens by drift and shift

In the course of their constant duel with the immune system, viruses are continually changing the structure of their surface antigens. They do so by processes termed 'antigenic drift' and 'antigenic shift'. For example, the surface of the influenza A virus contains a hemagglutinin (H), by which it adheres to cells prior to infection, and a neuraminidase (N), which releases newly formed virus from the surface sialic acid of the infected cell; of these, the hemagglutinin is the more important for the establishment of protective immunity. Minor changes in antigenicity of the hemagglutinin occur through point mutations in the viral genome (**drift**), but major changes (**shift**) arise through wholesale swapping of genetic material with reservoirs of dif-

ferent viruses in other animal hosts such as avian species (e.g. chickens, turkeys and ducks) and pigs (figure 12.17). When alterations in the hemagglutinin are sufficient to render previous immunity ineffective, new influenza pandemics break out, as occurred in 1888, 1918, 1957 and 1968 following antigenic shifts in the influenza A virus. In 1997, the avian H5N1 virus infected humans in Hong Kong and is now in circulation across much of the globe and proving fatal in some cases. There has since been a number of other avian influenza viruses causing illness or occasionally death in humans, including H9N2 in Hong Kong in 1999 and 2003, H7N7 in the Netherlands in 2003 and H7N3 in Canada in 2004.

Mutated viruses can be favored by selection pressure from antibody. In fact, one current strategy for generating mutants in a given epitope is to grow the virus in tissue culture in the presence of a monoclonal antibody which reacts with that epitope; only mutants which do not bind the monoclonal will escape and grow out. This principle underlies the antigenic variation characteristic of the common cold rhinoviruses. The site on the virus for attachment to the viral receptor ICAM-1 on mucosal cells is a hydrophobic pocket lying on the floor

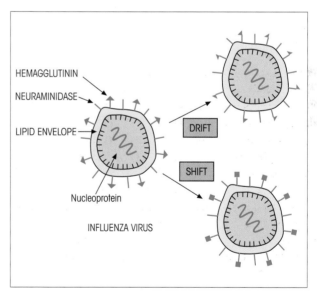

Figure 12.17. Antigenic drift and shift in influenza virus. The changes in hemagglutinin structure caused by drift may be small enough to allow protection by immunity to earlier strains. This may not happen with radical changes in the antigen associated with antigenic shift and so new virus epidemics break out. There have been 31 documented influenza pandemics (widespread epidemics occurring throughout the population) since the first well-described pandemic of 1580. In the last century there were three, associated with the emergence by antigenic shift of the Spanish flu in 1918 with the structure H1N1 (the official nomenclature assigns numbers to each hemagglutinin and neuraminidase major variant), Asian flu in 1957 (H2N2) and Hong Kong flu in 1968 (H3N2); note that each new epidemic was associated with a fundamental change in the hemagglutinin. The pandemic in 1918 killed an estimated 40 million people.

of a canyon. Following binding, ICAM-1 catalyzes the penetration of the virus by forcing the viral capsid into an expanded open state with subsequent release of viral RNA. Antibodies produced in response to rhinovirus infection are often too large to penetrate the canyon, many of them reacting with the rim of the viral canyon. Mutations in the rim would thus enable the virus to escape from the host immune response without affecting the conserved site for binding to the target cell. However, some neutralizing monoclonal antibodies have been identified which contact a significant proportion of the canyon directly overlapping with the ICAM-1-binding site. Hydrophobic drugs have been synthesized which fit the rhinovirus canyon and cause a change in conformation which prevents binding to cells and, since host proteins have very different folds to those of the viral capsid molecule, the drugs have limited cytotoxicity. A more recent drug has been designed to slot into the substrate-binding site of the neuraminidase, so inhibiting its biological activity.

Mutation can produce antagonistic T-cell epitopes

A number of infectious agents, including hepatitis B and C viruses, HIV and malaria, are capable of mutating their T-cell epitopes to exhibit TCR antagonistic activity which inhibits the activity of antiviral cytotoxic T-cells. Mutations which modify residues critical for recognition by MHC or TCR may generate partial agonists that can induce a profound and long-lasting state of T-cell anergy (cf. p. 241 and figure 8.8). Either strategy can lead to persistent infection.

Some viruses can affect antigen processing

Virtually every step in processing and presentation by MHC class I to cytotoxic T-cells can be sabotaged by one virus or another (figure 12.18). Human cytomegalovirus (HCMV) is particularly adept at this, producing a whole gamut of proteins that interfere with antigen processing and presentation. The MHC class II pathway is not exempt from viral interference. HIV Nef affects vesicle traffic and endocytic processing involved in the genera-

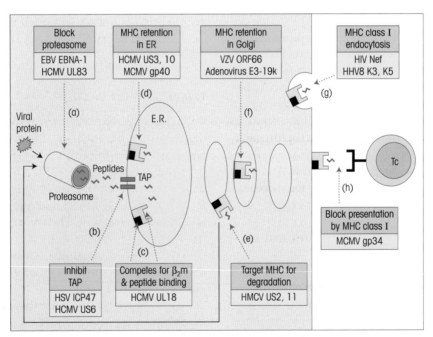

Figure 12.18. Viral interference with antigen processing and presentation by MHC class I. (a) The Epstein–Barr virus (EBV) nuclear antigen-1 (EBNA-1) contains glycine–alanine repeats which inhibit proteasome-mediated processing of the virus, whilst the *unique long* region protein 83 (UL83) of human cytomegalovirus (HCMV) causes viral proteins to become phosphorylated which is thought to block their proteasomal access. (b) Peptide binding to TAP is inhibited by the infected cell protein 47 (ICP47) of herpes simplex virus (HSV), and the *unique short* region protein 6 (US6) protein of HCMV prevents peptide transport through the TAP pore. (c) UL18 is an MHC class I homolog which not only competes with MHC class I molecules for β_2-microglobulin and peptide binding but potentially also could engage NK inhibitory receptors to prevent NK-mediated lysis. (d) HCMV US3

and US10 prevent or delay MHC class I export from the endoplasmic reticulum, as does gp40 of murine CMV (MCMV). (e) The US2 and US11 proteins of HCMV redirect the class I molecules to the cytosol for degradation by the proteasome. (f) Both the varicella zoster virus open reading frame 66 (VZV ORF 66) protein and the E3-19k protein of adenovirus cause retention of MHC class I molecules in the Golgi, the latter by inhibiting glycosylation. (g) Even if it makes it to the cell surface, the MHC class molecule is not safe. The K3 and K5 proteins of Kaposi's sarcoma associated human herpesvirus 8 (HHV8) can remove it from the cell surface, as can the Nef protein of HIV, by a process involving endocytosis and ubiquitination. (h) Finally the gp34 protein of MCMV interferes with recognition of the peptide–MHC complex by the TCR on the CD8[+] cytotoxic T-cell.

tion of peptides, whilst the EIA protein of adenovirus interferes with IFNγ-mediated upregulation of MHC class II expression.

Viruses can interfere with immune effector mechanisms

Playing games with the host's humoral responses

Just as bacteria possess proteins capable of binding the Fc region of antibody (cf. p. 267), so certain viruses also possess Fcγ receptors. Herpes simplex virus (HSV) types 1 and 2, pseudorabies virus, varicella-zoster virus and murine cytomegalovirus all bear such molecules which, by binding antibody 'the wrong way round', may inhibit Fc-mediated effector functions.

As we saw for bacteria (cf. p. 260), viruses can block complement-mediated induction of the inflammatory response and thereby prevent viral killing. The vaccinia virus complement control protein (VCP) binds C3b and C4b, making both the classical (C4b2a) and alternative (C3bBb) C3 convertases susceptible to factor I-mediated destruction. For its part, herpes simplex type 1 subverts the complement cascade by virtue of its surface glycoprotein C which binds C3b, interfering with its interaction with C5 and properdin.

Several viruses utilize complement receptors to gain entry into cells, especially since engagement of the complement receptor alone on a macrophage is a feeble activator of the respiratory burst. EBV infects B-cells by binding to the CR2 surface receptors, whilst flavivirus coated with iC3b enters through the CR3 receptors. Ominously, HIV coated with antibody and complement can be more virulent than unopsonized virus. Members of the regulators of complement activation (RCA) family are also used as cellular receptors for various viruses, such as CD46 (membrane cofactor protein) by measles virus and human herpes virus-6 (HHV-6), and CD55 (decay accelerating factor) by echoviruses and coxsackie viruses.

Cell-mediated immunity can also be manipulated

Parainfluenza virus type 2 strongly inhibits Tc cells by downregulating granzyme B expression (cf. p. 198). Viral homologs of host cytokines and their receptors act as immunosuppressants. The EBV protein BCRF1 (vIL-10) has an 84% homology to human IL-10 and helps the virus to escape the antiviral effects of IFNγ by downregulating Th1 cells. Poxviruses encode soluble homologs of both the IFNα/β receptor and the IFNγR, thereby competitively inhibiting the action of all three interferons. Human orthopoxvirus produces an IL-18 binding protein (IL-18BP) which inhibits IL-18-induced IFNγ production and NK responses. Herpesviruses and poxviruses possess several genes encoding chemokine-like and chemokine receptor-like proteins which can subvert the action of numerous chemokines. The list just goes on and on. Anti-IFN strategies are particularly abundant, with many viruses producing proteins able to block IFN-induced JAK/STAT pathway activation. A prime viral target is also the activation of the double-stranded RNA-dependent protein kinase (PKR) and other components of the cell involved in setting up an antiviral state following exposure to IFN. When the African swine fever virus (ASFV) infects macrophages, its A238L protein inhibits both NFκB and calcineurin-dependent cell activation pathways. The ASFV genome also encodes a homologue of the CD2 antigen (vCD2) which interferes with lymphocyte function.

Apoptosis of a cell could be considered bad news for a virus living very comfortably inside that cell. Therefore it is yet again not surprising that viruses have come up with ways of preventing apoptosis. Just a couple of examples; HHV8 produces a viral FLICE-inhibitory protein (vFLIP) which is a homolog of the prodomain of caspase 8 and thereby protects cells against apoptosis, whilst ASFV produces homologs of IAP and bcl2 in order to inhibit apoptosis. By contrast, some viral proteins including HIV-1 Vpr and HBV HBx are pro-apoptotic, in this case perhaps aiding dissemination of virus particles.

Protection by serum antibody

Antibodies can neutralize viruses by a variety of means. They may stereochemically inhibit combination with the receptor site on cells, thereby preventing penetration and subsequent intracellular multiplication, the protective effect of antibodies to influenza hemagglutinin providing a good example. Similarly, antibodies to the measles hemagglutinin prevent entry into the cell, but the spread of virus from cell to cell is stopped by antibodies to the fusion antigen. Antibody may destroy a free virus particle directly through activation of the classical complement pathway or produce aggregation, enhanced phagocytosis and intracellular death by the mechanisms already discussed. As far as any antibody-mediated effects are concerned, infected cells will need to rely upon ADCC (p. 32) as has been reported with herpes-, vaccinia- and mumps-infected target cells.

The most clear-cut protection by antibody is seen in diseases with long incubation times where the virus has to travel through the bloodstream before it reaches the tissue which it finally infects. For example, in poliomyelitis, the virus gains access to the body via the gastrointestinal tract and eventually passes through the circulation to reach the brain cells which become infected. Within the blood, the virus is neutralized

tion of the respiratory burst by catalase, mannitol and melanin. Following inhalation of *Aspergillus fumigatus* the alveolar macrophages phagocytose and destroy conidia (spores), although fungal proteases may help protect the spores from such activities. In the lungs the conidia can germinate into branching hyphae which are probably dealt with by the release of oxidants and fungicidal granule contents from neutrophils.

NK cells have been shown to have constitutive antifungal activity against, for example, *Cryptococcus neoformans*, whereas such activity against this organism needs to be induced in CTL. In the case of *A. fumigatus* the adaptive immune response becomes activated following uptake of conidia and hyphae by local dendritic cells and subsequent presentation to T-cells in the draining lymph nodes. Fungal cell wall components can signal dendritic cells through a number of pattern recognition receptors (figure 12.21), resulting in the release of IL-12 which drives a Th1 response. The role of antibody is complex and not always advantageous, although there are clear examples of protective effects such as the antibodies to *Candida albicans* heat-shock protein 90 (hsp90) which are protective against disseminated disease in patients with AIDS. Mannose-binding protein is able to agglutinate *Candida albicans* and subsequently activate the complement system.

The production of phospholipases, proteases and elastases by many fungi function as virulence factors. Dimorphic fungi such as *Blastomyces dermatitidis*, *Coccidiodes immitis* and *Histoplasma capsulatum* transform from filamentous moulds to unicellular yeasts, whilst some species of *Candida*, including *Candida albicans*, can take on the form of yeasts, blastospores, pseudohyphae or hyphae depending on the site of the infection. The antigenic changes which accompany such morphological changes are presumed to act as virulence factors, although this remains to be formally established. Recent studies have shown that adhesins on the fungal surface also behave as virulence factors since their neutralization by antibody variable region fragments can block infection in an animal model of vaginal candidiasis.

IMMUNITY TO PARASITIC INFECTIONS

The diverse organisms responsible for some of the major parasitic diseases are listed in figure 12.22. The numbers affected are truly horrifying and the sum of misery these organisms engender is too large to comprehend. The consequences of parasitism could be, at one extreme, a lack of immune response leading to overwhelming superinfection, and, at the other, an exaggerated life-threatening immunopathological response. To be successful, a parasite must steer a course *between* these extremes, avoiding wholesale killing of the human host and yet at the same time escaping destruction by the immune system.

The host responses

A wide variety of defensive mechanisms are deployed by the host, but the rough generalization may be made

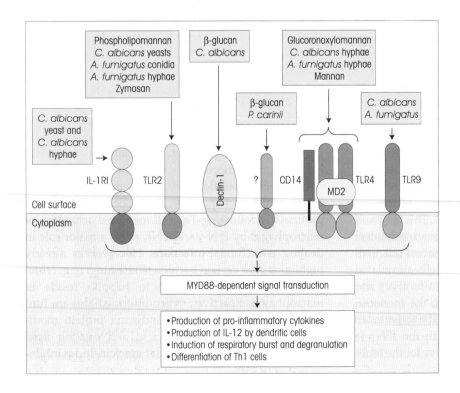

Figure 12.21. Pattern recognition receptor (PRR) mediated activation of immunity to fungi. A number of different pathogen-associated molecular patterns present on fungal cell walls can activate both the innate and adaptive immune response through the canonical MYD88 pathway following their recognition by PRRs on the host cells. IL-1RI, Interleukin-1 receptor type I; TLR, Toll-like receptor. (Modified from Romani L. (2004) *Nature Reviews Immunology* **4**, 1–23, with permission from the publishers.) *A. fumigatus*, *Aspergillus fumigatus*; *C. albicans*, *Candida albicans*; *P. carinii*, *Pneumocystis carinii*.

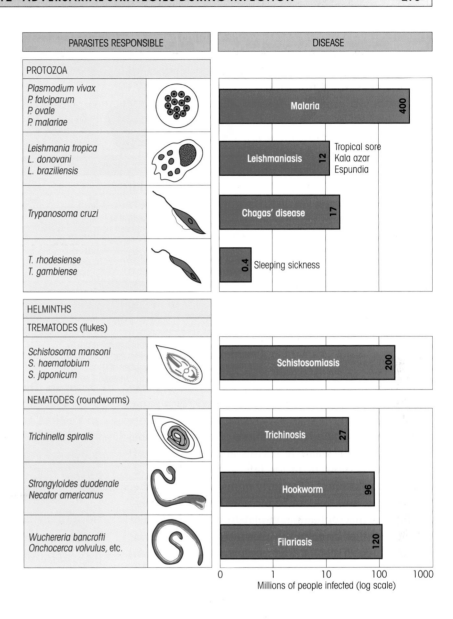

Figure 12.22. Some major parasites in humans and the sheer enormity of the numbers of people infected. (Data from World Health Organization, www.who.int)

that a humoral response develops when the organisms invade the bloodstream (malaria, trypanosomiasis), whereas parasites which grow within the tissues (e.g. cutaneous leishmaniasis) usually elicit CMI (table 12.2). Often, a chronically infected host will be resistant to reinfection with fresh organisms, a situation termed **concomitant immunity**. This is seen particularly in schistosomiasis but also in malaria. The resident and the infective forms must differ in some way yet to be pinpointed.

Humoral immunity

Antibodies of the right specificity present in adequate concentrations and affinity are reasonably effective in providing protection against blood-borne parasites, such as *Trypanosoma brucei*, and the sporozoite and merozoite stages of malaria. Thus, individuals receiving IgG from solidly immune adults in malaria endemic areas are themselves temporarily protected against infection, the effector mechanisms being opsonization and phagocytosis, and complement-dependent lysis.

A marked feature of the immune reaction to helminthic infections, such as *Trichinella spiralis* in humans and *Nippostrongylus brasiliensis* in the rat, is the eosinophilia and the high level of IgE antibody produced. In humans, serum levels of IgE can rise from normal values of around 100 ng/ml to as high as 10 000 ng/ml. These changes have all the hallmarks of response to Th2-type cytokines (cf. p. 191) and it is notable that, in animals infected with helminths, injection of anti-IL-4 greatly reduces IgE production and anti-IL-5 suppresses the eosinophilia. IL-13 in the skin, which together with IL-4 is a switch factor for IgE production, seems to play an important role in protection against schistosomes. Antigen-specific triggering of IgE-coated mast cells leads to exudation of serum pro-out becoming exposed to antibody are combated by CMI. Infected cells express a processed viral antigen peptide on their surface in association with MHC class I a short time after entry of the virus, and rapid killing of the cell by cytotoxic αβ T-cells prevents viral multiplication which depends upon the replicative machinery of the intact host cell. γδ Tc recognize native viral coat protein on the target cell surface. NK cells are also cytotoxic.

• T-cells and macrophages producing IFNγ and TNF bathe the contiguous cells and prevent them from becoming infected by lateral spread of virus.

Immunity to fungi

• Opportunistic fungal infections are common in immunosuppressed hosts.
• Phagocytosis plays a major role in dealing with fungi.
• CTL and NK cells exhibit anti-fungal activities.
• Antibody is not always advantageous, but does appear to help protect against systemic candida infections in patients with AIDS.

Immunity to parasitic infections

• Diseases involving *protozoal parasites* and *helminths* affect hundreds of millions of people. Antibodies are usually effective against the blood-borne forms. IgE production is increased in worm infestations and can lead to mast cell-mediated influx of Ig and eosinophils; schistosomes coated with IgG or IgE are killed by adherent eosinophils through extracellular mechanisms involving the release of cationic proteins and peroxidase.
• Organisms such as *Leishmania* spp., *Trypanosoma cruzi* and *Toxoplasma gondii* hide from antibodies inside macrophages, use the same strategies as intracellular parasitic bacteria to survive, and like them are killed when the macrophages are activated by Th1 cytokines produced during cell-mediated immune responses. NO· is an important killing agent.

• CD8 T-cells also have a protective role.
• Expulsion of intestinal worms usually depends on Th2 responses and requires the coordinated action of antibody, the release of mucin by cytokine-stimulated goblet cells and the production of intestinal contraction and diarrhea by mast cell mediators.
• Some parasites avoid recognition by disguising themselves as the host, either through molecular mimicry or by absorbing host proteins to their surface.
• Other organisms such as *Trypanosoma brucei* and various malarial species have the extraordinary ability to cover their surface with a dominant antigen which is changed by genetic switch mechanisms to a different molecule as antibody is formed to the first variant.
• Most parasites also tend to nonspecifically suppress host responses.
• Chronic persistence of parasite antigen in the face of an immune response often produces tissue-damaging immunopathological reactions such as immune complex nephrotic syndrome, liver granulomas and autoimmune lesions of the heart. Generalized immunosuppression increases susceptibility to bacterial and viral infections.
• As the features of the response to infection are analysed, we see more clearly how the specific acquired response operates to amplify and enhance innate immune mechanisms; the interactions are summarized in figure 12.27.

Prion diseases

• Scrapie, BSE and vCJD are transmissible spongiform encephalopathies caused by prions.
• Abnormally folded, protease-resistant forms of host prion protein (PrP) develop.
• FDCs in lymphoid tissues become infected prior to spread of the infectious agent to the CNS.

FURTHER READING

Bieniasz P.D. (2004) Intrinsic immunity: a front-line defense against viral attack. *Nature Immunology* **5**, 1109–1115.
Brinkmann V., Reichard U., Goosmann C. *et al.* (2004) Neutrophil extracellular traps kill bacteria. *Science* **303**, 1532–1535.
Janeway C.A. Jr. & Medzhitov R. (2002) Innate immune recognition. *Annual Review of Immunology* **20**, 197–216.
Kaufmann S.H.E. (2004) New issues in tuberculosis. *Annals of Rheumatic Diseases* **63** (Suppl. II), ii50–ii56.
Lewis D.B. (2006) Avian flu to human influenza. *Annual Review of Medicine* **57**, 139–154.
Mims C.A., Dockrell H., Goering R. *et al.* (2005) *Medical Microbiology*, 3rd edn. Mosby, London.
Portnoy D.A. (2005) Manipulation of innate immunity by bacterial pathogens. *Current Opinion in Immunology* **17**, 25–28.
Rappuoli R. (2004) From Pasteur to genomics: progress and challenges in infectious diseases. *Nature Medicine* **10**, 1177–1185.

Romani L. (2004) Immunity to fungal infections. *Nature Reviews Immunology* **4**, 1–23.
Tortorella D., Gewurz B.E., Furman M.H., Schust D.J. & Ploegh H.L. (2002) Viral subversion of the immune system. *Annual Review of Immunology* **18**, 861–926.
Weyrich A.S. & Zimmerman G.A. (2004) Platelets: signaling cells in the immune continuum. *Trends in Immunology* **25**, 489–495.

The following websites of the Centers for Disease Control and Prevention contain a large body of information:
Viral diseases: http://www.cdc.gov/ncidod/dvrd/disinfo/disease.htm
Bacteria and fungal diseases: http://www.cdc.gov/ncidod/dbmd/diseaseinfo/default.htm
Parasitic diseases: http://www.cdc.gov/ncidod/dpd/parasites/listing.htm

13 Vaccines

INTRODUCTION

The control of infection is approached from several directions. Improvements in public health—water supply, sewage systems, education in personal hygiene—prevent the spread of cholera and many other diseases. Antibiotics have had a major impact on bacterial diseases. Another strategy is to give the immune response a helping hand. This can be achieved by administering individual components of the immune response, such as defensins or antibodies, by using immunopotentiating agents such as cytokines, or more commonly by exposing the immune system to an antigen in order to stimulate the acquired immune response to generate memory cells—a procedure referred to as vaccination (Milestone 13.1). Vaccines have traditionally been aimed at generating responses against infectious agents, but increasingly they are also being explored in areas such as malignancy.

PASSIVELY ACQUIRED IMMUNITY

Temporary protection against infection or toxins can be established by giving preformed antibody from another individual of the same or a different species (table 13.1; figure 13.1). Prior to the introduction of antibiotics, horse serum containing antitetanus or antidiphtheria toxins was extensively employed prophylactically, but nowadays it is used less commonly because of the complication of serum sickness (a type III hypersensitivity) and immediate (type I) hypersensitivity developing in response to the foreign protein. Furthermore, as the acquired antibodies are utilized by combination with antigen or are catabolized in the normal way, this protection is lost. The use of passive immunization is currently largely restricted to anti-venoms where an immediate therapeutic effect is required for a usually rare event such as a snake bite. However, with the emergence of antibiotic strains of bacteria, and concerns about possible bioterrorism, there is a renewed interest in passive immunization against infectious agents.

Maternally acquired antibody

In the first few months of life, while the baby's own lymphoid system is slowly getting under way, protection is afforded to the fetus by maternally derived IgG antibodies acquired by placental transfer and to the neonate by intestinal absorption of colostral immunoglobulins (figure 13.1). The major immunoglobulin in milk is secretory IgA (SIgA) and this is not absorbed by the baby but remains in the intestine to protect the mucosal surfaces. In this respect it is quite striking that the SIgA antibodies are directed against bacterial and viral antigens often present in the intestine, and it is presumed that IgA-producing cells, responding to gut antigens, migrate and colonize breast tissue (as part of the mucosal immune system; see p. 163), where the antibodies they produce appear in the milk. The case for mucosal vaccination of future mothers against selected infections is inescapable.

Polyclonal and monoclonal antibodies for passive immunization

Intravenous immunoglobulin (IVIg) is a preparation of IgG obtained by large scale fractionation of plasma pooled from thousands of healthy blood donors. The preparations are given to individuals with immunodeficiencies associated with reduced or absent circulating antibody. IVIg is also of value in the treatment of a number of infection-associated conditions such as

Milestone 13.1—Vaccination

The notion that survivors of serious infectious disease seldom contract that infection again has been embedded in folklore for centuries. In an account of the terrible plague which afflicted Athens, Thucydides noted that, in the main, those nursing the sick were individuals who had already been infected and yet recovered from the plague. Deliberate attempts to ward off infections by inducing a minor form of the disease in otherwise healthy subjects were common in China in the Middle Ages. There, they developed the practice of inhaling a powder made from **smallpox** scabs as protection against any future infection. The Indians inoculated the scab material into small skin wounds, and this practice of **variolation** (Latin *varus*, a pustular facial disease) was introduced into Turkey where the inhabitants were determined to prevent the ravages of smallpox epidemics interfering with the lucrative sale of their gorgeous daughters to the harems of the wealthy.

Voltaire, in 1773, tells us that the credit for spreading the practice of variolation to Western Europe should be attributed to Lady Wortley Montague, a remarkably enterprising woman who was the wife of the English Ambassador to Constantinople in the time of George I. With little scruple, she inoculated her daughter with smallpox in the face of the protestations of her Chaplain who felt that it could only succeed with infidels, not Christians. All went well however and the practice was taken up in England despite the hazardous nature of the procedure which had a case fatality of 0.5–2%. These dreadful risks were taken because, at that time, as Voltaire recorded '. . . three score persons in every hundred have the smallpox. Of these three score, twenty die of it in the most favorable season of life, and as many more wear the disagreeable remains of it on their faces so long as they live.'

Edward Jenner (1749–1823), a country physician in Gloucestershire, suggested to one of his patients that she might have smallpox, but she assured him that his diagnosis was impossible since she had already contracted cowpox through her chores as a milkmaid (folklore again!). This led Jenner to the series of experiments in which he showed that prior inoculation with cowpox, which was nonvirulent (i.e. nonpathogenic) in the human, protected against subsequent challenge with smallpox (cf. p. 30). His ideas initially met with violent opposition but were eventually accepted and he achieved world fame; learned societies everywhere elected him to membership, although it is intriguing to note that the College of Physicians in London required him to pass an examination in classics and the Royal Society honored him with a Fellowship on the basis of his work on the nesting behavior of the cuckoo. In the end he inoculated thousands in the shed in the garden of his house in Berkeley, Gloucestershire, which now functions as a museum and venue for small symposia (rather fun to visit if you get the chance).

The next seminal development in vaccines came through the research of Louis Pasteur who had developed the germ theory of disease. A culture of chicken cholera bacillus, which had accidently been left on a bench during the warm summer months, lost much of its ability to cause disease; nonetheless, birds which had been inoculated with this old culture were resistant to fresh virulent cultures of the bacillus. This **attenuation** of **virulent** organisms was reproduced by Pasteur for anthrax and rabies using abnormal culture and passage conditions. Recognizing the relevance of Jenner's research for his own experiments, Pasteur called his treatment **vaccination**, a term which has stood the test of time.

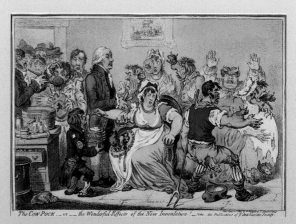

The Cow-Pock _ or _ the Wonderful Effects of the New Inoculation! _ vide _ the Publications of y* Anti-Vaccine Society.

Figure M13.1.1. Edward Jenner among patients in the Smallpox and Inoculation Hospital at St Pancras. Etching after J. Gillray, 1802. (Kindly supplied by The Wellcome Centre Medical Photographic Library, London.)

streptococcal toxic shock syndrome. Indeed, separate pools of polyclonal IgG with raised titers to selected organisms are available for hepatitis B, rabies, tetanus, cytomegalovirus (CMV) and varicella-zoster viruses, amongst others. Curiously, IVIg also has efficacy in the treatment of several autoimmune and inflammatory diseases such as idiopathic thrombocytopenic purpura, chronic inflammatory demyelinating polyneuropathy and Guillain–Barré syndrome. The mechanism of action in these nonimmunodeficient patients remains unclear, although it appears to act as an immunomodulating agent, possibly through anti-idiotypic mechanisms.

Monoclonal antibodies specific for individual organisms offer a better defined and consistent therapeutic agent and one such antibody, Palivizumab, is licensed for the prevention of respiratory syncytial virus infection in children and babies. Products under development include a chimeric anti-lipoteichoic acid for the

Table 13.1. Examples of passive therapy against infection and toxins.

Condition	Source of antibody	Use
Tetanus infection	Human polyclonal	Antitoxin. Management of tetanus-prone wounds in patients where immunization is incomplete or uncertain
Botulism	Horse polyclonal	Antitoxin. Post-exposure prophylaxis of botulism
Snake bites (various)	Horse polyclonal	Antivenom. Treatment following venomous snake bite
Spider bites (various)	Horse polyclonal, rabbit polyclonal	Antivenom. Treatment following venomous spider bite
Paralysis tick bite	Dog polyclonal	Antivenom. Treatment following bite from paralysis tick
Stonefish sting	Horse polyclonal	Antivenom. Treatment following stonefish sting
Jellyfish sting	Sheep polyclonal	Antivenom. Treatment following venomous jellyfish sting
Hepatitis B infection	Human polyclonal	Antiviral. Prevention of infection in laboratory and other personnel accidentally inoculated with hepatitis B virus, and in infants of mothers infected during pregnancy or who are high-risk carriers
Rabies	Human polyclonal	Antiviral. Following bite from a possibly infected animal
Varicella-zoster virus infection	Human polyclonal	Antiviral. Seronegative individuals at increased risk of severe varicella (chickenpox)
Cytomegalovirus infection	Human polyclonal	Antiviral. Prophylaxis in immunosuppressed patients
Respiratory syncytial virus infection	Humanized mouse IgG1 monoclonal	Antiviral. Prevention of serious lower respiratory tract disease in high risk children and infants

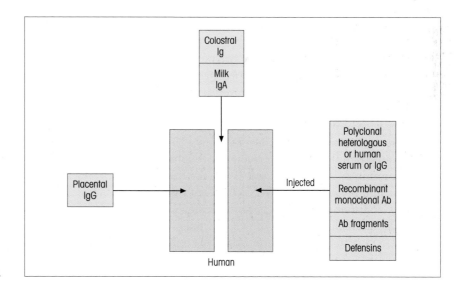

Figure 13.1. Passive immunization produced by: transplacental passage of IgG from mother to fetus, acquisition of IgA from mother's colostrum and milk by the infant, and injection of polyclonal antibodies, recombinant monoclonal antibodies, antibody fragments (Fab or scFv) derived from phage libraries and, perhaps in the future, synthetic neutrophil defensins.

prevention of staphylococcal infections by effective opsonization of staphylococci for neutrophil killing, and a recombinant human IgG1 anti-RhD antibody for prevention of hemolytic disease of the newborn. Antibody therapy which could act immediately against potential bioterrorism organisms such as smallpox and anthrax is also becoming available. Human and llama heavy chain domain antibody fragments specific for cellular adhesins on rotavirus and *Candida albicans* can block adherence to intestinal and vaginal epithelium, respectively, and have been shown to accelerate clearance of infection in experimental models.

Defensins

Never neglect innate immune mechanisms. Defensins, the broad-range antimicrobial peptides present in neutrophil granules, (cf. p. 9), as well as in other cells of the immune system, are now being investigated as therapeutic agents for the treatment of fungal and bacterial infections which become refractory to conventional antibiotics. Rather unexpectedly, the human neutrophil protein (HNP-1) defensin could directly protect mice from the lethal toxin of *Bacillus anthracis*, providing a potential antidote to any mischievous use of anthrax. The activities of the defensins extend to anti-viral effects, recombinant α-defensin-1 being harmful to both HIV-1 and herpes simplex virus (HSV)-1.

Adoptive transfer of cytotoxic T-cells

This is a labor-intensive operation and will be restricted to autologous cells or instances where the donor shares an MHC class I allele. Adoptive transfer of autologous cytotoxic T lymphocytes has been shown to be effective in enhancing EBV-specific immune responses and in reducing the viral load in patients with post-transplant lymphoproliferative disease.

VACCINATION

Herd immunity

In the case of tetanus, active immunization is of benefit to the individual but not to the community since it will not eliminate the organism which is found in the feces of domestic animals and persists in the soil as highly resistant spores. Where a disease depends on human transmission, immunity in just a proportion of the population can help the whole community if it leads to a fall in the reproduction rate (i.e. the number of further cases produced by each infected individual) to less than one; under these circumstances the disease will die out: witness, for example, the disappearance of diphtheria from communities in which around 75% of the children have been immunized (figure 13.2). But this figure must be maintained; there is no room for complacency. In contrast, focal outbreaks of measles have occurred in communities which object to immunization on religious grounds, raising an important point for parents in general. Each individual must compare any perceived disadvantage associated with vaccination in relation to the increased risk of disease in their unprotected child.

Strategic considerations

The objective of vaccination is to provide effective immunity by establishing adequate levels of antibody and a primed population of memory cells which can rapidly expand on renewed contact with antigen and so provide protection against infection. Sometimes, as

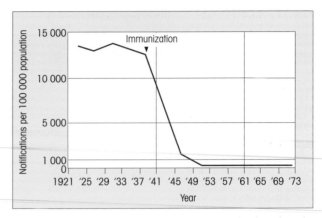

Figure 13.2. Notification of diphtheria in England and Wales per 100 000 population showing dramatic fall after immunization. (Reproduced from Dick G. (1978) *Immunisation*. Update Books; with kind permission of the author and publishers.)

with tetanus infection, a high blood titer of antibody is required; in mycobacterial diseases, such as tuberculosis (TB), a macrophage-activating cell-mediated immunity (CMI) is most effective, whereas with influenza virus infection, cytotoxic T-cells play a significant role. The site of the immune response evoked by vaccination may also be most important. For example, in cholera, antibodies need to be in the gut lumen to inhibit adherence to and colonization of the intestinal wall.

Eradication of the infectious agent is not always the most practical goal. To take the example of malaria, the blood-borne form releases molecules which trigger tumor necrosis factor (TNF) and other cytokines from monocytes, and the secretion of these mediators is responsible for the unpleasant effects of the disease. Accordingly, an antibody response targeted to these released antigens with structurally conserved epitopes may be a realistic holding strategy, while the search for a global vaccine aimed at the more elusive antigen-swapping parasite itself is grinding forward. Under these circumstances life with the parasite might be acceptable.

In addition to an ability to engender effective immunity, a number of mundane but nonetheless crucial conditions must be satisfied for a vaccine to be considered successful (table 13.2). The antigens must be readily available, and the preparation should be stable, cheap and certainly, safe, bearing in mind that the recipients are most often healthy children. Clearly, the first contact with antigen during vaccination should not be injurious and the maneuver is to avoid the pathogenic effects of infection, while maintaining protective immunogens.

KILLED ORGANISMS AS VACCINES

The simplest way to destroy the ability of microbes to

Table 13.2. Factors required for a successful vaccine.

FACTOR	REQUIREMENTS
Effectiveness	Must evoke protective levels of immunity: at the appropriate site of relevant nature (Ab, Tc, Th1, Th2) of adequate duration
Availability	Readily cultured in bulk or accessible source of subunit
Stability	Stable under extreme climatic conditions, preferably not requiring refrigeration
Cheapness	What is cheap in the West may be expensive in developing countries but the Bill and Melinda Gates Foundation and governments help
Safety	Eliminate any pathogenicity

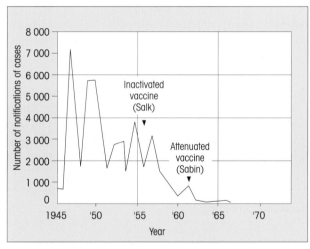

Figure 13.3. **Notifications of paralytic poliomyelitis in England and Wales** showing the beneficial effects of community immunization with killed and live vaccines. (Reproduced from Dick G. (1978) *Immunisation*. Update Books; with kind permission of the author and publishers.)

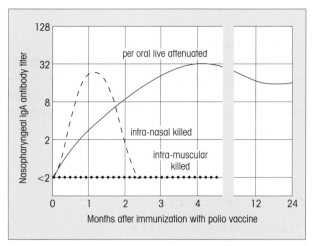

Figure 13.4. **Local IgA response to polio vaccine.** Local secretory antibody synthesis is confined to the specific anatomical sites which have been directly stimulated by contact with antigen. (Data from Ogra P.L. *et al.* (1975) In Notkins A.L. (ed.) *Viral Immunology and Immunopathology*, p. 67. Academic Press, New York.)

cause disease, yet maintain their antigenic constitution, is to prevent their replication by killing in an appropriate manner. Parasitic worms and, to a lesser extent, protozoa are extremely difficult to grow up in bulk to manufacture killed vaccines. This problem does not arise for many bacteria and viruses and, in these cases, the inactivated microorganisms have generally provided safe antigens for immunization. Examples are influenza, cholera and inactivated poliomyelitis (Salk) vaccines (figure 13.3). Care has to be taken to ensure that important protective antigens are not destroyed in the inactivation process.

LIVE ATTENUATED ORGANISMS HAVE MANY ADVANTAGES AS VACCINES

The objective of attenuation is to produce a modified organism which mimics the natural behavior of the original microbe without causing significant disease. In many instances the immunity conferred by killed vaccines, even when given with adjuvant (see below), is often inferior to that resulting from infection with live organisms. This must be partly because the replication of the living microbes confronts the host with a **larger and more sustained dose of antigen** and that, with budding viruses, infected cells are required for the establishment of good **cytotoxic T-cell memory**. Another significant advantage of using live organisms is that the immune **response takes place largely at the site of the natural infection**. This is well illustrated by the nasopharyngeal IgA response to immunization with polio vaccine. In contrast with the ineffectiveness of parenteral injection of killed vaccine, intranasal administration evoked a good local antibody response; however, whereas this declined over a period of 2 months or so, per oral immunization with *live attenuated* virus established a persistently high IgA antibody level (figure 13.4).

There is in fact a strong upsurge of interest in strategies for mucosal immunization. Remember, the mucosal immune system involves mucous membranes covering the aerodigestive and urogenital tracts as well as the conjunctiva, the ear and the ducts of all exocrine glands whose protection includes SIgA antibodies. Resident T-cells in these tissues produce large amounts of transforming growth factor-β (TGFβ), and the interleukins IL-10 and IL-4, which promote the B-cell switch to IgA, and note also that human intestinal epithelial cells themselves are major sources of TGFβ and IL-10.

Classical methods of attenuation

The objective of attenuation, that of producing an organism which causes only a very mild form of the natural disease, can be equally well attained if one can identify heterologous strains which are virulent for another species, but avirulent in humans. The best example of this was Jenner's seminal demonstration that cowpox would protect against smallpox. Subsequently, a truly remarkable global effort by the World Health Organization (WHO), combining extensive vaccination and selective epidemiological control methods, **completely eradicated the human disease**—a wonderful achievement. Emboldened by this success, the WHO embarked upon a program to eradicate polio using attenuated polio vaccine to block transmission of the virus and, despite setbacks such as a temporary halt in vaccination in Northern Nigeria following unfounded rumours regarding the safety of the vaccine, it is hoped that this goal will be achieved in the not too distant future. One can even follow the progress of this campaign on http://www.polioeradication.org.

Attenuation itself was originally achieved by empirical modification of the conditions under which an organism grows. Pasteur first achieved the production of live but nonvirulent forms of chicken cholera bacillus and anthrax (cf. Milestone 13.1) by such artifices as culture at higher temperatures and under anerobic conditions, and was able to confer immunity by infection with the attenuated organisms. A virulent strain of *Mycobacterium tuberculosis* became attenuated by chance in 1908 when Calmette and Guérin at the Institut Pasteur, Lille, added bile to the culture medium in an attempt to achieve dispersed growth. After 13 years of culture in bile-containing medium, the strain remained attenuated and was used successfully to vaccinate children against tuberculosis. The same organism, BCG (bacille Calmette–Guérin), is widely used today in many countries for the immunization of infants and of tuberculin-negative children and adolescents. However, its efficacy varies widely from, for example, protection in 80% of vaccinated individuals in the UK, to a total lack of efficacy in Southern India. This variability is not fully understood but is thought to be due to a number of factors including local differences in the antigenic composition of the vaccine and in the environmental mycobacterial strains, and differences in MHC alleles and other genetic factors in the various human populations. Attenuation by cold adaptation has been applied to influenza and other respiratory viruses; the organism can grow at the lower temperatures (32–34°C) of the upper respiratory tract, but fails to produce clinical disease because of its inability to replicate in the lower respiratory tract (37°C). An intranasal vaccine containing cold-adapted attenuated influenza virus strains was licensed for use in the USA in 2003.

Attenuation by recombinant DNA technology

It must be said that many of the classical methods of attenuation are somewhat empirical and the outcome is difficult to control or predict. With knowledge of the genetic makeup of these microorganisms, we can apply the molecular biologist's delicate scalpel to deliberately target the alterations which are needed for successful attenuation. Thus genetic recombination is being used to develop various attenuated strains of viruses, such as influenza, with not only a lower virulence for humans but also an increased multiplication rate in eggs (enabling newly endemic strains of influenza to be adapted for rapid vaccine production). Not surprisingly, strains of HIV-1, with vicious deletions of the regulatory genes, are being investigated as protective vaccines. The potential is clearly quite enormous.

The **tropism** of attenuated organisms for **the site** at which **natural infection** occurs is likely to be exploited dramatically in the near future to establish gut immunity to typhoid and cholera using attenuated forms of *Salmonella typhi* and *Vibrio cholerae* in which the virulence genes have been identified and modified by genetic engineering.

Microbial vectors for other genes

An ingenious trick is to use a virus as a 'piggy-back' for genes encoding a vaccine immunogen. Incorporation of such 'foreign' genes into attenuated recombinant viral vectors, such as fowlpox and canarypox virus and the modified vaccinia Ankara (MVA) strain virus, which infect mammalian hosts but are unable to replicate effectively, provides a powerful vaccination strategy with many benefits. The genes may be derived from organisms which are difficult to grow or inherently dangerous, and the constructs themselves are replication deficient, nonintegrating, stable and relatively easy to prepare. The proteins encoded by these genes are appropriately expressed *in vivo* with respect to glycosylation and secretion, and are processed for MHC presentation by the infected cells, thus effectively endowing the host with both humoral and cell-mediated immunity.

A wide variety of genes have been expressed in vaccinia virus vectors, and it has been demonstrated that the products of genes coding for viral envelope proteins, such as influenza virus hemagglutinin, vesicular stomatitis virus glycoprotein, HIV-1 gp120 and herpes simplex virus glycoprotein D, could be correctly

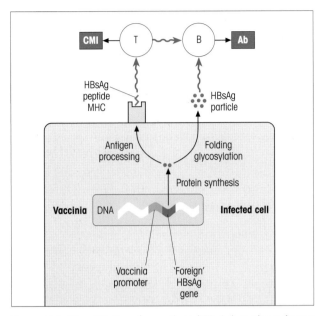

Figure 13.5. Hepatitis B surface antigen (HBsAg) vaccine using an attenuated vaccinia virus carrier. The HBsAg protein is synthesized by the machinery of the host cell: some is secreted to form the HBsAg 22 nm particle which stimulates antibody (Ab) production, and some follows the antigen processing pathway to stimulate cell-mediated immunity (CMI) and T-helper activity.

processed and inserted into the plasma membrane of infected cells. Hepatitis B surface antigen (HBsAg) was secreted from recombinant vaccinia virus-infected cells as the characteristic 22 nm particles (figure 13.5). It is an impressive approach and chimpanzees have been protected against the clinical effects of hepatitis B virus, while mice inoculated with recombinant influenza hemagglutinin generated cytotoxic T-cells and were protected against influenza infection.

Attention has also been paid to BCG as a vehicle for antigens required to evoke CD4-mediated T-cell immunity. The organism is avirulent, has a low frequency of serious complications, can be administered any time after birth, has strong adjuvant properties and gives long-lasting CMI after a single injection.

The ability of *Salmonella* to elicit **mucosal responses by oral immunization** has been exploited by the design of vectors which allow the expression of any protein antigen linked to *E. coli* enterotoxin, a powerful mucosal immunostimulant. There is an attractive possibility that the oral route of vaccination may be applicable not only for the establishment of gut mucosal immunity but also for providing systemic protection. For example, *Salmonella typhimurium* not only invades the mucosal lining of the gut, but also infects cells of the mononuclear phagocyte system throughout the body, thereby stimulating the production of humoral and secretory antibodies as well as CD4 and CD8 cell-mediated immunity. Since attenuated *Salmonella* can be made to express proteins from *Shigella*, cholera, malaria sporozoites and so on, it is entirely feasible to consider these as potential oral vaccines. *Salmonella* may also carry 'foreign genes' within separate DNA plasmids and, after phagocytosis by antigen-presenting cells, the plasmids can be released from the phagosome into the cytosol if the plasmid bears a recombinant lysteriolysin gene or the bacterium is a mutant whose cell walls disintegrate within the phagosome; the plasmid then moves to the nucleus where it is transcribed to produce the desired antigen. Quite strikingly, these attenuated organisms are very effective when inhaled and can elicit substantive mucosal and systemic immune responses comparable to those obtained by the parenteral route. Vaccinologists are still confidently predicting **'the age of the nose'** and we should soon hear more of human trials with this wide variety of attenuated vectors.

Constraints on the use of attenuated vaccines

Attenuated vaccines for poliomyelitis (Sabin), measles, mumps, rubella, varicella-voster and yellow fever have gained general acceptance. However, with live viral vaccines there is a possibility that the nucleic acid might be incorporated into the host's genome or that there may be reversion to a virulent form. Reversion is less likely if the attenuated strains contain several mutations. Another disadvantage of attenuated strains is the difficulty and expense of maintaining appropriate cold-storage facilities, especially in out-of-the-way places. In diseases such as viral hepatitis, AIDS and cancer, the dangers associated with live vaccines are daunting. With most vaccines there is a very small, but still real, risk of developing complications and it cannot be emphasized too often that this **risk must be balanced against the expected chance of contracting the disease with its own complications**. Where this is minimal, some may prefer to avoid general vaccination and to rely upon a crash course backed up if necessary by passive immunization in the localities around isolated outbreaks of infectious disease.

It is important to recognize those children with immunodeficiency before injection of live organisms; a child with impaired T-cell reactivity can become overwhelmed by BCG and die. It is also inadvisable to give live vaccines to patients being treated with steroids, immunosuppressive drugs or radiotherapy or who have malignant conditions such as lymphoma and leukemia; pregnant mothers must also be included here because of the vulnerability of the fetus.

Use in a veterinary context

For veterinary use, of course, there is a little less concern about minor side-effects and excellent results have been obtained using existing vaccinia strains with rinderpest in cattle and rabies in foxes, for example. In the latter case, a recombinant vaccinia virus vaccine expressing the rabies surface glycoprotein was distributed with bait from the air and immunized approximately 80% of the foxes in that area. No cases of rabies were subsequently seen, but epidemiological considerations indicate that, with the higher fox density that this leads to, the higher the percentage which have to be made immune; thus, either one has to increase the efficacy of the vaccine, or culling of the animals must continue—an interesting consequence of interference with ecosystems. Less complicated is the use of such immunization to control local outbreaks of rabies in rare mammalian species, such as the African wild dog, which are threatened with extinction by the virus in certain game reserves.

SUBUNIT VACCINES CONTAINING INDIVIDUAL PROTECTIVE ANTIGENS

A whole parasite or bacterium usually contains many antigens which are not concerned in the protective response of the host but may give rise to problems by suppressing the response to protective antigens or by provoking hypersensitivity, as we saw in the last chapter. Vaccination with the isolated protective antigens may avoid these complications, and identification of these antigens then opens up the possibility of producing them synthetically in circumstances where bulk growth of the organism is impractical or isolation of the individual components too expensive.

Identification of protective antigens is greatly facilitated if one has an experimental model. If protection is antibody-mediated, one can try out different monoclonal antibodies and use the successful ones to pull out the antigen. Where antigenic variation is a major factor, desperate attempts are being made to identify some element of constancy which could provide a basis for vaccination, again using monoclonal antibodies with their ability to recognize a single specificity in a highly complex mixture. If protection is based primarily on T-cell activity, the approach would then be through the identification of individual T-cell clones capable of passively transferring protection. Switching back to humans, one seeks encouragement that the experimental models have kept the focus on the right target by confirming that the immune response to the antigen identified in the models correlates with protection in naturally infected individuals.

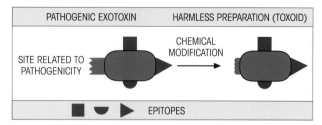

Figure 13.6. Modification of toxin to harmless toxoid without losing many of the antigenic determinants. Thus antibodies to the toxoid will react well with the original toxin.

The use of purified components

Bacterial exotoxins such as those produced by diphtheria and tetanus bacilli have long been used as immunogens. First, they must of course be detoxified and this is achieved by formaldehyde treatment, which fortunately does not destroy the major immunogenic determinants (figure 13.6). Immunization with the **toxoid** will therefore provoke the formation of protective antibodies, which neutralize the toxin by stereochemically blocking the active site, and encourage removal by phagocytic cells. The toxoid is generally given after adsorption to aluminum hydroxide which acts as an adjuvant and produces higher antibody titers. In addition to their use as vaccines to generate a protective antibody response against tetanus and diphtheria, the toxoids are often conjugated to other proteins, peptides or polysaccharides to provide helper T-cell epitopes for these antigens. Nontoxic variants of the toxins themselves, such as the CRM197 variant of diphtheria toxin, can also be used to provide helper T-cell epitopes for antigens such as the *Haemophilus influenzae* type-b (Hib) polysaccharide.

The emphasis now is to move towards gene cloning of individual proteins once they have been identified immunologically and biochemically. In general, a protein subunit used in a vaccine should contain a sufficient number of T-cell epitopes to avoid HLA-related unresponsiveness within the immunized population. In order to maintain a pool of memory B-cells over a reasonable period of time, persistence of antigen on the follicular dendritic cells in a form resistant to proteolytic degradation with retention of the native three-dimensional configuration is needed. Glycosylation of the protein contributes to this stability, but by the same token might not give a good T-cell response, so that the vaccine may need to be supplemented with a separate denatured source of T-cell epitopes. Purified polysaccharide vaccines are in a different category in that they normally require coupling to some immunogenic carrier protein, such as tetanus toxoid or mycobacterial heat-shock protein (figure 13.7), since they fail to

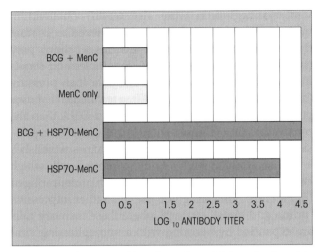

Figure 13.7. The carrier effect of mycobacterial heat-shock protein (hsp70) without adjuvant. Antibody responses to group C meningococcal polysaccharide (MenC) conjugated to hsp70 injected into mice with and without priming to the attenuated *Mycobacterium* BCG. (From Lambert P.-H., Louis J.A. & del Giudice G. (1992) In Gergely *et al.* (eds) *Progress in Immunology* **VIII**, pp. 683–689. Springer-Verlag, Budapest.)

stimulate T-helpers or induce adequate memory. This maneuver can give respectable antibody titers, but these will only be boosted by a natural infection if the carrier is derived from or related to the infecting agent itself.

Antigens can be synthesized through gene cloning

Recombinant DNA technology enables us to make genes encoding part or the whole of a protein peptide chain almost at will, and express them in an appropriate vector. We have already ruminated upon vaccinia virus and other recombinant vectors. Another strategy is to fuse the gene with the Ty element of yeast which self-assembles into a highly immunogenic virus-like particle. In a similar fashion, peptides can be fused with the core antigen of hepatitis B virus (HBcAg), which spontaneously polymerizes into 27 nm particles capable of eliciting strong T-cell help. A HBcAg-based vaccine incorporating *Plasmodium falciparum* circumsporozoite (CS) protein epitopes is currently undergoing clinical trials.

It is often desirable to develop vaccines which utilize the gene product on its own, incorporated in an adjuvant. Baculovirus vectors in moth cell lines produce large amounts of glycosylated recombinant protein, while yeast cells are used to express the hepatitis B surface antigen (HBsAg) used as a commercial vaccine. Stably transformed transgenic potatoes and tomatos are now being developed to express protein vaccines. Nearly two-thirds of volunteers who ate raw potato expressing HBsAg responded by producing increased

titers of antibodies to the hepatitis antigen. It is a sobering thought that a few hectares of fruit or veg could satisfy the annual global requirement for a single dose of oral immunogen.

DNA vaccines

Teams working with J. Wolff and P. Felgner experimented with a new strategy for gene therapy which involved binding the negatively charged DNA to cationic lipids which would themselves attach to the negatively charged surface of living cells and then presumably gain entry. The surprise was that controls injected with DNA without the lipids actually showed an *even higher uptake of DNA* and expression of the protein it encoded, so giving rise to the whole new technology of **DNA vaccination**. As Wolff put it: 'We tried it again and it worked. By the fourth or fifth time we knew we were onto something big. Even now I get a chill down my spine when I see it working.' Well, there is the real excitement of a blockbuster finding, even if, as usually happens to be the case, it arises from serendipity. It was quickly appreciated that the injected DNA functions as a source of immunogen *in situ* and can induce strong immune responses. So, now, vaccinologists everywhere are scurrying around trying to adapt the new technology. The DNA used in this procedure is sometimes referred to as **naked DNA** to reflect the fact that the nucleic acid is stripped bare of its associated proteins.

The transcription unit composed of the cDNA gene with a poly A terminator is stitched in place in a DNA plasmid with a promoter such as that from cytomegalovirus and a CpG bacterial sequence as a very potent adjuvant. It is usually injected into muscle where it can give prolonged expression of protein. Undoubtedly, the pivotal cell is the dendritic antigen-presenting cell which may be transfected directly, could endocytose soluble antigen secreted by the muscle cells into the interstitial spaces of the muscle, and could take up cells that have been killed or injured by the vaccine. The CpG immunostimulatory sequences engage toll-like-receptor-9 (TLR9) and thereby provoke the synthesis of IFNα and β, IL-12 and IL-18 which promote the formation of Th1 cells; this in turn generates good cell-mediated immunity, helps the B-cell synthesis of certain antibody classes (e.g. IgG2a in the mouse) and induces good cytotoxic T-cell responses, presumably reflecting the cytosolic expression of the protein and its processing in the MHC class I pathway. Let's look at an example. It will be recalled that frequent point mutations (drift; p. 274) in the gene encoding influenza surface hemagglutinin give rise to substantial antigenic variation,

bodies if it could be extracted from the molecular 'woodwork' so to speak.

Bearing in mind the many different circumstances we have discussed, the requirement may arise for a vaccine in which the good protective epitopes can be brought into the front line and dissociated from the molecular environment of the 'bad guys' which compromise the protective responses. In other words, we need to construct **epitope-specific vaccines**, preferably based on conserved regions, which provide broad defense. Several approaches are possible.

Epitopes can be mimicked by synthetic peptides

B-cell epitopes

Small peptide sequences corresponding to important epitopes on a microbial antigen can be synthesized readily and economically; long ones are rather expensive to manufacture. One might predict that, although the synthetic peptide has the correct linear *sequence* of amino acids, its random structure would make it a poor model for the *conformation* of the parent antigen and hence a poor vaccine for evoking humoral immunity. Curiously, this does not always seem to be a serious drawback. The 20-amino acid peptide derived from the foot and mouth virus-specific protein (VP1) evokes a good neutralizing response. The explanation has been forthcoming from X-ray structural analysis which shows the peptide sequence to be in a 'loop' region with blurred electron density indicative of dramatic disorder. In this case, the epitope is linear and evidently the flexibility of the loop structure may approach that of the free peptide which can thus mimic the epitope on the native VP1 molecule and stimulate a protective antibody response when used as a vaccine (figure 13.11a,b). Where the epitope is linear but is restricted in conformation by adjacent structures in the intact protein, immunization with free peptide tends to produce antibodies of disappointing affinity for the protein itself for the reasons outlined in figure 13.11c.

T-cell epitopes

Although short peptides may not have the conformation to stimulate adequate B-cell responses, they can prime antigen-specific T-cells as these recognize the primary sequence rather than the tertiary configuration of the protein. If the primed T-cells mediate CMI and possibly act to help B-cells make antibody, they could enable the host to have a head start in mounting an effective response on subsequent exposure to natural infection, and this would prove to be a useful prophylactic strategy.

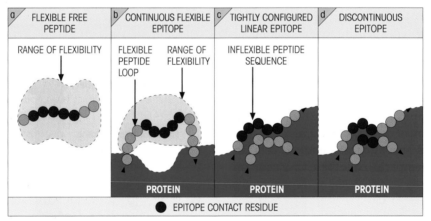

Figure 13.11. Structural basis for peptide mimicry of protein epitopes. (a) The free peptide is very flexible and can adopt a large number of structures in solution. (b) If the peptide sequence is present as a linear epitope on a part of a protein which is a flexible loop or chain, this will also exist in a variety of structures resembling the free peptide to a fair extent, and will behave comparably as an antigen and as an immunogen (vaccine) so that the peptide will raise antibodies which react well with the native protein. (c) If the linear epitope on the protein is structurally constrained (i.e. inflexible), it represents only one of the many structures adopted by the free peptide; thus if this peptide is used for immunization, only a minority of the B-cells stimulated will be complementary in shape to the native protein, so the peptide would be a poor vaccine for humoral immunity to microbes containing the protein antigen. (Note, however, that the antibodies produced would be good for Western immunoblots where the protein has been denatured after sodium dodecyl sulfate (SDS) treatment and the peptide structure is relatively free.) Preformed antibodies to the protein would react with the peptide, albeit with lower affinity, because energy must be used to constrain the peptide to the one structure which fits the antibody—just like the force used to restrain a madman in a strait-jacket. Where the sequence has a comparable degree of constraint in both peptide and protein, as in the disulfide-bonded loops in diphtheria toxin and hepatitis B surface antigen, antipeptide sera react reasonably well with the native protein. (d) Most commonly, the epitopes are discontinuous and, even if with difficulty we can predict the contact residues, the techniques for designing a peptide with appropriate structure are not robust, although some progress is being made using antibody to select from a random bacteriophage library in which the peptides are constrained on a structural scaffold, such as that supporting the Ig CDR3 loop.

We have already alluded to T-cell epitopes, often dominant and subject to high mutation rates, which can downregulate or subvert protective CMI responses. Under these circumstances, conserved peptide sequences which form **subdominant or cryptic epitopes** (cf. p. 211) **can function as effective vaccines**. The ineffectiveness of these sequences in providing adequate MHC–peptide levels to *prime* resting T-cells when the whole protein is processed by antigen-presenting cells can be side-stepped by immunizing with adequate doses of the preformed synthetic peptide. Because **primed**, as compared with **resting**, T-cells can be stimulated by much lower concentrations of MHC–peptide and do not necessarily require major costimulatory signals, they will react with infected cells which have processed and presented the cryptic epitopes; furthermore, because the primed T-cells will be directed against conserved sequences, they will therefore provide broad CMI protection against mutated strains.

A major worry about peptides as T-cell vaccines is the variation in ability to associate with the different polymorphic forms of MHC molecules present in an outbred population, which contributes to the immune response (*Ir*) gene effect described earlier (see p. 221). This is not quite as serious as it might be owing to groupings of HLA types into **supertypes** with common structural and functional features which enable them to recognize very similar peptide motifs. Given the huge number of allelic variants such groupings cannot be based on experimentally generated data for each allele and is therefore estimated from *in silico* analyses. So far, 11 class I supertypes (four HLA-As, five HLA-Bs, two HLA-Cs) and 12 class II supertypes (five HLA-DRs, three HLA-DQs, four HLA-DPs) have been identified using such approaches, covering the vast majority of individuals. Some peptide sequences are virtually universal T-cell epitopes in that they bind to multiple MHC supertypes. Examples include residues 326–345 of the malaria circumsporozoite protein, residues 106–130 and 166–193 of the mycobacterial MPB70 protein and residues 830–843 and 947–967 in tetanus toxin. These sequences can provide promiscuous (i.e. HLA-independent) T-cell helper epitopes to conjugate with peptide vaccines.

Making the peptides immunogenic

The immunogenicity of peptides for B-cells is invariably bound up with a dependence on T-cell help, and failure to provide linked T-cell epitopes is thought to be responsible for poor antibody responses to the foot and mouth disease VP1 loop peptide in cattle and pigs, and to polymers of the tetrapeptide asparagylalanylasparagylproline (NANP) of malarial circumsporozoite antigens in humans (cf. p. 306). When the general T-cell carrier, peptide 326–345 of the circumsporozoite protein (see above), was coupled to a (NANP)$_3$ tetramer repeat, good antibody responses were obtained in all strains of mice tested. Furthermore, after priming with this synthetic peptide, whole sporozoites would boost antibody titers. This brings up two points: first, as we have already noted, in order for the natural infection to boost, the T- and B-cell epitopes must both be present and, second, they must be linked so that the T-cell epitope is taken up for processing by the lymphocyte which recognizes the B-cell epitope (figure 8.12). This does not always imply that the link in the infectious agent must be covalent, since mice primed with the core antigen of hepatitis B virus gave excellent responses to the surface antigen when challenged with whole virions, i.e. an interstructural relationship may function in this regard as well as an intramolecular one. By contrast, animals immunized with an HBsAg B-cell peptide coupled with a streptococcal peptide T-cell carrier require boosting with the original vaccine but do not receive a boost from natural infection. Mycobacterial heat-shock proteins are excellent carriers for peptides even in the absence of adjuvants and irrespective of BCG priming (figure 13.7). In some cases, responses induced by protein carriers might suppress the ability of a second injection of the vaccine to boost peptide antibody levels through antigenic competition and, in this respect, peptides providing the carrier T-cell epitope have a distinct advantage. It is worth noting that the presentation of a peptide, such as the foot and mouth disease virus VP1 loop, in the form of an octamer coupled to a poly-L-lysine backbone produces responses of far greater magnitude than the monomer, a strategy which has proved successful when multiple clusters of peptides are linked to a small central oligolysine core as a multiple antigen peptide (MAP) in which the multiple peptide units may act as carriers for each other.

Notwithstanding these considerations, **the majority of protein determinants are discontinuous**, i.e. involve amino acid residues far apart in the primary sequence but brought close to each other by peptide folding (figure 13.11d; cf. p. 298). In such cases, peptides which represent linear sequences of the primary structure will, at best, only mimic part of a determinant and will generate low affinity responses. Defining a discontinuous determinant by X-ray crystallography, site-related mutagenesis and computer modeling takes a long time. Even when armed with this information, synthesis of a configured peptide which will topographically mimic the contact residues that constitute such an epitope still remains a serious challenge. Progress is being made in using monoclonal antibodies to select peptide epitopes binding with higher affinity from bacteriophage libraries of random hexa- or heptapeptides, which are constrained on a structural scaffold such as that holding the CDR3 loop in the immunoglobulin variable region. Well, we have already encountered this type of epitope. Since it would be selected by an antibody we would class it as an **anti-idiotype** and, likewise, if we used it as an immunogen it would be acting as an **idiotype**.

Anti-idiotypes can be exploited as epitope-specific vaccines

Internal image anti-idiotypes provide surrogates for discontinuous B-cell epitopes because, by definition, they possess a structure capable of binding with the antigen combining site of the idiotype antibody. Knowledge of the contact residues within the epitope is not necessary. Thus, from the spectrum of millions of different antibody shapes available, one selects those that have a closely complementary three-dimensional topographical configuration which facilitates effective binding (cf. figure 10.12). The antibodies can be selected from hybridoma clones (cf. p. 112) or phage display libraries of, for example, scFvs (cf. p. 115) (figure 13.12). Internal image anti-Ids could provide useful potential vaccines, particularly for carbohydrates which are notoriously poor immunogens in the very young. A number of examples of mimicry of epitopes on molecules such as hepatitis B surface antigen and yeast killer toxins have been reported.

Mutants which have lost unwanted epitopes can correctly fold desired discontinuous B-cell epitopes

The most natural way to achieve a correctly configured discontinuous B-cell epitope is to allow the protein to fold spontaneously. If the gene encoding the protein antigen is mutated so that the unwanted epitope is eliminated by replacement of its amino acid side-chains, without affecting the folding of the protein chain which generates the epitopes we wish to preserve, our object is achieved. Preservation of the desired epitopes and destruction of the 'bad' epitopes by 'genetic sandpapering' can obviously be monitored by following the reactivity of the mutants with the appropriate monoclonal antibody (figure 13.13). It will be apparent that 'bad' T-cell epitopes can also be eliminated by targeted mutations.

Sometimes, it is possible to mask an undesirable epitope by introducing additional glycosylation sites into the sequence. This approach has been used to mask epitopes on HIV-1 gp120 which provoke the production of antibodies which do not effectively neutralize the virus, the aim being to force the immune system to concentrate its efforts on those B-cell epitopes which elicit broadly neutralizing antibodies. In other cases, one can eliminate large unwanted segments of the antigen if the remaining peptide sequence can still fold correctly. Thus, immunization with the highly conserved extracellular domain of the influenza virus M2 antigen fused

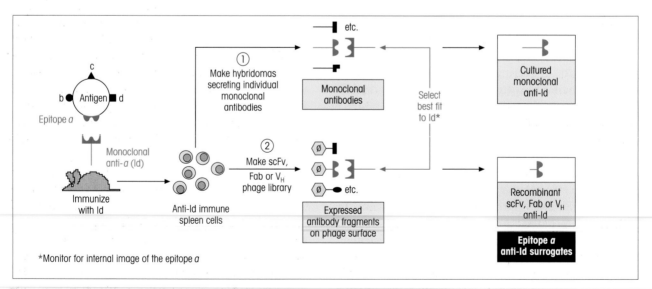

Figure 13.12. Derivation of anti-idiotypic mimics of a B-cell epitope. A high affinity monoclonal antibody (idiotype; Id) specific for the *a* epitope on the antigen is injected to generate an anti-Id response. Spleen cells from the immunized mice are used to make (1) a range of hybridomas, each secreting an individual monoclonal antibody, a small proportion of which will be internal image anti-Id, or (2) a phage library expressing surface antibody fragments. These are screened with the original monoclonal Id to select the best fitting anti-Id monoclonals or antibody fragments. These, in turn, are monitored for behavior as internal image of *a* through ability to block binding of the original Id to *a*, to bind to other anti-*a* monoclonals and to be recognized by a polyclonal antiserum raised against the antigen in other species. A successful candidate can then be produced in bulk to provide a surrogate vaccine for epitope *a*.

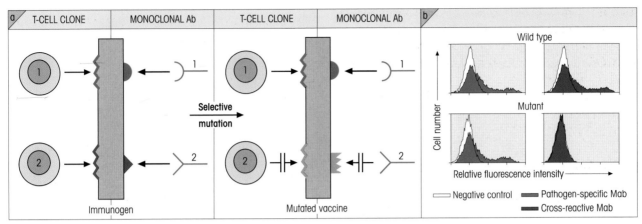

Figure 13.13. (a) Selective mutation of unwanted (dark blue) with retention of desirable (green) epitopes in a protein vaccine. Success of the mutation strategy can be monitored by reactivity with monoclonal antibodies (B-epitopes) and T-cell clones (T-epitopes). In this example, undesirable cross-reactive epitopes (such as might be shared between a pathogen and a self antigen) are mutated (orange) to avoid the unwanted cross-reactivity. For simplicity, the T-cell recognition of MHC–peptide has been ignored. (b) FACS analysis of cells transfected with the protein expressed on their surface, showing a mutant which retains the pathogen-specific epitope but has lost the cross-reactive epitopes characteristic of the wild-type protein.

to the N-terminus of the hepatitis B core protein gave 90–100% protection against lethal viral challenge and, bearing in mind the conserved nature of the antigen, this ought to cover a variety of influenza strains. Likewise, the isolated 19 kDa C-terminal fragment of the merozoite-specific protein MSP-1 confers antibody-mediated protection on monkeys to challenge with the blood stage of the malaria parasite.

CURRENT VACCINES

The established vaccines in current use and the schedules for their administration are set out in tables 13.3 and 13.4. Regional differences in immunization schedules reflect not only different degrees of perceived risk of infection but also other local considerations. Children under 2 years of age make inadequate responses to the T-independent *H. influenzae* capsular polysaccharide, so they are now routinely immunized with the antigen conjugated with tetanus toxoid or the CRM197 nontoxic variant of diphtheria toxin. The considerable morbidity and mortality associated with hepatitis B infection, its complex epidemiology and the difficulty in identifying high-risk individuals have led to routine vaccination in the USA from the time of birth. In the UK, BCG vaccination is routinely given. However, this is not the case in the USA where the fact that vaccination leads to individuals becoming positive to the Mantoux skin test, thus resulting in an inability to use this test as a means of excluding tuberculosis during the investigation of suspected infection, is seen as too much of a disadvantage. Due to the constant antigenic drift and occasional antigen shift that occurs with the influenza virus, a new

vaccine has to be produced each year for each hemisphere (figure 13.14).

VACCINES UNDER DEVELOPMENT

As with outer pharmaceutical agents, the development of vaccines comprises several stages. Successful preclinical studies in animal models are followed by phase I clinical trials in volunteers to initially evaluate safety and the immune response. If all goes well, phase II trials are then carried out in a small number of individuals to gain an indication of efficacy. If the phase II trial is successful, and the company and regulatory authorities decide to proceed, this is followed by a much larger (phase III) study to fully establish efficacy and safety, after which regulatory approval for distribution is given. Phase IV clinical trials finally establish efficacy and safety in large numbers of people. This whole process typically takes 12–15 years and hundreds of millions of dollars.

There are many vaccines currently under development for diseases where there is at present no vaccine available or where the vaccines that are available are left wanting (table 13.5). **Tuberculosis** is a good example of the latter situation. The Bacille Calmette-Guérin (BCG) vaccine has been in use for over 80 years but is only efficacious in protecting children and adolescents against disseminated and meningeal TB, and then only in some areas of the world, and is largely ineffective against the pulmonary TB which is the commonest form of the disease in adults. Indeed, TB remains a truly major problem in developing countries, and cases have also increased dramatically in Western countries. The

Table 13.3. Current licensed vaccines for use in USA and Europe.

Vaccine	Antigenic component	Use
Bacterial infections (+ viral in some combinations)		
Anthrax	Alum adsorbed protective antigen (PA) from *B. anthracis*	Individuals who handle infected animals or animal products. Laboratory staff working with *Bacillus anthracis*
BCG	Bacillus Calmette-Guérin live attenuated strain of *Mycobacterium bovis*	Children and adolescents in geographical regions where the vaccine has been shown to be effective, including UK. Not routinely used in the USA
Cholera	Inactivated *Vibrio cholerae* together with recombinant B-subunit of the cholera toxin	Drinkable oral vaccine for travelers to endemic or epidemic areas
Diphtheria, tetanus, pertussis, poliomyelitis, hepatitis B	Alum-adsorbed diphtheria toxoid, tetanus toxoid, acellular pertussis, inactivated poliomyelitis virus and recombinant hepatitis B virus surface antigen	Routine immunization of children
Diphtheria, tetanus, pertussis, poliomyelitis, *Haemophilus influenzae* type b	Another pentavalent combination vaccine, including *Haemophilus influenzae* type b capsular polysaccharides conjugated to tetanus toxoid or to the CRM197 nontoxic variant of diphtheria toxin	Routine immunization of children
Meningococcal group C	Four serotypes of meningococcus polysaccharide conjugated to diphtheria toxoid	Routine immunization of children in UK. As nearly all cases of childhood meningococcal disease in the UK are caused by groups B and C, the vaccine used for routine immunization contains only group C. A vaccine against meningococcal groups A, C, W-135 and Y is also available
Pneumococcal	Polysaccharide from either each of the 23 or from each of seven capsular types of pneumococcus, conjugated to diphtheria toxoid and adsorbed onto alum	Routine immunization of children (USA). Individuals at risk of pneumococcal infection, e.g. elderly, persons undergo splenectomy or with various chronic diseases (UK)
Typhoid fever	Vi polysaccharide antigen of *Salmonella typhi*	Travelers to countries with poor sanitation, laboratory workers handling specimens from suspected cases
Viral infections		
Hepatitis A	Alum-adsorbed inactivated hepatitis A virus	At risk individuals, e.g. laboratory staff working with the virus, patients with hemophilia, travelers to high-risk areas
Hepatitis B	Alum-adsorbed recombinant hepatitis B virus surface antigen (HBsAg)	Routine immunization of children (USA). Individuals at high risk of contracting hepatitis B (UK)
Influenza (inactivated)	Inactivated trivalent WHO recommended strains of influenza virus	Routine immunization of infants (USA). Individuals at high risk of complications from contracting influenza virus (UK)
Influenza (live attenuated)	Attenuated trivalent WHO recommended strains of influenza virus	Individuals aged 5–49 at high risk of complications from contracting influenza virus
Japanese encephalitis virus	Inactivated Japanese encephalitis virus	Individuals at risk of contracting Japanese encephalitis virus
Measles, Mumps and Rubella (MMR)	Live attenuated measles, mumps and rubella viruses	Routine immunization of children
Polio (Inactivated, Salk)	Inactivated poliovirus types 1, 2 & 3	Routine immunization of children. Protects against polio paralysis but does not prevent spread of wild polio virus (for which the oral polio vaccine [Sabin] containing live attenuated types 1, 2 & 3 virus is used)
Rabies	Inactivated rabies virus	At risk individuals
Tick-borne encephalitis	Inactivated tick-borne encephalitis virus	At risk individuals, e.g. working, walking or camping in infected areas
Varicella–zoster	Live attenuated varicella–zoster virus	Seronegative healthy children over 1 year old who come into close contact with individuals at high risk of severe varicella infections. Seronegative healthcare workers who come into direct contact with patients
Yellow fever	Live attenuated yellow fever virus	Those traveling or living in areas where infection is endemic, and laboratory staff who handle the virus or clinical samples from suspected cases

Vaccines separately containing the individual components of the polyvalent vaccines are also licensed.

Table 13.4. Recommended (by CDC in USA, NHS in UK) childhood and adolescent immunization schedules.

Vaccine	Immunization schedule
USA	
Hepatitis B	Three injections given at 0, 1 and 6 months old
Diphtheria (high dose), tetanus, acellular pertussis (DTaP)	Five injections given at 2, 4, 6 and 15 months old, and at 4–6 years old
Inactivated poliovirus (IPV)	Four injections given at 2, 4 and 6 months old, and at 4–6 years old
Haemophilus influenzae type b (Hib)	Two to three injections (depending on vaccine formulation) given at 2 and 4 (and 6) months old
Measles, mumps and rubella (MMR)	Two injections given at 12 months and 4–6 years old
Varicella	One injection at 12 months old in children that have not had chickenpox
Heptavalent pneumococcal conjugate vaccine (PCV)	Four injections given at 2, 4, 6 and 12 months old
Influenza	Annual injection in children aged 6–23 months old
Diphtheria (low dose), tetanus (Td)	One injection given at 11–12 years old
UK	
Diphtheria (high dose), tetanus, pertussis, inactivated poliovirus, *Haemophilus influenzae* type b (DTaP/IPV/Hib)	Three injections given at 2, 3 and 4 months old
Meningococcal group C (MenC)	Three injections given at 2, 3 and 4 months old
Measles, mumps and rubella (MMR)	Two injections given at 13 months and 3 years old
Diphtheria (low [d] or high [D] dose), tetanus, pertussis, inactivated poliovirus (dTaP/IPV or DTaP/IPV)	One injection given at 3 years old
BCG	One injection given at 10–14 years old (if skin test negative). Also given shortly after birth to at risk infants
Diphtheria (low dose), tetanus, inactivated poliovirus (Td/IPV)	One injection given at 13–18 years old

Figure 13.14. Influenza vaccine production timeline (Northern Hemisphere). The World Health Organization (WHO) Global Influenza Surveillance Network comprises 112 National Influenza Centres in 83 countries which continually isolate the local influenza viruses, carry out preliminary antigenic characterization, and send the viruses to four WHO Collaborating Centers in the USA, UK, Australia and Japan for detailed analysis. The information obtained forms the basis for the biannual WHO recommendations on which strains of virus are most likely to be dominant during the next northern and southern hemisphere winters. Two subtypes of influenza A and one of influenza B are selected for the next annual vaccine and in most cases one or two of the three virus strains will be the same as in the previous year. In the USA vaccine production by the manufacturers is coordinated by the Centers for Disease Control and Prevention (CDC) and the US Food and Drug Administration (FDA).

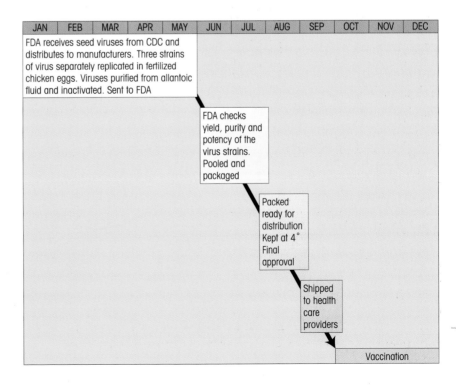

Table 13.5. Some examples of vaccines in the pipeline.

Vaccine	Antigenic component	Use
Bacterial infections (+ viral in some combinations)		
Borrelia burgdorferi	Recombinant outer surface proteins (Osp)	Lyme disease prophylaxis
Clostridium difficile	Toxoids A and B	Prophylaxis of *Clostridium difficile* infections
Diphtheria, tetanus, pertussis, poliomyelitis, *Haemophilus influenzae* type B, hepatitis B	Hexavalent combined vaccine containing the components of current pentavalent vaccine plus recombinant HBsAg	Infants, to minimize number of injections required. Some possible safety concerns have been raised
Meningococcus group B	Outer membrane proteins from multiple strains of group B meningococcus	Meningitis prophylaxis in infants
Neisseria meningitidis	Group A and C polysaccharide conjugated to tetanus toxoid	Meningitis prophylaxis
Salmonella typhi	Attenuated vaccine for oral immunization	Typhoid prophylaxis
Streptococcus group B	Pentavalent polysaccharide conjugated to streptococcal C protein	Prophylaxis against sepsis and meningitis caused by group B streptococcal infection in infants
Streptococcus pneumoniae	11-valent vaccine based on outer membrane protein D	Disease prophylaxis for children
Viral infections		
Cytomegalovirus	Trivalent DNA vaccine encoding phosphoprotein 65, glycoprotein B and immediate early 1 gene product	Prevention of congenital infection
Dengue	Attenuated tetravalent (serotype 1–4 viruses)	Prophylaxis of Dengue virus infections
Epstein–Barr virus	Recombinant gp220/350	EBV prophylaxis, including protection against infectious mononucleosis, Burkitt's lymphoma, nasopharyngeal carcinoma and other EBV-associated diseases
Hepatitis C virus	Recombinant E1	Hepatitis C prophylaxis
Hepatitis E virus	Recombinant ORF2	Hepatitis E prophylaxis
Herpes simplex virus	Attenuated virus	Genital herpes prophylaxis
Papillomavirus	Tetravalent virus-like particles (VLPs) 6, 11, 16 and 18	Prophylaxis against human papillomavirus infections, including prevention of cervical carcinoma
Ross river virus	Inactivated virus	Prophylaxis against epidemic polyarthritis caused by Ross river virus
Rotavirus	Attenuated virus	Oral, to prevent rotavirus-associated diarrhea and dehydration in infants. Replacement for withdrawn RotaShield vaccine which caused some cases of intussusception in vaccinated children (a condition in which one part of the intestine folds into itself)
Severe acute respiratory syndrome (SARS)-coronavirus	Recombinant spike protein (S protein)	SARS prophylaxis
Tick-borne encephalitis virus	Inactivated virus	Prophylaxis for at risk groups, particularly in areas of endemic infection including Russia, and Eastern and Central Europe
West Nile virus	Envelop genes in attenuated Yellow Fever virus vaccine replaced with West Nile virus envelop genes	Prophylaxis against West Nile virus

alarmingly heightened susceptibility to TB in individuals with HIV/AIDS has led to TB in up to half of HIV-infected individuals, and worldwide multidrug-resistant strains are appearing. This has led to an urgent search for improved vaccine candidates. Attempts have been made to increase the efficacy of BCG by either incorporating an additional copy of the Ag85B secretory protein gene or by inserting the gene for listeriolysin. In the latter case a potent CD8+ T-cell response was obtained in addition to the CD4+ T-cell response that is obtained with unmodified BCG. Other vaccine candidates utilize individual antigens isolated from *Mycobacterium tuberculosis* (Mtb), such as the 30 kDa major secretory protein (rBCG30). The Ag85A protein incorporated into modified vaccinia virus Ankara (MVA85A), currently undergoing clinical trials in the UK and Africa, induces enhanced CD4+ and CD8+ T-cell responses when used as a boost following priming with BCG. Other approaches include the use of fusion proteins constructed from two or more Mtb genes, for example between the Ag85B and TB10.4 antigens, or in the case of a vaccine candidate currently undergoing clinical trials in the USA, between the Mtb32 and Mtb39 antigens.

An extremely large number of vaccines against **HIV-1** (see Chapter 14) have undergone clinical trials in the hope of stemming the tide of this devastating disease. Immunogens that have been used include gp120, Env, Gag, Pol, Nef, reverse transcriptase, Tat, Rev, Vpu; in fact virtually every conceivable target, but so far the virus has continued to outwit the immune system by a variety of evasion strategies including a phenomenal rate of mutation.

VACCINES AGAINST PARASITIC DISEASES HAVE PROVED PARTICULARLY DIFFICULT TO DEVELOP

Malaria

Don't sneer at low technology. The major advance in malaria control has been the finding that the impregnation of bed nets with the insecticide pyrethroid reduces *Plasmodium falciparum* deaths by 40%. However, with the emergence of drug-resistant strains of mosquito, vaccines must be developed. The goal is achievable since, although children are very susceptible, adults resident in highly endemic areas acquire a protective but nonsterilizing immunity probably mediated by antibodies specific for the blood stages.

Antigen variation poses a big problem for vaccine development and a number of investigators in the malaria field have turned their attention to the invariant antigens of the **sporozoite**, which is the form with which the host is first infected; this rapidly reaches the liver to emerge later as merozoites which infect the red cells (figure 13.15). Because the sporozoite only takes 30

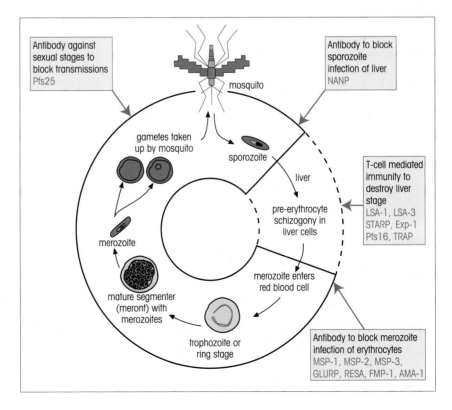

Figure 13.15. Strategies for malaria vaccines. Some examples of the many vaccine candidate molecules are shown. Eliciting the production of antibody against the NANP (Asn-Ala-Asn-Pro) repeats of the circumsporozoite antigen can block infection of hepatocytes. T-cell mediated responses, relying predominantly on IFNγ production, can target the liver stages. Vaccines which include merozoite surface antigens can be used to elicit antibodies able to block infection of the red blood cell. Finally, transmission blocking vaccines target gametocyte antigens such as Pfs25. AMA, apical membrane antigen; Exp1, exported protein-1; FMP, falciparum malaria protein; GLURP, glutamate-rich protein; LSA, liver stage antigen; MSP, merozoite surface protein; Pfs, *Plasmodium falciparum* surface protein; RESA, ring-infected erythrocyte surface antigen; STARP, sporozoite threonine and asparagine rich protein; TRAP, thrombospondin-related adhesive protein.

minutes to reach the liver, the antibody has to act fast, so that inactivation is limited by diffusion events and hence dependent on the concentration of antibody molecules. Other groups are focusing on blood stage antigens or specifically on antigens which elicit antibodies able to **block transmission**; these would be altruistic vaccines in that they only help the next guy down the line and finally the community as a whole.

Some of the different vaccine targets being deployed to counter this complex parasite are indicated in figure 13.15, and, ultimately, vaccines may contain antigens from all stages in the form of a DNA vaccine.

For the time being, a large number of malaria vaccines targeted at particular stages in the parasite life-cycle are in pre-clinical studies or undergoing clinical trials. As an amuse-bouche we will give you just a few examples to wet your appetite. The RTS,S pre-erythrocyte stage vaccine, designed to prevent parasite invasion of hepatocytes, contains most of the C-terminus of the *Plasmodium falciparum* circumsporozoite protein expressed with hepatitis B virus surface antigen (HBsAg). This malarial protein possesses 37 repeats of an immunodominant B-cell epitope, the tetrapeptide NANP (Asn-Ala-Asn-Pro). The RTS,S vaccine is the only malaria vaccine candidate that has so far prevented malaria in field trials. Thus, in a phase II trial involving approximately 2000 children in Mozambique, the vaccine led to a 37% lower prevalence of *P. falciparum* infection during a 6-month observation period. Another NANP-containing pre-erythrocyte stage vaccine candidate, ICC-1132, comprises a triple NANP repeat and two Th-cell epitopes, one of which is the previously mentioned 326–345 universal epitope able to bind a broad range of HLA class II alleles, incorporated into hepatitis B core antigen (HBcAg) which assembles into virus-like particles. The vaccine elicited *P. falciparum*-specific antibody and IFNγ-secreting malaria-specific T-cells in phase I trials. IFNγ is generally thought to be important in protection against the liver stage of the infection as, in various murine models, the level of protection is reduced by neutralizing antibody to the cytokine or in IFN-γR knock-out mice. The IFNγ may act by increasing MHC class I expression on hepatocytes, and by activating NK cells and macrophages to produce cytotoxic TNF and NO·. Also under development are vaccines containing multiple antigens, including a six pre-erythrocyte antigen polyprotein (LSA-1, LSA-3, STARP, Exp1, Pfs16 and TRAP) expressed in both MVA and fowlpox viruses and capable of inducing IFNγ-secreting T-cells specific for all six antigens. A blood stage vaccine comprising recombinant MSP1, MSP2 and RESA induced antibodies to all three antigens, stimulated IFNγ secreting MSP1-specfic T-cells, and led to a reduction of parasite

density in immunized children in Papua New Guinea. With so many candidate vaccines on the table it surely can only be a matter of time before effective vaccines for this major killer become available.

Schistosomiasis

The morbidity in this chronic and debilitating disease is related to the remarkable fecundity of the female worm which lays hundreds of eggs every day. These are deposited in numerous mucous membranes and tissues, and the granulomas which form around them (cf. figure 15.29) lead to the development of severe fibrotic and often irreversible lesions. Specific IgE can produce worm damage through *a*ntibody-*d*ependent *c*ellular *c*ytotoxicity (ADCC) mechanisms (cf. p. 31 and figure 12.23) involving eosinophils and possibly mononuclear phagocytes as effector cells, and may be regarded as a factor in recovery from infection together with Th1 CMI, schistosomes being susceptible to the lethal effects of NO· produced by activated macrophages. IgE, G and A antibodies correlate with resistance to reinfection in drug-cured patients, while IgA appears to control the reproductive capacity of the parasite as shown by passive transfer experiments. Our abilities to stimulate IgE and, to a lesser extent, IgA antibodies at will are, to put it mildly, still somewhat underdeveloped, but it is encouraging to note that a monoclonal antibody to the schistosomal glutathione-S-transferase inhibits the enzyme, protects against challenge and dramatically reduces the laying and viability of eggs. A vaccine based on the *Schistosoma haematobium* 28 kDa glutathione-S-transferase (Sh28-GST) vaccine has successfully undergone phase I clinical trials. Other vaccine candidates include the *Schistosoma mansoni* paramyosin (Sm97-paramyosin), a multiple antigen peptide (MAP) based on *S. mansoni* triose phosphatase isomerase (TPI), and a fusion protein of *S. mansoni* fatty acid-binding protein 14 (Sm14-FABP) fused to tetanus toxin fragment C.

Leishmaniasis

Approximately 1.5–2 million new cases of leishmaniasis occur annually, with increased rates of *Leishmania* infection being associated with HIV/AIDS. Candidate vaccine antigens include LmSTI1 (*Leishmania major* stress-inducible protein), TSA (*L. major* thiol-specific antioxidant protein) and LeIF (*L. major* initiation factor 4A). These have been combined into a polyprotein referred to as Leish-111f which, formulated with the TLR4 agonist monophosphoryl lipid A as an adjuvant, activates macrophages and dendritic cells and the secretion of IL-1, IL-12, TNF and GM-CSF resulting in strong Th1 responses. A phase I trial of the vaccine is currently underway in the USA.

VACCINES FOR PROTECTION AGAINST BIOTERRORISM

Biological warfare has a long and dark history. One early example occurred in 1346 when Tartars catapulted plague-infected bodies and heads over the city walls of the Black Sea town of Kaffa in an attempt to re-capture the town from the Genovese. In 1763, the British were fighting Delaware Indians and, as a supposed gesture of 'goodwill', donated smallpox-infected blankets to the Indians resulting in the death of many of the native tribes. Throughout the last century many countries throughout the world had biological weapons programs. Particularly alarming for citizens of the USA were the anthrax cases that occurred in late 2001 following exposure to mail items deliberately contaminated with anthrax spores and sent to news media offices in New York City and Boca Raton, Florida, and to two US Senators in Washington, DC. Aside from the anthrax (*Bacillus anthracis*), smallpox (variola) and plague (*Yersinia pestis*) mentioned above, many other infectious agents can potentially be used for bioterrorism including *Clostridium botulinum* toxin (botulism), *Francisella tularensis* (tularemia) and the Ebola, Marburg, Lassa and South American hemorrhagic fever viruses. Efforts are therefore underway to develop vaccines against these diseases in those cases where effective vaccines are not currently available. Following the eradication of smallpox, routine vaccination against smallpox was discontinued. Concern that this agent could be used as a biological weapon has led to calls for the re-introduction of routine vaccination against smallpox. Currently only a small number of laboratory researchers, key healthcare workers and military personnel are vaccinated because it is felt that routine vaccination of the entire population would inevitably lead to a small number of vaccine-related deaths, a scenario accepted when a disease is endemic but not for a currently 'extinct' disease. However, the vaccine is being stockpiled just in case. Incidentally, vaccination against smallpox would also protect against the related monkeypox virus.

IMMUNIZATION AGAINST CANCER

The realization that several different types of human cancer are closely associated with infectious agents rather obviously suggests that vaccination against agents such as human papilloma viruses (cervical cancer), Epstein–Barr virus (Burkitt's and other lymphomas, nasopharyngeal carcinoma), *Helicobacter pylori* (stomach cancer), hepatitis B virus (liver cancer), HTLV-1 (adult T-cell leukemia) and human herpesvirus 8 (Kaposi's sarcoma) should lead to a substantial reduction in the incidence of such tumors. Cancer vaccines have also been developed against a number of tumor-associated antigens including carcinoembryonic antigen (colorectal cancer), immunoglobulin idiotypes (B-cell lymphoma), MAGE (melanoma) and so on. Results to date have been somewhat less than spectacular using tumor-associated self antigens but there is hope that strategies such as targeted activation of dendritic cells will lead to improved response rates.

OTHER APPLICATIONS FOR VACCINES

A vaccine based on the human chorionic gonadotropin hormone, which is made by the preimplantation blastocyst and is essential for the establishment of early pregnancy, has undergone phase II clinical trials as an immunological contraceptive. The vaccine was highly effective in preventing pregnancy in the 80% of females who made sufficient levels of antibodies to bioneutralize the hormone, and since the effect of the vaccine was short lived in the absence of booster vaccination it could provide a reversible family planning option. Vaccines are also being developed for the treatment of allergies and autoimmune diseases. These are generally aimed at re-setting the Th1/Th2 balance, activating T regulatory cells, or re-establishing tolerance by clonal deletion or anergy. A vaccine for the treatment of addiction to tobacco consists of nicotine coupled to a bacteriophage Qb protein which assembles into a complex of 180 protein monomers to form virus-like particles (VLPs). The vaccine has shown efficacy in a phase II clinical trial in which there was a strong correlation between the levels of antibody induced against nicotine and continuous abstinence from smoking. An anti-cocaine vaccine consisting of a derivate of cocaine conjugated to recombinant cholera toxin B with alum adjuvant is also undergoing phase II clinical trials.

ADJUVANTS

For practical and economic reasons, prophylactic immunization should involve the minimum number of injections and the least amount of antigen. We have referred to the undoubted advantages of replicating attenuated organisms in this respect, but nonliving organisms, and especially purified products, frequently require an adjuvant which, by definition, is a substance incorporated into or injected simultaneously with antigen which potentiates the immune response (Latin *adjuvare*—to help). It is interesting that bacterial structures provide the major source of immunoadjuvants, presumably because they provide danger signals of infection, and it is no accident that the 'piggy-back' incorporation of the gene encoding an immunogen into attenuated *Salmonella* and BCG can be so effective. In a sense, the basis of adjuvanticity is often the recognition of these signals by pattern recognition receptors on accessory cells. The mode of action of adjuvants may be considered under several headings.

Depot effects

Free antigen usually disperses rapidly from the local tissues draining the injection site, and an important function of the so-called repository adjuvants is to counteract this by providing a long-lived reservoir of antigen, either at an extracellular location or within macrophages. The most common adjuvants of this type used in humans are **aluminum compounds** (phosphate or hydroxide). Empirically, it has long been realized that hydrophobic substances tend to augment immune responses, and Freund's incomplete adjuvant, in which the antigen is incorporated in the aqueous phase of a stabilized water-in-paraffin oil emulsion, usually produces higher and far more sustained antibody levels with a broadening of the response to include more of the epitopes in the antigen preparation. However, because of the lifelong persistence of oil in the tissues and the occasional production of sterile abscesses this adjuvant is not usually used in vaccines for use in humans except in the case of experimental anti-cancer vaccines where the possibility of such side effects is clearly more acceptable than with vaccines given to healthy children for infectious disease prophylaxis. Montanide ISA 720 and ISA51 are examples of more recently developed water-in-oil emulsions with improved safety profiles which make them more suitable for use in human vaccines.

Activation of antigen-presenting cells

Under the influence of the repository adjuvants, macrophages form granulomas which provide sites for interaction with antibody-forming cells. The maintenance by the depot of consistent antigen concentrations ensures that, as antigen-sensitive cells divide within the granuloma, their progeny are highly likely to be further stimulated by antigen. Virtually all adjuvants deliver antigens to antigen-presenting cells and stimulate them by improving immunogenicity through an increase in the concentration of processed antigen on their surface

and the efficiency of its presentation to lymphocytes, by the provision of accessory costimulatory signals to direct lymphocytes towards an immune response rather than tolerance, and by the secretion of soluble stimulatory cytokines which influence the proliferation of lymphocytes. For example, quite apart from the ability of mycobacterial hsp70 to act as a powerful carrier, its innate adjuvanticity (figure 13.7) is mediated through amino acids within the region 407-426 which bind to CD40 on dendritic cells and monocytes and thereby upregulate expression of CC chemokines and the proinflammatory cytokines TNF and IL-12. One of the most potent stimulators of antigen-presenting cells is lipid A from Gram-negative bacterial lipopolysaccharide (LPS), but it has many side-effects and interest has shifted to its derivative, monophosphoryl lipid A (MLA), which is less toxic. The **Ribi adjuvant**, a commonly used formulation in experimental work, is a water-in-oil emulsion incorporating MLA and mycobacterial trehalose dimycolate (TDM).

Effects on lymphocytes

In mice, alum tends to stimulate helper cells of the Th2 family, whereas complete Freund's adjuvant favors the Th1 subset. It will be recalled that complete Freund's is made from the incomplete adjuvant by addition of killed mycobacteria (cf. p. 203), but the immunopathological effects of the mycobacterial component in complete Freund's are so striking that its use in humans is not normally countenanced; fortunately, the active component has been identified as the water-soluble **muramyl dipeptide** (MDP; *N*-acetyl-muramyl-L-alanyl-D-isoglutamine) and a number of acceptable derivatives are now available. Hydrophilic MDP analogs with aqueous antigen preferentially stimulate antibody responses, but if administered in a hydrophobic microenvironment, such as mineral oil, or incorporated into liposomes, CMI is the major outcome.

The role of modulatory cytokines in these early immunologic interactions is important, and several experimental approaches are exploring the effect of cytokines administered simultaneously with antigen. In one study, a construct of the macrophage stimulator granulocyte–macrophage colony-stimulating factor (GM-CSF), linked to a monoclonal immunoglobulin, successfully induced anti-idiotypic responses relevant to the treatment of chronic lymphocytic leukemia. IL-2 has an adjuvant activity in unresponsive leprosy patients and a single injection in dialysis patients effectively induced their seroconversion to hepatitis B surface antigen. The potential of IL-12 to encourage Th1 responses is also being actively pursued.

Mucosal adjuvants

The need for adjuvants which stimulate mucosal immunity is being met by exploiting the ability of *E. coli* heat-labile enterotoxin (LT) and cholera toxin to target intestinal cells. LT is very immunogenic when given by the oral route and a nontoxic mutant with an arginine to glycine substitution at amino acid position 192 (LT_{R192G}) of comparable potency as an adjuvant has been developed for ultimate use in humans. Coupling a protein antigen to cholera toxin B subunit targets the vaccine to the epithelial cells of the intestinal tract and usually produces good IgG and IgA antibodies which appear also in the saliva, tears and milk, indicating that the antigen-specific IgA precursor cells become disseminated throughout the mucosal immune system. Synthetic oligonucleotides containing unmethylated CpG dinucleotide motifs have also been shown to act as effective mucosal adjuvants, stimulating the immune system by interacting with TLR9 and thereby promoting Th1 responses.

Newer approaches to the presentation of antigen

Recent interest has centered on the use of small lipid membrane vesicles (**liposomes**) as agents for the presentation of antigen to the immune system. It may be that the liposome acts as a storage vacuole within the macrophage or perhaps fuses with the macrophage membrane to provide a suitably immunogenic complex. The differing pathways for processing peptides within antigen-presenting cells can be turned to advantage by encapsulating antigen in acid-resistant liposomes so that they can only enter the MHC class I route and stimulate CD8 T-cells. Antigens within acid-sensitive liposomes become associated with both class I and class II molecules. Proteins anchored in the lipid membrane by hydrophobic means give augmented CMI. Short synthetic peptides coupled covalently to monophosphoryl lipid A or tripalmitoyl-*S*-glyceryl-cysteinyl-seryl-serine (P3CSS) have high priming efficiency. One can readily envisage the possibility of a single-shot liposome vaccine with multiple potentialities which incorporate several antigens, different adjuvants and specialized targeting molecules (figure 13.16).

Another innovation is the **Iscom** (immunostimulating complex), a hydrophobic matrix of the surfactant saponin, with antigen, cholesterol and phosphatidylcholine. Antigens with a transmembrane hydrophobic region, such as surface molecules of lipid-containing viruses, are powerfully immunogenic in this vehicle and may engender cytotoxic T-cell responses. Iscoms are extremely resistant to acid and bile salts and are

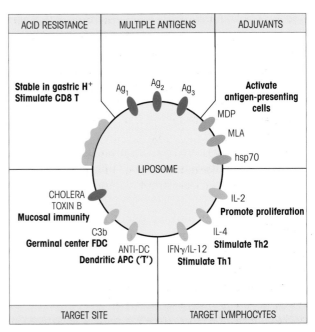

Figure 13.16. The 'do-it-all-in-one' omnipotent liposome particle illustrating some possible ways to build immunogenic flexibility into a single-shot liposome vaccine. The interior of the liposome may also contain depots of certain components. MDP, muramyl dipeptide; MLA, monophosphoryl lipid A; hsp70, mycobacterial heat-shock protein 70.

immunogenic by the oral route, producing systemic immunity and good local secretory IgA. Intranasal exposure established protective immunity to influenza in mice. Saponin itself, initially purified from the bark of the tree *Quillaja saponaria*, is too toxic for human use. A less toxic derivative, Quil A, is widely used for veterinary vaccines, but an even less toxic derivative, QS21, is being evaluated for safety and efficacy in clinical trials. Another group of surfactants, the nonionic block copolymers, which consist of blocks (chains) of hydrophobic polyoxypropylene attached to blocks of hydrophilic polyoxyethylene, are likely to be acceptable for use in humans. It may be useful to focus on the notion floated earlier that polymeric antigens tend to be more immunogenic, and to note a novel form of solid matrix of the Cowan strain of *S. aureus* which can bind several molecules of monoclonal antibody, which can, in turn, immobilize several molecules of antigen. Using a variety of monoclonals, one can purify onto their binding sites appropriate antigens from a mixture to give a multivalent subunit vaccine. One could also incorporate the *E. coli* enterotoxin mutants mentioned above to give good mucosal immunity.

With respect to the practicability and convenience of administration of vaccines, we should not ignore the use of the **biolistics gun** (cf. p. 147) to introduce gold microspheres coated with plasmids of the gene encoding the vaccine antigen or antigens (cf. p. 295). There have been some very important advances in the design of controlled-release systems for antigen delivery *in vivo*. Polymers of polylactic–polyglycolic esters are nontoxic biodegradable vehicles which can be prepared in a mixture of different formulations to provide **slow release** of an antigen (or any active drug or hormone) for periods up to several months.

Getting away from needles and guns, we have already mentioned intra-nasal immunization and edible vaccines. Another noninvasive option is transcutaneous immunization. Rather remarkably, addition of a CTL epitope from the model protein chicken ovalbumin to an ointment containing imiquimod, a chemical effective in the treatment of superficial basal cell carcinoma, led to potent activation of lymphocyte proliferation, IFNγ-production and CTL responses in mice. The fact that transcutaneous immunization allows direct access of antigens to the dendritic cells (Langerhans' cells) of the skin, and that imiquimod acts as an agonist of TLR7 and thereby induces the production of IL-12 and TNF, is unlikely to be purely coincidental.

There are exciting times ahead for vaccine development, but it should always be borne in mind that no matter how successful these clever strategies prove to be in experimental animals, the acid test which destroys so many promising approaches is their effectiveness in the human.

SUMMARY

Passively acquired immunity

• Passive immunity can be acquired by maternal antibodies or from IVIg.

• Horse antisera are more restricted because of the danger of serum sickness.

• Human monoclonal antibodies are being constructed to order using recombinant DNA technology.

Vaccination

• Active immunization provides a protective state through contact with a harmless form of the disease organism.

• A good vaccine should be based on antigens which are easily available, cheap, stable under extreme climatic conditions and nonpathogenic.

Killed organisms as vaccines

• Killed bacteria and viruses have been widely used.

Live attenuated organisms

• The advantages are: replication gives a bigger dose, the immune response is produced at the site of the natural infection.

• Attenuated fowlpox and modified vaccinia Ankara can provide a 'piggy-back' carrier for genes from other organisms which are difficult to attenuate.

• BCG is a good vehicle for antigens requiring CD4 T-cell immunity and salmonella constructs may give oral and systemic immunity. Intranasal immunization is fast gaining popularity.

• The risk with live attenuated organisms is reversion to the virulent form and danger to immunocompromised individuals.

Subunit vaccines

• Whole organisms have a multiplicity of antigens, some of which are not protective, may induce hypersensitivity or might even be immunosuppressive.

• It makes sense in these cases to use purified components.

• There is greatly increased use of recombinant DNA technology to produce these antigens. Expression in edible plants provides a very cheap way of achieving oral immunization.

• DNA encoding the vaccine subunit can be injected directly into muscle, where it expresses the protein and produces immune responses. The advantages are stability, ease of production and cheapness.

• Epitope-specific vaccines based on conserved structures have the advantage that they can provide broad protection and may avoid the possible deleterious effects of other epitopes (autoimmunity, T-downregulation, original antigenic sin, escape by mutation of immunodominant epitopes) when certain whole antigens are used for immunization.

• Epitope-specific vaccines can be based on peptides, internal image anti-idiotypes or epitope-loss mutants.

• Peptides may only usefully mimic the native protein for vaccination to produce antibody if the epitope is linear and relatively unconstrained in structure. Carriers such as tetanus toxoid or mycobacterial heat-shock proteins are needed to make the peptide immunogenic. Linear peptides can mimic T-cell epitopes in the whole protein.

• Epitope-loss mutants have undesirable epitopes replaced but still fold correctly to produce the wanted discontinuous B-cell epitope(s).

Current vaccines

• Children in both the USA and UK are routinely immunized with diphtheria and tetanus toxoids and acellular pertussis (DTP triple vaccine), attenuated strains of measles, mumps and rubella (MMR), inactivated polio, and the

(Continued p.311)

capsular polysaccharide of *H. influenzae* type b (Hib) linked to a carrier.

• Whilst in the UK and many other countries BCG is given at 10–14 years of age, or for high risk infants, immediately after birth, it is not used routinely in the USA.

• Vaccines against anthrax, Japanese encephalitis virus, hepatitis A, yellow fever, cholera and rabies, amongst others, are not given routinely but are available for travelers and high-risk groups.

Vaccines in development

• Vaccines against dengue, CMV, EBV, rotavirus, SARS, West Nile virus and a host of other infectious agents are currently at various stages in the development process.

• In malaria, experimental vaccines targeted at the pre-erythrocyte stage include those containing repeats of the circumsporozoite NANP tetrapeptide or aimed at the blood stage using merozoite surface proteins.

• Attempts are underway to make an improved vaccine against TB, either by enhancing the properties of BCG or using subunits from MTb such as the Ag85A protein inserted in modified vaccinia Ankara.

• Vaccines based upon a number of HIV-1 antigens including gp120, gag and pol have been tried, so far without success.

• Recombinant glutathione-*S*-transferase is a promising candidate for a vaccine against schistosomiasis.

• An oral vaccine composed of cholera toxin B subunit and killed vibrios induced good mucosal immunity to cholera.

• Where infectious agents are associated with the development of cancer, there is a clear potential for vaccination. It has so far proven more difficult to develop effective vaccines against tumor-associated self antigens.

• Autoimmunization against human chorionic gonadotropin, which is required for successful implantation of the fertilized ovum, can block fertility.

• Vaccines against nicotine and cocaine are undergoing clinical trials as anti-addiction agents.

Adjuvants

• Adjuvants work by producing depots of antigen, and by activating macrophages; they sometimes have direct effects on lymphocytes.

• Adjuvants such as the muramyl dipeptide analogs derived from mycobacterial cell walls and the monophosphoryl lipid A derivative from Gram-negative LPS may soon be in general use.

• Repetitive CpG dinucleotide sequences act as adjuvants for Th1 responses by stimulating through TLR9.

• New methods of delivery include linking the antigen to small lipid membrane vesicles (liposomes) or a special glycoside matrix (Iscom). These delivery particles can be furnished with many factors which improve their immunogenicity and flexibility. One can build in several antigens into the same particle, adjuvants such as MDP and MLA, cytokines to influence lymphocyte subset responses and molecules such as cholera toxin B and *E. coli* enterotoxin to target particular sites in the body.

• Antigens built into biodegradable polymers of varying half-life can provide single-shot vaccines which mimic a conventional course of immunization requiring several injections.

The overall strategies for vaccination are summarized in figure 13.17.

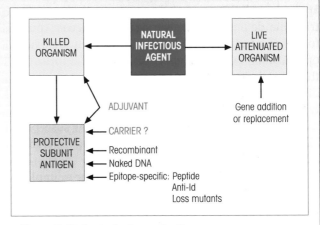

Figure 13.17. Strategies for vaccination.

FURTHER READING

Casadevall A., Dadachova E. & Pirofski L-A. (2004) Passive antibody therapy for infectious diseases. *Nature Reviews Microbiology* **2**, 695–703.

Donnelly J.J., Wahren B. & Liu M.A. (2005) DNA vaccines: progress and challenges. *Journal of Immunology* **175**, 633–639.

Mims C.A., Dockrell H.M., Goering R.V. *et al.* (2004) *Medical Microbiology*, 3rd edn. Mosby, London.

Moorthy V.S., Good M.F. & Hill A.V.S. (2004) Malaria vaccine developments. *Lancet* **363**, 150–156.

Neutra M.A. & Kozlowski P.A. (2006) Mucosal vaccines: the promise and the challenge. *Nature Reviews Immunology* **6**, 148–155.

Nossal G.J.V. (2000) The global alliance for vaccines and immunization—a millennial challenge. *Nature Immunology* **1**, 5.

Petrovsky N. & Aguilar J.C. (2004) Vaccine adjuvants: current state and future trends. *Immunology and Cell Biology* **82**, 488–496.

Plotkin S.A. & Orenstein W.A. (eds) (2004) *Vaccines* 4th edn. Saunders, Philadelphia, PA.

Zinkernagel R.M. (2003) On natural and artificial vaccinations. *Annual Review of Immunology* **21**, 515–546.

ated through the formation of fluid phase alternative pathway C3 convertase from the spontaneous hydrolysis of the internal thiolester of C3. There are several regulatory components on the red cell surface to deal with this. The C3 convertase complex is dissociated by decay accelerating factor (DAF; CD55) and by CR1 complement receptors (not forgetting factor H from the fluid phase; cf. p. 10), after which the C3b is dismembered by factor I in concert with CR1, membrane cofactor protein (MCP) or factor H (figure 14.3). There are also two inhibitors of the membrane attack complex, homolo-

gous restriction factor (HRF) and the abundant protectin molecule (CD59) which, by binding to C8, prevent the unfolding of the first C9 molecule needed for membrane insertion. DAF, HRF and CD59 bind to the membrane through glycosyl phosphatidylinositol anchors. In a condition known as **paroxysmal nocturnal hemoglobinuria (PNH)**, there is a defect in the ability to synthesize these anchors, caused by a mutation in the X-linked *PIG-A* gene encoding the enzyme required for adding *N*-acetylglucosamine to phosphatidylinositol. In the absence of these complement regulators, lysis of the red cells occurs. In the less severe type II PNH, there is a defect in DAF, but in the type III form, associated also with deficiency of CD59 and HRF, susceptibility to spontaneous complement-mediated lysis is greatly increased (figure 14.3). The erythrocytes can be normalized by adding back the deficient factors.

Factor H polymorphism, specifically the possession of a histidine rather than a tyrosine in the C-reactive protein and heparin-binding region at residue 402, predisposes towards the development of **age-related macular degeneration**.

An inhibitor of active C1 is grossly lacking in **hereditary angioedema** and this can lead to recurring episodes of acute circumscribed noninflammatory edema mediated by a vasoactive C2 fragment (figure 14.4). The patients are heterozygotes and synthesize small amounts of the inhibitor which can be raised to useful levels by administration of the synthetic anabolic steroid danazol or, in critical cases, of the purified

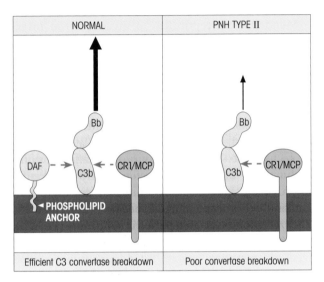

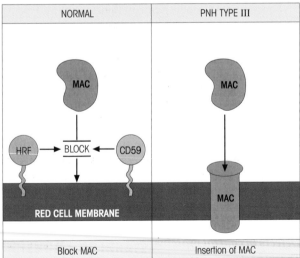

Figure 14.3. Paroxysmal nocturnal hemoglobinuria (PNH). A mutation in the *PIG-A* gene, which encodes α-1,6-*N*-acetyl glucosaminyltransferase, results in an inability to synthesize the glycosyl phosphatidylinositol anchors, deprives the red cell membrane of complement control proteins and renders the cell susceptible to complement-mediated lysis. Type II is associated with a DAF defect and the more severe type III with additional CD59 and HRF deficiency. DAF, decay accelerating factor; CR1, complement receptor type 1; MCP, membrane cofactor protein; HRF, homologous restriction factor; MAC, membrane attack complex.

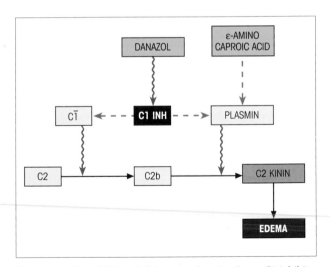

Figure 14.4. C1 inhibitor deficiency and angioedema. C1 inhibitor stoichiometrically inhibits C1, plasmin, kallikrein and activated Hageman factor and deficiency leads to formation of the vasoactive C2 kinin by the mechanism shown. The synthesis of C1 inhibitor can be boosted by methyltestosterone or preferably the less masculinizing synthetic steroid, danazol; alternatively, attacks can be controlled by giving ε-aminocaproic acid to inhibit the plasmin.

inhibitor itself. ε-Aminocaproic acid, which blocks the plasmin-induced liberation of the C2 kinin, provides an alternative treatment.

Deficiency of components of the complement pathway

Deficiencies in C1q, C1r, C1s, C4 and C2 predispose to the development of immune complex diseases such as SLE (cf. p. 435), perhaps due to a decreased ability to mount an adequate host response to infection with a putative etiologic agent or, more probably, to eliminate antigen–antibody complexes effectively (cf. p. 352). Bearing in mind the focus of the autoimmune response in SLE on the molecular constituents of the blebs appearing on the surface of apoptotic cells (cf. p. 436), the importance of C1q in binding to and clearing these apoptotic bodies becomes paramount. So it is that C1q-deficient mice develop high titer antinuclear antibodies and die with severe glomerulonephritis.

Permanent deficiencies in C5, C6, C7, C8 and C9 can all occur in humans, yet in virtually every case the individuals are healthy and not particularly prone to infection, apart from an increased susceptibility to disseminated *Neisseria gonorrhoeae* and *N. meningitidis*. Thus full operation of the terminal complement system does not appear to be essential for survival, and adequate protection must be largely afforded by opsonizing antibodies and the immune adherence mechanism.

Approximately 5% of individuals have mutations that lead to reduced levels of mannose-binding lectin (MBL). Although in some studies these individuals have been reported to have an increased incidence of both bacterial and viral infections, other studies have failed to find an association. In most instances complement activation by other mammalian lectins such as ficolin, or indeed by the antibody-mediated classical pathway, compensates for the absence of the MBL-mediated pathway. Deficiency of MBL-associated serine protease-2 (MASP-2) has been reported to increase susceptibility to infection with *Streptococcus pneumoniae*.

PRIMARY B-CELL DEFICIENCY

X-Linked (Bruton-type) agammaglobulinemia is due to early B-cell maturation failure

X-linked agammaglobulinemia (XLA) is one of several immunodeficient syndromes which have been mapped to the X chromosome (figure 14.5). The defect occurs at the pre-B-cell stage and the production of immunoglobulin in affected males is grossly depressed, there being few lymphoid follicles or plasma cells in lymph node

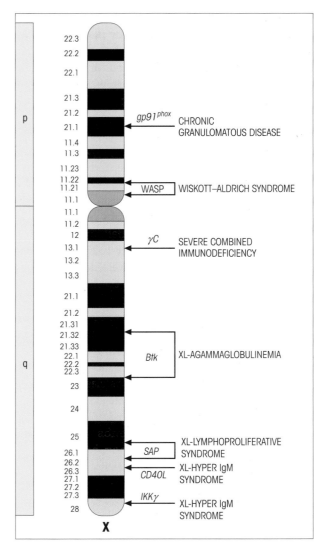

Figure 14.5. Loci of the X-linked (XL) immunodeficiency syndromes. Males are more likely to be affected by X-linked recessive genes because, unlike the situation with females where there are two X chromosomes, homozygosity is not needed. In some cases the precise location of the relevant gene is still to be ascertained.

biopsies. Mutations occur in Bruton's tyrosine kinase (*Btk*) gene, as is also seen in *xid* mice. The children are subject to repeated infection by pyogenic bacteria— *Staphylococcus aureus*, *Streptococcus pyogenes* and *S. pneumoniae*, *Neisseria meningitidis*, *Haemophilus influenzae* — and by a protozoan, *Pneumocystis carinii*, which produces a strange form of pneumonia. Cell-mediated immune responses are normal and viral infections are readily brought under control.

Mutations in either the μ heavy chain or the $λ_5$ chain, which contribute to the surrogate IgM receptor on pre-B-cells (cf. p. 247), result in a phenotype similar to that seen in XLA with arrest at the pro-B stage. The implication would be that *Btk* provides the signal for pro- to pre-B differentiation through this pre-B-cell receptor complex. Other mutations which cause a similar phenotype include those in the genes for the Igα (CD79a) signal transducing protein and for the BLNK B-cell *link*er protein which is again required for the transition from pro-B to pre-B-cells.

IgA deficiency and common variable immunodeficiency (CVID) have a similar genetic basis

These diseases, which are the first and second most common primary immunodeficiencies, represent the extreme ends of a spectrum of immunoglobulin deficiencies. IgA deficiency, which may include IgG2, and CVID often occur within the same family, and individual family members may gradually convert from one disease to the other. The major CVID/IgA deficiency susceptibility locus, *IGAD1*, maps to the HLA-DQ/DR region of the MHC. Most patients have a defect in T-cell priming by antigen which might be attributable to an antigen-presenting cell dysfunction. They also have a pattern of raised CD8 IFNγ production, increased expression of HLA-DR and Fas by CD4 cells and an increased rate of apoptosis. Restrictions in the T-cell repertoire can occur, and autoantibodies are often present. A few patients with adult onset CVID have been shown to have a homozygous loss of ICOS, the *in*ducible *co*stimulator involved in T-cell activation. CVID patients can be protected against recurrent pyogenic infections with intravenous gammaglobulin.

Transient hypogammaglobulinemia is seen in early life

A degree of immunoglobulin deficiency occurs naturally in human infants as the maternal IgG level wanes, and may become a serious problem in very premature babies. A more protracted **transient hypogammaglobulinemia of infancy**, characterized by recurrent respiratory infections, is associated with low IgG levels which often return to normal by 4 years of age. There is a deficiency in the number of circulating lymphocytes and in their ability to generate help for Ig production by B-cells activated by pokeweed mitogen, but this becomes normal as the disease resolves spontaneously.

PRIMARY T-CELL DEFICIENCY

Patients with no T-cells or poor T-cell function are vulnerable to opportunistic infections and, since B-cell function is to a large extent T-dependent, T-cell deficiency also impacts negatively on humoral immunity. Dysfunctional T-cells often permit the emergence of allergies, lymphoid malignancies and autoimmune syndromes, the latter presumably arising from ineffi-

cient negative selection in the thymus or the failure to generate appropriate regulatory cells.

Some deficiencies affect early T-cell differentiation

The **DiGeorge** and **Nezelof syndromes** are characterized by a failure of the thymus to develop properly from the third and fourth pharyngeal pouches during embryogenesis (DiGeorge children also lack parathyroids and have severe cardiovascular abnormalities). Consequently, stem cells cannot differentiate to become T-lymphocytes and the 'thymus-dependent' areas in lymphoid tissue are sparsely populated; in contrast, lymphoid follicles are seen but even these are poorly developed (figure 14.6). Cell-mediated immune responses are undetectable and, although the infants can deal with common bacterial infections, they may be overwhelmed by live attenuated vaccines such as measles or bacille Calmette–Guérin (BCG) if given by mistake. Antibodies can be elicited, but the response is subnormal, reflecting the need for the cooperative involvement of T-cells. (The similarity of this condition to neonatal thymectomy and of B-cell deficiency to neonatal bursectomy in the chicken should not go unmentioned.) Treatment by grafting neonatal thymus leads to restoration of immunocompetence, but some matching between the MHC on the nonlymphocytic thymus cells and peripheral cells is essential for the proper functioning of the T-lymphocytes (p. 236). Complete absence of the thymus is pretty rare and more often one is dealing with a 'partial DiGeorge' in which the T-cells may rise from 6% at birth to around 30% of the total circulating lymphocytes by the end of the first year (compared to 60–70% in normal one year olds); antibody responses are adequate.

Mutation of the gene encoding the purine degradation enzyme, **purine nucleoside phosphorylase**, results in the accumulation of the metabolite deoxy-GTP which is toxic to T-cell precursors through its ability to inhibit ribonucleotide reductase, an enzyme required for DNA synthesis. Targeting of the T-cell lineage by this deficiency could well be linked to a relatively low level of 5'-nucleotidase. Some T-cells 'leak through' but they give inadequate protection against infection and the disease is usually fatal unless a bone marrow transplant lifeline is offered. In addition to recurrent infections, patients usually suffer from neurologic dysfunction and autoimmunity.

Mutations in the recombinase enzymes, RAG-1 and RAG-2 (cf. figure 3.24), which initiate *VDJ* recombination events, usually result in complete failure to generate mature antigen-specific lymphocyte receptors and give rise to the severe combined immunodeficiency

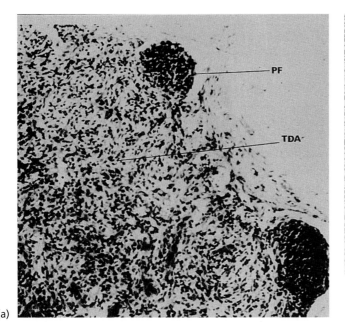

(a)

(b)

Figure 14.6. Lymph node cortex. (a) From patient with DiGeorge syndrome showing depleted thymus-dependent area (TDA) and small primary follicles (PF); (b) from normal subject: the populated T-cell area and the well-developed secondary follicle with its mantle of small lymphocytes (M) and pale-staining germinal center (GC) provide a marked contrast. (DiGeorge material kindly supplied by Dr D. Webster; photograph by Mr C.J. Sym.) In the murine model, the athymic nude mouse, there is an abnormality in the winged helix protein.

(SCID) phenotype (see below). In **Omenn syndrome**, the particular mutations in RAG allow some T-cells, apparently mostly of the Th2 phenotype, to sneak through because VDJ recombination is not completely abolished, although they are not capable of preventing a failure to thrive and relatively early death. Patients often exhibit eosinophilia and raised IgE, and sometimes have autoimmune disease affecting the skin and gut. **MHC class II deficiency**, 'bare lymphocyte syndrome', is associated with recurrent bronchopulmonary infections and chronic diarrhea occurring within the first year of life, with death from overwhelming viral infections at a mean age of 4 years. The condition arises from mutations affecting the *class II transactivator* (CIITA), RFXB, RFX5 and RFXAP promoter proteins that bind to the 5'-untranslated region of the class II genes. Feeble expression of class II molecules on thymic epithelial cells grossly impedes the positive selection of CD4 T-helpers, and those that do leak through will not be encouraged by the lack of class II on antigen-presenting cells. Note also that rare patients with mutations in *TAP-1* or *TAP-2* have an MHC class I bare lymphocyte syndrome.

Deficiencies leading to dysfunctional T-cells

Cell-mediated immunity (CMI) is depressed in immunodeficient patients with **ataxia telangiectasia** or with thrombocytopenia and eczema (**Wiskott–Aldrich syndrome**). The *Wiskott–Aldrich syndrome protein* (**WASP**) plays a critical role in linking signal transduction pathways and the actin-based cytoskeleton by clustering physically with actin through the GTPase Cdc42 and the Arp2/3 (*actin-related protein*) complex which regulate actin polymerization. Mutations in the *WASP* gene thus adversely affect T-cell motility, phagocyte chemotaxis, dendritic cell trafficking and the polarization of the T-cell cytoskeleton towards the B-cells during T–B collaboration. Poor cell-mediated immunity and impaired antibody production in affected boys are hardly surprising consequences.

Ataxia telangiectasia, a **chromosomal breakage syndrome,** is a human autosomal recessive disorder of childhood characterized by progressive cerebellar ataxia with degeneration of Purkinje cells, a hypersensitivity to X-rays and an unduly high incidence of cancer. The *ataxia telangiectasia mutated* (*ATM*) gene encodes the Atm protein kinase, a member of the phosphatidylinositol 3-kinase family. Following ultraviolet or ionizing radiation, the normal gene acts through the tumor suppressor protein p53 and thence p21 to arrest the cell cycle at the G1–S border, and through the Chk2 kinase and Cdc25 to block the G2–M transition. Presumably, the cellular DNA repair mechanisms now have a chance to operate. Furthermore, the Atm kinase is required for hematopoietic stem cell self-renewal by inhibiting oxidative stress in these cells. Another disease characterized by immune dysfunction, radiation sensitivity and increased incidence of cancer is the **Nijmegen breakage syndrome** where a mutation in the *NBS1* gene leads to a defect in a component, nibrin, of a double-stranded DNA repair complex. Both Atm and nibrin are required for efficient class switch recombination in B-cells.

It is exciting to see the molecular basis of diseases being unraveled and an excellent example of nature yielding its secrets has been provided by studies on the **hyper-IgM syndrome**, a rare disorder characterized by recurrent bacterial infections, very low levels or absence of IgG, IgA and IgE and normal to raised concentrations of serum IgM and IgD. Most patients have an X-linked form of the disease involving point mutations and deletions in the T-cell CD40L (CD154). These mutations largely map to the part of the molecule involved in the interaction with B-cell CD40 (cf. p. 183), thereby rendering the T-cells incapable of transmitting the signals needed for Ig class switching in B-cells. Less commonly, mutation of the X-linked IKK (*i*nhibitor of *k*appa light chain enhancer *k*inase) γ chain gene, or the autosomal *CD40*, activation-induced cytidine deaminase (*AID*) or uracil-DNA glycosylase (*UNG*) genes are responsible. In these cases it is the B-cells rather than the helper T-cell that are defective.

'Immunodeficiency' affecting regulatory or tolerance mechanisms will result in an undesirable enhancement of particular types of immune response. Thus, given the critical role of Foxp3 in the induction of regulatory T-cells, it will come as no surprise to hear that loss-of-function mutations in the Foxp3 gene have a profound effect, being responsible for the IPEX (*i*mmune dysregulation, *p*olyendocrinopathy, *e*nteropathy, *X*-linked) syndrome in which unregulated T-cell activity leads to multisystemic and often fatal autoimmune disease. The somewhat less severe clinical condition referred to as APECED (*a*utoimmune *p*olyendocrinopathy-candidiasis-*e*ctodermal *d*ystrophy) is due to mutations in the *AIRE* gene leading to inadequate central tolerance of T-cells.

Rare cases of T-cell functional deficiency arise from mutation in the γ chain of the CD3 complex and the ZAP-70 kinase (p. 174).

COMBINED IMMUNODEFICIENCY

In the primary T-cell deficiencies described above there are at least some mature T-cells present, albeit functionally defective. However, in severe combined immunodeficiency disease (SCID) there is normally an absolute failure in T-cell development and therefore SCID represents the most severe form of primary immunodeficiency, affecting one child in approximately every 80 000 live births. These infants exhibit profound defects in cellular and humoral immunity, with death occurring within the first year of life due to severe and recurrent opportunistic infections. Prolonged diarrhea resulting from gastrointestinal infections and pneumonia due to *Pneumocystis carinii* are common; *Candida albicans* grows vigorously in the mouth or on the skin. If vaccinated with attenuated organisms these infants usually die of progressive infection.

Several different gene defects can be responsible for the development of SCID

Mutations in several different genes can cause SCID, which involves a block in T-cell development together with a direct or indirect B-cell deficiency. In some cases NK cells also fail to develop (figure 14.7).

Cytokine signaling pathway defects
Approximately 40% of patients with SCID have mutations in the **common γ (γ_c) chain** of the receptors for interleukins IL-2, -4, -7, -9, -15 and -21. Of these, IL-7R is

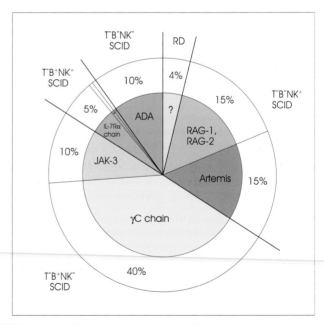

Figure 14.7. Genetic defects responsible for severe combined immunodeficiency (SCID). There may be a few rare cases of SCID in which other genes are mutated. Mutations in CD45 [*] or either CD3δ or CD3ε [†] each account for <1% of SCID cases. The SCID phenotype is dependent upon the particular gene defect that is responsible. Thus in the 15% of SCID cases caused by mutation of the artemis gene there is a complete lack of both T- and B-cells but NK cells are present (i.e. T⁻B⁻NK⁺ SCID). The gene defect responsible for reticular dysgenesis (RD), a condition in which T, B, NK, myeloid cells and platelets are all affected to varying degrees, has yet to be identified.

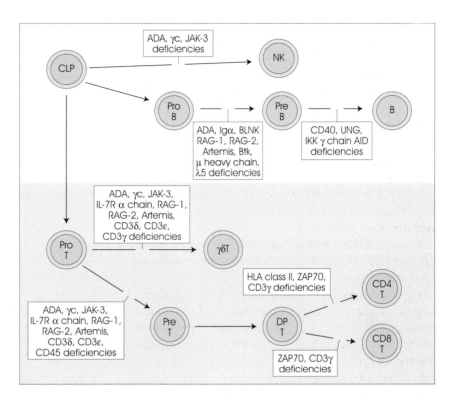

Figure 14.8. Blocks in lymphocyte development result in immunodeficiency. The site and nature of the mutation will determine the extent to which the function of the gene product is compromised. Thus, although homozygous inheritance of the mutated gene will often lead to an absolute block in development of the relevant lymphocyte populations, some mutations only cause a partial block in development. Furthermore, even some loss of function mutations will only partially abrogate lymphocyte differentiation. This is the case with CD3 γ chain and HLA class II deficiencies where the consequences are usually less severe than in many other immunodeficiencies. CLP, common lymphoid progenitor; DP, double positive.

the most crucial for lymphocyte differentiation, and mutations in the interleukin-specific **IL-7R α chain**, or in **JAK-3** which transduces the γ_c signal, also result in SCID (figure 14.8).

SCID can arise from grossly deficient VDJ recombination

Unlike the sneak through of immunocompetent T-cells which accompanies the partial *RAG* deficiency in Omenn syndrome, grossly dysfunctional mutations in the recombinase enzymes, which catalyze the introduction of the double-stranded breaks permitting subsequent recombination of the *V, D* and *J* segments, prevent the emergence of any mature lymphocytes (figure 14.8). Failure of the VDJ recombination mechanism is also a feature of the radiosensitive cells from those SCID patients with a defective Artemis gene. Artemis is an essential component of the DNA-dependent protein kinase complex which realigns and repairs the free coding ends created by the RAG enzymes.

Other causes of SCID

Ten percent of SCID patients have a genetic deficiency of the purine degradation enzyme, adenosine deaminase (ADA), which results in the accumulation of the metabolite, dATP, which is toxic to early lymphoid progenitor cells (figure 14.8). If either the CD3 δ or ε chain of the T-cell receptor complex is mutated there is a block in T-cell development, in marked contrast to the CD3 γ

chain deficiency mentioned previously which does not prevent T-cell differentiation but does result in defective T-cell activation. Mutations of the CD45 protein tyrosine phosphatase can also give rise to SCID in very rare instances. **Reticular dysgenesis**, the genetic basis of which remains unclear, is a rapidly fatal variant of severe combined immunodeficiency associated with a lack of both myeloid and lymphoid cell precursors.

Combined immunodeficiency resulting from inherited defective control of lymphocyte function

X-linked lymphoproliferative disease (XLP), or Duncan's syndrome, is a progressive immunodeficiency disorder characterized by fever, pharyngitis, lymphadenopathy and dysgammaglobulinemia (i.e. a selective deficiency of one or more, but not of all, the classes of antibody). Patients are particularly vulnerable to Epstein–Barr viral infection. Mutations occur in the *SH2DIA/SAP* gene encoding SAP (*s*ignaling lymphocytic *a*ctivation molecule (SLAM)-*a*ssociated *p*rotein) which binds to SLAM through its SH2 domain. Since triggering of SLAM leads to strong induction of IFNγ in T-cells and acts on B-cells to enhance proliferation and increase susceptibility to apoptosis, mutations in SAP which adversely affect the activation of SLAM will weaken the immune response, especially with regard to EBV infection where viral replication in B-cells is heavily controlled by host T-cells.

RECOGNITION OF IMMUNODEFICIENCIES

Defects in immunoglobulins can be assessed by quantitative estimations; levels of 2 g/l arbitrarily define the practical lower limit of normal. The humoral immune response can be examined by first screening the serum for natural antibodies (A and B isohemagglutinins, heteroantibody to sheep erythrocytes, bactericidins against *E. coli*) and then attempting to induce active immunization with diphtheria, tetanus, pertussis and killed poliomyelitis—but no live vaccines. CD19, CD20 and CD22 are the main markers used to enumerate B-cells by immunofluorescence.

Patients with T-cell deficiency will be hypo- or unreactive in skin tests to such antigens as tuberculin, *Candida* and mumps. Active skin sensitization with dinitrochlorobenzene may be undertaken. The reactivity of peripheral blood mononuclear cells to the phytohemagglutinin mitogen is a good indicator of T-lymphocyte reactivity as is also the one-way mixed lymphocyte reaction (see Chapter 16). Enumeration of T-cells is most readily achieved by cytofluorimetry using CD3 monoclonal antibody.

In vitro tests for complement and for the bactericidal and other functions of neutrophils are available, while the reduction of nitroblue tetrazolium (NBT) or the stimulation of superoxide production provides a measure of the oxidative enzymes associated with active phagocytosis.

TREATMENT OF PRIMARY IMMUNODEFICIENCIES

Early intervention with antibiotics is of immediate importance, with the option of long-term low dose prophylactic antibiotics to prevent reinfection and subsequent complications such as hearing loss following otitis media (infection of the middle ear). As already mentioned above, if a suitable matched donor is available then bone marrow or hematopoietic stem cell transplantation is the treatment of choice and has led to reconstitution of immune responses in patients with various primary immunodeficiencies including SCID, leukocyte adhesion deficiency, Chediak–Higashi disease and Wiskott–Aldrich syndrome. In patients with ADA⁻ SCID for whom no matched donor is available, the missing enzyme can be replaced by weekly intramuscular injections of bovine ADA conjugated to polyethylene glycol, the latter phenomenally improves the biological half-life of ADA from a few minutes for the free enzyme to 48–72 hours for the conjugate.

Deficiencies affecting humoral responses can to some extent be compensated for by intravenous immunoglobulin (IVIg) given every 3–4 weeks. Where innate responses are compromised, cytokine therapy can be helpful, for example by stimulating the defective phagocytes in chronic granulomatous disease by injections of interferon gamma.

The ideal treatment where a matched transplant is not available is correction of the gene defect. The first gene therapy trials for primary immunodeficiencies were initiated over 15 years ago and there has been a steady improvement in this approach, with some setbacks along the way. The majority of patients treated by this procedure have been those with ADA⁻ SCID in which the normal gene for ADA is inserted into a retroviral vector which is then used to introduce the functional gene into the patient's own CD34⁺ stem cells (figure 14.9). More recently this approach has been extended to the replacement of the defective γ_c cytokine receptor gene in patients with this form of SCID, although in this case more caution is required as a very small number of these patients have developed leukemia following treatment. However, in both types of SCID the gene therapy approach has led to a sustained clinical benefit with restoration of immune responses to common pathogens. Future progress will depend upon improvements in vector design to enhance the efficiency and safety of the gene transfer, and a more precise targeting of the gene integration sites. The use of self-inactivating lentiviral vectors (lentiviruses, which include HIV, are a subfamily of retroviruses) incorporating tissue-specific promoters has been proposed, although their efficacy and safety remain to be established.

SECONDARY IMMUNODEFICIENCY

Immune responsiveness can be depressed nonspecifically by many factors. CMI in particular may be impaired in a state of malnutrition, even of the degree which may be encountered in urban areas of the more affluent regions of the world. Iron deficiency is particularly important in this respect, as are zinc and selenium deficiencies.

Viral infections are not infrequently immunosuppressive, and the profound fall in cell-mediated immunity which accompanies **measles infection** has been attributed to specific suppression of IL-12 production by viral cross-linking of monocyte surface CD46 (membrane cofactor protein; cf. p. 314). The most notorious immunosuppressive virus, human immunodeficiency virus (HIV), will be elaborated upon in the next section. In lepromatous leprosy and malarial infection there is evidence for a constraint on immune responsiveness imposed by distortion of the normal lymphoid traffic pathways and, additionally, in the latter instance,

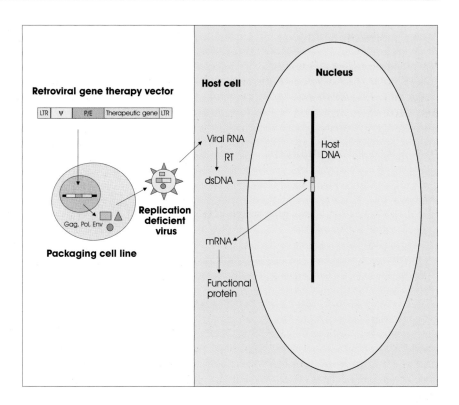

Figure 14.9. Gene therapy. In a typical retroviral vector the Gag (core protein), Pol (reverse transcriptase [RT]) and Env (viral envelope) genes are replaced with the therapeutic gene, together with appropriate promoter (P) and enhancer (E) regulatory sequences. The 5' and 3' long terminal repeats (LTR) include sequences involved in gene integration, and the ψ (psi) sequence directs packaging of the viral nucleic acid. The essential Gag, Pol and Env proteins are available in the packaging cell line into which the vector is introduced, but the virus particles that are produced will lack the genes for these proteins and therefore cannot go on to produce further infectious particles following delivery of the therapeutic gene to the host T-cells. In the patient's cells the viral RNA is reverse transcribed into double-stranded DNA which subsequently integrates into the host chromosomal DNA. The therapeutic gene can then be transcribed into mRNA for production of a functional form of the previously defective protein.

macrophage function appears to be aberrant. Skewing of the balance between Th1 and Th2 cells as a result of infection may also depress the subset most appropriate for immune protection.

Many therapeutic agents, such as X-rays, cytotoxic drugs and corticosteroids, can have dire effects on the immune system (see p. 394). **B-lymphoproliferative disorders**, such as chronic lymphocytic leukemia, myeloma and Waldenström's macroglobulinemia, are associated with varying degrees of hypogammaglobulinemia and impaired antibody responses. Their common infections with pyogenic bacteria contrast with the situation in Hodgkin's disease where the patients display all the hallmarks of defective CMI— susceptibility to tubercle bacillus, *Brucella*, *Cryptococcus* and herpes zoster virus.

ACQUIRED IMMUNODEFICIENCY SYNDROME (AIDS)

Acquired immunodeficiency syndrome (AIDS) is a devastating illness that had killed more than 20 million people by the end of 2005. According to the 2005 UNAIDS report, approximately 40 million people are currently living with human immunodeficiency virus (HIV), the agent responsible for AIDS (figure 14.10). There were approaching 5 million new infections in 2005 alone. The epicentre of the plague is sub-Saharan Africa with nearly two-thirds of worldwide HIV infec-

tions and an adult infection rate estimated at about 7%. As of the end of 2003, 12 million children had been orphaned because of AIDS. Although the numbers are worst in Africa, the incidence of HIV infection is increasing in most regions, particularly in Eastern Europe and Central Asia. There are growing epidemics in India and China, which have an estimated 1–2% prevalence of infected pregnant women. Increasingly, HIV/AIDS has a female face; females over 16 years of age account for nearly 50% of all people living with HIV or AIDS (closer to 60% in sub-Saharan Africa) and their rate of infection is increasing. The other key demographic is young people 15–24 years old, who account for about one-third of all infected individuals.

The first reported case of AIDS was in 1981. The syndrome was characterized by a predisposition to opportunistic infections, i.e. those easily warded off by a normally functioning immune system; the incidence of an aggressive form of Kaposi's sarcoma or B-cell lymphoma; and the concurrent depletion of CD4+ T-cells. It was suspected that AIDS was caused by a previously unknown virus since it spread through contact with bodily fluids, and in 1983, HIV-1 was isolated and identified. There are in fact two closely related HIVs, HIV-1 and the less virulent HIV-2, which differ both in origin and sequence. The majority of AIDS cases are caused by HIV-1. HIV-2 is found predominantly in West Africa.

Both HIV-1 and HIV-2 have their origins in non-human primates. Based on sequence similarities (figure

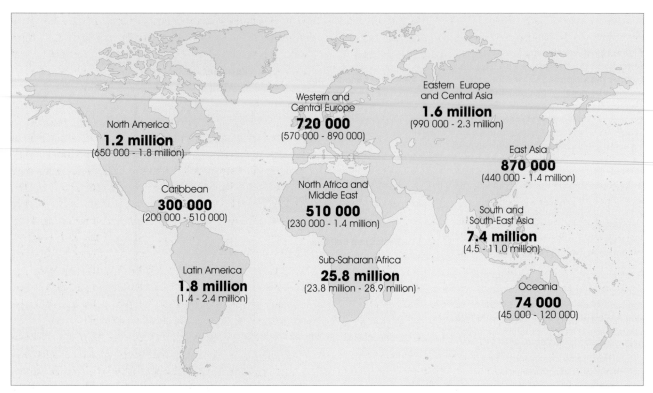

Figure 14.10. Adults and children estimated to be living with HIV as of the end of 2005 across the regions of the world. It is estimated that a total of 40.3 (36.7–45.3) million individuals are infected (from the UNAIDS website, www.unaids.org).

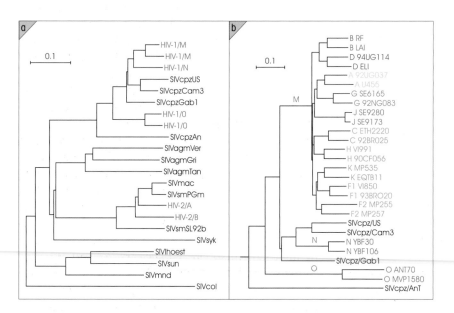

Figure 14.11. Evolution of AIDS viruses. Two evolutionary trees are shown in which the scale bar indicates 10% protein sequence divergence. (a) Tree showing the origins of primate lentiviruses. SIV strains have a suffix indicating their species of origin, e.g. SIV$_{cpzUS}$ is SIV from a chimpanzee in captivity in the USA. The distinct origins of HIV-1 and HIV-2 (shown in red) are apparent. This tree was derived using Pol protein sequences. (b) Tree showing the relationship between HIV-1 groups and clades and SIV$_{cpz}$. This tree was derived from Env protein sequences. (Kindly provided by Paul Sharp; after P.M. Sharp (2002) Origins of human virus diversity, *Cell* **108**, 305–312.)

14.11) with simian immunodeficiency viruses (SIV), HIV is likely the evolutionary product of closely related SIVs that crossed from their non-human primate hosts into humans in the early to mid part of the twentieth century. The closest relative of HIV-1 is SIVcpz, the natural host of which is the chimpanzee, *Pan troglodytes*. HIV-2 is more closely related to SIVsmm from the sooty mangabey, *Cercocebus atys*. Phylogenetic mapping and sequence analyses indicate several independent zoonoses of SIVcpz and SIVsmm within the past century. The leading hypothesis is that SIVcpz and SIVsmm were transmitted to humans through cutaneous or mucosal membrane exposure to infected animal blood. This scenario is consistent with regular direct exposure of hunters in the bushmeat trade to primate blood.

Based on viral sequences, HIV-1 is categorized into three groups: M (main), O (outlier) and N (non-M, non-O), each representing separate zoonoses (figure 14.11). HIV-2 is similarly categorized into eight groups, A through H. HIV-1 from group M has spread throughout the world and is further subcategorized into clades A through K, which predominate in different geographical regions. The other two groups, N and O, are mainly confined to Gabon, Cameroon and neighboring countries in West Africa.

The evolution of the different group M clades most probably occurred within the human population following one cross-species transmission event. The discovery of an HIV-1 isolate from 1959 that appears to be an ancestor of clades B and D is consistent with this viewpoint. The oldest common ancestor of group M has been estimated to date to 1915–1941, suggesting that HIV-1 has been infecting humans longer than originally thought, unnoticed clinically among populations in West Central Africa. The early spread of AIDS may have resulted from various economic, social and behavioral factors (e.g. use of nonsterilized needles for parenteral injections and vaccinations) that facilitated virus transmission.

HIV does not usually cause AIDS immediately and controversy still remains as to precisely how the virus damages the immune system and whether all HIV-1 infected individuals will necessarily develop disease. Great strides have been made since the identification of HIV but much remains a puzzle and a cure or a vaccine are elusive.

The clinical course of disease: from infection to AIDS

Initial infection generally occurs by exposure to bodily fluids from an infected individual. HIV is found as free virus particles and infected cells in semen, vaginal fluid and mother's milk. Currently, the most common route of transmission worldwide is through sexual intercourse. The use of contaminated needles for intravenous drug delivery and the use of blood or blood products for therapeutic purposes are also common means of infection with HIV. Screening the blood supply for HIV has virtually eliminated transmission via the inadvertent administration of infected human blood in developed countries. Another important route of transmission is from infected mothers to their children. Mothers can pass HIV to their child either during birth or by breastfeeding. In Africa, the perinatal transmission rate is around 25%. The chance of perinatal transmission can be significantly reduced if the mother is undergoing antiretroviral therapy.

Two to eight weeks after infection (figure 14.12), 80%

of individuals experience acute viremia. Symptoms are reminiscent of a bout of influenza and include a high spiking fever, sore throat, headaches and swollen lymph nodes. This is referred to as the acute retroviral syndrome, the symptoms of which usually subside spontaneously in 1–4 weeks. During this acute phase, there is an explosion of viral replication, particularly in CD4$^+$ T-cells in the gut, and a corresponding marked decline in circulating CD4$^+$ T-cells. At this time, most individuals also launch a strong HIV-specific CD8$^+$ T-cell response (figure 14.12) that kills infected cells, followed by the production of HIV-specific antibodies (seroconversion). CD8$^+$ T-cells are thought to be important for controlling primary viremia. Virus levels spike, then fall as CD4$^+$ T-cell counts rebound but to levels still below normal (800 cells/μl compared to 1200 cells/μl). The baseline level of virus persisting in the blood after the symptoms of acute viremia subside (the "set point") is currently the best indicator for an individual's prognosis.

Following primary infection, a period of clinical latency (no or few symptoms) follows during which time HIV continues to replicate while CD4$^+$ T-cells gradually decline in function and number. There are three main mechanisms thought to be responsible for the depletion of CD4$^+$ T-cells during HIV infection. First, there are the direct cytopathic effects of the virus on its host T-cell. Second, infected cells have an increased susceptibility to the induction of apoptosis. Finally, there is the elimination of infected CD4$^+$ T-cells by CD8$^+$ T-cells that recognize viral peptides displayed by MHC class I.

The great majority of HIV-infected individuals will, over the course of years, progress to AIDS. The asymptomatic period typically lasts somewhere between 2 and 15 years; however, the number of functional CD4$^+$ T-cells eventually drops below a threshold (about 400 cells/μl) and opportunistic infections begin to appear. Once the CD4$^+$ T-cell count has dropped below 200 cells/μl, the individual is classified as having AIDS.

In the earlier stages of HIV-1 disease, typical opportunistic microbes to evade the impaired cellular immune system are oral *Candida* species and *Mycobacterium tuberculosis*, which manifest as oral thrush and tuberculosis respectively. Later, patients often suffer from shingles due to the activation of latent varicella zoster virus from a previous case of chickenpox. Also common is the development of EBV-induced B-cell lymphomas and Kaposi's sarcoma, a cancer of endothelial cells, likely due to the effects of cytokines secreted in response to both the existing HIV infection and a new herpes virus (HHV-8) found in these tumors. Hepatitis C/HIV co-infection is also common and disease progression due to hepatitis C is accelerated. Pneumonia caused by the fungus *Pneumocystis carinii* is a frequent

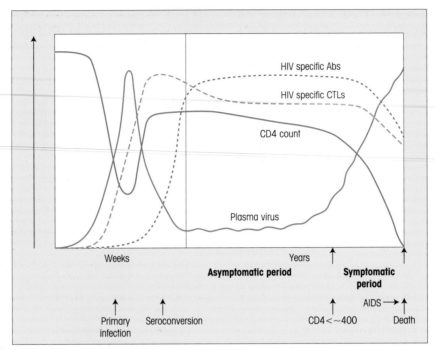

Figure 14.12. The typical course of HIV infection. Primary infection is characterized by a rapid rise in plasma virus and a rapid decline in circulating CD4+ T-cells. The plasma virus levels peak and decline to a low roughly constant level ('the set point'), which is predictive of the time of progression to disease. The CD4+ T-cell count recovers somewhat but to a lower level than prior to infection. The HIV-specific CD8+ T-cell response is activated as virus peaks and is probably important in controlling primary infection. The HIV-specific antibody response takes somewhat longer to initiate and results in seroconversion. The neutralizing antibody response is yet slower to initiate (see figure 14.20). Clinical latency follows primary infection for a period of the order of a decade. No symptoms are apparent but depletion of CD4+ T-cells in lymphoid tissues continues. Eventually, CD4+ T-cell depletion is so pronounced that resistance to opportunistic infections begins to wane, leading ultimately to a complete collapse of a functioning immune system and death. Drug intervention can take plasma viral loads below the level of detection and prevent CD4+ T-cell depletion.

occurrence in patients and was often fatal prior to the introduction of effective antifungal therapy. In the final stages of AIDS, the prominent pathogens causing infection are *Mycobacterium avium* and cytomegalovirus. Respiratory infections are the major cause of death for AIDS sufferers. Although the above-mentioned infections and cancers are typical, not all AIDS patients will develop these illnesses and a number of other tumors and infections, though less prominent, are still of note.

The time of progression from HIV infection to AIDS varies greatly due to genetic variations in virus and/or host. For example, some viruses are naturally attenuated and are associated with slower disease progression. The HLA type of the host can be important. Homozygosity of HLA class I is linked to faster progression, probably due to a less diverse T-cell response to the infection. Certain HLA types are associated with different prognoses: HLA-B57 and HLA-B27 are associated with slower progression while HLA-B35 is associated with more rapid progression. There are also individuals who are highly resistant to HIV infection because they have a mutation in the chemokine receptor CCR5, which serves as a coreceptor for HIV, as discussed later.

Two small groups of people are of particular interest to researchers due to their ability to remain disease-free after exposure to HIV. The first group, long-term non-progressors, are clearly infected with virus but control virus replication at very low levels and have not progressed to disease. The second group, highly exposed seronegative individuals, have been repeatedly exposed to HIV yet remain disease-free and have no detectable virus. Intriguingly, some of this latter group appear to possess HIV-specific CD8+ T-cells suggesting previous exposure to the virus or at least to noninfectious viral antigens. Whether the immune response seen in these individuals is responsible for clearing an HIV infection is unclear. Nonetheless, these individuals are the focus of much interest for vaccine design and development. We will now review key aspects of the virus itself including its cellular tropism, genome and life cycle.

HIV-1 genome

HIV-1 is a retrovirus, which means that it has an RNA genome but that replication passes through DNA with the involvement of the enzyme reverse transcriptase. It belongs to a group of retroviruses called the lentiviruses, from the Latin lentus, meaning 'slow viruses' because of the slow course of disease associated with infection by these viruses. The HIV-1 genome is composed of approximately 9 kb of RNA, which consists of nine different genes encoding 15 proteins. Two copies of the single-stranded genome are packaged in the virus particle along with additional enzymes and accessory proteins. Three of the reading frames encode Gag (group specific antigen), Pol (polymerase) and Env (envelope) polyproteins, which are proteolytically cleaved into individual structural proteins and enzymes (figure 14.13). Gag is cleaved into four structural proteins, MA (matrix), CA (capsid), NC (nucleocapsid) and p6, while Env is cleaved into two, SU (surface gp120) and TM (transmembrane gp41). Pol cleavage produces the enzymes PR (protease), RT (reverse transcriptase) and IN (integrase), which are encapsulated in the virus particle. Several accessory proteins are also encoded, three of which—Vif, Vpr and Nef—are packaged inside the virus particle. The remaining accessory proteins are Tat, Rev and Vpu. The functions of the 15 HIV proteins are summarized in figure 14.13 and discussed in relation to the HIV life cycle below.

The life cycle of HIV-1

Viral entry

Initial virus-cell attachment is believed to be mediated primarily through nonspecific interactions between the envelope spikes that decorate the surface of the virus and target T-cell surface molecules. The envelope spike is a putative trimer of heterodimers composed of noncovalently associated surface glycoprotein (gp120) and transmembrane glycoprotein (gp41) subunits. The sugar moieties and positively charged patches on gp120 probably mediate binding to cell surface lectins and negatively charged heparan sulfate proteoglycans, respectively.

The first receptor-specific binding event occurs when gp120 on the viral envelope spike engages CD4 on the target T-cell surface (figure 14.14). HIV-1 specifically

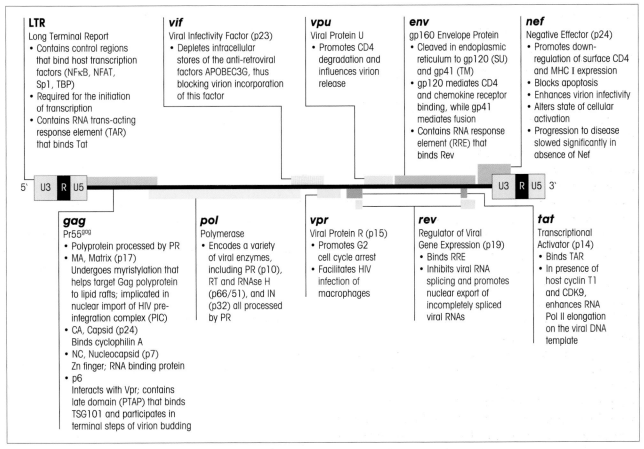

Figure 14.13. The HIV-1 genome. The organization of the genome is shown and the functions of the gene products summarized. (Kindly provided by Warner Greene; after Greene W.C. & Peterlin B.M. (2002) Charting HIV's remarkable voyage through the cell: basic science as a passport to future therapy. *Nature Medicine* **8**, 673–680.)

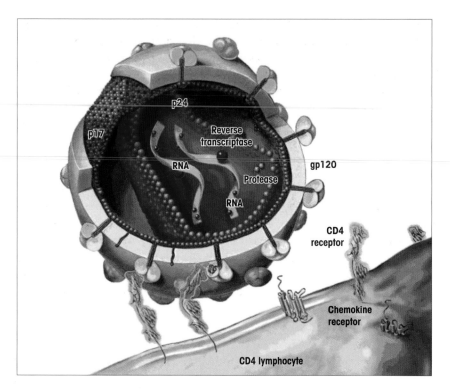

Figure 14.14. HIV-1 and viral entry receptors. Two copies of the RNA genome are present inside the viral capsid, together with the reverse transcriptase, integrase and viral protease enzymes. Matrix protein encases the capsid, which is contained within the viral envelope membrane. The surface of the virus is decorated with spikes, heterotrimers formed by the gp120 surface glycoprotein and the gp41 transmembrane protein. The spikes interact with CD4 molecules on the surface of target T-cells. Conformational changes are induced in gp120 that permit interaction with chemokine receptor and the reaction fusing viral and cell membranes is triggered. This permits entry of viral genomes into the target T-cell.

infects cells expressing CD4, including T lymphocytes, macrophages and dendritic cells. CD4 binds with high affinity to a recessed cavity of gp120 as revealed by a structure of gp120 in complex with CD4. This binding event triggers multiple conformational changes in gp120 that expose and form the coreceptor binding site. The coreceptor is most often the chemokine receptor CCR5 or CXCR4. These receptors normally function in chemoattraction, in which immune cells move along gradients of chemokine molecules to sites of inflammation. HIV-1s are often grouped by their coreceptor usage. R5 viruses use CCR5, X4 viruses use CXCR4 and dual tropic R5X4 viruses use both CCR5 and CXCR4. R5 viruses only require low levels of CD4 expressed on the surface of target T-cells, whereas X4 viruses require higher levels. Thus, differential expression of CD4 and coreceptors makes different T-cell types (or subtypes) more susceptible to infection by either X4 or R5 viruses: X4 viruses infect naive CD4+ T-cells and mature DCs while the preferred *in vivo* targets of R5 viruses include immature dendritic cells, macrophages and activated effector or memory CD4+ T-cells. Initially, R5 variants were labeled as 'macrophage-tropic' when variants were classified based on the cell lines in which they could grow *in vitro* and likewise, X4 viruses were labeled as 'lymphocyte-tropic'. These former designations for HIV variants are misleading, since R5 viruses do infect lymphocytes, and therefore the designations were changed to reflect coreceptor usage.

Coreceptor binding induces conformational changes in the transmembrane glycoprotein, gp41, that result in the exposure of the highly hydrophobic N-terminal fusion peptide of gp41, previously buried in the spike structure. The fusion peptide inserts into the host T-cell membrane like a harpoon, both destabilizing the target T-cell membrane and generating an extended alpha-helical gp41 fusion intermediate, designated the 'pre-hairpin intermediate.' This intermediate is unstable and readily collapses back onto itself forming a six-helix bundle, or 'hairpin,' comprising three internal α-helices arranged antiparallel to three external α-helices. The only high-resolution structure of gp41 available to date is of gp41 in this putative postfusion form. The collapse of gp41 into this extremely stable six-helix bundle is thought to provide the thermodynamic driving force for fusion. Six-helix bundles are a common structural motif among other viral and cellular fusion proteins; other viruses having surface proteins with structural similarities to gp41 include influenza virus, SARS and Ebola virus. Although it is not well understood how six-helix bundle formation enables the merging of cellular and viral membranes, if bundle formation is prevented using peptide analogs that compete for the occupancy of the external α-helices, fusion is also abrogated. One such peptide has been developed into an HIV drug, the first of a new class of drugs—viral entry inhibitors.

Fusion is a highly cooperative process that occurs on a time scale of minutes and may require the interaction of several spikes with corresponding receptors and coreceptors to be an efficient process, although this is controversial.

Following fusion, the virus particle has lost its enveloped exterior, and the viral core, or reverse transcription complex, remains. This complex is composed of two viral RNAs, RT, IN, tRNA^{Lys}, matrix (p17), nucleocapsid (p7), capsid protein (p24) and Vpr.

Reverse transcription and integration

En route to the nucleus, RT uses the two single-stranded RNA molecules enclosed within the viral core as a template to convert the viral genome into a double-stranded cDNA copy of the viral genome. RT has no proofreading mechanism and introduces approximately one mutation per genome per reverse transcription. RNAse H degrades the RNA template as the minus strand DNA is

synthesized and DNA polymerase catalyzes the generation of a double-stranded viral cDNA genome.

Upon reverse transcription, the complex contains essentially the same factors as before, except that the RNA genome has been replaced with a newly synthesized cDNA genome. This complex is referred to as the preintegration complex, which translocates to the nucleus, possibly via microtubules by a mechanism only partially understood, given the large size of the complex.

Integration of the viral cDNA genome into the host T-cell genome is mediated by integrase and the actions of several host proteins (figure 14.15). It requires the viral LTR sequence and is preferentially targeted to areas of active transcription. Integration can lead to latent or transcriptionally active viral cDNA referred to as a provirus. Active provirus serves as the template for viral replica-

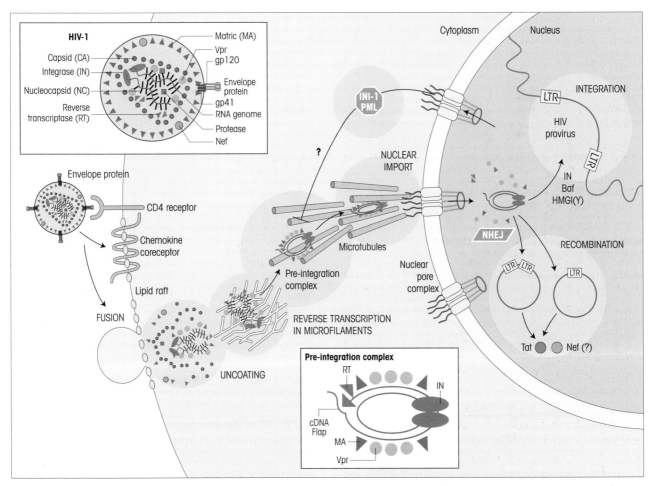

Figure 14.15. Viral entry, reverse transcription and integration. Interaction of the viral spikes with CD4 and chemokine receptors triggers fusion and the injection of the nucleocapsid into the cytoplasm of the host T-cell (cf. figure 14.14). Uncoating of the nucleocapsid is followed by reverse transcription and the formation of the pre-integration complex (PIC) containing viral cDNA. The PIC is transported into the nucleus and the viral cDNA integrated into host chromosomes to produce provirus. Some PICs produce LTR circles as shown. (Kindly provided by Warner Greene; after Greene W.C. & Peterlin B.M. (2002) Charting HIV's remarkable voyage through the cell: basic science as a passport to future therapy. *Nature Medicine* **8**, 673–680.)

tion and transcription. Latency explains the inability of viral therapies employed to date to eliminate virus completely from infected individuals and is the great challenge to a complete cure to HIV. The number of latently infected cells in an infected individual is very small, of the order of 10^5–10^6.

Replication

Replication of the virus commences postintegration with the production of nascent viral transcripts by cellular RNA polymerases (figure 14.16). Transcription is regulated by proteins that bind within the LTR sequences, which flank the genome of the virus. For example, activation of T-cells results in the expression of transcription factor NFκB. NFκB binds to several cellular promoters including those within the 5' LTR.

Production of the viral proteins is biphasic. During the early phase (also called the Rev-independent phase), the viral transcripts are completely processed (i.e. all internal splice sites are utilized), polyadenylated and exported to the cytoplasm as all other cellular transcripts. Translation of these transcripts results in three gene products: Tat, Rev and Nef. Like other viruses, HIV-1 makes full use of a single template and therefore, in order for the other genes to be expressed, alternative splicing patterns are utilized (four different 5' splice sites, eight different 3' splice sites); however, this cannot occur until a critical threshold of Rev is achieved in the nucleus. A nuclear localization signal in the N-terminus of Rev guides it back to the nucleus post-translation with the help of cellular factor Importin β. This arginine-rich domain also serves as a binding site for an RNA target, the Rev response element (RRE), which is located within the env intron of all incompletely spliced mRNAs. Splicing of HIV transcripts by cellular splicing factors is an inefficient process, and this allows time for Rev to bind the RRE. Rev cooperatively multimerizes (up to 12 additional Rev monomers) along the RNA and

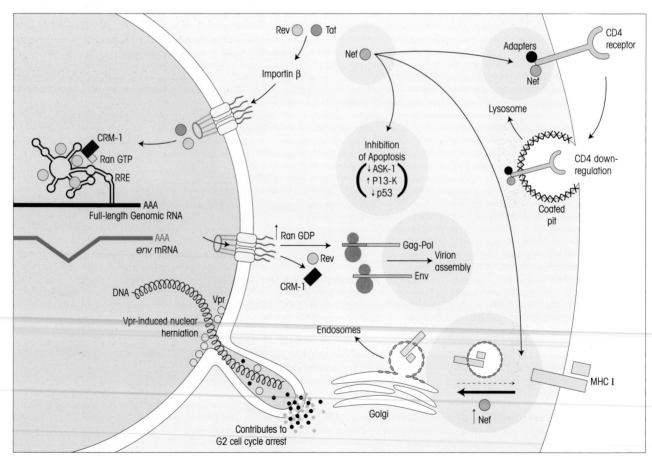

Figure 14.16. Optimization by viral proteins of the intracellular environment for viral transcription. Nef downregulates CD4 and MHC class I and inhibits apoptosis. Vpr contributes to G2 cell-cycle arrest. Rev promotes nuclear export of incompletely spliced viral transcripts that encode the structural and enzymatic proteins as well as the viral genome of new virions. (Kindly provided by Warner Greene; after Greene W.C. & Peterlin B.M. (2002) Charting HIV's remarkable voyage through the cell: basic science as a passport to future therapy. *Nature Medicine* **8,** 673–680.)

this Rev–RRE complex associates with Exportin/Crm-1 via a nuclear export signal in the C-terminus of Rev. This allows for efficient transport of the partially spliced or unspliced transcripts from the nucleus to the cytoplasm before the splicing factors are able to process the transcripts.

These actions by Rev permit the second phase of gene expression to commence and the partially spliced and unspliced mRNAs are translated into Env, Vif, Vpr and Vpu and Gag and Gag-Pol, respectively. This is a crucial adaptation on the part of the virus as transcripts with introns are normally retained and degraded if they cannot be processed. Without Rev, HIV-1 is not able to transport its genetic material (containing multiple introns) to the cytoplasm where newly synthesized virus particles assemble; indeed, in experiments where Rev is removed from the genome, the resulting virus clones are replication incompetent.

Tat and Nef are also crucial in HIV replication. In the absence of Tat, transcription begins but the polymerase fails to elongate efficiently along the viral genome. Tat binds to a well-defined structure on the RNA, recruits positive elongation factors and promotes the rate of viral replication. Nef acts differently to Tat and Rev; it does not bind directly to viral RNA but rather acts upon the environment of the infected cell to favor replication. The activities of Nef include the ability to affect signal-ing cascades, downregulate CD4 expression at the infected cell surface and promote the generation of more infectious virions as well as virus dissemination. In addition, Nef impairs immunological responses to HIV and inhibits apoptosis, thereby prolonging the life of the infected cell and increasing viral replication.

The number of mechanisms by which HIV promotes its own reproduction is staggering. It reflects the rapid turnover and inherent infidelity in HIV replication. The virus has sampled a huge number of different protein–protein and protein–nucleic acid interactions in its dance with humans and selection pressure has brought forth those interactions that favor virus survival and expansion. This is evolution on a time scale far shorter than normally experienced.

Virus assembly, budding and maturation

New virus particle assembly occurs at the plasma membrane of the infected cell (figure 14.17). One of the viral proteins translated in the cytosol during the late phase of gene expression is the Gag precursor protein p55. p55 traffics to the plasma membrane or late endosomes and attaches to lipid bilayer where Env glycoproteins are attached via the transmembrane anchor of gp41. Assembly is dependent on the cellular protein HP68 that binds p55 and promotes the formation of an immature viral core. Other structural viral proteins assemble at the cell

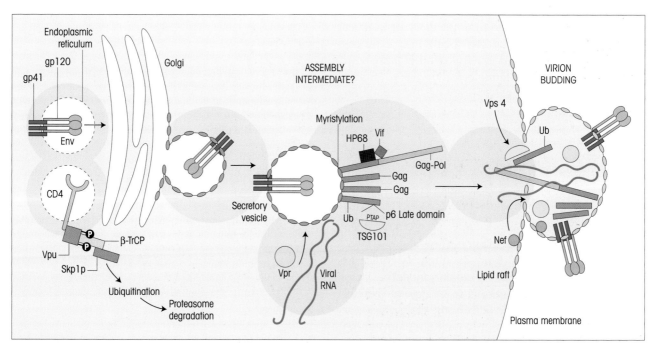

Figure 14.17. Assembly of new virions. Assembly occurs principally at the plasma membrane but may be initiated on secretory vesicles destined for the plasma membrane, as suggested by the critical roles played by proteins of the vesicular protein sorting machinery such as TSG101. (Kindly provided by Warner Greene; after Greene W.C. & Peterlin B.M. (2002) Charting HIV's remarkable voyage through the cell: basic science as a passport to future therapy. *Nature Medicine* **8**, 673–680.)

membrane with two copies of the viral RNA genome, RT, protease, and integrase to be integrated into an immature virus particle. One of the key structural proteins present is p6, which connects the virus core to components of the endosomal sorting complex at sites of budding in the plasma membrane and late endosomes. Just before budding, other host factors including cytoplasmic viral restriction factors such as APOBEC3G can be incorporated into the virion. Coincident with budding of the immature virion from the plasma membrane, proteolytic processing of capsid occurs, generating the mature viral particle.

APOBEC3G is an interesting molecule that can restrict viral replication by cysteine deamination of DNA and resultant loss of functionality of viral genomes. The HIV-1 protein vif binds to APOBEC3G and by targeting it for professional degradation reduces its incorporation into virions. APOBEC3G is expressed in cells that do not permit HIV replication. Another important HIV-1 restriction factor is Trim5α, which is responsible for the resistance of primate cells to diverse retrovirus infection. It targets the capsid protein and blocks an early step of retroviral infection prior to reverse transcription.

Finally, it is important to note that much propagation of infection in HIV-1 *in vivo* probably occurs by cell to cell spread of virus rather than by free virus particles. Env proteins on the infected cell surface engage receptors on neighboring target T-cells, but HIV-1 transfer still requires viral budding. It appears that HIV-1 particles transfer directionally through sites of contact between infected and uninfected T-cells in an arrangement that has been termed the virological synapse with similarities to the immunological synapse found between T-cells and DCs. Nef promotes the formation of such synapses between infected macrophages and T-cells.

Vaginal transmission of HIV and the early stages of infection

Most HIV infections are now acquired through heterosexual transmission, most frequently by women through vaginal intercourse. There has therefore been an increased focus on understanding how vaginal transmission takes place and how one might intervene to prevent transmission. The SIV/monkey model has been very useful in this area (figure 14.18). It appears that the virus struggles against the odds in the early phases of infection, but once it gains a foothold, circumstances rapidly change in favor of the virus to the point that progression to disease is virtually inevitable without drug intervention.

The first problem the virus encounters is the mucosal

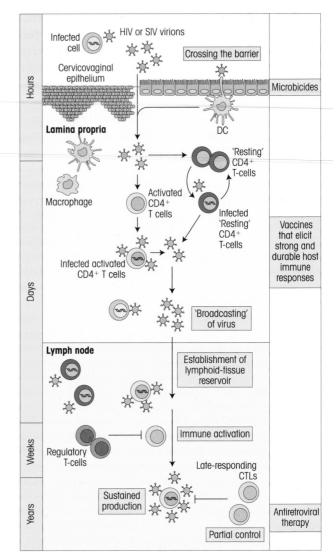

Figure 14.18. Vaginal transmission of HIV and SIV and subsequent stages of infection. Virus and/or infected cells cross the cervicovaginal mucosal barrier in the first hours after infection either through breaks in the barrier or with the help of DCs. Virus then infects CD4+ T-cells, macrophages and DCs in the lamina propria. Infection is suggested to occur mainly in resting CD4+ T-cells because they are the most numerous target T-cells in the lamina propria. Activated CD4+ T-cells sustain infection much more effectively but are less common. Small founder populations of infected cells release enough virus to seed infection in distant lymphoid tissues. Here, larger numbers of activated CD4+ T-cells in close proximity lead to an explosive production of virus and primary viremia. Microbicides and vaccines that could reduce the size of founder populations of infected cells might abort infection at the point of entry or prevent the efficient viral seeding of distant sites required for the establishment of a systemic infection. (Kindly provided by Ashley Haase; after Haase A.T. (2005) Perils at mucosal front lines for HIV and SIV and their hosts. *Nature Reviews Immunology* **5**, 783–792.)

barrier. If this barrier is damaged, e.g by ulcerative genital diseases, bacterial vaginosis or after the use of some microbicides such as nonoxynol-9, then transmission rates are greatly increased. If the barrier is largely intact, then very few viruses will make it across, probably via small breaks or by transport on DCs. DCs express C-type lectins, such as DC-SIGN and DC-SIGNR, which bind high mannose glycans displayed on the surface of gp120, thereby capturing virions which may be internalized into a low-pH, nonlysosomal compartment, where they remain infectious. Once across the barrier, free virus infects target T-cells such as CD4$^+$ T-cells, macrophages and DCs in the lamina propria. Infectious virus inside DCs can enter resting and activated CD4$^+$ T-cells via DC–T-cell conjugates as bursts of viral replication are observed at DC–T-cell synapses. In addition, HIV-1 Nef-induced upregulation of DC-SIGN and β chemokines in DCs may promote lymphocyte clustering and viral spread. Other studies suggest that Nef may also alter the physiological characteristics of infected macrophages so as to enhance conditions for viral dissemination.

Nevertheless, at this point in time, there is only a small founder population of infected cells, which must spread infection to the relatively few number and spatially dispersed susceptible cells in the mucosa. Infection is still fragile and probably susceptible to intervention at this time. Then sometime between a day and a week, the virus finds its way to lymphoid tissue, a rich source of activated CD4$^+$ T-cells. Now conditions favor the virus since access is provided to large numbers of closely packed target T-cells leading to an extremely rapid rise in virus production to give peak viral loads in plasma. One very important lymphoid tissue compartment is the lamina propria of the gut where massive killing of CD4$^+$ memory T-cells occurs either via direct killing or via apoptosis. The counter-attack by the host's immune system has been described as 'too little, too late.'

HIV-1 therapy

Great advances have been made in recent years in the containment of HIV replication in infected individuals and the slowing down or blocking of the progression to AIDS. Many new drugs are available. Many steps in the virus life cycle are potential targets for drugs, including: (i) entry; (ii) fusion; (iii) reverse transcription; (iv) integration; (v) transcription/transactivation; (vi) assembly; and (vii) maturation.

Currently, four classes of drugs targeting three steps are in clinical use. The first antiretroviral class to become available was the nucleoside/nucleotide reverse transcription inhibitors. These nucleoside/nucleotide analogs are incorporated into the growing strand of viral DNA leading to chain termination and the production of noninfectious virus. Reverse transcription can also be inhibited by a second class of drugs, the non-

nucleoside/nucleotide reverse transcription inhibitors, which bind allosterically to a site distant from the substrate-binding site. Viral protease inhibitors inhibit cleavage of the gag and pol polyproteins. Finally, the first fusion inhibitor, enfuvirtide, was approved by the Federal Drug Administration (FDA) in the United States in 2003, and is a peptide that binds to gp41 to inhibit fusion.

A major problem in HIV therapy is the development of drug resistance. The error-prone nature of reverse transcription, the large viral load and the rapid rate of virus replication in many infected individuals means that they typically harbor a very large number of HIV variants. Administration of drugs may select for a variant that has resistance. Drug resistance against many protease inhibitors and some of the more potent nucleoside analogs develops within a few days since a single mutation in the target enzyme confers resistance to many of these drugs. Resistance to other antiretrovirals, such as zidovudine (AZT), requires multiple mutations (three or four for AZT) and correspondingly longer to develop. Due to the relatively rapid development of resistance to all HIV drugs used singly, successful suppression of HIV currently necessitates combination therapy. Antiretroviral therapy (ART) involves the administration of a combination of nucleotide and non-nucleotide RT inhibitors and/or protease inhibitors and, in some cases, the fusion inhibitor, enfuvirtide.

ART has proven very effective in the management of viral levels in infected individuals. During the first 2 weeks of treatment, plasma virus loads decrease very rapidly reflecting the inhibition of virus production from infected cells and the rapid clearance of free virus from the circulation (half-life about 6 hours). The results indicate that the half-life of productively infected cells is about 2 days. At the end of 2 weeks, viral plasma levels have decreased by more than 95%, signifying a nearly complete loss of productively infected CD4$^+$ T-cells. There is a concomitant rise in CD4$^+$ T-cell counts in the peripheral blood as HIV replication and infection is controlled. This rise has been attributed to three mechanisms: redistribution of CD4$^+$ memory cells from lymphoid tissues into the circulation; reduction in the abnormal levels of immune activation associated with reduced CD8$^+$ T-cell killing of infected cells; and the emergence of new naive T-cells from the thymus.

After the initial rapid and almost complete clearance of free virus, a second slow phase of viral decay reflects the very slow decay of virus production in longer-lived reservoirs, such as in dendritic cells and macrophages, from latently infected memory CD4$^+$ T-cells that have been activated. A third phase has been postulated, which is even slower, resulting from reactivation of integrated provirus in memory T-cells and other long-lived reservoirs of infection. Follicular DCs store virus in the form of immune complexes, making them potential long-term sources of infectious virus. These latent reservoirs may persist for years and are resistant to current HIV drug therapy.

HIV-1 vaccines

Most epidemiologists agree that the most efficient means to control the HIV-1 pandemic would be an effective vaccine. Unfortunately, the development of such a vaccine faces some major hurdles intimately associated with features of the virus. These include the variability of the virus, the nature of the envelope spikes of the virus and the ability of the virus to integrate into host chromosomes and become latent.

Most viral vaccines appear to be effective because they mimic natural infection and elicit neutralizing antibody responses. Long-lived plasma cells in the bone marrow secrete neutralizing antibodies that are present in serum and can act immediately to inactivate virus particles (figure 14.19). Indeed, the likelihood that a vaccine will be effective is often assessed by looking at serum neutralizing antibody levels. Additionally on contact with virus, vaccine-induced memory B-cells are stimulated to secrete neutralizing antibodies. Studies in monkeys show that neutralizing antibodies can protect against HIV. If neutralizing antibodies are administered at relatively high doses and then the monkeys challenged with a hybrid human (HIV)/monkey (SIV) virus, they show no signs of infection, i.e. they exhibit sterilizing immunity. However, achieving such levels of neutralizing antibodies by vaccination appears to be very difficult. In addition, there is a requirement that the neutralizing antibodies elicited by vaccination be active against a wide spectrum of different HIV variants (so called broadly neutralizing antibodies). Such antibodies are known to exist but the design of immunogens to elicit them has not yet been achieved. Indeed, natural HIV infection elicits relatively weak broadly neutralizing antibody responses, highlighting the difficulties of finding an appropriate immunogen. Natural infection tends to elicit type-specific neutralizing antibodies (figure 14.20). When these antibodies reach a critical threshold, a resistant virus emerges. Eventually, a neutralizing antibody response to this virus develops and a new resistant virus emerges and so on. Apparently the virus always stays one step ahead of the neutralizing antibody response.

For the reasons outlined above, it appears that it will be challenging to design an HIV vaccine that will provide sterilizing immunity through elicitation of broadly neutralizing antibodies. In fact, most current vaccines effective against other viruses are not thought to provide sterilizing immunity. Rather they elicit sufficient serum titers of neutralizing antibody to blunt infection, which is then contained by cellular or innate immunity and overt symptoms are avoided. In other words, vaccination protects against disease rather than infection.

Studies in animal models have shown that protection against disease for a number of viruses can be achieved by eliciting a cellular immune response through vaccination. In the absence of effective methods to elicit broadly neutralizing antibodies, much HIV vaccine research has targeted cellular immune responses. The primary rationale has been that if potent T-cellular immune responses can be elicited in vaccinees, the response may reduce the damage to CD4$^+$ T-cells following primary infection and lower the viral set point.

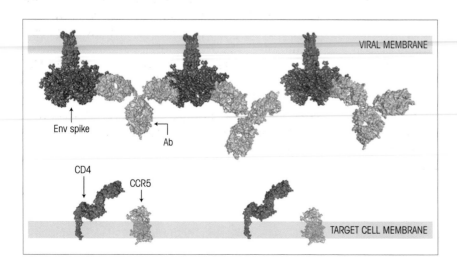

Figure 14.19. Model for neutralization of HIV by antibody. The antibody molecule has a molecular volume approaching that of an HIV envelope spike. Therefore the attachment of an antibody molecule to a spike is expected to show strong steric interference with virus attachment and/or fusion. (After Poignard *et al.* (2001) *Annual Review of Immunology*, **19**, 253–274.)

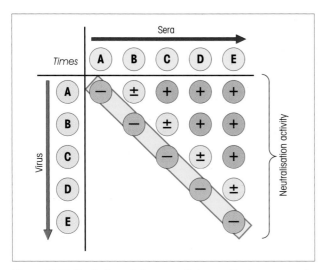

Figure 14.20. Evolution of the neutralizing antibody response in HIV infection. A–E refer to virus and sera from time points A–E during the course of infection of an individual. Serum taken at time point A has no significant neutralizing activity against virus isolated from the plasma of the infected individual at time point A. Serum taken at time point B has some weak activity. Serum taken at time point C and points thereafter clearly neutralizes virus from time point A. Once the serum neutralizing antibody concentration has reached a certain threshold following exposure to a given predominant virus variant, selection pressure is exerted such that a new neutralization-resistant variant emerges from the huge pool of variants present in the infected individual. A neutralizing antibody response develops to this new variant and the cycle is repeated. (Courtesy of Doug Richman; after Richman D.D. *et al.* (2003) Rapid evolution of the neutralization antibody response to HIV-1 infection. *Proceedings of the National Academy of Sciences of the USA* **100**, 4144–4149.)

Table 14.1. Protection against SIV in macaques by different vaccines. Published data is included from challenge experiments in Indian rhesus macaques using various pathogenic SIVs and various challenge routes. The attenuated (Δ) viruses are: Δ*nef*, nef-deleted SIV; Δ3, nef and vpr-deleted SIV; Δ5G, an SIV in which asparagines were mutated in order to remove five out of the 22 N-glycans from gp120. (Table courtesy of Wayne Koff; after W.C. Koff *et al.* (2006) HIV vaccine design: insights from live attenuated SIV vaccines. *Nature Immunology* **7**, 19–39).

Vaccine	Monkeys protected*
Live attenuated: Δ*nef*	59 of 63
Live attenuated: Δ3	12 of 12
Live attenuated: Δ5*G*	3 of 3
Live attenuated summary	74 of 78 (95%)
All other vaccine strategies†	18 of 256 (7%)†

*Protection is considered as suppression of viral load of more than 3 logs sustained over at least 6 months and generally much longer. In early studies, before plasma virus load assays were available, protection was judged by low or negative PCR results in peripheral blood mononuclear cells and/or failure of isolation of virus from peripheral blood mononuclear cells after challenge.
†The 256 monkeys here are distributed among the following vaccine categories: DNA alone (n = 11), DNA plus vector (n = 22), poxvirus vectors (n = 101), other vectors (n = 93), vector combinations (n = 8) and whole-inactivated SIV or proteins and/or peptides (n = 21). Of the 256 monkeys immunized with protein or vectored vaccines, 200 (78%) had a plasma load reduction of less than 1 log.

Since viral set point has been correlated with time of progression to AIDS, this would provide direct benefit to vaccinees. Furthermore, reduction of average plasma viral loads in vaccinated individuals should reduce transmission rates since transmission correlates with plasma viral load. Thus, vaccination should provide benefit to the population at large. Finally, reducing the damage to CD4$^+$ T-cells in primary infection may help to maintain immunity against many pathogens over a long period.

Most studies on so-called 'T-cell vaccines' have been carried out in monkeys. The results have been mixed. The best CD8$^+$ T-cell responses, at least in terms of Elispot measurements, have been achieved using recombinant viral vectors to express HIV/SIV gene products. In particular, adenovirus vectors, either alone or in combination with other vectors or DNA vaccina-

tion, have elicited significant T-cellular responses. These responses have shown some protection in some monkey models but not in others. The T-cell vaccine concept is now being evaluated in human clinical trials.

One regime that has protected against SIV challenge in monkeys is vaccination with live attenuated SIV (table 14.1). Attenuation can be achieved by deletion of the nef or multiple accessory genes or by engineering of Env. The protection is most apparent for homologous challenge, i.e. the live attenuated SIV is from the same strain as the challenge SIV, and matures over time. These features argue that the origin of protection lies in adaptive rather than innate immunity but the mechanism(s) remain an enigma.

Overall, it is clear that the development of an HIV vaccine is one of the major challenges facing modern medicine. Many believe that success will require the development of immunogens that can elicit both potent broadly neutralizing antibody and cellular immune responses.

SUMMARY

Primary immunodeficiency states (table 14.2)

• These occur, albeit somewhat rarely, as a result of a defect in almost any stage of differentiation in the whole immune system.

• Rare X-linked mutations produce disease in males.

• Defects in phagocytic cells, the complement pathways or the B-cell system lead in particular to infection with bacteria which are disposed of by opsonization and phagocytosis.

• Patients with T-cell deficiencies are susceptible to viruses and fungi which are normally eradicated by CMI.

• A lack of functional T-cells will impair B-cell responses, this effect being particularly pronounced in severe combined immunodeficiency (SCID) where there is a complete block in T-cell development.

Secondary immunodeficiency

• Immunodeficiency may arise as a secondary consequence of malnutrition, lymphoproliferative disorders, agents such as X-rays and cytotoxic drugs, and viral infections.

DEFECTIVE GENE PRODUCT(S)	DISORDER
COMPLEMENT DEFICIENCIES	
MBL, MASP-2	Reccurent bacterial infections
C1 inhibitor	Angioedema
PIG-A glycosyltransferase	Paroxysmal nocturnal hemoglobinuria
C3, Factor H, Factor I	Reccurent pyogenic infections
C5, C6, C7, C8	Reccurent *Neisseria* infections
PHAGOCYTIC DEFECTS	
NADPH oxidase	Chronic granulomatous disease
CD18 (β_2-integrin β chain)	Leukocyte adhesion deficiency
CHS	Chediak-Higashi disease
IFNγR1/2, IL-12 p40, IL-12Rβ1	Mendelian susceptibility to mycobacteria infection
PRIMARY T-CELL DEFICIENCY	
?	DiGeorge and Nezelof syndromes; failure of thymic development
RAG-1, RAG-2	Omenn's syndrome; partial *VDJ* recombination
MHC class II promoters	MHC class II deficiency (Bare lymphocyte syndrome)
Atm	Ataxia telangiectasia; defective DNA repair
CD154 (CD40L)	Hyper-IgM syndrome
CD3γ, ZAP-70	Severe T-cell deficiency
PNP	Purine nucleoside phosphorylase deficiency toxic to T-cells
WASP	Wiskott-Aldrich syndrome, defective cytoskeletal regulation
SEVERE COMBINED IMMUNODEFICIENCY	
γC, JAK-3	TB$^+$NK SCID
RAG-1, RAG-2, Artemis	TB$^-$NK$^+$ SCID
ADA	TB$^-$NK$^-$ SCID
IL-7Rα, CD45, CD3δ, CD3ϵ	TB$^+$NK$^+$ SCID

Table 14.2. Summary of the major primary immunodeficiency states.

(Continued p.335)

Acquired immunodeficiency syndrome (AIDS)

- AIDS results from infection with the lentiviruses HIV-1 or HIV-2, with HIV-1 being much more prevalent worldwide.
- HIV-1 infects CD4$^+$ cells, including CD4$^+$ T-cells, macrophages and dendritic cells.
- Depletion of CD4$^+$ T-cells, dramatically in primary infection particularly in the gut and then more slowly over a period of years during clinical latency, leads to damage to the immune system, which renders an individual susceptible to opportunistic pathogens (AIDS).
- HIV-1 is a retrovirus, which gains entry to cells by interaction of envelope spikes with CD4 and the chemokine receptors, CCR5 or CXCR4. The RNA genome is reverse transcribed and the resulting viral cDNA integrated into host T-cell chromosomes.
- Integrated proviral DNA can remain latent in cells for very long times, posing enormous problems for complete elimination of the virus from an individual and therefore hampering a complete cure for HIV-1 infection.
- Proviral DNA can be transcribed to generate new viral particles with the aid of several viral accessory proteins, which act to aid viral replication and/or adapt the host T-cell machinery to virus production.
- A major hallmark of HIV is the enormous diversity of the virus, present even in a single infected individual, because of the inherent errors involved in transcribing from an RNA genome, the rapid turnover of the virus and the high viral burden typically carried by the individual.
- Viral diversity and latency present major challenges to drug therapy but nevertheless drug design has been highly successful and combination drug regimes can hold the virus in check for many years, if not indefinitely.
- Vaccine design has also struggled with viral diversity and no immunogens that elicit broadly neutralizing antibodies or sufficiently potent T-cell responses to significantly contain challenge with a wide diversity of HIVs have yet been designed, although efforts are intense and there are promising leads.

See the accompanying website (**www.roitt.com**) for multiple choice questions.

FURTHER READING

Austen K.F., Burakoff S.J., Rosen F.S. & Strom T.B. (eds) (2001) *Therapeutic Immunology*, 2nd edn. Blackwell Science, Oxford.

Bonilla F.A. & Geha R.S. (2006) Update on primary immunodeficiency diseases. *Journal of Allergy and Clinical Immunology* **117** (2 suppl):S435–441.

Buckley R.H. (2002) Primary immunodeficiency diseases: dissectors of the immune system. *Immunological Reviews* **185**, 206–219.

Burton D.R. *et al.* (2004) HIV vaccine design and the neutralizing antibody problem. *Nature Immunology* **5**, 233–236.

Cavazzana-Calvo M., Lagresle C., Hacein-Bey-Abina S. & Fischer A. (2005) Gene therapy for severe combined immunodeficiency. *Annual Review of Medicine* **56**, 585–602.

Chapel H., Haeney M., Misbah S. & Snowden N. (2006) *Essentials of Clinical Immunology*, 5th edn. Blackwell Publishing, Oxford.

Daar E.S. & Richman D.D. (2005) Confronting the emergence of drug-resistant HIV type 1: impact of antiretroviral therapy on individual and population resistance. *AIDS Research Human and Retroviruses* **21**, 343–357.

Davis C.W. & Doms R.W. (2004) HIV transmission: closing all the doors. *Journal of Experimental Medicine* **199**, 1037–1040.

Goulder P.J. & Watkins D.I. (2004) HIV and SIV CTL escape: implications for vaccine design. *Nature Reviews Immunology* **4**, 630–640.

Greene W.C. (2004) The brightening future of HIV therapeutics. *Nature Immunology* **5**, 867–871.

Greene W.C. & Peterlin B.M. (2002) Charting HIV's remarkable voyage through the cell: basic science as a passport to future therapy. *Nature Medicine* **8**, 673–680.

Haase A.T. (2005) Perils at mucosal front lines for HIV and SIV and their hosts. *Nature Reviews Immunology* **5**, 783–792.

Johnson W.E. & Desrosiers R.C. (2002) Viral persistence: HIV's strategies of immune system evasion. *Annual Review of Medicine* **53**, 499–518.

Kaufmann S.H. & McMichael A.J. (2005) Annulling a dangerous liaison: vaccination strategies against AIDS and tuberculosis. *Nature Medicine* **11**, S33–S44.

Koff W.C. *et al.* (2006) HIV vaccine design: insights from live attenuated SIV vaccines. *Nature Immunology* **7**, 19–23.

Letvin N.L. & Walker B.D. (2003) Immunopathogenesis and immunotherapy in AIDS virus infections. *Nature Medicine* **9**, 861–866.

McMichael A.J. & Hanke T. (2003) HIV vaccines 1983–2003. *Nature Medicine* **9**, 874–880.

Ochs H.D., Smith C.I.E. & Puck J.M. (eds) (2000) *Primary Immunodeficiency Diseases—A Molecular and Genetic Approach.* Oxford University Press, Oxford.

Shattock R.J. & Moore J.P. (2003) Inhibiting sexual transmission of HIV-1 infection. *Nature Reviews Microbiology* **1**, 25–34.

Simonte S.J. & Cunningham-Rundles C. (2003) Update on primary immunodeficiency: defects of lymphocytes. *Clinical Immunology* **109**, 109–118.

Stiehm E.R., Ochs H.D. & Winkelstein J.A. (eds) (2004) *Immunological Disorders in Infants and Children*, 5th edn. W.B. Saunders, Philadelphia.

Stevenson M. (2003) HIV-1 pathogenesis. *Nature Medicine* **9**, 853–860.

15 Hypersensitivity

INTRODUCTION

When an individual has been immunologically primed, further contact with antigen leads to secondary boosting of the immune response. However, the reaction may be excessive (hypersensitivity) and lead to gross tissue changes if the antigen is present in relatively large amounts or if the humoral and cellular immune state is at a heightened level. It should be emphasized that the mechanisms underlying these **inappropriate immune responses leading to tissue damage**, which we speak of as **hypersensitivity reactions**, are those normally employed by the body in combating infection as discussed in Chapter 12. Hypersensitivity can also arise from direct interaction of the inciting agent with elements of the innate immune system without intervention by acquired responses.

ANAPHYLACTIC HYPERSENSITIVITY (TYPE I)

The phenomenon of anaphylaxis

The earliest accounts of inappropriate responses to foreign antigens relate to **anaphylaxis** (Milestone 15.1). The phenomenon can be readily reproduced in guinea-pigs which, like humans, are a highly susceptible species. A single injection of 1mg of an antigen such as egg albumin into a guinea-pig has no obvious effect. Repeat the injection 2–3 weeks later and the sensitized animal reacts very dramatically with the symptoms of generalized anaphylaxis; almost immediately, the guinea-pig begins to wheeze and within a few minutes dies from asphyxia. Examination shows intense constriction of the bronchioles and bronchi and generally there is: (i) contraction of smooth muscle, and (ii) dilatation of capillaries. Similar reactions do occur in human

subjects highly allergic to insect stings, pollens, foods, drugs such as penicillin, or other agents which have the potential to cause life-threatening anaphylactic responses. In many instances only a timely injection of epinephrine, which rapidly reverses the action of histamine on smooth muscle contraction and capillary dilatation, can prevent death. Individuals known to be at risk are given self administration preloaded epinephrine syringes.

Sir Henry Dale recognized that histamine mimics the systemic changes of anaphylaxis and, furthermore, that exposure of the uterus from a sensitized guinea-pig to antigen induces an immediate contraction associated with an explosive degranulation of mast cells (figure 1.14) responsible for the release of histamine and a number of other mediators (figure 1.15).

Anaphylaxis is triggered by clustering of IgE receptors on mast cells through cross-linking

In rodents two main types of **mast cell** have been recognized, those in the intestinal mucosa and those in the peritoneum and other connective tissue sites. They differ in a number of respects, for example in the type of protease and proteoglycan in their granules, and in their ability to proliferate and differentiate in response to stimulation by IL-3 (table 15.1). The two types have common precursors and are interconvertible depending upon the environmental conditions, with the mucosal MC_t (*t*ryptase) phenotype favored by IL-3 and connective tissue MC_{tc} (both *t*ryptase and *c*hymase) being promoted by relatively high levels of stem cell factor (c-kit ligand). In humans most mast cells in the intestinal mucosa and lung alveoli are tryptase-only positive, whilst those in skin, intestinal submucosa and other connective tissues are tryptase, chymase and

Milestone 15.1 — The Discovery of Anaphylaxis

Hypersensitive reactions in some individuals to normally innocuous environmental agents have been observed from time immemorial. Scientific interest in such reactions was aroused by the observations of Charles Richet and Paul Portier. During a South Sea cruise on Prince Albert of Monaco's yacht, the Prince, presumably smarting from an encounter with *Physalia* (the jelly-fish known as the Portugese-Man-of-War with very nasty tentacles), suggested that toxin production by the fish might be of interest. Let Richet and Portier take up the story in their own words (1902):

'On board the Prince's yacht, experiments were carried out proving that an aqueous glycerin extract of the filaments of *Physalia* is extremely toxic to ducks and rabbits. On returning to France, I could not obtain *Physalia* and decided to study comparatively the tentacles of *Actinaria* (sea anemone). While endeavouring to determine the toxic dose (of extracts), we soon discovered that some days must elapse before fixing it;

for several dogs did not die until the fourth or fifth day after administration or even later. We kept those that had been given insufficient to kill, in order to carry out a second investigation upon these when they had recovered. At this point an unforeseen event occurred. The dogs which had recovered were intensely sensitive and died a few minutes after the administration of small doses. The most typical experiment, that in which the result was indisputable, was carried out on a particularly healthy dog. It was given at first 0.1 ml of the glycerin extract without becoming ill: 22 days later, as it was in perfect health, I gave it a second injection of the same amount. In a few seconds it was extremely ill; breathing became distressful; it could scarcely drag itself along, lay on its side, was seized with diarrhea, vomited blood and died in 25 minutes.'

The development of sensitivity to relatively harmless substances was termed by these authors **anaphylaxis**, in contrast to **prophylaxis**.

Table 15.1. Comparison of two types of mast cell.

CHARACTERISTICS	MUCOSAL MAST CELL	CONNECTIVE TISSUE MAST CELL
GENERAL		
Abbreviation*	MC_t	MC_{tc}
Distribution	Gut & lung	Most tissues**
Differentiation favored by	IL-3	Stem cell factor
T-cell dependence	+	−
High affinity Fcε receptor	2×10^5/cell	3×10^4/cell
GRANULES		
Alcian blue and Safranin staining	Blue & brown	Blue
Ultrastructure	Scrolls	Gratings/lattices
Protease	Tryptase	Tryptase & chymase
Proteoglycan	Chondroitin sulfate	Heparin
DEGRANULATION		
Histamine release	+	++
LTC_4 : PGD_2 release	25 : 1	1 : 40
Blocked by disodium cromoglycate/theophylline	−	+

*Based on protease in granules.

**Predominate in normal skin and intestinal submucosa.

carboxypeptidase positive. A third, less frequent, population are chymase-only positive and are found in the nasal mucosa and intestinal submucosa.

Mast cells, and their circulating counterpart the basophil, abundantly display the FcεRI high affinity (K_a 10^{10} M^{-1}) receptor for IgE (cf. table 3.2). The receptor is also expressed, albeit at considerably lower levels, on Langerhans cells, monocytes, platelets and eosinophils. On basophils and mast cells (and possibly eosinophils) the receptor consists of an α chain, a tetraspan β chain

and two disulfide-linked γ chains, whereas on the other cell types the β chain is absent. The α chain possesses two external Ig-type domains responsible for binding the Cε3 region of IgE (figure 15.1), whereas the γ chains and β chain each contain a cytoplasmic *i*mmunorecep-tor *t*yrosine-based *a*ctivation *m*otif (ITAM) for cell signaling. In the absence of bound IgE the level of FcεRI drops substantially. However, in its presence there is upregulation of the receptor on mast cells and, because the γ chain is shared with the mast cell FcγRIIIA, a consequent competitive downregulation of the Fc receptor for IgG. Anaphylaxis is mediated by the reaction of the allergen with the IgE antibodies held on the surface of the mast cell, cross-linking of these antibodies triggering mediator release (figure 15.2). The critical event is aggregation of the receptors by cross-linking as clearly shown by the ability of divalent antibodies reacting directly with the receptor to trigger the mast cell.

Aggregation of the FcεRI α chains activates the Lyn protein tyrosine kinase associated with the β chains and, if the aggregates persist, this leads to transphosphorylation of the β and γ chains of other FcεRI receptors within the cluster and recruitment of the Syk kinase (figure 15.3). The subsequent series of phosphorylation-induced activation steps ultimately leads to mast cell degranulation with release of preformed mediators and the synthesis of arachidonic acid metabolites formed by the cyclo-oxygenase and lipoxygenase pathways (cf. figure 1.15). To recapitulate, the preformed mediators released from the granules include histamine, heparin, tryptase, chymase, carboxypeptidase, eosinophil, neutrophil and monocyte chemotactic factors, platelet

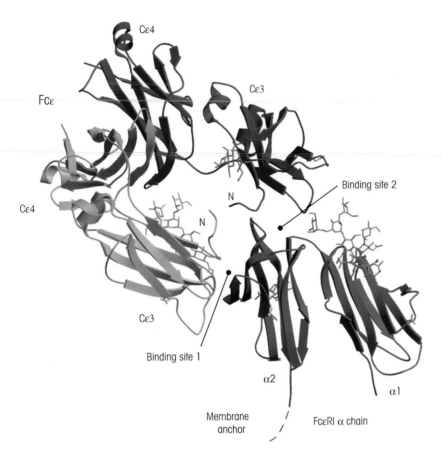

Figure 15.1. The structural basis of the binding of IgE to the high affinity mast cell receptor FcεRI. Side view of the complex with the two Fc chains in yellow and red and the FcεRI α chain in blue; carbohydrate residues are shown as sticks. The two Cε3 domains of the heavy chain dimer of IgE bind asymmetrically to two distinct interaction sites on the α chain of the receptor. The β-turn loop on one Cε3 binds along one side of the α2 domain, while surface loops plus the Cε2–Cε3 linker region on the other Cε3 interact with the top of the α1–α2 interface. The 1:1 stoichiometry of this asymmetric binding precludes the linkage of one IgE to two receptor molecules and ensures that triggering due to α–α aggregation only occurs through multivalent binding to surface IgE (see figure 15.2). (Photograph kindly provided by Dr Ted Jardetzky and reproduced by permission of the Nature Publishing Group.)

activating factor and, in rodents but apparently not in humans, serotonin. By contrast, leukotrienes LTB_4, LTC_4 and LTD_4, the prostaglandin PGD_2 and thromboxanes are all newly synthesized. The Th2 type cytokines IL-4, IL-5, IL-6, IL-9, IL-10, IL-13, as well as IL-1, IL-3, IL-8, IL-11, granulocyte–macrophage colony-stimulating factor (GM-CSF), TNF, CCL2 (monocyte chemotactic protein-1, MCP-1), CCL5 (RANTES) and CCL11 (eotaxin), are all also released. Under normal circumstances, these mediators help to orchestrate the development of a defensive acute inflammatory reaction (and in this context let us not forget that complement fragments C3a and C5a can also trigger mast cells through complement receptors). When there is a massive release of these mediators under abnormal conditions, as in atopic disease, their bronchoconstrictive and vasodilatory effects predominate and become distinctly threatening.

Atopic allergy

Clinical responses to extrinsic allergens

It has been claimed that in Westernized countries up to 30% of adults and 45% of children may suffer to a greater or lesser degree with allergies involving localized IgE-mediated anaphylactic reactions to allergens such as

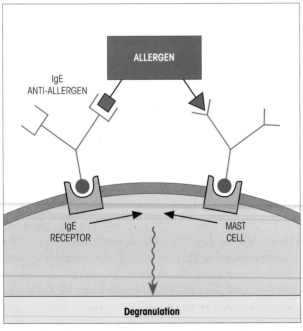

Figure 15.2. Clustering of IgE receptors either by multivalent allergen or antibody to the receptors themselves leads to mast cell degranulation.

Figure 15.3. Mast cell triggering.
Simplified scheme of some of the signaling events through the high affinity IgE receptor, FcεRI. Aggregation of the FcεRI α chains in lipid rafts through cross-linking of bound IgE by multivalent antigen (allergen) alerts the β and γ chains of the receptor, leading to activation of the linked Lyn and Syk protein tyrosine kinases. They in turn phosphorylate and activate the membrane adaptor protein LAT which recruits phospholipase Cγ1 (PLCγ1) and adaptor molecules concerned in the activation of GTPase/kinase cascades. Activation of PLCγ1 generates diacylglycerol (DAG) which targets protein kinase C, while inositol $(1,4,5)P_3$ (IP_3) elevates cytoplasmic Ca^{2+} by depleting the ER stores. The raised calcium concentration activates transcriptional factors and causes granule exocytosis. The Grb-2/Sos and Slp-76/Vav complexes are also associated with the LAT adaptor and trigger the Ras and Rac/Rho GTPase-induced serial kinase cascades, respectively, leading to the activation of transcription factors and rearrangements of the actin cytoskeleton. (Figure essentially designed by Dr Helen Turner, based on the article by Turner H. & Kinet J.-P. (1999) *Nature* (Supplement on Allergy and Asthma) **402**, B24.)

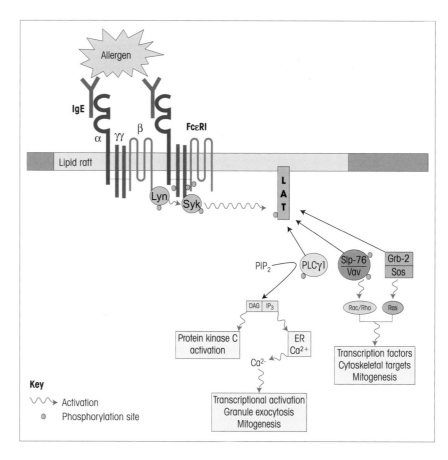

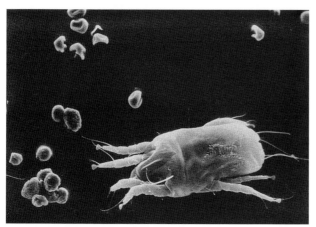

Figure 15.4. House dust mite—a major cause of allergic disease. The electron micrograph shows the rather nasty looking mite graced by the name *Dermatophagoides pteryonyssinus* and fecal pellets on the bottom left. A typical double bed can contain up to 200 million mites, each mite producing approximately 20 fecal pellets/day and each pellet containing 0.2 ng of proteolytically active Der p1 allergen. The biconcave pollen grains (top left) shown for comparison indicate the size of particle which can become airborne and reach the lungs. The mite itself is much too large for that. (Reproduced by courtesy of Dr E. Tovey.)

grass pollens, animal danders, the feces from mites in house dust (figure 15.4) and so on. Even if these are over-estimates, it is clear that allergies affect a large number of people and that they are on the increase. A large number

of allergens have now been cloned and expressed (table 15.2), several of which turn out to be enzymes. For example, Der p1 is a cysteine protease which increases the permeability of the bronchial mucosa, thereby facilitating its own passage along with other allergens across the epithelium and allowing access to and sensitization of cells of the immune system. The CD23 low affinity receptor for IgE (FcεRII) on B-cells downregulates IgE synthesis upon antigen-mediated cross-linking of the bound IgE. However, Der p1 proteolytically cleaves CD23 and thereby reduces its negative impact on IgE synthesis. Furthermore, Der p1 also cleaves CD25 (the IL-2 receptor α chain) on T-cells and thus limits the activation of Th1 cells, biasing the immune response to Th2-dependent IgE production. Short cuts to allergen purification can be achieved by screening cDNA expression libraries with IgE. This was a godsend for the purification of the allergen from the venom of the Australian jumper ant, *Myrmecia pilosula*; just think of trying to accumulate ants by the kilogram to isolate the allergen using conventional protein fractionation.

The local anaphylactic reaction to injection of antigen into the skin of atopic patients is manifest as a wheal and flare (figure 15.5) which is maximal at 30 minutes or so and resolves within about an hour; it may be succeeded by a late phase response involving eosinophil infiltrates

Table 15.2. Some examples of allergens.

Category	Origin	Allergens	Example
Insect	House dust mite (*Dermatophagoides pteronyssinus*) feces	Der p 1–Der p 14	Der p 1: cysteine protease
	Honeybee (*Apis mellifera*) venom	Api m 1–7	Api m 1: phospholipase A$_2$
	German cockroach (*Blattella germanica*)	Bla g 1–6	Bla g 2: aspartic protease
Companion animals	Cat (*Felis domesticus*)	Fel d 1–7	Fel d 4: lipocalin
	Dog (*Canis domesticus*)	Can f 1–4	Can f 3: albumin
Trees	Birch (*Betula verrucosa*)	Bet v 1–7	Bet v 7: cyclophilin
	Hazel (*Corylus avellana*)	Cor a 1–11	Cor a 8: lipid transfer protein
Grasses and plants	Timothy grass (*Phleum pretense*)	Phl p 1–13	Phl p 13: polygalacturonase
	Perennial ryegrass (*Lolium perenne*)	Lol p 1–11	Lol p 11: trypsin inhibitor
	Short ragweed (*Ambrosia artemisiifolia*)	Amb a 1–7	Amb a 5: neurophysin
Molds	*Aspergillus fumigatus*	Asp f 1–23	Asp f 12: heat shock protein p90
	Cladosporium herbarum	Cla h 1–12	Cla h 3: aldehyde dehydrogenase
Foods	Peanut	Ara h 1–8	Ara h 1: vicilin
	Cows' milk (*Bos domesticus*)	Bos d 1–8	Bos d 4: α-lactalbumin
	Chicken's eggs (*Gallus domesticus*)	Gal d 1–5	Gal d 2: ovalbumin
Drugs	Penicillin	–	Amoxicillin
	Fluoroquinolone	–	Ciprofloxacin
Occupational allergens	Toluene diisocyanate	–	–
	Latex (derived from the rubber tree, *Hevea brasiliensis*)	Hev b 1–13	Hev b 1: elongation factor

For a complete list see International Union of Immunological Societies Allergen Nomenclature Sub-Committee http://www.allergen.org/List.htm

which peak at around 5 hours. Contact of the allergen with cell-bound IgE in the bronchial tree, the nasal mucosa and the conjunctival tissues releases mediators of anaphylaxis and produces the symptoms of **asthma** or **allergic rhinitis and conjunctivitis** (hay fever) as the case may be. A proportion of the patients who experience late phase responses after bronchial challenge with allergen eventually develop chronic **asthma**. Three hundred million individuals worldwide suffer from asthma and it costs over $6 billion a year to treat in the USA alone. Indeed, according to the World Health Organization, the worldwide economic costs associated with asthma are estimated to exceed those of tuberculosis and HIV/AIDS combined. Asthma can be associated with agents encountered in the workplace, and is then described as **occupational asthma**. Allergens here include toluene diisocyanate in spray paints, colophony fumes from solders used in the electronics industry and danders (particles of old skin on animal hair) encountered by animal handlers. Although the majority of asthma patients have **extrinsic asthma** associated with **atopy** (from the Greek *atopos*, meaning 'out of place'), i.e. the genetic predisposition to synthesize inappropriate levels of IgE specific for external allergens, some patients are nonatopic and therefore are said to have **intrinsic or idiopathic asthma**.

Bronchial biopsy and lavage of asthmatic patients reveal an unequivocal involvement of **mast cells and eosinophils** as the major mediator-secreting effector cells, while T-cells provide the microenvironment required to sustain the chronic inflammatory response which is an essential feature of the histopathology

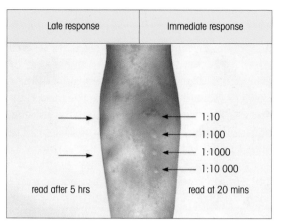

Figure 15.5. Atopic allergy. Skin prick tests with grass pollen allergen in a patient with typical summer hay fever. Skin tests were performed 5 hours (left) and 20 minutes (right) before the photograph was taken. The tests on the right show a typical titration of a type I immediate wheal and flare reaction. The late phase skin reaction (left) can be clearly seen at 5 hours, especially where a large immediate response has preceded it. Figures for allergen dilution are given.

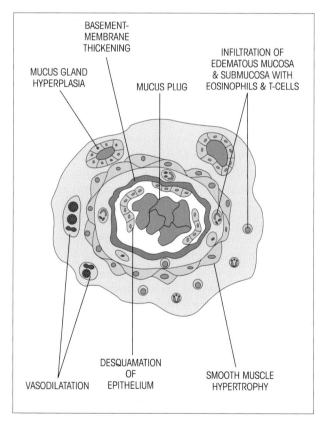

Figure 15.6. Pathological changes in asthma. Diagram of cross-section of an airway in severe asthma.

(figure 15.6). The resulting variable airflow obstruction and bronchial hyper-responsiveness are the cardinal clinical and physiological features of the disease.

The atopic trait can also manifest itself as an **atopic**

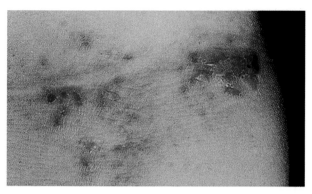

Figure 15.7. An atopic eczema reaction on the back of a knee of a child allergic to rice and eggs. (Kindly provided by Professor J. Brostoff.)

dermatitis (figure 15.7), with house dust mite, domestic cats and German cockroaches often proving to be the environmental offenders. Recalling the inflammation in asthma, skin patch tests with Der p1 in these eczema patients produce an infiltrate of eosinophils, T-cells, mast cells and basophils. The number of individuals affected is comparable to the number affected by asthma. The beneficial effect of the calcineurin inhibitors cyclosporine and, more recently, topical tacrolimus in patients with eczema highlights the important role of T-cells in the pathogenesis of this disease.

Awareness of the importance of IgE sensitization to **food allergens** in the gut has increased dramatically. Contact with allergens such as those present in cows' milk, eggs, nuts and shellfish before mucosal protective mechanisms, especially IgA, are reasonably established leads to an increase in the incidence of atopy in the newborn. Although, overall, children who are breastfed have a lower incidence of allergies, sensitization to dietary allergens can also occur in early infancy through breast-feeding, with antigen passing into the mother's milk. One could argue that breast-feeding mothers should limit their intake of common allergens. Allergy to peanuts is seen in approximately 1% of children and, as with other allergens, reactions are sometimes life threatening or even occasionally fatal. Food additives such as sulfiting agents can also cause adverse reactions. Contact of the food with specific IgE on mast cells in the gastrointestinal tract may produce local reactions resulting in abdominal pain, cramps, diarrhea and vomiting, or may allow the allergen to enter the body by causing a change in gut permeability through mediator release; the allergen may complex with antibodies and cause distal lesions by depositing in the joints, for example, or it may diffuse freely to other sensitized sites, such as the skin (figure 15.7) or lungs, where it will cause a further local anaphylactic reaction. Thus eating strawberries may produce urticarial reactions (hives, raised

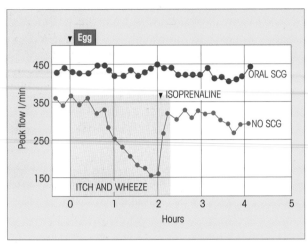

Figure 15.8. The role of gut sensitivity in the development of asthma to food allergens. A patient challenged by feeding with egg developed asthma within hours, as shown here by the depressed lung function test of measuring peak air flow; the symptoms at the end-organ stage were counteracted by the β-adrenoreceptor agonist, isoprenaline. However, oral sodium cromoglycate (SCG), which prevents antigen-specific mast cell triggering, also prevented the onset of asthma after oral challenge with egg. Note that SCG taken orally has no effect on the response of an asthmatic to inhaled allergen. (From Brostoff J. (1986) In Brostoff J. & Challacombe S.J. (eds) *Food Allergy*, p. 441. Baillière Tindall, London, reproduced with permission.)

areas of itchy skin) and egg may precipitate an asthmatic attack in appropriately sensitized individuals. The role of the sensitized gut in acting as a 'gate' to allow entry of allergens is strongly suggested by experiments in which oral sodium cromoglycate, a mast cell stabilizer, prevented subsequent asthma after ingestion of the provoking food (figure 15.8).

Anaphylactic drug allergy is manifest in the dramatic responses to drugs such as **penicillin** which haptenate body proteins by covalent coupling to induce IgE synthesis. In the case of penicillin, the β-lactam ring links to the ε-amino of lysine to form the penicilloyl determinant. The fine specificity of the IgE antibodies permits discrimination between closely similar drugs, such that some patients may be allergic to amoxicillin but tolerate benzylpenicillin which differs by only very minor modifications of the side-chains.

Pathological mechanisms in asthma

We should now look in more depth at those events which generate the chronicity of asthma. Remember that there is an *early phase* bronchial response to inhaled antigen essentially involving mast cell mediators, and an inflammatory *late phase* dominated by eosinophils. **Both phases are IgE-dependent** as shown by their marked attenuation in asthmatics treated with the humanized monoclonal anti-IgE antibody Omalizumab (Xolair, RhuMAb-E25) which reduces IgE to almost

undetectable levels. Activated mast cells produce IL-11 which is thought to contribute towards the development of the asthma-associated structural changes referred to as airway remodeling; thickening of the airway walls, and increases in the adventitia, submucosal tissue and smooth muscle. The mast cells also contribute to eosinophil recruitment by secretion of tryptase which can activate coagulation Factor II receptor-like 1 (F2RL1, protease-activated receptor-2 [PAR-2]) on the surface of endothelial and epithelial cells, fibroblasts and smooth muscle. Activation of the receptor leads to TNF, IL-1 and IL-4 production, promoting the expression of the vascular endothelial adhesion molecules VCAM-1, ICAM-1 and P-selectin which recruit eosinophils and basophils. An important trigger of the late phase reaction is the **activation of alveolar macrophages** through the interaction of allergen with IgE bound to the low affinity FcεRII leading to a significant increase in the production of TNF and IL-1β. These cytokines stimulate the release of the powerful **eosinophil chemoattractants** eotaxin (CCL11), RANTES (CCL5) and MCP5 (CCL12) (cf. p. 196) from bronchial epithelial cells and fibroblasts. Note also that eotaxin and RANTES can contribute directly to local inflammation by IgE-independent degranulation of basophils.

A new player now enters the field: primed T-cells traffic into the inflamed site and are strongly attracted by eotaxin. Since the T-cell response is heavily skewed towards the **Th2 subset in asthma** (figure 15.9), encounter with allergen-derived peptides on antigen-presenting cells will promote the synthesis of IL-4, -5 and -13. IL-4 stimulates further eotaxin release, while IL-5 upregulates chemokine receptors on eosinophils, maintains their survival through an inhibitory effect on natural apoptosis and is involved in their longer term recruitment from bone marrow.

Things now look bad for the bronchial tissues and a multitude of factors contribute to allergen-induced airway dysfunction: (i) a virtual soup of bronchoconstrictors, the leukotrienes being especially important, bathe the smooth muscle cells, (ii) edema of the airway wall, (iii) altered neural regulation of airway tone through binding of eosinophil major basic protein (MBP) to M2 autoreceptors on the nerve endings with increased release of acetylcholine, (iv) airway epithelial cell desquamation due to the toxic action of MBP, there being a strong correlation between the number of desquamated cells in bronchoalveolar lavage fluid and the concentration of MBP, (v) mucus hypersecretion due to IL-13 and, to a lesser extent, IL-4, leukotrienes and platelet activating factor acting on submucosal glands and their controlling neural elements, and finally (vi) a

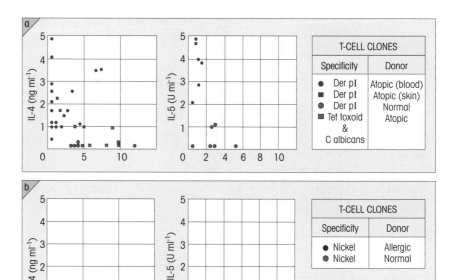

Figure 15.9. Th2 dominance in atopic allergy shown by cytokine profiles of antigen-specific CD4⁺ T-cell clones from (a) patients with type I atopic allergy and (b) subjects with type IV contact sensitivity, compared with normal controls. Each point represents the value for an individual clone. Archetypal Th1 clones have high IFNγ and IL-2 and low IL-4 and IL-5; Th2 clones show the converse. The high level of IL-4 drives the switch to IgE production by B-cells and further promotes the Th2 bias. (Data from Kapsenberg M.L., Wierenga E.A., Bos J.D. & Jansen H.M. (1991) *Immunology Today* **12**, 392.)

repair-type response involving the production of fibroblast growth factor, TGFβ and platelet-derived growth factor, the laying down of collagen, scar and fibrous tissue and hypertrophy of smooth muscle, leading to an exaggerated narrowing of the airways in response to a variety of environmental stimuli (figure 15.6). The wide range of cytokines and mediators produced by lung epithelial and endothelial cells, fibroblasts and smooth muscle cells may account for the persistence of airway inflammation and the permanent structural changes in chronic disease sufferers, even in the absence or apparent absence of ongoing exposure to inhalant allergens to which subjects are sensitized, a state where conventional immunotherapy might not be expected to be beneficial.

Unlike atopic asthmatics, **intrinsic asthmatics** have negative skin tests to common aeroallergens, no clinical or family history of allergy, normal levels of serum IgE and no detectable specific IgE antibodies to common allergens. Nonetheless, they resemble the atopics in important respects: bronchial biopsies show enhanced expression of IL-4, IL-13, RANTES and eotaxin, and of the mRNA for the ε heavy chain, suggestive of local IgE synthesis. Is there a role for virus-specific IgE or for IgE autoantibodies to the FcεRI?

The inflammatory infiltrate in **atopic dermatitis** resembles that in asthma and includes mast cells, basophils, eosinophils and T-cells. Epidermal dendritic cells express FcεRI, and incoming allergens are taken up as allergen–IgE complexes and passed to the MHC class II processing pathway for presentation to Th2 cells. CC

chemokines produced by keratinocytes and fibroblasts preferentially attract eosinophils and the skin-homing CLA⁺ memory Th2-cells. The latter comprise 80–90% of the T-cells in the infiltrate and account for the specific response to the offending allergen.

Etiological factors in the development of atopic allergy

There is a strong familial predisposition to the development of atopic allergy (figure 15.10). One factor is undoubtedly the overall ability to synthesize the IgE isotype—the higher the level of IgE in the blood, the greater the likelihood of becoming atopic (figure 15.10). Genetic studies have provided evidence that many different genes contribute to susceptibility to develop asthma (figure 15.11), including polymorphisms in a number of pattern recognition receptors (PRR). What relevance might this have for atopic disease? Well, the PRR-mediated recognition of pathogens by dendritic cells is important in developing the correct balance between Th1 and Th2 responses. Current thinking goes along the following lines. At the time of birth the neonatal immune system is skewed towards Th2-type responses, but in the face of a hostile microbial environment there is a shift towards Th1 responses. This shift extends to inhaled allergens, and is sometimes referred to as immune deviation. However, in the absence of repeated infections with common pathogens (due to a 'cleaner' environment and widespread early use of antibiotics) the immune system maintains a Th2 phenotype which will favor the secretion of IL-4 (promoting

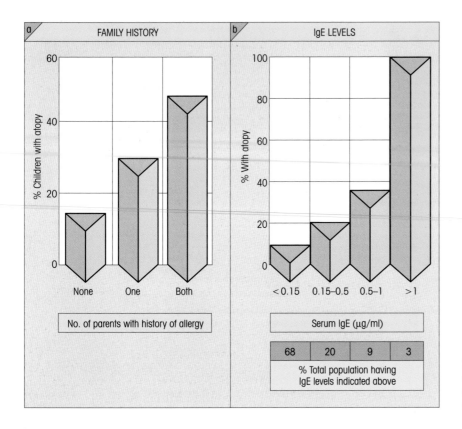

Figure 15.10. Risk factors in allergy: (a) family history; (b) IgE levels—the higher the serum IgE concentration, the greater the chance of developing atopy.

IgE production) and IL-5 (promoting eosinophilia). This idea forms the basis of the hygiene hypothesis put forward to explain the rise in allergies seen in Westernized countries, and even more tellingly in countries that *become* Westernized, such as the former East Germany where levels of atopic allergy started to catch up with those in West Germany following re-unification. The overall picture relating to Westernization is, however, complex—let us not forget that a finger has been pointed at environmental pollutants such as tobacco smoke and diesel exhaust particles as cofactors for asthma attacks. At the molecular level, expression of the GATA-3 transcription factor, c-maf and the presence of prostaglandin E_2 all promote Th2 development. Yet another piece of the jigsaw relates to the role of regulatory T-cells in atopic disease. Evidence is accumulating that indicates a deficit of these cells in patients with allergy, although which of the various T-reg populations (TGFβ-secreting Th3 cells, IL-10 secreting Tr1 cells, $CD4^+CD25^+$ contact-dependent T-regs, NKT regulatory cells, and so on) are the most critical in preventing allergic responses is still under investigation. The T-regs may themselves be influenced by interactions with distinct dendritic cell subsets. Watch this space, as they say.

Clinical tests for allergy

Sensitivity is normally assessed by the response to intra-dermal challenge with antigen. The release of histamine and other mediators rapidly produces a **wheal and erythema** (figure 15.5), maximal within 30 minutes and then subsiding. These immediate wheal and flare reactions may be followed by a late phase reaction (cf. figure 15.5) which sometimes lasts for 24 hours, redolent of those seen following challenge of the bronchi and nasal mucosa of allergic subjects and similarly characterized by dense infiltration with eosinophils and T-cells.

The correlation between skin prick test responses and the **radioallergosorbent test** (RAST, see p. 136) for allergen-specific serum IgE is fairly good. In some instances, intranasal challenge with allergen may provoke a response even when both of these tests are negative, probably as a result of local synthesis of IgE antibodies.

The presence of proteins secreted from mast cells or eosinophils in the serum or urine could provide important surrogate markers of disease and might predict exacerbations.

Therapy

If one considers the sequence of reactions from initial exposure to allergen right through to the production of atopic disease, it can be seen that several points in the chain provide legitimate targets for therapy (figure 15.12).

Allergen avoidance. Avoidance of contact with *potential* allergens is often impractical, although, to give one

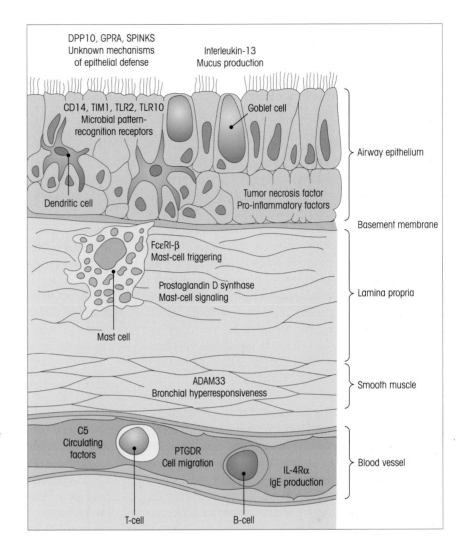

Figure 15.11. Gene products that influence susceptibility to asthma. Multiple genes have been implicated that act at various stages in the type I hypersensitivity response. (Modified from Cookson W. & Moffatt M. (2004) *New England Journal of Medicine* **351**, 1794–1796, with permission from the publishers.)

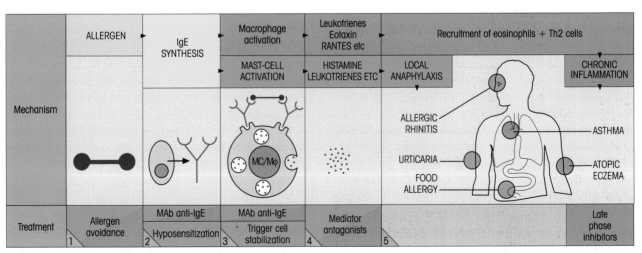

Figure 15.12. Atopic allergies and their treatment: sites of local responses and possible therapies. Events and treatments relating to local anaphylaxis are in green and to chronic inflammation in red.

example, feeding infants cows' milk at too early an age is discouraged. After sensitization, avoidance where possible is obviously worthwhile, but the reluctance of some parents to dispose of the family cat to stop little Algernon's wheezing is sometimes quite surprising.

Modulation of the immunological response. Attempts to desensitize patients immunologically by repeated subcutaneous injection of small amounts of allergen can lead to worthwhile improvement in individuals subject to insect venom anaphylaxis or hay fever, but are less effective in asthma. Sublingual allergen immunotherapy (SLIT) also appears to be effective and carries less risk of severe systemic reactions than subcutaneous administration. Injection of naked DNA coding for house dust mite allergen directly into the muscle, or oral administration of chitosan (a naturally occuring polysaccharide)-coated plasmid DNA containing a dominant peanut allergen gene, reduced IgE synthesis and gave good protection against anaphylactic challenge in mice, but the long-term endogenous expression of allergen in sensitized humans might lead to precarious situations. The purpose of allergen hyposensitization therapy was originally to boost the synthesis of IgG 'blocking' antibodies, whose function was to divert the allergen from contact with tissue-bound IgE. While this may well prove to be a contributory factor, downregulation of IgE synthesis by engagement of the FcγRIIB receptor (cf. p. 47) on B-cells by allergen-specific IgG linked to allergen molecules bound to surface IgE receptors also seems likely (cf. p. 212; see Chapter 10 on IgG regulation of Ab production). Additionally, T-lymphocyte cooperation is important for IgE synthesis and eosinophil-mediated pathogenesis, and therefore the beneficial effects of antigen injection may also be mediated through induction of anergic or regulatory T-cells and a switch from Th2 to Th1 cytokine production. Injection of heat-killed *Mycobacterium vaccae* induces IL-10 and TGFβ secretion by regulatory T-cells with a resultant decrease in Th2 activity. Inhibition of the Th2-associated transcription factor GATA-3 using PPAR (peroxisome proliferator-activated receptor) agonists, or stimulating Th1-associated T-bet expression with CpG motifs, may provide future therapeutic options for promoting Th1 rather than Th2 responses. The administration of tolerizing or antagonist peptide epitopes represents another possible therapeutic modality. Fortunately, most patients respond to a remarkably limited number of T-cell epitopes on any given allergen, and so it may not be necessary to tailor the therapeutic peptide to each individual. Clinical trials with high doses of Fel d 1-derived peptides from cat allergen have resulted in decreased sensitivity, although isolated late

responses to allergen by direct T-cell activation may be induced. A case can be made for future prophylactic hyposensitization of children with two asthmatic parents who have an approximately 50% probability of developing the disease.

Blocking the action of IgE. We have already mentioned the humanized monoclonal Omalizumab directed against the FcεRI-binding Cε3 domain of IgE (cf. p. 338) which provides an exciting new therapy for severe forms of asthma. It reduces the circulating IgE levels almost to vanishing point by direct neutralization, and as a secondary effect this decreases the IgE-dependent expression of the FcεRI receptor on mast cells. Thus there are far fewer receptors on the mast cell to bind IgE, and virtually no IgE to be bound anyway. It is not surprising therefore that this antibody successfully completed phase II clinical trials and was subsequently approved by the FDA for use in those adults and adolescents with moderate or severe persistent atopic asthma whose symptoms are inadequately controlled with inhaled corticosteroids.

Stabilization of the triggering cells. Much relief has been obtained with agents such as inhalant isoprenaline and **sodium cromoglycate** (cromolyn sodium) which render mast cells resistant to triggering. Sodium cromoglycate blocks chloride channel activity and maintains cells in a normal resting physiological state, which probably accounts for its inhibitory effects on a wide range of cellular functions, such as mast cell degranulation, eosinophil and neutrophil chemotaxis and mediator release, and reflex bronchoconstriction. Some or all of these effects are responsible for its anti-asthmatic actions.

The triggering of macrophages through allergen interaction with surface-bound IgE is clearly a major initiating factor for late reactions, as discussed above, and resistance to this stimulus can be very effectively achieved with corticosteroids. Unquestionably, **inhaled corticosteroids** have revolutionized the treatment of asthma. Their principal action is to suppress the transcription of multiple inflammatory genes, including in the present context those encoding several cytokines.

Mediator antagonism. **Histamine H₁-receptor antagonists** have for long proved helpful in the symptomatic treatment of atopic disease. Newer drugs of this class such as loratadine and fexofenadine are effective in rhinitis and in reducing the itch in atopic dermatitis, although they have little benefit in asthma. Cetirizine additionally has useful effects on eosinophil recruitment in the late phase reaction. Short acting selective β₂-

agonists such as Ventolin, the active ingredient of which is albuterol (salbutamol), are inhaled to alleviate mild to moderate symptoms of asthma. Such β-adrenergic receptor agonist drugs increase cAMP levels leading to relaxation of bronchial smooth muscle and inhibition of mast cell degranulation. An important advance has been the introduction of **long-acting β₂-agonists** such as salmeterol and formoterol which protect against bronchoconstriction for over 12 hours. Potent **leukotriene receptor antagonists** such as pranlukast also block constrictor challenges and show striking efficacy in certain patients, particularly aspirin-sensitive asthmatics.

Theophylline was introduced for the treatment of asthma over 50 years ago and, as a **phosphodiesterase (PDE) inhibitor,** it increases intracellular cAMP, thereby causing bronchodilatation, inhibition of IL-5-mediated eosinophil survival and probably suppression of eosinophil migration into the bronchial mucosa. Good news for the patient.

Attacking chronic inflammation. Certain drugs impede atopic disease at more than one stage. **Cetirizine** is a case in point with its dual effects on the histamine receptor and on eosinophil recruitment. **Corticosteroids** seem to do almost everything; apart from their role in stabilizing macrophages, they solidly inhibit the activation and proliferation of Th2 cells, which are the dominant underlying driving force in chronic asthma, and may call a halt to the development of irreversible narrowing of the airways. So it is that inhaled steroids (e.g. budesonide, mometasone furoate, fluticasone propionate) with high anti-inflammatory potency but minimal side-effects due to hepatic metabolism, provide first-line therapy for most chronic asthmatics, with supplementation by long-acting β₂-agonists and theophylline.

ANTIBODY-DEPENDENT CYTOTOXIC HYPERSENSITIVITY (TYPE II)

Where an antigen is present on the surface of a cell, combination with antibody will encourage the demise of that cell by promoting contact with phagocytes by **opsonic adherence** to Fcγ receptors and, often, to C3b receptors following activation of complement by the classical pathway. Cell death may also occur through activation of the full complement system up to C8 and C9 producing **direct membrane damage** (figure 15.13), although this will have to overcome the protective effect of cell surface complement regulatory proteins.

A quite distinct cytotoxic mechanism, **antibody-dependent cellular cytotoxicity (ADCC),** occurs when target cells coated with IgG or IgE antibody are killed through an extracellular nonphagocytic process involving leukocytes which bind to the target by their specific Fc receptors (figures 15.13 and 15.14). ADCC can be mediated by a number of different types of leukocyte including NK cells (see p. 18), monocytes, neutrophils and eosinophils. Although readily observed as a phenomenon *in vitro*, e.g. schistosomules coated with either IgG or IgE can be killed by eosinophils (cf. figure 12.23), whether ADCC plays a role *in vivo* remains a tricky question. Functionally this extracellular cytotoxic mechanism would be expected to be of significance where the target is too large for ingestion by phagocytosis, e.g. large parasites and solid tumors. It could also act as a back-up system for T-cell mediated killing.

Type II reactions between members of the same species (alloimmune)

Transfusion reactions
Of the many different polymorphic constituents of the

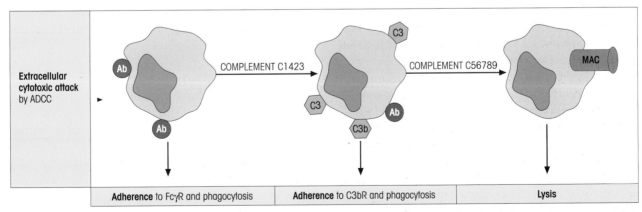

Figure 15.13. Antibody-dependent cytotoxic hypersensitivity (type II). Antibodies directed against cell surface antigens cause cell death not only by complement-dependent lysis using the C5b–C9 membrane attack complex (MAC) but also by Fcγ and C3b adherence reactions leading to phagocytosis, or through nonphagocytic extracellular killing by certain lymphoid and myeloid cells (antibody-dependent cellular cytotoxicity).

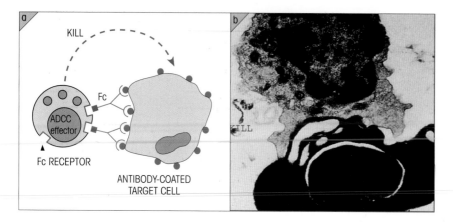

Figure 15.14. Killing of Ab-coated target by antibody-dependent cellular cytotoxicity (ADCC). Fcγ receptors bind the effector to the target which is killed by an extracellular mechanism. Human monocytes and IFNγ-activated neutrophils kill Ab-coated tumor cells using their FcγRI receptors; NK cells kill hybridoma targets through FcγRIII receptors. (a) Diagram of effector and target cells. (b) Electron micrograph of attack on Ab-coated chick red cell by a mouse NK cell showing close apposition of effector and target and vacuolation in the cytoplasm of the latter. ((b) Courtesy of P. Penfold.)

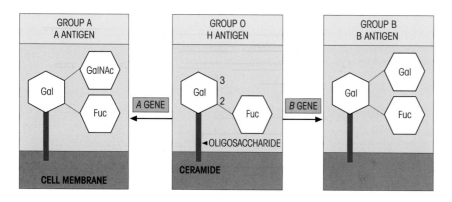

Figure 15.15. The ABO system. The allelic genes A and B code for transferases which add either N-acetylgalactosamine - (GalNAc) or galactose (Gal), respectively, to H substance. The oligosaccharide is anchored to the cell membrane by coupling to a sphingomyelin called ceramide. Eighty-five per cent of the population secrete blood group substances in the saliva, where the oligosaccharides are present as soluble polypeptide conjugates formed under the action of a secretor (se) gene. Fuc, fucose.

human red cell membrane, **ABO blood groups** form the dominant system. The antigenic groups A and B are derived from H substance (figure 15.15) by the action of glycosyltransferases encoded by A or B genes, respectively. Individuals with both genes (group AB) have the two antigens on their red cells, while those lacking these genes (group O) synthesize H substance only. Antibodies to A or B occur spontaneously when the antigen is absent from the red cell surface; thus a person of blood group A will possess anti-B and so on. These **isohemagglutinins** are usually IgM and probably belong to the class of 'natural antibodies'; they would be boosted through contact with antigens of the gut flora which are structurally similar to the blood group carbohydrates, so that the antibodies formed cross-react with the appropriate red cell type. If an individual is blood group A, she/he would be tolerant to antigens closely similar to A and would only form cross-reacting antibodies capable of agglutinating B red cells; similarly an O individual would make anti-A and anti-B (table 15.3). On transfusion, mismatched red cells will be coated by the isohemagglutinins which will cause severe complement-mediated intravascular hemolysis.

Clinical refractoriness to platelet transfusions is frequently due to HLA alloimmunization, but one can

Table 15.3. ABO blood groups and serum antibodies.

BLOOD GROUP (PHENOTYPE)	GENOTYPE	ANTIGEN	SERUM ANTIBODY
A	AA, AO	A	ANTI-B
B	BB, BO	B	ANTI-A
AB	AB	A and B	NONE
O	OO	H	ANTI-A ANTI-B

usually circumvent this problem by depleting the platelets of leukocytes.

Rhesus incompatibility

The **rhesus (Rh) blood groups** form the other major antigenic system, the RhD antigen being of the most consequence for isoimmune reactions. A mother with an RhD–ve blood group (i.e. dd genotype) can readily be sensitized by red cells from a baby carrying RhD antigens (DD or Dd genotype). This occurs most often at the birth of the first child when a placental bleed can release a large number of the baby's erythrocytes into the mother. The antibodies formed are predominantly of the IgG class and are able to cross the placenta in any

Figure 15.16. Hemolytic disease of the newborn due to rhesus incompatibility. (a) RhD+ve red cells from the first baby sensitize the RhD−ve mother. (b) The mother's IgG anti-D crosses the placenta and coats the erythrocytes of the second RhD+ve baby causing type II hypersensitivity hemolytic disease. (c) IgG anti-D given prophylactically at the first birth removes the baby's red cells through phagocytosis and prevents sensitization of the mother.

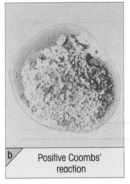

Figure 15.17. The Coombs' test for antibody-coated red cells used for detecting rhesus antibodies and in the diagnosis of autoimmune hemolytic anemia (cf. table 18.2, note 5, p. 415). (Photographs courtesy of Professor A. Cooke.)

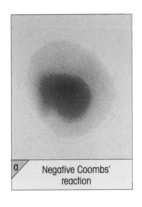
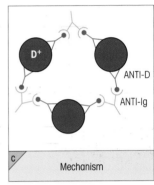

subsequent pregnancy. Reaction with the D-antigen on the fetal red cells leads to their destruction through opsonic adherence, giving hemolytic disease of the newborn (figure 15.16).

These anti-D antibodies fail to agglutinate RhD+ve red cells *in vitro* ('incomplete antibodies') because the low density of antigenic sites does not allow sufficient antibody bridges to be formed between the negatively charged erythrocytes to overcome the electrostatic repulsive forces. Erythrocytes coated with anti-D can be made to agglutinate by addition of an anti-immunoglobulin serum (Coombs' reagent; figure 15.17).

If a mother has natural isohemagglutinins which can react with any fetal erythrocytes reaching her circulation, sensitization to the D-antigens is less likely due to 'deviation' of the red cells away from the antigen-sensitive cells. For example, a group O RhD−ve mother with a group A RhD+ve baby would destroy any fetal erythrocytes with her anti-A before they could immunize to produce anti-D. In an extension of this principle, **RhD−ve mothers are treated prophylactically** with small amounts of IgG anti-D at the time of birth of the first child, and this greatly reduces the risk of sensitization. Another success for immunology.

Another disease resulting from transplacental passage of maternal antibodies is **neonatal alloimmune thrombocytopenia**. The fall in platelet numbers is greatly ameliorated by i.v. injections of pooled human IgG (IVIg), thought by some to involve anti-idiotype networks (cf. p. 218), although the efficacy of Fcγ fragments and anti-FcγR rather point the finger at blockade of the Fcγ receptors.

Organ transplants

Allografts can evoke humoral antibodies in the host directed against surface transplantation antigens. These may be directly cytotoxic or cause adherence of phagocytic cells or attack by ADCC. The antibodies may also lead to platelet adherence when they bind antigens on the surface of the vascular endothelium (figure 16.6, p. 369). Hyperacute rejection is mediated by preformed antibodies in the graft recipient.

Autoimmune type II hypersensitivity reactions

Autoantibodies to the patient's own red cells are produced in **autoimmune hemolytic anemia**. They react at 37°C with epitopes on antigens of the rhesus complex distinct from those which incite transfusion reactions.

Erythrocytes coated with these antibodies have a short-ened half-life, largely through their adherence to phago-cytic cells in the spleen. Similar mechanisms account for the anemia in patients with cold hemagglutinin disease who have monoclonal anti-I after infection with *Mycoplasma pneumoniae*, and in some cases of paroxys-mal cold hemoglobinuria associated with the actively lytic Donath–Landsteiner antibodies specific for blood group P. These antibodies are primarily of IgM isotype and only react at temperatures well below 37°C. IgG autoantibodies against platelet surface glycoproteins are responsible for the depletion of platelets in **idio-pathic thrombocytopenic purpura**; primarily through Fcγ receptor-mediated clearance by tissue macrophages in spleen and liver.

Patients with Hashimoto's thyroiditis have autoanti-bodies which, in the presence of complement, are directly cytotoxic for isolated human thyroid cells in culture. In Goodpasture's syndrome, autoantibodies recognize the noncollagenous (NC1) domain of the α3 chain of type IV collagen in kidney glomerular basement membrane. Biopsies show these antibodies, together with complement components, bound to the basement membranes where the action of the full complement system leads to serious damage (figure 15.18a). One could also include the stripping of acetylcholine receptors from the muscle endplate by autoantibodies in myasthenia gravis as a further example of type II hypersensitivity.

Type II drug reactions

Drugs may become coupled to body components and thereby undergo conversion from a hapten to a full antigen which will sensitize certain individuals. If IgE antibodies are produced, anaphylactic reactions can result. In some circumstances, particularly with topi-cally applied ointments, cell-mediated hypersensitivity may be induced. In other cases where coupling to serum proteins occurs, the possibility of type III immune complex-mediated reactions may arise. In the present context, we are concerned with those instances in which the drug appears to form an antigenic complex with the surface of a formed element of the blood and evokes the production of antibodies which are cytotoxic for the cell–drug complex. When the drug is withdrawn, the sensitivity is no longer evident. Examples of this mecha-nism occur in the **hemolytic anemia** sometimes associ-ated with continued administration of chlorpromazine or phenacetin, in the **agranulocytosis** associated with the taking of amidopyrine or of quinidine, and the now classic situation of **thrombocytopenic purpura** which may be produced by sedormid, a sedative of yesteryear. In the latter case, freshly drawn serum from the patient

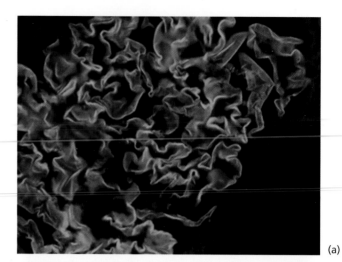

(a)

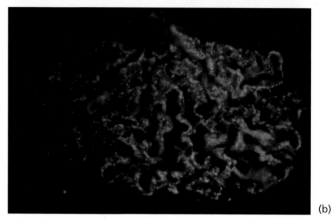

(b)

Figure 15.18. Glomerulonephritis: (a) in Goodpasture's syndrome due to a type II hypersensitivity with linear deposition of antibody to glomerular basement membrane, here visualized by staining the human kidney biopsy with a fluorescent anti-IgG; and in contrast to (b) in systemic lupus erythematosus (SLE, cf. p. 435) where a type III hypersensitivity is associated with deposition of antigen–antibody complexes, which can be seen as discrete masses lining the glomerular basement membrane following immunofluorescent staining with anti-IgG. Similar patterns to these are obtained with a fluorescent anti-C3. (Courtesy of Dr S. Thiru.)

will lyse platelets in the presence, but not in the absence, of sedormid; inactivation of complement by preheating the serum at 56°C for 30 minutes abrogates this effect.

IMMUNE COMPLEX-MEDIATED HYPERSENSITIVITY (TYPE III)

The body may be exposed to an excess of antigen over a protracted period in a number of circumstances: persist-ent infection, autoimmunity to self-components and repeated contact with environmental agents. The union of such antigens and antibodies to form a complex within the body may well give rise to acute inflamma-tory reactions through a variety of mechanisms (figure

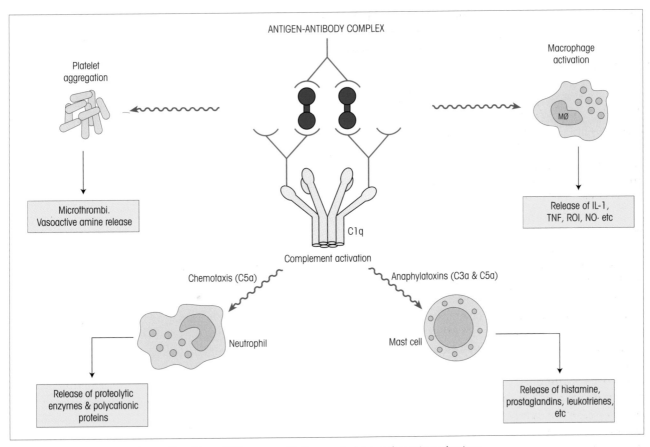

ANTIGEN-ANTIBODY COMPLEX

Platelet aggregation

Microthrombi. Vasoactive amine release

Macrophage activation

MØ

Release of IL-1, TNF, ROI, NO· etc

C1q

Complement activation

Chemotaxis (C5a)

Anaphylatoxins (C3a & C5a)

Neutrophil

Mast cell

Release of proteolytic enzymes & polycationic proteins

Release of histamine, prostaglandins, leukotrienes, etc

Figure 15.19. Immune complex-mediated (type III) hypersensitivity—underlying pathogenic mechanisms.

15.19). For a start, complexes can stimulate macrophages through their Fcγ receptors to generate the release of proinflammatory cytokines IL-1 and TNF, reactive oxygen intermediates and nitric oxide (figure 15.19). Complexes which are insoluble often cannot be digested after phagocytosis by macrophages and so provide a persistent activating stimulus. If complement is fixed, the anaphylatoxins C3a and C5a will be generated and these will cause release of mast cell mediators with vascular permeability changes. The chemotactic factors also produced will lead to an influx of neutrophils which begin the phagocytosis of the immune complexes; this in turn results in the extracellular release of the neutrophil granule contents, particularly when the complex is deposited on a basement membrane and cannot be phagocytosed (so-called 'frustrated phagocytosis'). The proteolytic enzymes (including neutral proteinases and collagenase), kinin-forming enzymes, polycationic proteins and reactive oxygen and nitrogen intermediates which are released will of course damage local tissues and intensify the inflammatory responses. Further havoc may be mediated by reactive lysis in which activated C5,6,7 becomes adventitiously attached to the surface of nearby cells and

binds C8,9. Intravascular complexes can aggregate platelets with two consequences: they provide yet a further source of vasoactive amines and may also form microthrombi which can lead to local ischemia. The need for the system of inhibitors present in the body should be absolutely clear.

The outcome of the formation of immune complexes *in vivo* depends not only on the absolute amounts of antigen and antibody, which determine the intensity of the reaction, but also on their *relative* proportions, which govern the nature of the complexes (cf. figure 6.24, p. 133) and hence their distribution within the body. Between **antibody excess** and **mild antigen excess**, the complexes are rapidly precipitated and tend to be localized to the site of introduction of antigen, whereas in **moderate** to **gross antigen excess**, soluble complexes are formed.

Covalent attachment of C3b prevents the Fc–Fc interactions required to form large insoluble aggregates, and these small complexes bind to CR1 complement receptors on the human erythrocyte and are transported to fixed macrophages in the liver where they are safely inactivated. This is an important role of the erythrocyte, a cell often unfairly ignored in discussion of the immune system. If there are defects in this process, for example deficiencies in classical pathway components, or perhaps if the system is overloaded, then widespread disease involving deposition in the kidneys, joints, skin and choroid plexus may result.

Inflammatory lesions due to locally formed complexes

The Arthus reaction

Maurice Arthus found that injection of soluble antigen intradermally into hyperimmunized rabbits with high levels of precipitating antibody produced an erythematous and edematous reaction reaching a peak at 3–8 hours which then usually resolved. The lesion was characterized by an intense infiltration with neutrophils (cf. figure 15.20a and b). The injected antigen precipitates with antibody often within the venule, too fast for the classical complement system to prevent it; subsequently, the complex binds complement and, using fluorescent reagents, antigen, immunoglobulin and complement components can all be demonstrated in this lesion, as illustrated by the inflammatory response to deposits of immune complexes containing hepatitis B surface antigen in a patient with periarteritis nodosa (figure 15.20c). Anaphylatoxin production, mast cell degranulation, macrophage activation, platelet aggregation and influx of neutrophils all make their contribution. The Arthus reaction can be attenuated by depletion of neutrophils by nitrogen mustard or of complement by anti-C5a; soluble forms of the complement regulatory

proteins CD46 (membrane cofactor protein) and CD55 (delay accelerating factor) are also inhibitory.

Reactions to inhaled antigens

Intrapulmonary Arthus-type reactions to exogenous inhaled antigen are responsible for a number of hypersensitivity disorders. The severe respiratory difficulties associated with **farmer's lung** occur within 6–8 hours of exposure to the dust from mouldy hay. The patients are found to be sensitized to thermophilic actinomycetes which grow in the mouldy hay, and extracts of these organisms give precipitin reactions with the subject's serum and Arthus reactions on intradermal injection. Inhalation of bacterial spores in dust from the hay introduces antigen into the lungs and an immune complex-mediated hypersensitivity reaction occurs. Similar situations arise in pigeon-fancier's disease, where the antigen is probably serum protein present in the dust from dried feces, in rat handlers sensitized to rat serum proteins excreted in the urine (figure 15.21) and in many other quaintly named cases of **extrinsic allergic alveolitis** resulting from continual inhalation of organic particles, e.g. cheese washer's disease (*Penicillium casei* spores), furrier's lung (fox fur proteins) and maple bark stripper's disease (spores of *Cryptostroma*). Evidence that an immediate anaphylactic type I response may sometimes be of importance for the initiation of an Arthus reaction comes from the study of patients with allergic bronchopulmonary aspergillosis who have high levels of IgE and precipitating IgG antibodies to *Aspergillus* species.

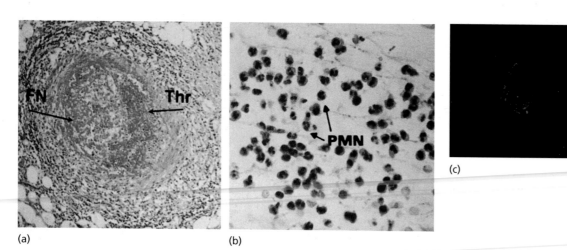

(a)   (b)

Figure 15.20. Histology of acute inflammatory reaction in polyarteritis nodosa associated with immune complex formation with hepatitis B surface (HBs) antigen. (a) A vessel showing thrombus (Thr) formation and fibrinoid necrosis (FN) is surrounded by a mixed inflammatory infiltrate, largely neutrophils. (b) High-power view of acute inflammatory response in loose connective tissue of patient with polyarteritis nodosa—polymorphonuclear neutrophils (PMN) are prominent. (c) Immunofluorescence studies of immune complexes in

the renal artery of a patient with chronic hepatitis B infection stained with fluoresceinated antihepatitis B antigen (left) and rhodaminated anti-IgM (right). The presence of both antigen and antibody in the intima and media of the arterial wall indicates the deposition of the complexes at this site. IgG and C3 deposits are also detectable with the same distribution. ((a) and (b) provided by courtesy of Professor N. Woolf; (c) kindly provided by Professor A. Nowoslowski.)

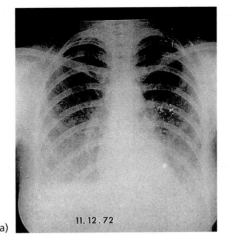

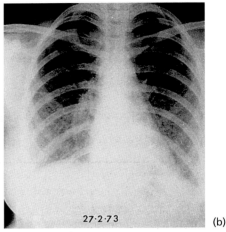

(a) 11.12.72

(b) 27.2.73

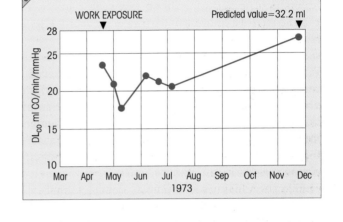

WORK EXPOSURE   Predicted value=32.2 ml

Figure 15.21. Extrinsic allergic alveolitis due to rat serum proteins in a research assistant handling rats (type III hypersensitivity). Typical systemic and pulmonary reactions on inhalation and positive prick tests were elicited by rat serum proteins; precipitins against serum proteins in rat urine were present in the patient's serum. (a) Bilateral micronodular shadowing during acute episodes. (b) Marked clearing within 11 days after cessation of exposure to rats. (c) Temporary fall in pulmonary gas exchange measured by DL_{CO} (gas transfer, single breath) following a 3-day exposure to rats at work (arrowed). (From Carroll K.B. *et al.* (1975) *Clinical Allergy* **5**, 443; figures by courtesy of Professor J. Pepys.)

Reactions to internal antigens

Type III reactions are often provoked by the local release of antigen from infectious organisms within the body; for example, living filarial worms, such as *Wuchereria bancrofti*, are relatively harmless, but the dead parasite found in lymphatic vessels initiates an inflammatory reaction thought to be responsible for the obstruction of lymph flow and the ensuing, rather monstrous, elephantiasis. Microbial cell death following chemotherapy may cause an abrupt release of microbial antigens and in individuals with high antibody levels produce quite dramatic immune complex-mediated reactions, such as **erythema nodosum leprosum** in the skin of dapsone-treated lepromatous leprosy patients (figure 15.22) and the Jarisch–Herxheimer reaction in syphilitics on penicillin.

An interesting variant of the Arthus reaction is seen in rheumatoid arthritis where complexes are formed locally in the joint due to the production of self-associating IgG anti-IgG by synovial plasma cells (cf. p. 439).

Complexes could also be generated at a local site by a quite different mechanism involving nonspecific adherence of an antigen to tissue structures followed by the binding of soluble antibody—in other words, the

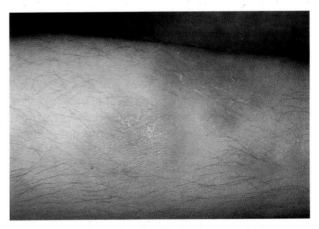

Figure 15.22. Erythema nodosum leprosum, forearm. The patient has lepromatous leprosy with superimposed erythema nodosum leprosum. These acutely inflamed nodules were extremely tender and the patient was pyrexial. (Photograph kindly provided by Dr G. Levene.)

antigen becomes fixed in the tissue *before* not *after* combining with antibody. Although it is not clear to what extent this mechanism operates in patients with immune complex disease, let us describe the experimental observation on which it is based. After injection with bacterial endotoxin, mice release DNA into their circulation which binds specifically to the collagen in the basement membrane of the glomerular capillaries; the endotoxin also polyclonally activates B-cells making anti-DNA which gives rise to antigen–antibody complexes in the kidney.

Disease resulting from circulating complexes

Immune complex glomerulonephritis

The deposition of complexes is a dynamic affair and long-lasting disease is only seen when the antigen is persistent, as in chronic infections and autoimmune diseases. Experimentally, Dixon produced chronic glomerular lesions by repeated administration of foreign proteins to rabbits. Not all animals showed the lesion, and perhaps only those genetically capable of producing low affinity antibody or antibodies to a restricted number of determinants formed soluble complexes in the right size range. The **smallest complexes reach the epithelial side**, but progressively **larger complexes are retained in or on the endothelial side of the glomerular basement membrane** (figure 15.23). They build up as 'lumpy' granules staining for antigen, immunoglobulin and complement (C3) by immunofluorescence (figure 15.18b), and appear as large amorphous masses in the electron microscope (cf. figure 18.22). The inflammatory process damages the base-

ment membrane through engagement of the complexes with effector cells bearing Fcγ receptors, as revealed by the absence of glomerulonephritis despite immune complex deposition in the kidneys of FcγR-knockout New Zealand (B×W) F1 hybrids (a murine model of human systemic lupus erythematosus, SLE; p. 435). Proteinuria results from the leakage of serum proteins through the damaged membrane and serum albumin, being small, appears in the urine (figure 15.24, lane 3).

Many cases of glomerulonephritis are associated with circulating complexes, and biopsies give a fluorescent staining pattern similar to that of figure 15.18b, which depicts DNA/anti-DNA/complement deposits in the kidney of a patient with SLE (cf. p. 436). Well known is the disease which can follow infection with certain strains of so-called 'nephritogenic' streptococci and the nephrotic syndrome associated with malaria, where complexes with antigens of the infecting organism have been implicated. Immune complex nephritis can arise in the course of chronic viral infections; as seen in individuals co-infected with HIV and hepatitis C virus.

Deposition of immune complexes at other sites

The choroid plexuses (networks of capillaries in the walls of the ventricles in the brain) are a major filtration site and therefore also favored for immune complex deposition. This could account for the frequency of

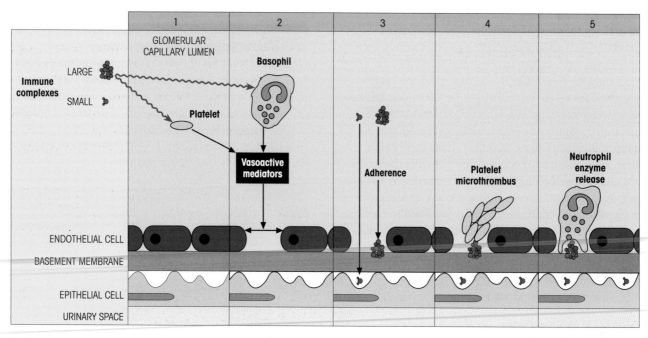

Figure 15.23. Deposition of immune complexes in the kidney glomerulus. (1) Complexes induce release of vasoactive mediators from basophils and platelets which cause (2) separation of endothelial cells. (3) Attachment of larger complexes to exposed basement membrane, with smaller complexes passing through to the epithelial side. (4) Complexes induce platelet aggregation. (5) Chemotactically attracted neutrophils release granule contents in 'frustrated phagocytosis' to damage basement membrane and cause leakage of serum proteins. Complex deposition is favored in the glomerular capillary because it is a major filtration site and has a high hydrodynamic pressure. Deposition is greatly reduced in animals depleted of platelets or treated with vasoactive amine antagonists.

central nervous disorders in SLE. Neurologically affected patients tend to have depressed complement component C4 in the cerebrospinal fluid (CSF) and, at post-mortem, SLE patients with neurologic disturbances and high titer anti-DNA were shown to have scattered deposits of immunoglobulin and DNA in the choroid plexus. Subacute sclerosing panencephalitis is associated with a high CSF to serum ratio of measles antibody, and deposits containing Ig and measles Ag may be found in neural tissue.

Vasculitic skin rashes are also characteristic of systemic and discoid lupus erythematosus (figure 15.25),

and biopsies of the lesions reveal amorphous deposits of Ig and C3 at the basement membrane of the dermo–epidermal junction (cf. figure 18.23).

Another example of immune complex hypersensitivity is the hemorrhagic shock syndrome found in South-East Asia during a second infection with dengue virus. There are four types of virus, and antibodies to one type produced during a first infection may not neutralize a second strain but rather facilitate its entry into, and replication within, human monocytes by attachment of the complex to Fc receptors. The enhanced production of virus leads to immune complex formation and a massive intravascular activation of the classical complement pathway. In some instances drugs such as penicillin become antigenic after conjugation with body proteins and form complexes which mediate hypersensitivity reactions.

It should be said that persistence of circulating complexes does not invariably lead to type III hypersensitivity (e.g. in many cancer patients and in individuals with idiotype–anti-idiotype reactions). Perhaps in these cases the complexes lack the ability to initiate the changes required for complex deposition, but some hold the view that complexes detected in the serum may sometimes be artifacts released from their *in vivo* attachment to the erythrocyte CR1 receptors by the action of factor I during processing of the blood.

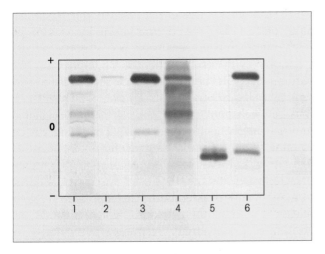

Figure 15.24. Proteinuria demonstrated by electrophoresis. Lane 1: Normal serum as reference. The major band nearest to the cathode is albumin. Lane 2: Normal urine showing a trace of albumin. Lane 3: Glomerular proteinuria showing a major albumin component. Lane 4: Proteinuria resulting from tubular damage with a totally different electrophoretic pattern. Lane 5: Bence Jones proteinuria representing excreted paraprotein light chains (cf. p. 397). Lane 6: Bence-Jones proteinuria with a trace of the intact paraprotein. Some of the samples have been concentrated. (Electropherograms kindly supplied by T. Heys.)

Treatment

The avoidance of exogenous inhaled antigens inducing type III reactions is obvious. Elimination of microorganisms associated with immune complex disease by chemotherapy may provoke a further reaction due to copious release of antigen. Suppression of the accessory factors thought to be necessary for the deposition of complexes would seem logical. Sodium cromoglycate,

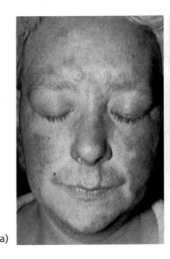

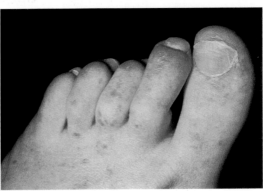

Figure 15.25. Vasculitic skin rashes due to immune complex deposition.
(a) Facial appearance in systemic lupus erythematosus (SLE). Lesions of recent onset are symmetrical, red and edematous. They are often most pronounced on the areas of the face which receive most light exposure, i.e. the upper cheeks and bridge of the nose, and the prominences of the forehead.
(b) Vasculitic lesions in SLE. Small purpuric macules are seen.

(a)

(b)

heparin and salicylates are often used, the latter being an effective platelet stabilizer as well as a potent anti-inflammatory agent. Corticosteroids are particularly powerful inhibitors of inflammation and are immuno-suppressive. In many cases, particularly those involv-ing autoimmunity, conventional immunosuppressive agents may be justified.

CELL-MEDIATED (DELAYED-TYPE) HYPERSENSITIVITY (TYPE IV)

Delayed-type hypersensitivity (DTH) is encountered in many allergic reactions to infectious agents, in the contact dermatitis resulting from sensitization to certain simple chemicals and in transplant rejection. Perhaps the best known example is the **Mantoux reaction** obtained by injection of tuberculin into the skin of an individual in whom previous infection with the mycobacterium had induced a state of cell-mediated immunity (CMI). The reaction is characterized by ery-thema and induration (figure 15.26a) which appears only after several hours (hence the term 'delayed') and reaches a maximum at 24–48 hours, thereafter subsid-ing. Histologically, the earliest phase of the reaction is seen as a perivascular cuffing with mononuclear cells followed by a more extensive exudation of mono- and polymorphonuclear cells. The latter soon migrate out of the lesion leaving behind a predominantly mononu-clear cell infiltrate consisting of lymphocytes and cells of the monocyte–macrophage series (figure 15.26b). This contrasts with the essentially 'neutrophil' character of the Arthus reaction (figure 15.20b).

Comparable reactions to soluble proteins are obtained when sensitization is induced by incorpora-tion of the antigen into complete Freund's adjuvant (see p. 308). In some, but not all cases, if animals are primed with antigen alone or in incomplete Freund's adjuvant (which lacks the mycobacteria present in the complete adjuvant), the delayed hypersensitivity state is of shorter duration and the dermal response more tran-sient. This is known as 'Jones–Mote' sensitivity but has more recently been termed **cutaneous basophil hyper-sensitivity** on account of the high proportion of basophils infiltrating the skin lesion.

The cellular basis of type IV hypersensitivity

Unlike the other forms of hypersensitivity which we have discussed, delayed-type reactivity cannot be transferred from a sensitized to a nonsensitized individual with serum antibody; T-lymphocytes are required. It cannot be stressed too often that the hyper-sensitivity lesion results from an exaggerated interac-tion between antigen and the *normal* cell-mediated immune mechanisms (cf. p. 194). Following earlier priming, memory T-cells recognize the antigen peptide together with MHC class II molecules on an antigen-presenting cell and are stimulated into blast cell trans-formation and proliferation. The stimulated T-cells release a number of cytokines which mediate the ensuing hypersensitivity response, particularly by attracting and activating macrophages if they belong to the Th1 subset, or eosinophils if they are Th2; they also help Tc precursors to become killer cells which can cause damage to virally infected target cells (figure 15.27), the CD8 TCRαβ cytotoxic cells being activated by

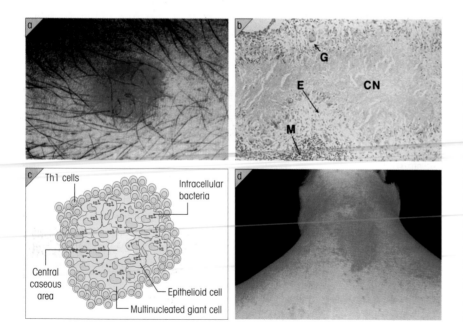

Figure 15.26. Cell-mediated (type IV) hypersensitivity reactions. (a) Mantoux test showing cell-mediated hypersensitivity reaction to tuberculin, characterized by induration and erythema. (b) Chronic type IV inflammatory lesion in tuberculous lung showing caseous necrosis (CN), epithelioid cells (E), giant cells (G) and mononuclear inflammatory cells (M). (c) Highly diagrammatic representation of a granuloma with central caseous ('cheesy') necrosis. (d) Type IV contact hypersensitivity reaction to nickel caused by the clasp of a necklace. ((a) Kindly provided by Professor J. Brostoff and (b) by Professor R. Barnetson; (d) reproduced from the British Society for Immunology teaching slides with permission of the Society and the Dermatology Department, London Hospital.)

recognition of MHC class I complexes with processed viral proteins and TCRγδ killers operating through binding to native viral proteins on the surface of the infected cells.

Tissue damage produced by type IV reactions

Infections

The development of a state of cell-mediated hypersensitivity to bacterial products is probably responsible for the lesions, such as the cavitation, caseation and general toxemia, seen in human tuberculosis and the granulomatous skin lesions found in patients with the borderline form of leprosy. When the battle between the replicating bacteria and the body defenses fails to be resolved in favor of the host, persisting antigen provokes a chronic local delayed hypersensitivity reaction. Continual release of cytokines from sensitized T-lymphocytes leads to the accumulation of large numbers of macrophages, many of which give rise to arrays of epithelioid cells, while others fuse to form multinucleated giant cells. Macrophages presenting peptides derived from bacterial antigens using their surface MHC class I molecules may become targets for cytotoxic

T-cells and be destroyed. Further tissue damage will occur as a result of indiscriminate cytotoxicity by cytokine-activated macrophages. Morphologically, this combination of cell types with proliferating lymphocytes and fibroblasts associated with areas of fibrosis and necrosis is termed a **chronic granuloma** and represents an attempt by the body to wall off a site of persistent infection (figures 15.26b,c and 15.27). It should be noted that granulomas can also arise from the persistence of indigestible antigen–antibody complexes or inorganic materials, such as talc, within macrophages, although nonimmunological granulomas may be distinguished by the absence of lymphocytes.

The skin rashes in measles and the lesions associated with herpes simplex infection may be largely attributed to delayed-type reactions with extensive Tc-mediated damage to virally-infected cells. By the same token, specific cytotoxic T-cells can cause extensive destruction of liver cells infected with hepatitis B virus. Cell-mediated hypersensitivity has also been demonstrated in the fungal diseases candidiasis, dermatomycosis, coccidioidomycosis and histoplasmosis, and in the parasitic disease leishmaniasis.

Crohn's disease and ulcerative colitis are the two

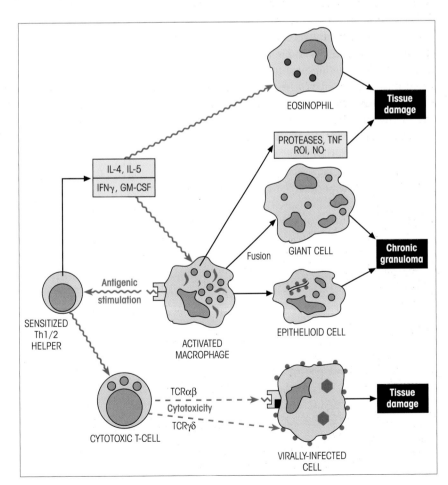

Figure 15.27. The cellular basis of type IV hypersensitivity. Th1 cells will activate macrophages and cytotoxic T-cells, whereas Th2 cells will recruit eosinophils.

main forms of **inflammatory bowel disease** (IBD) and are distinct entities, although both probably result from dysregulated mucosal immune responses to microbial antigens in the gut. **Crohn's disease** is characterized by transmural granulomatous inflammation involving the entire bowel wall from mucosa to serosa, and the development of fibrosis, microperforations and fistulas. Inflammation can occur throughout the gastrointestinal tract. By contrast, in ulcerative colitis there is a more superficial inflammation which is confined to the colon and rectum. Mutations in the *NOD2* gene, encoding a cytoplasmic pattern recognition receptor for the muramyl dipeptide of bacterial cell wall peptidoglycan, are strongly associated with susceptibility to Crohn's disease. IBD can be induced in severe combined immunodeficient (SCID) mice by the transfer of CD45RB^{hi} (naive) CD4 T-cells, but the colitis which develops can be cured by the subsequent transfer of CD4$^+$, CD25$^+$, CD45RB^{lo} regulatory T-cells. The aggressor cells belong to the IL-12-driven Th1 population producing TNF and IFNγ, which are highly toxic for enterocytes, whereas the regulators secrete the suppressor cytokines TGFβ and IL-10. Monoclonal anti-TNF is a very effective therapy; probiotic treatment with lactobacilli and *Streptococcus salivarius* would appear to maintain remission in severe colitis, is less Draconian and is easier on the budget (remember the friendly yoghurt adverts). Clinical trials to establish the efficacy of such treatments in large cohorts of patients are underway.

Experimental colitis induced in SJL/J mice by administration of oxazolone presents as a relatively superficial inflammation resembling human **ulcerative colitis.** It is initially mediated by IL-4-producing Th2 cells but rapidly superceded by an atypical Th2 response involving IL-13-producing NKT cells. The inflamed tissue in patients with ulcerative colitis has also recently been shown to contain increased numbers of IL-13-producing nonclassical NKT cells (unlike most NKT

cells, these do not bear an invariant TCR) which have the potential to be cytotoxic for human epithelial cells.

Sarcoidosis

Sarcoidosis is a disease of unknown etiology affecting lymphoid tissue and involving the formation of chronic granulomas. A chronic inflammatory Th1 response to an infectious, environmental or autoantigen is thought to be responsible. Increased numbers of activated B-cells and hypergammaglobulinemia are often present. Evidence for atypical mycobacteria has been obtained, but delayed-type hypersensitivity is depressed and the patients are anergic on skin testing with tuberculin, perhaps due to the presence of increased numbers of CD4$^+$CD25$^+$ regulatory T-cells in those patients with active disease. Patients develop a granulomatous reaction a few weeks after intradermal injection of spleen extract from another sarcoid patient—the **Kveim reaction**.

Contact dermatitis

The epidermal route of inoculation tends to favor the development of a Th1 response through processing by class II-rich dendritic Langerhans' cells (cf. figure 2.6f) which migrate to the lymph nodes and present antigen to T-lymphocytes. Thus, delayed-type reactions in the skin are often produced by foreign low molecular weight materials capable of binding to peptides within the groove of MHC molecules on the surface of Langerhans' cells, to form new antigens. The reactions are characterized by a mononuclear cell infiltrate peaking at 12–15 hours, accompanied by edema of the epidermis with microvesicle formation (figure 15.28). There is a most unusual twist to this story, however, possibly because the inciting reagent is a reactive hapten. The late mononuclear reaction is entirely dependent upon very early events (1–2 hours) mediated by hapten-specific IgM produced by B-1 cells which, together with complement, activates local vessels to permit T-cell recruit-

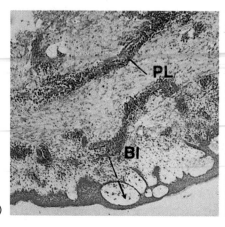

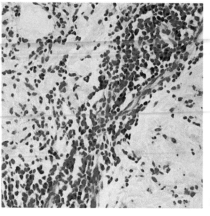

(a)   (b)

Figure 15.28. Contact sensitivity. (a) Perivascular lymphocytic infiltrates (PL) and blister (Bl) formation characterize a contact sensitivity reaction of the skin. (b) High-power view to show the lymphocytic nature of the infiltrate in a contact hypersensitivity reaction. (Photographs kindly provided by Professor N. Woolf.)

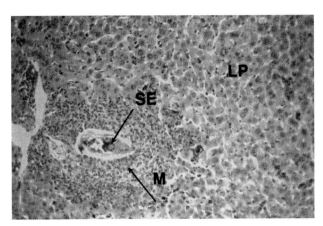

Figure 15.29. Th2-mediated response to schistosome egg. Th2-type hypersensitivity lesion of inflammatory cells (M) around a schistosome egg (SE) within the liver parenchyma (LP). (Photograph by courtesy of Professor M. Doenhoff.)

ment. Contact hypersensitivity can occur in people who become sensitized while working with chemicals, such as picryl chloride and chromates, or who repeatedly come into contact with the substance urushiol from the poison ivy plant. *p*-Phenylene diamine in certain hair dyes, neomycin in topically applied ointments, and nickel salts formed from articles such as nickel jewellery clasps (figure 15.26d) can provoke similar reactions. T-cell clones specific for nickel salts isolated from the latter group produce a Th1-type profile of cytokines (IFNγ, IL-2) on antigen stimulation (figure 15.9b).

Other examples
Excessive responses by Th2 cells can damage tissues through activation of eosinophils (figure 15.27). As recounted earlier, T-cells synthesizing IL-5 are largely responsible for the sustained influx of eosinophils in asthma and atopic dermatitis (cf. p. 342). Th2 cells also account for the liver pathology in schistosomiasis which has been attributed to a reaction against soluble enzymes derived from the eggs which lodge in the capillaries (figure 15.29).

It has been suggested that the relatively mixed Th1–Th2 DTH response induced by bites from blood-feeding insects such as sand flies (*Phlebotomus papatasi*) might represent an adaptation of the insect to direct the host immune response to its own advantage. Thus, it was shown that the increased blood flow associated with the DTH sites allowed sand flies to feed twice as fast relative to feeding from normal skin sites.

The contribution of DTH reactions to allograft rejection is covered in Chapter 16, whilst the potential role of Tc cells for the control of cancer cells is discussed in Chapter 17. In certain organ-specific autoimmune diseases, such as type I diabetes, cell-mediated hypersensi-

tivity reactions undoubtedly provide the major engine for tissue destruction.

The intestinal inflammation in **celiac disease**, an HLA-DQ2/8-associated enteropathy, is precipitated by exposure to dietary wheat gliadin. The disorder involves what is probably a genetically related increased mucosal activity of transglutaminase (the main target antigen of anti-endomysium autoantibodies; cf. p. 433). This enzyme deamidates the glutamine residues in gliadin and creates a new T-cell epitope that binds efficiently to DQ2 and is recognized by IFNγ-secreting intraepithelial CD4$^+$ Th1-cells. Local production of IL-15 also plays a role by increasing expression of nonclassical MHC class I molecules such as MICA on epithelial cells and receptors for these such as NKG2D on intraepithelial CD8$^+$ αβ T-cells, γδ T-cells and NK cells, leading to cytotoxic killing of the epithelial cells.

Psoriasis involves marked proliferation of epidermal keratinocytes and accelerated incomplete epidermal differentiation. For reasons that are not understood, in around 10% of patients the skin manifestations are associated with psoriatic arthritis involving joint inflammation and destruction. The skin inflammation involves neutrophils and both CD4 and CD8 T-cells which are CD45RO$^+$ indicating that they are antigen experienced. The release of IFNγ induces epidermal hyperplasia and, together with TNF, increases the expression of ICAM-1 on epidermal keratinocytes, thereby facilitating the adhesion of T-cells. Experiments in a skin xenograft model of psoriasis involving the transplantation of human skin onto severe combined immunodeficient (SCID) mice have identified that the activated form of the *s*ignal *t*ransducer and *a*ctivator of *t*ranscription 3 (STAT3) cell signaling molecule localizes to the nucleus of epidermal keratinocytes following the transfer of CD4 but not CD8 T-cells, indicating a central role for STAT3 signaling in the interactions between activated CD4 cells and keratinocytes. Efalizumab, a humanized IgG1 monoclonal antibody against CD11a (LFA-1) which functions both by decreasing T-cell activation and by interfering with T-cells trafficking to inflammatory sites, is effective in the treatment of psoriasis.

STIMULATORY HYPERSENSITIVITY (TYPE V)

When thyroid-stimulating hormone (TSH) binds to its receptor on the thyroid epithelial cells, adenyl cyclase is activated, and the cAMP 'second messenger' is generated to stimulate thyroid hormone production. Once sufficient levels of the hormones are produced a negative feedback loop shuts off the production of TSH. The **thyroid-stimulating antibody** present in patients with Graves' disease (cf. p. 432) is an autoantibody against

complexes with hepatitis B virus and an element of the synovial lesion in rheumatoid arthritis.
• In relative *antigen excess*, soluble complexes are formed which are removed by binding to the CR1 C3b receptors on red cells. If this system is overloaded or if the classical complement components are deficient, the complexes circulate in the free state and are deposited under circumstances of increased vascular permeability at certain preferred sites: the kidney glomerulus, the joints, the skin and the choroid plexus.
• Examples are: glomerulonephritis associated with systemic lupus erythematosus (SLE) or infections with streptococci, malaria and co-infection with HIV and hepatitis C virus; neurological disturbances in SLE and subacute sclerosing panencephalitis; and hemorrhagic shock in dengue viral infection.

Cell-mediated or delayed-type hypersensitivity (type IV)
• This is based upon the interaction of antigen with primed T-cells and represents tissue damage resulting from inappropriate cell-mediated immunity reactions.
• Cytokines, including IFNγ, are released which activate macrophages and account for the events that occur in a typical delayed hypersensitivity response such as the Mantoux reaction to tuberculin, that is, the delayed appearance of an indurated and erythematous reaction which reaches a maximum at 24–48 hours and is characterized histologically by infiltration with mononuclear phagocytes and lymphocytes.

• Continuing provocation of delayed hypersensitivity by persisting antigen leads to formation of chronic granulomas.
• Th2-type cells producing IL-5 can also produce tissue damage through their ability to recruit eosinophils.
• CD8 T-cells are activated by class I MHC antigens to become directly cytotoxic to target cells bearing the appropriate antigen.
• Examples are: tissue damage occurring in bacterial (tuberculosis, leprosy), viral (measles, herpes), fungal (candidiasis, histoplasmosis) and parasitic (leishmaniasis, schistosomiasis) infections, contact dermatitis from exposure to chromates and poison ivy, insect bites and psoriasis. Inflammatory bowel disease can result from Th1-type (Crohn's disease) or 'Th2-like' NKT (ulcerative colitis) reactions to intestinal bacteria. Celiac disease is an aberrant response to wheat gliadin.

Stimulatory hypersensitivity (type V)
• The antibody reacts with a key surface component such as a hormone receptor and 'switches on' the cell.
• An example is the thyroid hyper-reactivity in Graves' disease due to a thyroid-stimulating autoantibody. Features of these five types of acquired hypersensitivity are compared in table 15.4.

'Innate' hypersensitivity reactions
• Many infections provoke a 'toxic shock syndrome' involving excessive release of TNF, IL-1 and IL-6 and activation of the alternative complement pathway.

Table 15.4. Comparison of types of hypersensitivity involving acquired responses.

	Anaphylactic (I)	Cytotoxic (II)	Complex-mediated (III)	Cell-mediated (IV)	Stimulatory (V)
Antibody mediating reaction	Homocytotropic Ab Mast-cell binding	Humoral Ab ± CF*	Humoral Ab ± CF*	None (T-cell mediated)	Humoral Ab Non-CF*
Antigen	Usually exogenous (e.g. grass pollen)	Cell surface	Extracellular	Associated with MHC on macrophage or target cell	Cell surface
Response to intradermal antigen: Max. reaction Appearance	30 min (+ late reaction) Wheal and flare	–	3–8 h Erythema and edema	24–48 h Erythema and induration	–
Histology	Degranulated mast cells; edema; (late reaction cellular including eosinophils)	–	Acute inflammatory reaction; predominant neutrophils	Perivascular inflammation: polymorphs migrate out leaving predominantly mononuclear cells	–
Transfer sensitivity to normal subject	◄———————— Serum antibody ————————►			Lymphoid cells	Serum antibody
Examples:	Atopic allergy, e.g. hay fever	Hemolytic disease of newborn (Rh)	Complex glomerulonephritis Farmer's lung	Mantoux reaction to TB Granulomatous reaction to TB Contact sensitivity	Graves' disease

*CF, complement fixation.

(Continued p.363)

- Acute respiratory distress syndrome associated with Gram-negative bacteria is primarily due to the lipopolysaccharide (LPS) endotoxin provoking a massive invasion of the lung by neutrophils.
- Gram-positive organisms cause release of TNF and macrophage migration inhibitory factor (MIF) through direct action on macrophages and stimulation of selected T-cell families by the enterotoxin superantigens.

- Aberration of innate mechanisms may underlie idiopathic pulmonary fibrosis and contribute to the β-amyloid plaques in Alzheimer's disease.

See the accompanying website (**www.roitt.com**) for multiple choice questions.

FURTHER READING

The Allergy Report (2000) Published by the American Academy of Allergy, Asthma & Immunology. http://www.aaaai.org/ar/

Alasdair M., Gilfillan A.M. & Tkaczyk C. (2006) Integrated signalling pathways for mast-cell activation. *Nature Reviews Immunology* **6**, 218–230.

Blank U. & Rivera J. (2004) The ins and outs of IgE-dependent mast-cell exocytosis. *Trends in Immunology* **25**, 266–273.

Bruhns P., Fremont S. & Daeron M. (2005) Regulation of allergy by Fc receptors. *Current Opinion in Immunology* **17**, 662–669.

Busse W.W. & Lemanske R.F. (2001) Asthma. *New England Journal of Medicine* **344**, 350–362.

Chapel H., Haeney M., Misbah S. & Snowden N. (2006) *Essentials of Clinical Immunology*, 5th edn. Blackwell Publishing, Oxford.

Cines D.B. & Blanchette V.S. (2002) Immune thrombocytopenic purpura. *New England Journal of Medicine* **346**, 995–1008.

Coleman J.W. & Blanca M. (1998) Mechanisms of drug allergy. *Immunology Today* **19**, 196–198.

Gould H.J. *et al.* (2003) The biology of IgE and the basis of allergic disease. *Annual Reviews Immunology* **21**, 579–628.

Holgate S.T., Church M.K. & Lichtenstein L.M. (2001) *Allergy*, 2nd edn. Mosby, London.

Kay A.B. (2001) Allergy and allergic diseases. *New England Journal of Medicine* **344**, 30–37 (part 1); 109–113 (part 2).

Romagnani S. (2004) The increased prevalence of allergy and the hygiene hypothesis: missing immune deviation, reduced immune suppression, or both? *Immunology* **112**, 352–363.

Rothenberg M.E. & Hogon S.P. (2006) The eosinophil. *Annual Review of Immunology* **24**, 147–174.

grafting in 1962 of an unrelated cadaveric kidney under the immunosuppressive umbrella of azathioprine, the more effective derivative of 6-mercaptopurine devised by Hutchings and Elion.

This story is studded with Nobel Prize winners and readers of a historical bent will gain further insight into the develop-ment of this field and the minds of the scientists who gave medicine this wonderful prize in Terasaki P.I. (ed.) (1991) *History of Transplantation; Thirty-Five Recollections*, UCLA Tissue Typing Laboratory, Los Angeles, CA and, subsequently, Brent L. (1996) *A History of Transplantation Immunology*, Academic Press, London.

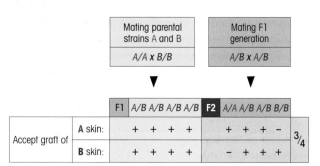

Figure 16.1. Graft rejection induces memory which is specific and can be transferred by T-cells. In experiment 1, an A strain recipient of T-cells from another A strain mouse, which had rejected a graft from strain B, will give accelerated (i.e. 2nd set) rejection of a B graft. Experiments 2 and 3 show the specificity of the phenomenon with respect to the genetically unrelated third party strain C.

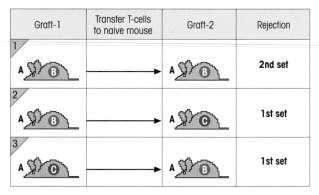

Figure 16.2. Inheritance of genes controlling transplantation antigens. *A* represents a gene expressing the A antigen and *B* the corresponding allelic gene at the same genetic locus. The pure strains are homozygous for *A/A* and *B/B* respectively. Since the genes are codominant, an animal with *A/B* genome will express both antigens, become tolerant to them and therefore accept grafts from either A or B donors. The illustration shows that, for each gene controlling a transplantation antigen specificity, three-quarters of the F2 generation will accept a graft of parental skin. For *n* genes the fraction is $(3/4)^n$. If F1 *A/B* animals are back-crossed with an *A/A* parent, half the progeny will be *A/A* and half *A/B*; only the latter will accept B grafts.

locus, three out of four of the F2 generation will accept parental strain grafts.

In the mouse around 40 such loci have been established but, as we have seen earlier, the complex set of loci termed H-2 (HLA in the human) predominates in the sense that it controls the 'strong' transplantation anti-gens which provoke intense allograft reactions. We have looked at the structure (cf. figure 4.13) and biology of this **major histocompatibility complex (MHC)** in some detail in previous chapters (see Milestone 4.2, p. 76). Given the Mendelian segregation and codominant expression of these genes, it should be evident that in outbred populations siblings have a 1:4 chance of identity with respect to MHC. The non-H-2 or 'minor' transplantation antigens, such as the male H-Y, are rec-ognized as processed peptides in association with the *m*ajor *h*istocompatibility *c*omplex (MHC) molecules on the cell surface by T-cells but not by B-cells. One should not be misled by the term 'minor' into thinking that these antigens do not give rise to serious rejection prob-lems, albeit more slowly than the MHC.

SOME OTHER CONSEQUENCES OF MHC INCOMPATIBILITY

Class II MHC differences produce a mixed lymphocyte reaction (MLR)

When lymphocytes from individuals of different class II haplotype are cultured together, blast cell transforma-tion and mitosis occur (MLR), the T-cells of each popula-tion of lymphocytes reacting against MHC class II determinants on the surface of the other population. The responding cells are predominantly CD4+ T-cells and are stimulated by the class II determinants present mostly on B-cells, macrophages and especially dendritic cells. Thus, the MLR is inhibited by antisera to class II determinants on the stimulator cells.

The graft-vs-host (g.v.h.) reaction

When competent T-cells are transferred from a donor to a recipient which is incapable of rejecting them, the grafted cells survive and have time to recognize the host antigens and react immunologically against them. Instead of the normal transplantation reaction of host against graft, we have the reverse, a graft-vs-host (g.v.h.) reaction. In the young rodent there can be inhibition of growth (runting), spleen enlargement and hemolytic anemia (due to the production of red cell antibodies). In

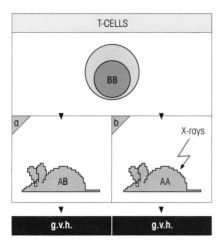

Figure 16.3. Graft-vs-host reaction. When competent T-cells are inoculated into a host incapable of reacting against them, the grafted cells are free to react against the antigens on the host's cells which they recognize as foreign. The ensuing reaction may be fatal. Two of many possible situations are illustrated: (a) the hybrid AB receives cells from one parent (BB) which are tolerated but react against the A antigen on host cells; (b) an X-irradiated AA recipient restored immunologically with BB cells cannot react against the graft and a g.v.h. reaction will result.

the human, fever, anemia, weight loss, rash, diarrhea and splenomegaly are observed, with cytokines, especially tumor necrosis factor (TNF), being major mediators of pathology. The 'stronger' the transplantation antigen difference, the more severe the reaction. Where donor and recipient differ at HLA or H-2 loci, the consequences can be fatal, although it should be noted that reactions to dominant minor transplantation antigens, or combinations of them, may be equally difficult to control.

Two possible situations leading to g.v.h. reactions are illustrated in figure 16.3. In the human this may arise in immunologically anergic subjects receiving bone marrow grafts, e.g. for combined immunodeficiency (see p. 318), for red cell aplasia after radiation accidents, or as a form of cancer therapy. Competent T-cells in blood or present in grafted organs given to immunosuppressed patients may also mediate g.v.h. reactions.

MECHANISMS OF GRAFT REJECTION

Lymphocytes can mediate rejection

A primary role of lymphoid cells in first set rejection would be consistent with the histology of the early reaction showing infiltration by mononuclear cells with very few polymorphonuclear cells or plasma cells (figure 16.4). The dramatic effect of neonatal thymectomy on prolonging skin transplants, and the long survival of grafts on children with thymic deficiencies, implicate the T-lymphocytes in these reactions. In the

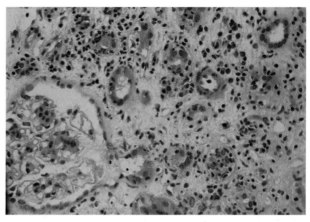

Figure 16.4. Acute rejection of human renal allograft showing dense cellular infiltration of interstitium by mononuclear cells. (Photograph courtesy of Drs M. Thompson and A. Dorling.)

chicken, homograft rejection and g.v.h. reactivity are influenced by neonatal thymectomy but not bursectomy. More direct evidence has come from *in vitro* studies showing that T-cells taken from mice rejecting an allograft could kill target cells bearing the graft antigens *in vitro*. Although CD8 cytotoxic T-cells play a major role in allograft rejection, a number of murine models have indicated that in the absence of CD4 T-cells allografts can be accepted indefinitely. Indeed, rejection can be mediated by CD4 T-cells in the absence of CD8 T-cells, perhaps because the CD4 cells sometimes have cytotoxic potential for class II targets. However, in intact animals, cytokine secretion from CD4 T-cells will recruit and activate CD8 T-cells, B-cells, NKT cells and macrophages which all have the potential to contribute to the rejection process. Futhermore, γ-interferon (IFNγ) upregulates antigen expression on the target graft cell, so increasing its vulnerability to CD8 cytotoxic cells.

The allograft response is powerful

Remember, we defined the MHC by its ability to provoke the most powerful rejection of grafts between members of the same species. This intensity of MHC mismatched rejection is a consequence of the **very high frequency of alloreactive T-cells** (i.e. cells which react with allografts) **present in normal individuals.** Whereas merely a fraction of a per cent of the normal T-cell population is specific for a given single peptide, upwards of 10% of T-cells react with alloantigens. Two main pathways of recognition have been described. In the **direct pathway** large numbers of recipient alloreactive T-cells recognize **allo- (i.e. graft) MHC** on the surface of donor cells, whereas in the **indirect pathway** a smaller number of recipient T-cells recognize peptides

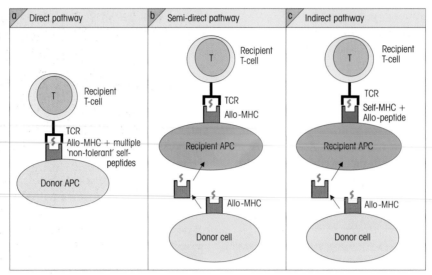

Figure 16.5. Recognition of graft antigens by alloreactive T-cells. (a) **Direct pathway.** T-cell receptors (TCR) on the recipient's T-cells directly recognize allogeneic MHC on the surface of donor antigen-presenting cells. Polymorphic differences between MHC allotypes largely affect peptide binding rather than TCR contact by the donor MHC. Under these circumstances, the donor allogeneic MHC molecule will be seen as if it were 'self' MHC by the recipient's T-cells but, unlike the self-MHC, the donor MHC groove on graft antigen-presenting cells will bind large numbers of processed serum and cellular peptides common to graft and recipient to which the responder host T-cells have not been rendered tolerant and which can therefore provoke a reaction in up to 10% of these host T-cells. This provides the intensity of the allograft response. This explanation for the high frequency of alloreactive T-cells is given further credibility by the isola- tion of individual T-cell clones which react with self- and allo-MHC, each binding a different peptide sequence. Direct recognition of donor MHC by recipient T-cells can also occur if the limited polymorphism in the α-helix adventitiously allows binding of TCRs to the allo-MHC independently of the associated peptide. Multiple bonds of this nature between the APC and T-cell may give rise to a strong enough interaction to permit T-cell activation. (b) **Semi-direct pathway.** It has recently been proposed that recipient dendritic cells can acquire intact MHC molecules from donor cells and then show these intact MHC molecules to the recipient's T-cells. (c) **Indirect pathway.** The recipient's APCs process donor MHC and donor minor histocompatibility molecules and then present the generated allogeneic peptides using their own, i.e. self, MHC. The initially small population of T-cells which are stimulated by the indirect pathway will expand with time.

derived from **allo-MHC** (and allo-minor transplantation antigens) presented by self MHC molecules on the recipient's own antigen-presenting cells (figure 16.5a and c). A third, **semi-direct**, pathway has also recently been proposed, in which intact MHC molecules are acquired from the donor cells by the dendritic cells of the recipient (figure 16.5b).

Allogeneic MHC differs from the recipient essentially in the groove residues which contact processed peptide, but much less so in the more conserved helical regions which are recognized by the TCR. Having a different groove structure, the allo-MHC will be able to bind a number of peptides derived from proteins common to donor and host which might be unable to fit the groove in the host MHC and therefore fail to induce self-tolerance. Thus the host T-cells which recognize allo-MHC plus common peptides will not have been eliminated, and will be available to react with the large number of different peptides binding to the allo-groove of the donor antigen-presenting cells (APCs) which migrate to the secondary lymphoid tissue of the graft recipient. In some cases, the polymorphic residues may lie within the regions of the MHC helices which contact

TCR directly and, by chance, a proportion of the T-cell repertoire cross-reacts and binds to the donor MHC with high affinity. Attachment of the T-cell to the APC will be particularly strong since the TCRs will bind to all the donor MHC molecules on the APC, whereas in the case of normal MHC–peptide recognition, only a small proportion of the MHC grooves will be filled by the specific peptide in question. These direct pathways of immunization by the allograft MHC which are usually initiated by the most powerful APC, the dendritic cell, dominate the early sensitization events, since this acute phase of rejection (see below) can be blocked by antibodies to the allo-MHC class II.

However, with time, as the donor APCs in the graft are replaced by recipient cells, another rejection mechanism based on an indirect pathway of sensitization involving the presentation of processed **allogeneic peptides** by **host MHC** (figure 16.5c) becomes possible. Although T-cells recognizing peptides derived from polymorphic graft proteins would be expected to be present in low frequency comparable to that observed with any foreign antigen, a graft which has been in place for an extended period will have the time to expand this small population significantly so that later rejection may depend progressively on this indirect pathway. In these circumstances, antirecipient MHC class II can now be shown to prolong renal allografts in rats.

The role of antibody

Allogeneic cells can be destroyed by cytotoxic (type II hypersensitivity) reactions involving humoral antibody. Consideration of the different ways in which kidney allografts can be rejected illustrates the contribution of antibody to the rejection process.

Hyperacute rejection within minutes of transplantation, characterized by sludging of red cells and microthrombi in the glomeruli, occurs in individuals with pre-existing humoral antibodies—either due to blood group incompatibility or presensitization to class I MHC through blood transfusion.

Acute early rejection occurring up to 10 days or so after transplantation is characterized by dense cellular infiltration (figure 16.4) and rupture of peritubular capillaries, and appears to be a cell-mediated hypersensitivity reaction mainly involving CD8 cytotoxic attack on graft cells whose MHC antigen expression has been upregulated by γ-interferon. Antibody does not play a role in this phase of the rejection process.

Acute late rejection, which occurs from 11 days onwards in patients suppressed with prednisolone and azathioprine, may be due to breakthrough of immunosuppression by the immune response, or can be caused by the binding of immunoglobulin (presumably graft-specific antibody) and complement to the arterioles and glomerular capillaries, where they can be visualized by immunofluorescent techniques. These immunoglobulin deposits on the vessel walls induce platelet aggregation in the glomerular capillaries leading to acute renal shutdown (figure 16.6). The possibility of damage to antibody-coated cells through antibody-dependent cellular cytotoxicity must also be considered.

Insidious and late rejection is associated with subendothelial deposits of immunoglobulin and C3 on the glomerular basement membranes which may sometimes be an expression of an underlying immune complex disorder (originally necessitating the transplant) or possibly of complex formation with soluble antigens derived from the grafted kidney.

The complexity of the action and interaction of cellular and humoral factors in graft rejection is therefore considerable and an attempt to summarize the postulated mechanisms involved is presented in figure 16.7.

There are also circumstances when antibodies may actually protect a graft from destruction, a phenomenon termed enhancement.

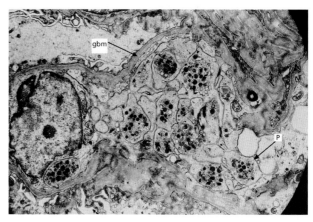

Figure 16.6. Acute late rejection of human renal allograft showing platelet aggregation in a glomerular capillary induced by deposition of antibody on the vessel wall (electron micrograph). gbm, glomerular basement membrane; P, platelet. (Photograph courtesy of Professor K. Porter.)

THE PREVENTION OF GRAFT REJECTION

Matching tissue types on graft donor and recipient

Since MHC differences provoke the most vicious rejection of grafts, a prodigious amount of effort has gone into defining these antigen specificities, in an attempt to minimize rejection by matching graft and recipient in much the same way that individuals are cross-matched for blood transfusions (incidentally, the ABO group provides strong transplantation antigens).

HLA tissue typing

HLA alleles are defined by their gene sequences and individuals can be typed by the *p*olymerase *c*hain *r*eaction (PCR) using discriminating pairs of primers. Molecules encoded by the class II *HLA-D* loci provoke CD4 T-cell responses, whereas HLA-A, -B and -C products are targets for alloreactive CD8 T-cells.

The polymorphism of the human HLA system

With so many alleles at each locus and several loci in each individual (figure 16.8), it will readily be appreciated that this gives rise to an exceptional degree of polymorphism. This is of great potential value to the species, since the need for T-cells to recognize their own individual specificities provides a defense against microbial molecular mimicry in which a whole species might be put at risk by its inability to recognize as foreign an organism which generates MHC–peptide complexes similar to self. It is also possible that in some way the existence of a high degree of polymorphism helps to maintain the diversity of antigenic recognition within the lymphoid system of a given species and also ensures heterozygosity (hybrid vigor).

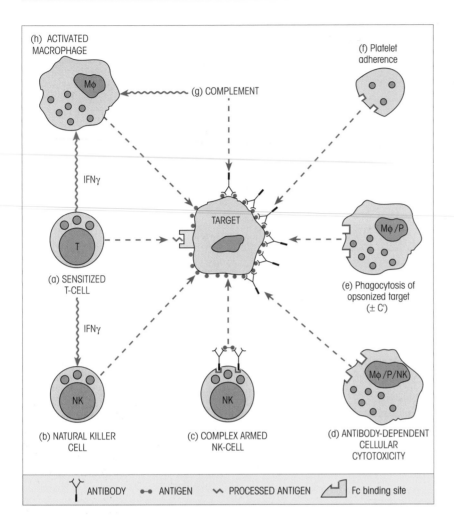

Figure 16.7. Mechanisms of target cell destruction. Mφ, macrophage; P, polymorphonuclear leukocyte; NK, natural killer cell. (a) Direct killing by Tc cells and indirect tissue damage through release of cytokines such as IFNγ and TNF from Th1-cells. (b) Direct killing by NK cells (see p. 18) enhanced by interferon. (c) Specific killing by immune complex-armed NK cell which recognizes the target through free antibody valencies in the complex. (d) Attack by antibody-dependent cellular cytotoxicity (in (a)–(d) the killing is extracellular). (e) Phagocytosis of target coated with antibody (heightened by bound C3b). (f) Sticking of platelets to antibody bound to the surface of graft vascular endothelium leading to formation of microthrombi. (g) Complement-mediated cytotoxicity. (h) Macrophages activated nonspecifically by agents such as IFNγ and possibly C3b can be cytotoxic for graft cells, perhaps through extracellular action of TNF and O_2^-· radicals generated at the cell surface (see p. 6).

The value of matching tissue types

Improvements in operative techniques and the use of drugs such as cyclosporine have diminished the effects of mismatching HLA specificities on solid graft survival but, nevertheless, most transplanters favor a reasonable degree of matching (see figure 16.17). Tissue typing can be carried out using serological methods which employ panels of antibodies each specific for a different HLA allele, and which enable the detection of the HLA variants on the cell surface of leukocytes. These techniques are increasingly being replaced by molecular genetics techniques, such as the use of sequence-specific oligonucleotide primers, to determine the variants. HLA-DR matching is the most critical, followed by HLA-B and then HLA-A. In fact, it is only these three loci that are usually typed, although recent studies have suggested that typing of HLA-C might also be advantageous in optimizing the success of some transplants. Mismatches at HLA-DQ are thought to generally be less important, and those at the HLA–DP loci appear to have minimal consequences. In addition to typing recipients and potential donors, cross-matching is carried out to ensure the absence of pre-existing antibodies to donor antigens in the proposed recipient. Hematopoietic stem cell grafts, including bone marrow grafts, require a very high degree of compatibility because of the increased potential for graft-versus-host disease in addition to host-versus-graft reactions; the greater accuracy of DNA typing methods and the inclusion of HLA-DQ typing can be most helpful in this respect.

Because of the many thousands of different HLA phenotypes possible (figure 16.8), it is usual to work with a large pool of potential recipients on a continental basis (Eurotransplant), so that when graft material becomes available the best possible match can be made. The position will be improved when the pool of available organs can be increased through the development of long-term tissue storage banks, but techniques are not good enough for this at present, except in the case of bone marrow and hematopoietic stem cells which can be kept viable even after freezing and thawing. With a paired organ such as the kidney, living donors may be used; siblings provide the best chance of a good match. However, the use of living donors poses difficult ethical

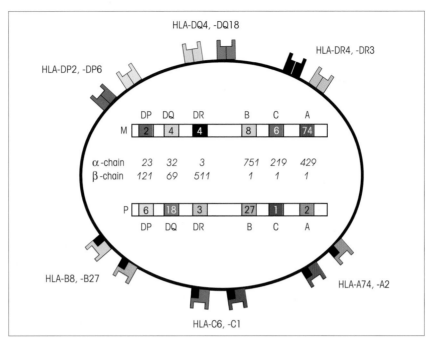

Figure 16.8. Polymorphic HLA specificities and their inheritance. Since there are several possible alleles at each locus, the probability of a random pair of subjects from the general population having identical HLA specificities is very low. Indeed, the class I and II MHC genes are the most polymorphic in the genome and the number of different allelic variants based upon nucleotide sequences assigned as of January 2006 are indicated by the numbers in italics in the center of the figure (data from http://www.anthonynolan.org.uk/HIG). In the example given the individual expresses the particular α- and β-chain alleles at the DP loci (see figure 4.18) on the maternal (M) chromosome which specify HLA-DP2, has inherited those for HLA-DP6 on the paternal (P) chromosome, and so on. These genes are codominantly expressed and therefore cells can express up to six different alleles of the main class I molecules and, on their professional antigen-presenting cells, additionally up to at least six different class II molecules. The fact that there are usually two DRβ genes inherited on both copies of chromosome 6, and the potential for *trans* pairing as well as *cis* pairing of some class II α and β-chains, further increases the HLA diversity in the individual. Conversely, homozygosity at any of the loci will reduce the number of variants. Note that not all polymorphisms in nucleotide sequence will result in a polymorphism at the protein level, and furthermore that not all polymorphisms in the polypeptide chain will affect binding of antigenic peptides or T-cell receptors to the MHC molecule and therefore impact upon transplant rejection. The MHC class I molecules all employ the same β-chain, β_2-microglobulin, which is nonpolymorphic, encoded outside of the MHC, and does not form part of the peptide-binding groove. There is a 1 : 4 chance that two siblings will be MHC identical because each group of specificities on a single chromosome forms a haplotype which will usually be inherited *en bloc*, giving four possible combinations of paternal and maternal chromosomes. Parent and offspring can only be identical (1 : 2 chance) if the mother and father have one haplotype in common.

problems and organs are most commonly obtained from brain dead donors in which there has been a loss of all brain function including that of the brain stem which controls respiration. There has also been encouraging progress in the use of cadaver material from nonheart-beating donors.

There is active interest in the possibility of using animal organs (see below) or mechanical substitutes, while some are even trying to prevent the disease in the first place!

Agents producing general immunosuppression

Graft rejection can be held at bay by the use of agents which nonspecifically interfere with the induction or expression of the immune response (figure 16.9). Because these agents are nonspecific, patients on immunosuppressive therapy tend to be susceptible to infections; they are also more prone to develop lymphoreticular cancers, particularly those of viral etiology.

Targeting lymphoid populations

Anti-CD3 monoclonals are in widespread use as anti-T-cell reagents to reverse acute graft rejection. Originally the mouse monoclonal antibody OKT3 was used and, although shown to have a beneficial effect, its efficacy was to some extent compromised by its immunogenicity in the human host. Furthermore, it possesses a mitogenic activity responsible for triggering a severe cytokine release syndrome involving 'flu-like' symptoms. These problems are circumvented by the use of engineered antibodies (see p. 115). The ChAglyCD3 antibody is a humanized non-mitogenic version of a rat monoclonal antibody in which position 297 in the heavy chain has been mutated to prevent glycosylation and consequently binding to Fc receptors and to comple-

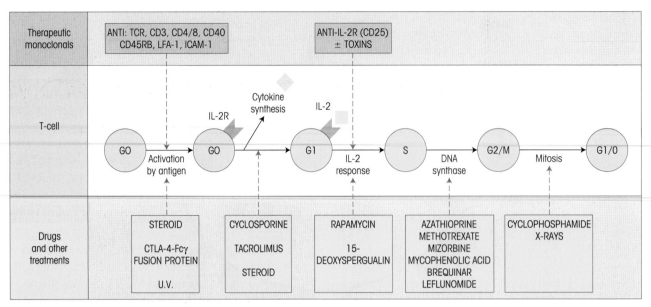

Figure 16.9. Immunosuppressive agents used to control graft rejection. Mycophenolate mofetil is a powerful immunosuppressant which, when metabolized into the purine analog mycophenolic acid, inhibits proliferation but also suppresses expression of CD25, -71, -154 (CD40L) and CD28. Another potent drug is 15-deoxyspergualin (DSG) which interferes with lymphocyte function by binding to heat shock protein and possibly thereby inhibiting NFκB translocation to the nucleus. Leflunomide (Arava), which is also effective as a disease-modifying antirheumatic drug (DMARD) for the treatment of rheumatoid arthritis, effectively blocks the proliferation of activated T-cells by inhibiting dihydroorotate dehydrogenase (DHODH)-mediated pyrimidine synthesis. Simultaneous treatment with agents acting at sequential stages in development of the rejection response would be expected to lead to strong synergy and this is clearly seen with cyclosporine and rapamycin.

ment. As an alternative, the humanized huOKT3γ1 Ala-Ala antibody in which leucines were replaced with alanines at positions 234 and 235 to eliminate FcγR binding is also non-mitogenic and efficacious.

The IL-2 receptor α chain (CD25), expressed by activated but not resting T-cells, represents another exploitable target. Daclizumab is a humanized monoclonal anti-IL-2Rα, and basiliximab a chimeric (mouse V region, human C region) antibody of similar specificity. They are of particular benefit in the prevention of acute kidney transplant rejection when used in combination with cyclosporine plus corticosteroids.

Immunosuppressive drugs

The development of an immunological response requires the active proliferation of a relatively small number of antigen-sensitive lymphocytes to give a population of sensitized cells large enough to be effective. Many of the immunosuppressive drugs now employed were first used in cancer chemotherapy because of their toxicity to dividing cells. Aside from the complications of blanket immunosuppression mentioned above, these antimitotic drugs are especially toxic for cells of the bone marrow and small intestine and must therefore be used with great care.

A commonly used drug in this field is **azathioprine** which inhibits nucleic acid synthesis and has a preferen-

tial effect on T-cell-mediated reactions. Another drug, **methotrexate**, through its action as a folic acid antagonist also inhibits synthesis of nucleic acid. The N-mustard derivative **cyclophosphamide** attacks DNA by alkylation and cross-linking, so preventing correct duplication during cell division. These agents appear to exert their damaging effects on cells during mitosis and, for this reason, are most powerful when administered after presentation of antigen at a time when the antigen-sensitive cells are dividing. An exciting group of fungal metabolites has had a dramatic effect in human transplantation and in the therapy of immunological disorders through their ability to target T-cells. **Cyclosporine** (Sandimmune, or its microemulsion version Neoral which exhibits increased bioavailability) is a neutral hydrophobic 11 amino acid cyclical peptide which selectively blocks the transcription of IL-2 in activated T-cells. Resting cells which carry the vital memory for immunity to microbial infections are spared and there is little toxicity for dividing cells in gut and bone marrow. The drug also directly affects dendritic cells, inhibiting a number of their functions including antigen processing, production of TNF and IL-12, expression of chemokine receptors and cell migration. Cyclosporine is firmly established as a first-line therapy in the prophylaxis and treatment of transplant rejection; figure 16.11 gives an example of its use in kidney transplantation. Another

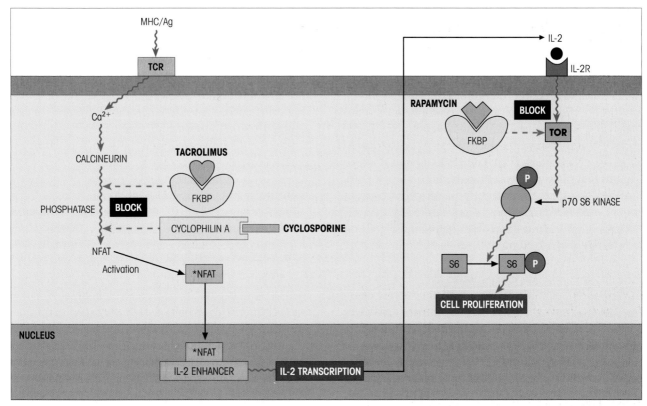

Figure 16.10. The mode of action of cyclosporine, tacrolimus and rapamycin. The complexes of cyclosporine with cyclophilin A and of tacrolimus with FKBP (*FK*506 [tacrolimus]-*b*inding *p*rotein) bind to and inactivate the phosphatase calcineurin responsible for activating the *n*uclear *f*actor of *a*ctivated *T*-cells (NFAT) transcription factor for IL-2 synthesis. Transfection with calcineurin decreases the inhibitory powers of cyclosporine and tacrolimus. On binding to cyclophilin A, cyclosporine undergoes a conformational change enabling it to exteriorize hydrophobic side-chains to form a patch which can bind calcineurin, rather like double-sided tape. The rapamycin–FKBP complex inhibits the TOR (*t*arget *of r*apamycin) kinase and thereby blocks the activation of p70 S6 kinase by transduced IL-2 signals, thus inhibiting cell proliferation.

T-cell-specific immunosuppressive drug, **tacrolimus** (FK506), isolated from a species of *Streptomyces*, also blocks various T-cell and dendritic cell activities. One of the latest additions to the stable is **rapamycin** (sirolimus), a product of the fungus *Streptomyces hygroscopicus*, which is a macrolide like tacrolimus but in contrast acts to block signals induced by combination of IL-2 with its receptor.

We now have greater insight into the mode of action of these drugs (figure 16.10). Cyclosporine complexes with cyclophilin A, a member of the **immunophilin** family, whilst tacrolimus complexes with another immunophilin family member, *FK-b*inding *p*rotein (FKBP). These complexes then interact with and inhibit the calcium- and calmodulin-dependent phosphatase, calcineurin, which activates the NFAT (*n*uclear *f*actor of *a*ctivated *T*-cells) transcription factor for IL-2 in activated T-cells. Although rapamycin also binds to FKBP, the complex has a quite different activity and inhibits the TOR (*t*arget *of r*apamycin) serine/threonine kinase. The immunosuppressive activity of rapamycin is at

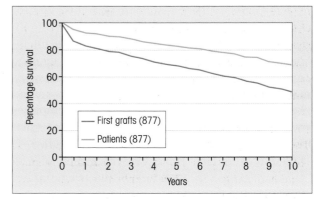

Figure 16.11. Actuarial survival of primary cadaveric kidney grafts in 877 patients treated at the Oxford Transplant Centre with triple therapy of cyclosporine, azathioprine and prednisolone. (Data kindly provided by Professor Peter J. Morris.)

least partially explained by the fact that TOR plays a central role in transducing proliferative signals, such as those through the IL-2 receptor. In addition to its role in transplantation, cyclosporine has also been evaluated in a wide range of disorders where T-cell-mediated hypersensitivity reactions are suspected. Indeed, the benefits of cyclosporine in diseases such as rheumatoid arthritis, psoriasis, idiopathic nephrotic syndrome, type 1 diabetes, Behçet's syndrome, active Crohn's disease, aplastic anemia and severe corticosteroid-dependent asthma have been interpreted to suggest or confirm a pathogenic role for the immune system. Inhibition of keratinocyte proliferation by cyclosporine may contribute to the favorable outcome in psoriasis. A rapid onset of benefit, and of relapse when treatment is stopped, are common features of cyclosporine therapy. There are, of course, side-effects, the most significant being nephrotoxicity. It has to be used at doses below those causing renal fibrosis due to stimulation of TGFβ production by several cell types.

Tacrolimus is greatly superior to cyclosporine on a molar basis *in vitro* but is not substantially more effective. Because they act at different stages in the activation of the T-cell, cyclosporine and rapamycin show an impressive degree of synergy which allows the two drugs to be used at considerably lower dose levels with correspondingly less likelihood of side-effects (figure 16.9). Another possible synergistic partner for cyclosporine is fludarabine which, unlike cyclosporine, blocks signaling by STAT-1, an intracellular intermediate activated by interferons and important for cell-mediated immunity. Combination therapies may also include mycophenolate mofetil and leflunomide which limit the availability of DNA precursors.

Steroids such as prednisolone intervene at many points in the immune response, affecting lymphocyte recirculation and the generation of cytotoxic effector cells, for example; in addition, their outstanding anti-inflammatory potency rests on features such as inhibition of neutrophil adherence to vascular endothelium in an inflammatory area and suppression of monocyte/macrophage functions such as microbicidal activity and response to cytokines. Corticosteroids form complexes with intracellular receptors which then bind to regulatory genes and block transcription of TNF, IFNγ, IL-1, -2, -3, -6 and MHC class II, i.e. they block expression of cytokines from both lymphocytes and macrophages, whereas cyclosporine has its main action on the former.

Inducing tolerance to graft antigens

If the disadvantages of blanket immunosuppression are to be avoided, we must aim at knocking out only the reactivity of the host to the antigens of the graft, leaving the remainder of the immunological apparatus intact — in other words, the induction of **antigen-specific tolerance**.

It turns out that bone marrow represents an excellent source of tolerogenic alloantigens, and the production of stable lymphohematopoietic mixed chimerism by bone marrow engraftment is proving to be a potent means of inducing robust specific transplantation tolerance to solid organs across major MHC mismatches. However, successful allogeneic bone marrow transplantation in immunocompetent adults normally requires cytoablative treatment of recipients with irradiation or cytotoxic drugs and this has tended to restrict its use to malignant conditions. A most encouraging recent study has shown the feasibility of inducing long-lasting tolerance not only to bone marrow cells but also to fully MHC-mismatched skin grafts in naive recipients receiving high-dose bone marrow transplantation and costimulatory blockade by single injections of monoclonal anti-CD154 (CD40L) plus a CTLA-4-Ig fusion protein (figure 16.12). A persistent hematopoietic macrochimerism is achieved with a significant proportion of donor-type lymphocytes in the thymus indicating intrathymic deletion of donor-reactive T-cells.

While this protocol permits long-term engraftment of bone marrow and solid organs, it seems that direct blockade with just anti-CD154 and CTLA-4-Ig is sufficient to induce tolerance to solid organ grafts. Stimulation of alloreactive T-cells by the graft in the presence of costimulatory blockade leads to apoptosis, a process promoted by rapamycin which improves the tolerant state. Bcl-X_L (cf. figure 10.5, p. 214) prevents both T-cell

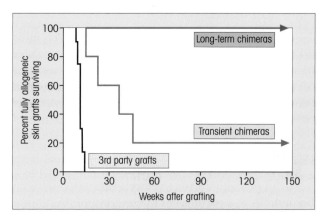

Figure 16.12. Induction of tolerance and macrochimerism by fully allogeneic bone marrow transplantation plus costimulatory blockade. B6 mice received bone marrow cells from the fully allogeneic B10.A strain with injections of anti-CD154 (CD40L) and the CTLA-4-Ig fusion protein which blocks CD80/CD86–CD28 interactions (CTLA-4 is a receptor for CD80 and CD86 which downregulates T-cell activation; cf. pp. 172 and 177). Eight mice showing long-term persistence of multilineage donor cells (macrochimerism) were fully tolerant to B10.A skin grafts. Five mice with transient chimerism showed moderate prolongation of skin graft survival relative to unrelated 3rd party grafts. (Data taken from Wekerle T. *et al.* (2000) *Nature Medicine* **6**, 464, with permission.)

apoptosis and tolerance induction by this treatment revealing the importance of apoptotic T-cell deletion for the establishment of antigen-specific unresponsiveness. In a further twist to the tale, the apoptotic T-cells 'reach from beyond the grave' by producing IL-10, so that their phagocytosis along with antigen leads to the presentation of the antigen in a tolerogenic form which maintains tolerance through the production of immunoregulatory cells.

Despite the role of the *mature* dendritic cell as the champion stimulator of resting T-cells, the dendritic cell *precursors* may present antigen in the absence of B7 costimulators and, by mechanisms echoing those described above in the costimulatory blockade experiments, would appear to have a powerful potential for tolerance induction. This concept is of particular relevance to the specific unresponsiveness generated by grafts of liver which, being a hematopoietic organ, continually exports large numbers of these immature dendritic cells.

Nondepleting anti-CD4 and -8 monoclonals, by depriving T-cells of fully activating signals, can render them anergic when they engage antigen through their specific receptors. These anergic cells can induce unresponsiveness in newly recruited T-cells ('infectious tolerance', p. 241) and so establish specific and indefinite acceptance of mouse skin grafts across class I or multiple minor transplantation antigen barriers (figure 16.13). It should be noted that skin allografts provide the most difficult challenge for tolerance induction, and transplants of organs such as the heart, which are less fastidious than skin, require less aggressive immunotherapy.

Given the wide variety of different peptide epitopes presented by the graft MHC, full-frontal attack on the alloreactive T-cells by administration of tolerogenic peptides represents quite a challenge, and the strategy of using costimulatory blockade with the antigens being provided by the graft itself looks to be a more promising route.

IS XENOGRAFTING A PRACTICAL PROPOSITION?

Because the supply of donor human organs for transplantation lags seriously behind the demand, a widespread interest in the feasibility of using animal organs is emerging. Pigs are more favored than primates as donors both on the grounds of ethical acceptability and the hazards of zoonoses. The first hurdle to be overcome is **hyperacute rejection** due to xenoreactive natural antibodies in the host. The sugar structure galactose α-1,3-galactose is absent in humans, apes and Old World monkeys due to a mutation in the gene encoding α-1,3-galactosyltransferase in these species. They are there-

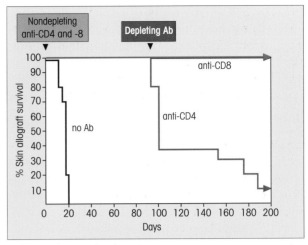

Figure 16.13. Induction of allograft tolerance by nondepleting anti-CD4 plus anti-CD8. Tolerance to skin grafts from donors with multiple minor transplantation antigen mismatches was achieved by concurrent injection of IgG2a monoclonal antibodies to CD4 and CD8 which do not induce cell depletion (green arrow). The maintenance of tolerance depends upon the continued presence of antigen which enables the unresponsive cells to interact with newly arising immunocompetent cells on the surface of the same antigen-presenting cells and render them unresponsive through an infectious tolerance mechanism (cf. figures 11.9 and 18.37). Loss of tolerance on depletion of CD4 but not CD8 cells (red arrows) shows that active tolerance is maintained by the CD4 subset. Indeed, tolerance can be transferred by CD4⁺ CD25⁺ T-regulatory cells. (Figure synthesized from data kindly provided by Dr S.P. Cobbold and Professor H. Waldmann.)

fore not immunologically tolerant to this non-self sugar structure. Furthermore, they have pre-existing antibodies to the Gal α-1,3-Gal epitope which is present on many common bacteria and expressed abundantly on the xenogeneic pig vascular endothelium. The natural antibodies bind to the endothelium and activate complement in the absence of regulators of the human complement system, such as decay accelerating factor, CD59 and MCP (cf. figure 14.3), precipitating the hyperacute rejection phenomenon. Novel genetic engineering strategies for the solution of this problem are outlined in figure 16.14.

The next crisis is **acute vascular rejection** occurring within 6 days as *de novo* antibody production is elicited in response to the xenoantigens on donor epithelium. Interleukin-12 and IFNγ inhibit acute vascular rejection of xenografts and, over the long term, IFNγ may protect the graft by promoting the formation of NO· which prevents constriction of blood vessels. Brequinar sodium (figure 16.9), an inhibitor of pyrimidine biosynthesis and suppressor of both B- and T-cell-mediated responses, has been evaluated for efficacy, but induction of tolerance would clearly be more desirable. A limited degree of success has been achieved using baboons as recipients of hearts or kidneys from α-1,3-galactosyltransferase

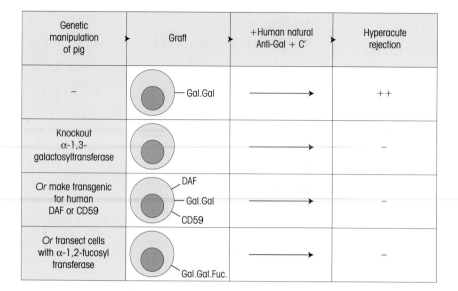

Figure 16.14. Strategies for avoiding complement-mediated hyperacute rejection of a xenograft caused by reaction of natural antigalactose antibodies with Galα-1,3-Gal on the surface of the pig graft cells. Heart or kidney xenografts from α-1,3-galactosyltransferase knockout pigs can function for reasonable periods of time in baboons, as can hearts from transgenic pigs expressing the human complement regulatory proteins decay accelerating factor (DAF) or CD59. Transfection of pig cells with α-1,2-fucosyl transferase converted the terminal sugars into the blood group H and rendered the cells resistant to lysis by the antigalactose. Other strategies involve transfection with genes encoding an α-galactosidase or intracellular recombinant scFv reacting with α-1,3-galactosyltransferase.

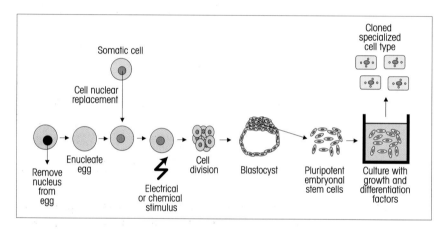

Figure 16.15. Cell nuclear replacement for therapeutic cloning. The nucleus of an egg is replaced with the nucleus from a body cell, such as a mammary gland cell or skin cell. The egg is then stimulated electrically or with chemicals to initiate cell division. Following its development into an embryo the stem cells can be isolated and are then encouraged to develop into the desired cell type by culture with appropriate growth and differentiation factors.

knockout pigs, although fairly hefty immunosuppressive regimens were employed together with, in the case of the kidney grafts, cotransplantation of thymic tissue with the aim of inducing tolerance in the recipient.

Even when the immunological problems are overcome, it remains to be seen whether the xenograft will be compatible with human life over a prolonged period. There is also concern over the presence of porcine endogenous retroviruses (PERVs) which are related to viruses associated with leukemias in a number of species. Given that the PERV-A receptors PAR-1 and PAR-2 are widely distributed in human tissues such concerns are warranted, although it is unclear if infection of human cells with such viruses would have detrimental consequences.

STEM CELL THERAPY

The ideal transplant is one created **entirely from cells of the recipient**, i.e. an autograft, which would eliminate the need for immunosuppression. It is possible to isolate stem cells from various adult organs including bone marrow. By way of an example, human bone marrow-derived multipotent stem cells have been shown to induce therapeutic neovascularization and cardiomyogenesis in a rat model of myocardial infarction. Recent advances in cell nuclear replacement have also opened up the possibility of therapeutic cloning using embryonic stem cells (figure 16.15). Knowledge is steadily accumulating concerning the various growth factors required to guide relatively undifferentiated stem cells into the desired mature form, for example pancreatic, nerve or liver cells for regenerative therapy, or erythrocytes for transfusion. An exciting development came from the cloning of 'Dolly' the sheep, the first cloned animal produced from a cell taken from an adult animal. Such reproductive cloning has led to concerns that cloned human embryos could be re-implanted and used in attempts to produce cloned humans. However, in therapeutic cloning the embryo is only allowed to grow for a few days in order to provide a source of stem cells for subsequent differentiation and expansion *in vitro*. A

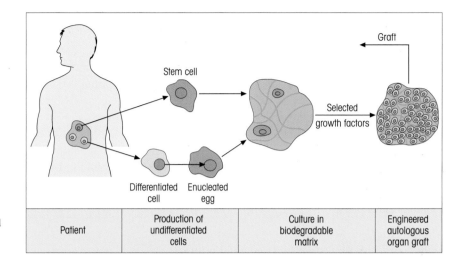

Figure 16.16. Anticipated production of autologous grafts by tissue engineering. Undifferentiated cells are obtained directly from the patient either as adult stem cells or by cell nuclear replacement into enucleated oocytes. They are cultured in a biodegradable matrix with appropriate growth factors to provide a tissue populated with differentiated cells which can function as an autologous graft.

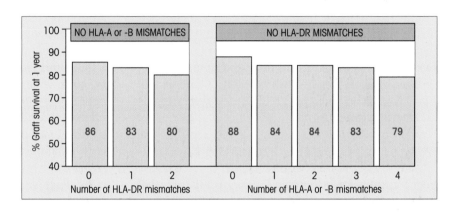

Figure 16.17. First cadaveric kidney graft survival in Europe for the period January 1993 to December 1997 ($n = 12584$) on the basis of mismatches for HLA-A, -B and -DR. There is a significant influence of matching, $p < 0.001$, for both sets of data. (Data kindly supplied by Drs Guido Persijn and Jacqueline Smits of the Eurotransplant International Foundation.)

major step in this direction was the announcement in 2005 that a team at the University of Newcastle in the UK had succeeded in their attempts to clone a human blastocyst. This powerful technology could revolutionize the treatment of neurodegenerative diseases, heart disease, diabetes, visual impairment and many other afflictions. The potential to grow stem cells on a matrix in order to engineer tissues or even whole organs provides further opportunities to circumvent the problem of allograft rejection (figure 16.16).

CLINICAL EXPERIENCE IN GRAFTING

Privileged sites

Corneal grafts survive without the need for immunosuppression. Because they are avascular they tend not to sensitize the recipient. This privileged protection is boosted by the local production of immunosuppressive factors such as TGFβ, IL-1Ra, limited expression of MHC and the strategic presence of FasL which can induce apoptosis in infiltrating lymphocytes. Nonetheless, they do become cloudy if the individual has been *presensitized*. Grafts of **cartilage** are successful in the

same way but an additional factor is the protection afforded the chondrocytes by the matrix. With bone and artery it doesn't really matter if the grafts die because they can still provide a framework for host cells to colonize.

Kidney grafts

Many thousands of kidneys have been transplanted and with improvement in patient management there is a high survival rate. In the long term (5 years or more), the desirability of reasonable matching at the HLA-A, -B and -D loci becomes apparent (figure 16.17).

Patients are partially immunosuppressed at the time of transplantation because uremia causes a degree of immunological nonresponsiveness. The **triple therapy** combination of a calcineurin inhibitor such as cyclosporine, azathioprine (now often replaced with mycophenolate mofetil) and a glucocorticoid such as prednisolone has been the mainstay for long-term management of kidney grafts (figure 16.11). One hopes that the synergy between cyclosporine and rapamycin, and possibly other immunosuppressants, will lead to the emergence of powerful new therapeutic regimens. If kidney function is poor during a rejection crisis, renal dialysis can be used. As mentioned above, there is active interest in the possibility of xenografting. When transplantation is performed because of immune complex-induced glomerulonephritis, the immunosuppressive treatment used may help to prevent a similar lesion developing in the grafted kidney. Patients with glomerular basement membrane antibodies (e.g. Goodpasture's syndrome) are likely to destroy their renal transplants unless first treated with plasmapheresis and immunosuppressive drugs.

Heart transplants

The overall 1-year organ survival figure for heart transplants has moved up to over 85% (figure 16.18), helped considerably by the introduction of combination immunosuppressive therapy of the type mentioned above. Aside from the rejection problem, it is likely that the number of patients who would benefit from cardiac replacement is much greater than the number dying with adequately healthy hearts. More attention will have to be given to the possibility of xenogeneic grafts and mechanical substitutes.

Liver transplants

Survival rates for orthotopic (in the normal or usual position) liver grafts are just slightly lower than those achieved with heart transplants (figure 16.18). The hepatotrophic capacity of tacrolimus is an added bonus which makes it the preferred drug for liver transplantation. Rejection crises are dealt with by high-dose steroids and, if this proves ineffective, antilymphocyte globulin. The use of a totally synthetic colloidal hydrox-

yethyl starch solution, containing lactobionate as a substitute for chloride, allows livers to be preserved for 24 hours or more and has revolutionized the logistics of liver transplantation. To improve the prognosis of patients with primary hepatic or bile duct malignancies, which were considered to be inoperable, transplantation of organ clusters with liver as the central organ has been designed, e.g. liver and pancreas, or liver, pancreas, stomach and small bowel or even colon. Nonetheless, the outcome is not very favorable in that up to three-quarters of the patients transplanted for hepatic cancer have recurrence of their tumor within 1 year. For the future we must look forward to the creation of autologous liver from adult cells when tissue engineering techniques have been developed sufficiently.

Experience with liver grafting between pigs revealed an unexpected finding. Many of the animals retained the grafted organs in a healthy state for many months without any form of immunosuppression and enjoyed a state of unresponsiveness to grafts of skin or kidney from the same donor. True tolerance is induced by the donor-type intrahepatic hematopoietic stem cells and immature dendritic cells (see above) and possibly also by the liver parenchyma itself, known to produce copious amounts of soluble MHC class I.

Work is in progress on the transfer of isolated hepatocytes attached to collagen-coated microcarriers injected i.p. for the correction of isolated deficiencies such as albumin synthesis. This attractive approach has much wider application as a general vehicle for gene therapy.

Bone marrow and hematopoietic stem cell grafts

Patients with certain immunodeficiency disorders and

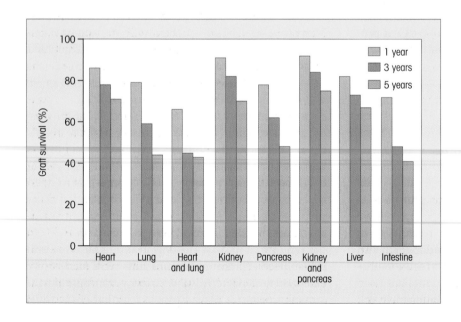

Figure 16.18. Graft survival rates for primary transplants performed 1995–2002 in the USA. Survival rates for repeat transplants are generally somewhat lower. (Data from the Organ Procurement and Transplantation Network http://www.optn.org/optn)

aplastic anemia are obvious candidates for treatment with **bone marrow** or with isolated peripheral **hematopoietic stem cells** with their potential to differentiate into all the formed elements of the blood; so, too, are patients with leukemia, lymphoma, myeloma and metastatic breast cancer treated radically with intensive chemotherapy and possibly whole-body irradiation in attempts to eradicate the neoplastic cells, as will be discussed in the next chapter.

Bone marrow contains not only hematopoietic but also mesenchymal stem cells which can give rise to cartilage, tendons and bone; after expansion in culture by a factor of 5–10 times, they provide an excellent treatment for children with osteogenesis imperfecta, a genetic disorder in which the osteoblasts produce defective type I collagen with resulting osteopenia and severe bony deformities. Favorable results have been obtained with stem cell transplantation *in utero* for severe combined immunodeficiency (SCID) using populations from paternal bone marrow enriched for the stem cell marker, CD34. From the practical standpoint, it has been recognized that cord blood contains sufficient hematopoietic stem cells for bone marrow replacement, but what is even more convenient is to use cytokines such as granulocyte colony-stimulating factor (G-CSF) to mobilize donor stem cells out of the bone marrow to increase the number of peripheral blood stem cells (PBSCs). Transplantation with either autologous (involving re-infusion of CD34$^+$ cells taken prior to myeloablative therapy) or allogeneic PBSCs results in a more rapid recovery in neutrophil and platelet numbers than that seen following bone marrow transplantation, and in many centers is rapidly replacing bone marrow as the source of such cells. Allogeneic cells can exhibit a graft-versus-tumor effect, although this needs to be weighed against the risk of graft-versus-host (g.v.h) disease (see below). Hematopoietic stem cell transplantation is also increasingly being explored as a mechanism of inducing tolerance to donor antigens in solid organ transplantation by creating a state of chimerism in the recipient, which would then lead to deletion or inactivation of the relevant alloreactive lymphocytes.

Graft-vs-host disease results from allogeneic T-cells in the graft

G.v.h. disease resulting from the recognition of recipient antigens by allogeneic T-cells in the bone marrow or peripheral blood-derived inoculum represents a serious, sometimes fatal, complication, and the incidence of g.v.h. disease is reduced if T-cells are first depleted with a cytotoxic cocktail of anti-T-cell monoclonals.

It is fondly hoped that successful engraftment and avoidance of g.v.h. reactions following allogeneic cell transplantation will be achieved in the clinic by strategies such as costimulatory blockade (figure 16.12) without a requirement for cytoablative treatment of graft or recipient. Until then, successful results are more likely with highly compatible donors, particularly if fatal g.v.h. reactions are to be avoided, and here siblings offer the best chance of finding a matched donor. Undoubtedly, non-HLA minor transplantation antigens are important and are more difficult to match. Acute g.v.h. disease occurring within the first 100 days following infusion of allogeneic cells primarily affects the skin, liver and gastrointestinal tract. Antibodies to TNF or IL-1R block mortality. Current therapy uses steroids such as prednisolone in combination with either cyclosporine or tacrolimus, but inclusion of methotrexate in this regimen is said to improve efficacy. Chronic g.v.h. disease (i.e. later than 100 days) has a relatively good prognosis if limited to skin and liver, but if multiple organs are involved, clinically resembling progressive systemic sclerosis, the outcome is poor. Patients are treated with cyclosporine and prednisolone. The pathogenesis of g.v.h. disease may initially involve secretion of IL-1, TNF and IFNγ from damaged host tissue, with both donor and recipient dendritic cells activating donor Th1 cells to secrete IL-2 and more IFNγ. The host is attacked by donor cytotoxic T-cells and NK cells using both the Fas-FasL and the perforin/granzyme B pathways to induce apoptotic cell death, with production of TNF also putting the boot in. There is hope that CD4$^+$CD25$^+$ Foxp3$^+$ Treg cells can be harnessed to limit this process, and experiments in animal models are in progress to evaluate the efficacy of such approaches.

Other organs and tissues

It is to be expected that improvement in techniques of control of the rejection process will encourage transplantation in several other areas, for example in type I diabetes where the number of transplants recorded is rising rapidly. The current 5-year organ-survival rate is around 75% for simultaneous transplantation of pancreas and kidney (figure 16.18). Transplantation with isolated islet cells is a more attractive option that avoids the need for major surgery and appears to require less immunosuppression than that required following transplantation of a pancreas. Collagenase is injected into the pancreatic duct in a brain dead donor and the recovered islets purified by density gradient centrifugation. These are then infused into the hepatic portal vein of the recipient from where they lodge in the liver sinusoids. Recently, the procedure has been sucessfully extended to using islets isolated from a fragment of pancreas removed from a living donor. The benefits of islet cell transplantation as an alternative to insulin injections do, of course, need to be weighed against the risks of the immunosuppression that is required.

The 5-year graft survival rate of 43–44% for lung and simultaneous heart–lung is improving but is still less than satisfactory (figure 16.18). Transplantation of intestine is also in need of improvement, with 5-year graft survival currently at 41% (figure 16.18). One also looks forward to the day when the successful transplantation of skin for lethal burns becomes more commonplace. The grafting of **neural tissues** has the potential to benefit patients with neurodegenerative conditions such as Parkinson's disease, Huntington's disease and stroke. Indeed, the transplantation of human fetal mesencephalic tissue into the brain of patients with Parkinson's disease has shown that dopaminergic neurons from such tissue can integrate into the brain's neuronal circuits. Some patients were able to discontinue treatment with L-dopa for a period of several years. However, such transplantation is far from routine and the results from clinical trials have been very mixed. Researchers are turning to stem cells as a source of neurons, although the optimal growth factors and culture conditions required to generate particular types of neurons require further evaluation.

Cryopreservation of sperm is a successful strategy in the management of adult cancer sufferers to protect the sperm from mutagenic cancer treatment. This is not available to prepubertal boys, but an alternative for them is cryopreservation of their spermatogonial stem cells for reintroduction post-treatment, since the Sertoli cells which support differentiation into mature spermatozoa will function normally. There is a potential for identifying and correcting genetic defects in the spermatogonia before their reintroduction, but ethical committees fight shy of this sort of 'Frankenstein' tinkering. More acceptably, in cases of male infertility due to dysfunctional Sertoli cells, it should be possible to develop mature spermatids by culture of the spermatogonia with Sertoli cells derived from a normal individual.

Coronary bypass surgery involves autografting with the saphenous vein from the leg, the internal mammary arteries or the radial artery from the arm. The blood vessel is grafted onto the heart to bypass a blocked or damaged coronary artery. Vascular grafts in other areas of the body can employ synthetic blood vessels, made of materials such as Dacron or polytetrafluroethylene (PTFE), autografts or, very rarely, allografts. Work proceeds on the generation of engineered blood vessels, for example by using human stem cells grown on biodegradable fibronectin-coated polymer scaffolds in the presence of appropriate mediators such as vascular endothelial growth factor.

THE FETUS IS A POTENTIAL ALLOGRAFT

A consequence of polymorphism in an outbred population is that mother and fetus will almost certainly have different MHCs. In the human hemochorial placenta, maternal blood with immunocompetent lymphocytes circulates in contact with the fetal trophoblast and we have to explain how the fetus avoids allograft rejection, despite the development of an immunological response in a proportion of mothers as evidenced by the appearance of anti-HLA antibodies and cytotoxic lymphocytes. In fact, prior sensitization with a skin graft fails to affect a pregnancy, showing that trophoblast cells are immunologically protected; indeed, they are resistant to most cytotoxic mechanisms although susceptible to IL-2-activated NK cells. Some of the many speculations which have been aired on this subject are summarized in figure 16.19.

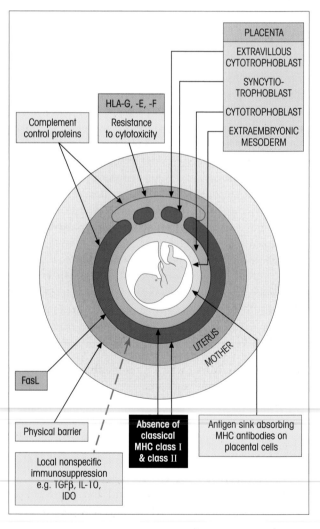

Figure 16.19. Mechanisms postulated to account for the survival of the fetus as an allograft in the mother. IDO, indoleamine 2,3-dioxygenase.

Undoubtedly, the most important factor is the well-documented lack of both conventional class I and class II MHC antigens on the placental syncytiotrophoblast and cytotrophoblast which protects the fetus from allogeneic attack. These fundamental changes in the regulation of MHC genes also lead to the unique expression of the nonclassical HLA-G, -E and -F proteins on the extravillous cytotrophoblast. These molecules, which show extremely limited polymorphism (6, 3 and 4 protein sequence variants have so far been described for HLA-G, -E and -F, respectively) may protect the trophoblast from killing by uterine endometrial NK cells which would normally attack cells lacking MHC class I molecules (cf. p. 73). Maternal IgG antipaternal MHC is found in 20% of first pregnancies and this figure rises to 75–80% in multiparous women. Some of these antibodies cross-react with HLA-G, but the vulnerability of the trophoblast cells to complement is blocked by the presence on their surface of the control proteins which inactivate C3 convertase (cf. p. 314). Mice in which the gene for the Crry complement regulatory protein has been knocked out develop placental inflammation and fetal loss. Immunohistochemical analysis revealed a deposition of complement components in the placenta of these mice, but if they were bred with mice in which complement component C3 has been knocked out then the detrimental effect of the absence of Crry was abrogated. This clearly indicates a role for inhibition of complement activation as one of the mechanisms that helps maintain the semi-allogeneic fetus, at least in mice. The presence of Fas-ligand at the trophoblast maternal–fetal interface may contribute towards limiting immunological aggression towards the fetus, although the fact that *gld* mice which lack FasL and *lpr* mice which lack Fas give birth to live offspring suggests that this mechanism is not essential for the maintenance of pregnancy. Suppression of T-cell, B-cell and NK cell activity also occurs through the generation of toxic tryptophan metabolites by the catabolic enzyme indoleamine 2,3-dioxygenase which is present in trophoblast cells and macrophages.

Cytokines seem to have a complex role in postimplantation pregnancy given the production of growth factors such as CSF-1 and GM-CSF, which have a trophic influence on the placenta, and of transforming growth factor-β (TGFβ), which could help to damp down any activation of NK cells by potentially abortive events such as intrauterine exposure to lipopolysaccharide (LPS) or to interferons. Indeed, production of immunosuppresive IL-10 and TGFβ by regulatory T-cells may play a central role in limiting any immunological attack on the fetus. Cells bearing the hallmark of naturally occurring regulatory T-cells, i.e. CD4$^+$ CD25$^+$ CTLA-4$^+$ GITR$^+$ FoxP3$^+$ cells, are present in increased numbers, both in the circulation and in the decidua, during the first and second trimester of human pregnancy. The absence of such T-regulatory cells in mice has been shown to result in immunologically mediated rejection of the fetus.

SUMMARY

Graft rejection is an immunological reaction
• It shows specificity, the second set response is brisk, it is mediated by lymphocytes and antibodies specific for the graft are formed.

Genetic control of transplantation antigens
• In each vertebrate species there is a *major histocompatibility complex* (MHC) which is responsible for provoking the most intense graft reactions.
• Parental MHC antigens are codominantly expressed on cell surfaces.
• Siblings have a 1 : 4 chance of identity with respect to MHC.

Other consequences of MHC incompatibility
• Class II MHC molecules provoke a mixed lymphocyte reaction of proliferation and blast transformation when genetically dissimilar lymphocytes interact.
• Class II differences are largely responsible for the reaction of tolerated grafted lymphocytes against host antigen (graft-vs-host (g.v.h.) reaction).

Mechanisms of graft rejection
• Preformed antibodies cause hyperacute rejection within minutes.
• CD8 lymphocytes play a major role in the acute early rejection of first set responses.
• The strength of allograft rejection is due to the surprisingly large number of allospecific precursor cells which directly recognize allo-MHC (the direct pathway); later rejection increasingly involves allogeneic peptides presented by self-MHC (the indirect pathway).
• Acute late rejection of organ grafts from 11 days onwards is caused by Ig and complement binding to graft vessels.
• Insidious and late rejection is associated with immune complex deposition.

(Continued p.382)

Prevention of graft rejection

• This can be minimized by cross-matching donor and graft for ABO and MHC tissue types. Individual MHC antigens are typed by serological or molecular genetic techniques.

• Rejection can be blocked by agents producing general immunosuppression such as antimitotic drugs (e.g. azathioprine), anti-inflammatory steroids and antilymphocyte monoclonals. Cyclosporine, tacrolimus and rapamycin represent T-cell-specific drugs; complexes of cyclosporine and tacrolimus, with their cellular ligands (cyclophilin A and FKBP, respectively), block calcineurin, a phosphatase which activates the IL-2 transcription factor NFAT, while rapamycin (which also complexes with FKBP) inhibits the TOR kinase involved in cell proliferation.

• Antigen-specific depression through tolerance induction can be achieved with injection of allogeneic bone marrow with costimulatory blockade by anti-CD154 (CD40L) plus a CTLA-4-Ig fusion protein. Dendritic cell precursors can also induce tolerance through antigen presentation in the absence of B7 costimulators.

Xenografting

• Strategies are being developed to prevent hyperacute rejection of pig grafts in humans due to reaction of natural antibodies in the host with galactose α-1,3-galactose epitopes on pig cells and acute vascular rejection by acquired antibodies produced by the xenogeneic antibody response.

Stem cell therapy

• Stem cells can be isolated from various adult tissues and have the potential to provide material for autografts. Cell nuclear replacement has been used to generate embryonic stem cells which can be differentiated in culture under the influence of specified growth factors.

Clinical experience in grafting

• Cornea and cartilage grafts are avascular, produce local immunosuppressive factors and are comparatively well tolerated.

• Kidney grafting gives excellent results and has been the most widespread, although immunosuppression must normally be continuous.

• High success rates are also being achieved with heart and liver transplants particularly helped by the use of cyclosporine. Lung is less successful. Isolated islets cells from the pancreas are increasingly being used for the treatment of patients with type I diabetes.

• Bone marrow grafts for immunodeficiency and aplastic anemia are accepted from matched siblings, but it is difficult to avoid g.v.h. disease with allogeneic marrow without first purging T-cells in the graft or preferably by inducing tolerance using costimulatory blockade. Stem cells isolated from peripheral blood following mobilization of these cells from the bone marrow using G-CSF can be used instead of bone marrow.

• Transplantation of neural tissue has met with some success in patients with Parkinson's disease.

• Various approaches to tissue engineering, including the production of engineered vascular grafts, have been described.

The fetus as an allograft

• Differences between MHC of mother and fetus imply that, as a potential graft, the fetus must be protected against transplantation attack by the mother.

• A major defense mechanism is the lack of classical class I and II MHC antigens on the syncytiotrophoblast and cytotrophoblast cells which form the outer layers of the placenta.

• The extravillous cytotrophoblast expresses the nonclassical MHC class I proteins, HLA-G, HLA-E and HLA-F, which may act to inhibit cytotoxicity by maternal NK cells.

• The trophoblast cells bear surface complement regulatory proteins which break down C3 convertase and so block any complement-mediated damage.

• Local production of IL-10 and TGFβ by CD4$^+$ CD25$^+$ Foxp3$^+$ regulatory T-cells, tryptophan degradation by indoleamine 2,3-dioxygenase, and the presence of FasL may all contribute towards the suppression of unwanted reactions.

FURTHER READING

Al-Khaldi A. & Robbins R.C. (2006) New directions in cardiac transplantation. *Annual Review of Medicine* **57**, 455–471.

Austen K.F., Burakoff S.J., Rosen F.S. & Strom T.B. (eds) (2001) *Therapeutic Immunology*, 2nd edn. Blackwell Science, Oxford.

Borel J.F. *et al.* (1996) *In vivo* pharmacological effects of cyclosporine and some analogues. *Advances in Pharmacology* **35**, 115–246. (An in-depth review of the field by the discoverer of cyclosporine and his colleagues.)

Fairchild P.J., Cartland S., Nolan K.F. & Waldmann H. (2004) Embryonic stem cells and the challenge of transplantation tolerance. *Trends in Immunology* **25**, 465–470.

Halloran P.F. (2004) Immunosuppressive drugs for kidney transplantation. *New England Journal of Medicine* **351**, 2715–2729.

Hwang W.S., Ryu Y.J., Park J.H. *et al.* (2004) Evidence of a pluripotent human embryonic stem cell line derived from a cloned blastocyst. *Science* **303**, 1669–1674.

Jiang S., Herrera O. & Lechler R.I. (2004) New spectrum of allorecognition pathways: implications for graft rejection and transplantation tolerance. *Current Opinion in Immunology* **16**, 550–557.

Ricordi C. & Strom T.B. (2004) Clinical islet transplantation: advances and immunological challenges. *Nature Reviews Immunology* **4**, 259–268.

Rocha P.N., Plumb T.J., Crowley S.D. & Coffman T.M. (2003) Effector mechanisms in transplant rejection. *Immunological Reviews* **196**, 51–64.

Sayegh M.H. & Carpenter C.B. (2004) Transplantation 50 years later—Progress, Challenges, and Promises. *New England Journal of Medicine* **351**, 2761–2766.

Shizuru J.A., Negrin R.S. & Weissman I.L. (2005) Hematopoietic stem and progenitor cells: clinical and preclinical regeneration of the hematolymphoid system. *Annual Review of Medicine* **56**, 509–538.

Starzl T.E. (2004) Chimerism and tolerance in transplantation. *Proceedings of the National Academy of Sciences of the USA* **101**, 14607–14614.

Trowsdale J. & Betz A.G. (2006) Mother's little helpers: mechanisms of maternal-fetal tolerance. *Nature Immunology* **7**, 241–246.

Walsh P.T., Taylor D.K. & Turka L.A. (2004) Tregs and transplantation tolerance. *Journal of Clinical Investigation* **114**, 1398–1403.

17 Tumor immunology

INTRODUCTION

The immune system has evolved to discriminate self from nonself based upon the pragmatic principle that anything recognized as nonself may be dangerous and therefore warrants expulsion from the body. In the relentless pursuit of nonself our well-meaning immune systems sometimes work against us, rejection of transplanted organs being a case in point, but there are also situations where self may give serious cause for concern; cancer being the pre-eminent example of this.

CELLULAR TRANSFORMATION AND IMMUNE SURVEILLANCE

Cancer represents a wide spectrum of conditions caused by a failure of the controls that normally govern cell proliferation, differentiation and cell survival. Cells that undergo **malignant transformation** escape normal growth controls, invade surrounding tissue, and may ultimately migrate to other sites in the body to establish secondary tumors. Cellular transformation is a multi-step process involving a combination of genetic lesions affecting genes that regulate cell cycle entry, cell cycle exit and cell death (apoptosis); typically such mutations act in concert to achieve the fully transformed state. Cancer is often associated with **activating mutations** in genes that promote cell proliferation, such as *MYC* and *RAS*, which results in increased activity, stability or expression of the protein products of these genes. In tandem with this, **inactivating mutations** in genes that promote cell cycle arrest, *P53* and *RB* being prime examples, are frequently observed. Deregulated expression of genes involved in the control of programed cell death (such as *BCL-2* or *ABL*) is also a common feature of many malignancies.

Depending on their tissue of origin and transformation stage, cancers may grow slowly, or rather rapidly, they may be poorly metastatic or highly aggressive, some cancers are relatively responsive to therapy, while others are refractory and refuse to give in to even the most protracted assaults. Cancer therapy typically involves surgery (for solid tumors) followed by cytotoxic drugs or radiation, either alone or in combination, to kill the errant cells while sparing as many normal (nonmalignant) cells as possible. It is the latter consideration that typically sets a limit on how much radiation or cytotoxic drug can be used in the hope of eradicating all of the tumor burden.

Unfortunately, some tumors are very resilient and manage to frustrate all efforts directed towards their elimination. While many forms of cancer do respond to currently available therapies, most conventional cancer therapeutics cannot discriminate between the tumor and healthy nontransformed cells: a handicap that our immune systems also seem to be afflicted with. And therein lies the problem; cancers often appear to be beyond the reach of the immune system, which seems powerless to deal with such cells. That is not to say that immune responses to tumors do not occur; they do, but they are frequently modest and seem to make little inroads in tumor growth. This may be attributed, at least in part, to evasive maneuvers on the part of the tumor and also due to an acquired state of immune tolerance to the tumor. Despite this, immunologists have long nurtured the view that there must be ways in which the immune system can be harnessed to repel transformed cells, akin to the way in which the immune system rejects transplanted tissue with remarkable efficiency.

The ability to reject transplants of tissue may be traced back a long way down the evolutionary tree—back even as far as the annelid worms. Long before the studies on the involvement of self-*major h*istocompatibility *c*omplex (MHC) in immunological responses, Lewis Thomas suggested that the allograft rejection mechanism represented a means by which the body's cells could be kept under **immunological surveillance** so that altered cells with neoplastic potential could be identified and summarily eliminated. For this to operate, cancer cells must display some new discriminating structure which can be recognized by the immune system; such molecules are frequently referred to as **tumor antigens**.

TUMOR ANTIGENS

For the immune system to mount an effective anti-tumor response the tumor must make its presence known by expressing molecules that are not normally found within the body, or conversely, by failing to express a molecule that is normally present on healthy cells (figure 17.1). A good example of the latter is the class I MHC molecules that are displayed on the surface of practically all nucleated cells; failure to express MHC molecules is one of the criteria used by NK cells to select target cells for attack (see p. 73), and as a result NK cells may play an important role in immune surveillance. The ideal tumor antigen would be expressed by cells of the tumor, but not by normal cells, and would be required for tumor growth, thereby preventing the tumor from losing expression of this antigen through immune-driven selection. It might also be acceptable to target antigens that are highly expressed by the tumor but are also expressed by a restricted-range of normal nontransformed cells, depending on whether the potential damage to normal tissue can be kept within an acceptable range. However, few of the tumor antigens identified to date fit this ideal profile; for the most part tumor proteins represent nonmutated proteins or other molecules that are aberrantly expressed by the tumor. Other tumor antigens represent mutant forms of proteins that appear due to the **genomic instability** that contributed to the formation of the tumor in the first instance. Many of the latter antigens will be specific to the tumor of a particular individual and will not be shared between individuals, thereby making it difficult to select candidate antigens that are likely to have widespread utility.

Identification of tumor antigens

A number of strategies have been used to identify tumor antigens. One approach involves isolating tumor-reactive T-cells from peripheral blood or tumor tissue of cancer patients and using these cells to screen autologous target cells transfected with genes from a tumor-derived cDNA library (figure 17.2). Expansion of T-cells in response to cells transfected with a particular cDNA identifies the protein encoded by this cDNA as a candidate tumor antigen. An alternative approach uses peptides eluted from tumor-derived MHC molecules to pulse APCs to test for their ability to elicit responses from tumor-reactive lymphocytes. Peptides eliciting positive responses in such assays can be subsequently identifed by purification and sequencing; not exactly a technically simple approach but feasible nonetheless.

Yet another strategy, **serological analysis of recombinant cDNA expression libraries** (SEREX), uses diluted antiserum from cancer patients to screen for antibodies that react against proteins expressed by cDNA libraries generated from cancer tissue (figure 17.3). This approach is predicated upon the assumption that anti-tumor antibodies are indicative of T-helper cells specific for such antigens. More than 1500 immunogenic proteins, which are all candidate tumor antigens, have been isolated using this method. So there is no shortage of candidates. But it is important to note that *in vitro* recognition assays may not select ideal or valid tumor antigens; validation of candidate tumor antigens is clearly essential, as proteins found to be immunogenic *in vitro* may exhibit little potency *in vivo*. These problems aside, it is clear that tumor antigens do indeed exist and some examples will now be discussed.

Virally controlled antigens

A substantial minority of tumors arise through infection with **oncogenic viruses**, Epstein–Barr virus (EBV) in lymphomas, *h*uman *T*-cell *l*eukemia *v*irus-1 (HTLV-1) in

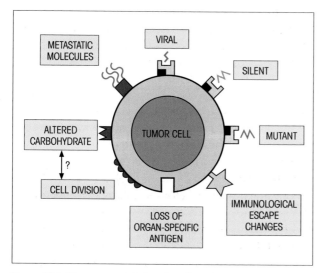

Figure 17.1. Tumor-associated surface changes.

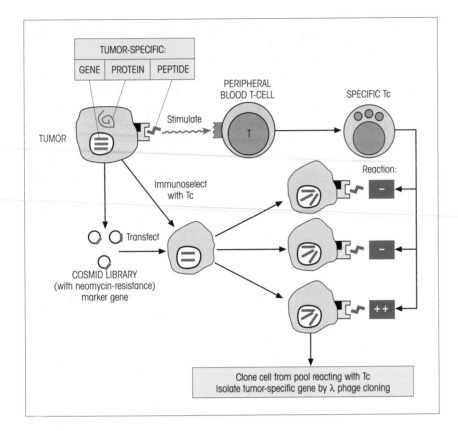

Figure 17.2. Identification of tumor-specific gene using tumor-specific cytotoxic T-cell (Tc) clones derived from mixed tumor–lymphocyte culture. A cosmid library incorporating the tumor DNA is transfected into an antigen-negative cell line derived from the wild-type tumor by immunoselection with the Tc. Small pools of transfected cells are tested against the Tc. A positive pool is cloned by limiting dilution and the tumor-specific gene (*MAGE-1*) cloned from the antigen-positive well(s). (Based on van der Bruggen P. *et al.* (1991) *Science* **254**, 1643. Copyright © 1991 by the AAAS.) The original **MAGE-1** belongs to a family of 12 genes. Further melanoma-specific genes, including *MART-1*, *gp100* and *tyrosinase*, have been discovered.

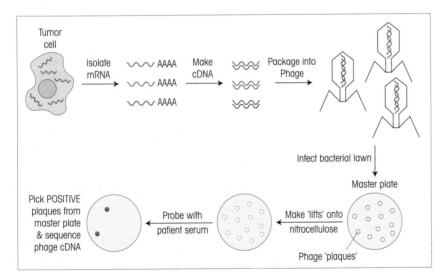

Figure 17.3. Identification of tumor antigens by serological identification of antigens expressed by recombinant cloning (SEREX). In the SEREX method, mRNA isolated from tumor biopsies is used to construct cDNA expression libraries that are then packaged into bacteriophage. A bacterial lawn is then infected with the phage library under conditions that permit expression of the tumor-derived proteins. Replica 'lifts' of the bacterial lawn are made using nitrocellulose membranes and these are then probed with diluted antisera from the cancer patient. Bacterial colonies expressing tumor-derived proteins that are detected by antibodies within the patient serum can then be identified by isolating the phage from the relevant colony and sequencing the cDNA harbored within this phage.

leukemia and human papilloma virus (HPV) in cervical cancers. After infection, the viruses express genes homologous with **cellular oncogenes** which encode factors affecting growth and cell division. Expression of these genes therefore leads to potentially malignant transformation. Virus-derived peptides associated with MHC on the surface of the tumor cell behave as powerful transplantation antigens which generate haplotype-specific cytotoxic T-cells (Tc). All tumors induced by a given virus should carry the same surface antigen, irrespective of their cellular origin, so that immunization with any one of these tumors would confer resistance to subsequent challenge with the others provided that there were no artful mutations by the virus (Milestone 17.1). Unfortunately, viruses are not innately friendly.

Expression of normally silent genes

The dysregulated uncontrolled cell division of the cancer cell creates a milieu in which the products of

Milestone 17.1 — Tumors Can Induce Immune Responses

The first convincing evidence for tumor-associated antigens came from the work of Prehn and Main who demonstrated quite clearly that **chemically induced cancers** can induce immune responses to themselves but not to other tumors produced by the same carcinogen (figure M17.1.1a). Tumors induced by **oncogenic viruses** are different in that processed viral peptides are present on the surface of all neoplastic cells bearing the viral genome so that Tc cells raised to one tumor will cross-react with all others produced by the same virus (figure M17.1.1b).

Dramatic advances were made by Boon and colleagues. First, they showed that random mutagenesis of transplantable tumors, i.e. tumors which can be passaged within a

pure mouse strain without provoking rejection, can give rise to mutant progeny with strong transplantation antigens. As a result they could not be grown in syngeneic animals with a normal immune system; accordingly they were referred to as **tum−** variants. Boon's team developed a powerful technology (cf. figure 17.2) which enabled them to use Tc clones specific for the tum− variant to screen cosmid clones for the mutant gene. These two breakthroughs, the recognition that mutation in tumors can generate strong transplantation reactions, and the development of the technique for identifying the relevant antigens with Tc cells, heralded really profound developments in tumor immunology and put it firmly on the map as a key area for cancer research.

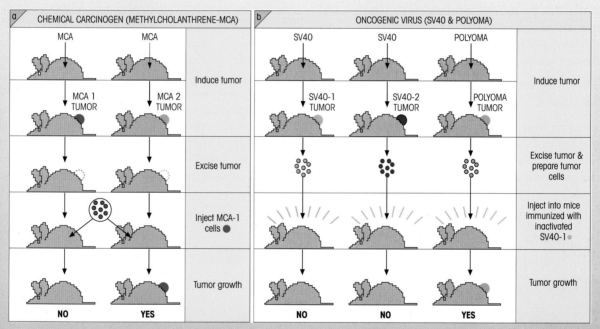

Figure M17.1.1. The specificity of immunity induced by tumors. (a) A chemically induced tumor MCA-1 can induce resistance to an implant of itself but not to a tumor produced in a syngeneic mouse by the same carcinogen. Thus each tumor has an individual antigen, now thought to be a processed mutant endogenous protein complexed with a heat-shock protein. More recent data suggest that, if immunized animals are challenged with much lower numbers of

tumor cells, a greater degree of cross-protection between tumors may be observed, which has been ascribed to a 44 kDa oncofetal antigen, possibly an immature version of a laminin receptor protein. (b) Tumors produced by a given oncogenic virus immunize against tumors produced in syngeneic mice by the same but not other viruses. Thus tumors produced by an oncogenic virus share a common antigen.

normally silent genes may be expressed. Sometimes these encode differentiation antigens normally associated with an earlier developmental stage. Thus tumors derived from the same cell type are often found to express such **oncofetal antigens** which are also present on embryonic cells. Examples would be α-fetoprotein in hepatic carcinoma and carcinoembryonic antigen (CEA) in cancer of the intestine. Certain monoclonal antibodies also react with tumors of neural crest origin

and fetal melanocytes. Another monoclonal antibody defines the SSEA-1 antigen found on a variety of human tumors and early mouse embryos but absent from adult cells with the exception of human granulocytes and monocytes.

But the exciting quantum leap forward stems from the original observation that cytosolic viral nucleoprotein could provide a target for Tc cells by appearing on the cell surface as a processed peptide associated with MHC class I (cf. p. 95). This established the general principle that the intracellular proteins which are not destined to be positioned in the surface plasma membrane can still signal their presence to T-cells in the outer world by the processed peptide–MHC mechanism. Cytotoxic T-cells specific for tumor cells, obtained from mixed cultures of peripheral blood cells with tumor, can be used to establish the identity of the antigen employing the strategy described in figure 17.2. By something of a *tour de force* a gene encoding a melanoma antigen, MAGE-1, was identified. It belongs to a family of 12 genes, six of which are expressed in a significant proportion of melanomas as well as head and neck tumors, nonsmall cell lung cancers and bladder carcinomas. MAGE-1 is *not* expressed in normal tissues except for germ-line cells in testis and gives rise to antigenic T-cell epitopes which, in the light of the absence of class I MHC on the testis cells, must be considered tumor-specific. This exciting research reveals the tumor-specific antigen as an expression of a normally silent gene.

Mutant antigens

The seminal work on tum– mutants (Milestone 17.1) has persuaded us that single point mutations in oncogenes can account for the large diversity of antigens found on carcinogen-induced tumors. The specific immunity provoked by chemically induced tumors can be elicited by **heat-shock protein** 70 (hsp70) and hsp90 isolated from the tumor cells, but their immunogenicity is lost when the associated low molecular weight peptides are removed. These peptides could, however, stimulate the specific CD8 cytotoxic T-cell clones generated by the tumors, and three possible mechanisms have been advanced to account for the enhancement of tumor immune responses by hsps. First, they can act as 'danger' signals by activating antigen-presenting cells. Second, necrotic tumor cells expressing the hsps can transfer hsp–peptide complexes to host antigen-presenting cells where they can cross-prime cytotoxic CD8 T-cells through the MHC class I endogenous presentation pathway. And last, the hsps may influence the capacity of the tumor cell itself to process and present endogenous mutated and, of course, 'silent' antigens as targets for specific T-cells (figure 17.4).

There is considerable evidence for the production of mutated peptides in human tumors. The gene encoding cell cycle checkpoint protein, p53, is a hotspot for mutation in numerous cancers. The mutant forms of p53 that are frequently found in tumors represent loss-of-function mutants that fail to arrest division of cells that have suffered DNA damage; such damage would normally trigger cell cycle arrest or apoptosis of the afflicted cell. The oncogenic human *ras* genes differ from their

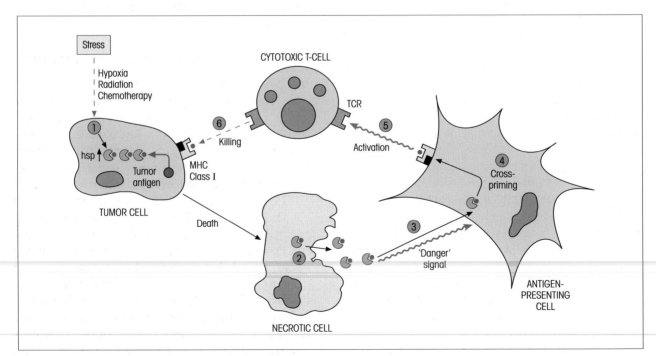

Figure 17.4. The role of heat-shock proteins (hsps) in tumor immunogenicity. (1) Stress factors upregulate hsps which can form complexes with processed tumor antigen and increase surface presentation of antigenic peptide by MHC class I. (2) They can also lead to necrosis and release of hsp–peptide complexes, which (3) can act as stimulatory danger signals to dendritic antigen-presenting cells and penetrate the cytoplasm, where (4) they can enter the MHC class I processing pathway by so-called cross-priming. (5) CD8 resting T-cells become activated and (6) kill the tumor cells. (Based on Wells A.D. & Malkowsky M. (2000) *Immunology Today* **21**, 129.)

normal counterparts by point mutations usually leading to single amino acid substitutions in positions 12, 13 or 61. Such mutations generate constitutively active forms of Ras that promote increased rates of cell division through activation of the MAPK pathway (see p. 174), and have been recorded in 40% of human colorectal cancers and in more than 90% of pancreatic carcinomas, as well as other malignancies. The mutated ras peptide can induce proliferative T-cell lines *in vitro*.

Changes in carbohydrate structure

The chaotic internal control of metabolism within neoplastic cells often leads to the presentation of abnormal carbohydrate structures on the cell surface. Sometimes one sees blocked synthesis, e.g. deletion of blood group A. In other cases there may be enhanced synthesis of structures absent in progenitor cells: thus some gastrointestinal cancers express the Lewis Le^a antigen in individuals who are Le(a$^-$,b$^-$) and others produce extended chains bearing dimeric Le^a or Le(a,b).

Abnormal mucin synthesis can have immunological consequences. Consider the mucins of pancreatic and breast tissue. These consist of a polypeptide core of 20-amino acid tandem repeats with truly abundant O-linked carbohydrate chains. A monoclonal antibody SM-3 directed to the core polypeptide reacts poorly with normal tissue where the epitope is masked by glycosylation, but well with breast and pancreatic carcinomas possessing shorter and fewer O-linked chains. Tc cells specific for tumor mucins are not MHC restricted and the slightly heretical suggestion has been made that the T-cell receptors (TCRs) are binding multivalently to closely spaced SM-3 epitopes on unprocessed mucins; alternatively, and closer to the party line, recognition is by $\gamma\delta$ cells.

Molecules related to metastatic potential

Changes in surface carbohydrates can have a dramatic effect on malignancy. For example, colonic cancers expressing sialyl Le^x have a poor prognosis and higher propensity to metastasize. Lung cancer patients whose tumors showed deletion of blood group A had a much worse prognosis than those with continuous A; the finding that patients expressing H/Le^y/Le^b also had a poorer prognosis than antigen-negative subjects is consistent with this observation.

The role of **CD44** (HERMES/Pgp-1) in cell trafficking, based on its interaction with vascular endothelium, has afforded it some prominence in the facilitation of metastatic spread. CD44 occurs in several isoforms with a varying number of exons between the transmembrane and common N-terminus. Normal epithelium expresses the CD44H isoform with hyaluran-binding domains, but lacking the intervening v1–v10 exons; expression of certain of these exons on tumors is indicative of a growth advantage, since they are present with higher frequency on more advanced cancers. Stable transfection of a nonmetastatic tumor with a CD44 cDNA clone encompassing exons v6 and v7 induced the ability to form metastatic tumors—a most striking effect. Further, injection of a monoclonal anti-CD44 v6 prevented the formation of lymph node metastases. Exons v6 and v10 have now been shown to bind blood group H and chondroitin 4-sulfate, respectively, and the latest hypothesis is that these carbohydrates can bind to CD44H on endothelium and thence homotypically to each other so generating a metastatic nidus.

Changes have quite frequently been observed in the expression of class I MHC molecules. For example, oncogenic transformation of cells infected with adenovirus 12 is associated with highly reduced class I as a consequence of very low levels of TAP-1 and -2 mRNA. Mutation frequently leads to diminished or absent class I expression linked in most cases to increased metastatic potential, presumably reflecting decreased vulnerability to T-cells but not NK cells. In breast cancer, for example, around 60% of metastatic tumors lack class I.

SPONTANEOUS IMMUNE RESPONSES TO TUMORS

Immune surveillance against strongly immunogenic tumors

When present, many of the antigens discussed in the previous section can provoke immune responses in experimental animals which lead to resistance against tumor growth, but they vary tremendously in their efficiency. Powerful antigens associated with tumors induced by oncogenic viruses or ultraviolet light generate strong resistance, while the transplantation antigens on chemically induced tumors (Milestone 17.1) are weaker and somewhat variable; disappointingly, tumors which arise spontaneously in animals produce little or no response. The **immune surveillance theory** would predict that there should be more tumors in individuals whose adaptive immune systems are suppressed. This undoubtedly seems to be the case for **strongly immunogenic tumors**. There is a considerable increase in skin cancer in immunosuppressed patients living in high sunshine regions north of Brisbane and, in general, transplant patients on immunosuppressive drugs are unduly susceptible to skin cancers, largely associated with papilloma virus, and EBV-positive lymphomas. The EBV-related Burkitt's lymphomas crop up with undue frequency in regions infested with malarial infection, known to compromise the efficacy of the immune system. Likewise, the lymphomas which arise in children with T-cell deficiency linked to Wiskott–Aldrich syndrome or ataxia telangiectasia express *EBV* genes; they show unusually restricted expression of EBV latent proteins which are the major potential target epitopes for immune recognition, while cellular adhesion molecules, such as *i*ntercellular *a*dhesion *m*olecule-1 (ICAM-1) and *l*ymphocyte *func*tion-*a*ssociated molecule-3 (LFA-3), which mediate conjugate formation with Tc cells, cannot be detected on their surface (figure 17.5). Knowing that most normal individuals have highly efficient EBV-specific Tc cells, this must be telling us that only by downregulating appropriate surface molecules can the lymphoma cells escape even the limited T-cell surveillance operating in these patients.

These examples aside, it must be acknowledged that the incidence of **spontaneous** tumor formation in mice lacking T- and B-lymphocytes is not substantially higher than in those with intact immune systems; the same is also true for immunodeficient humans. Such observations weaken arguments that adaptive immune responses have a significant role to play in cancer prevention. Nonetheless, while normal adaptive immune responses may be insufficient to deal with the establishment of many tumors, this does not necessarily mean that the immune system cannot be manipulated to deliver an effective response.

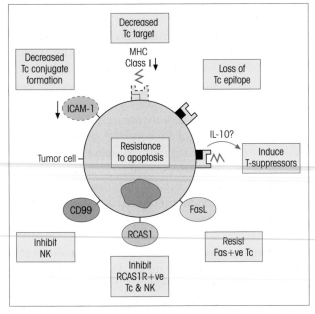

Figure 17.5. Tumor escape mechanisms.

A role for innate immunity?

Perhaps in speaking of immunity to tumors, one too readily thinks only in terms of acquired responses, whereas it is now accepted that innate mechanisms are of significance. Macrophages which often infiltrate a tumor mass can destroy tumor cells in tissue culture through the copious production of reactive oxygen intermediates (ROIs) and tumor necrosis factor (TNF) when activated by a diversity of factors, bacterial lipopolysaccharide, double-stranded RNA, T-cell γ-interferon (IFNγ), and so forth.

There is an uncommon flurry of serious interest in **natural killer (NK)** cells. It is generally accepted that they subserve a function as the earliest cellular effector mechanism against dissemination of blood-borne metastases. Let's look at the evidence. Patients with advanced metastatic disease often have abnormal NK activity and low levels appear to predict subsequent metastases. In experimental animals, removal of NK cells from mice with surgically resected B16 melanoma resulted in uncontrolled metastatic disease and death. Acute ethanol intoxication in rats boosted the number of metastases from an NK-sensitive tumor 10-fold, but had no effect on an NK-resistant cancer, hinting at a possible underlying cause for the association between alcoholism, infectious disease and malignancies. (Those who enjoy the odd Bacchanalian splurge should not be too upset—be comforted by the beneficial effect in heart disease, but no excesses please!) Powerful evidence implicating these cells in protection against cancer is provided by beige mice which congenitally lack NK cells. They die with spontaneous tumors earlier than their nondeficient +/bg littermates, and the incidence of radiation-induced leukemia is reduced by prior injection of cloned isogeneic NK cells which could be suppressing preleukemic cells. Note, however, that tumors induced chemically or with murine leukemia virus were handled normally.

Resting NK cells are spontaneously cytolytic for certain, but by no means all, tumor targets; cells activated by IL-2 and possibly by IL-12 and -18 display a wider lethality. As described earlier in Chapter 4, recognition of the surface structures on the target cell involves various activating and inhibitory receptors, but it is important to re-emphasize that recognition of class I imparts a **negative inactivating** signal to the NK cell. Conversely, this implies that downregulation of MHC class I, which tumors employ as a strategy to escape Tc cells (figure 17.5), would make them **more susceptible to NK attack**. The tumor cells can fight back by expressing CD99, which downregulates NK CD16, and the growth inhibitor RCAS1, which induces apoptosis in

NK as well as in Tc cells (figure 17.5). It is not clear whether surface FasL, which can repel attack by the Fas-positive cytolytic T-cells, is also effective against NK cells, but the relative resistance of tumor cells to apoptosis must be innately protective.

Divisions are surfacing in the NK ranks. The NK cells, which remarkably constitute up to 50% of the liver-associated lymphocytes in humans, have a higher level of expression of IL-2 receptor and adhesion molecules such as integrins compared with NK cells in peripheral blood. They are precursors of a subset of activated adherent NK cells (A-NK) which adhere rapidly to solid surfaces under the influence of IL-2 and are distinguished from their nonadherent counterparts by their superiority in entering solid tumors and in prolonging survival following adoptive transfer with IL-2 into animal models of tumor growth or metastasis. The nonadherent NK variety are better at killing antibody-coated cancer cells through antibody-dependent cellular cytotoxicity (ADCC), mediated by their CD16 FcγRIII receptor.

Be kind to your NK cells. Really late nights which involve major curtailment of slow-wave sleep lead to drastic falls in NK cells and levels of IL-2, quite apart from bleary eyes.

TUMOR ESCAPE MECHANISMS

Strong supporting evidence for a role for the immune system in surveillance against transformed cells comes from observations that tumors employ a range of strategies to evade and manipulate the immune system. Indeed, it could be said that tumors are positively brimming with various **immunological escape mechanisms** (figure 17.5) and thus they resemble successful infections. We have already referred to the fact that down-regulation of HLA class I molecules to make the tumor a less attractive target for cytolytic T-cells is a favorite ploy. This is a common feature of breast cancer metastases, and this is true also of cervical carcinoma where, prognostically, loss of HLA-B44 in premalignant lesions is an indicator of tumor progression. Rather than lose expression of all class I molecules and risk attracting the attentions of NK cells, tumors may lose just the expression of class I alleles that are capable of presenting antigenic peptides to T-cells.

Many tumors are also not particularly immunogenic to begin with, possibly because strongly immunogenic tumors may be readily weeded out and fail to develop to the point that they become clinically significant. In this way, the immune system may exert a darwinian selective pressure for cancer-causing mutations that are largely immunologically silent; a process that has been termed **immunoediting**. Subtle point mutations in oncogenes, such as *RAS*, that have profound effects on the function of the protein products of such genes and contribute to transformation, may completely fail to create any new epitopes that would result in immune attack. In a similar vein, complete loss of expression of important tumor suppressor genes, such as *P53 or RB*, through nonsense mutations would also fail to create any new epitopes.

Loss of tumor antigen epitopes, where they do arise, represents another escape mechanism and mutations in an oncogenic virus itself can increase its tumorigenic potential. Thus the frequent association of a high-risk variant of human papilloma virus with cervical tumors in HLA-B7 individuals is attributed to the loss of a T-cell epitope which would otherwise generate a protective B7-mediated cytolytic response. There is also an increasing appreciation that tumors may create a microenvironment where **active tolerization** of tumor-infiltrating lymphocytes occurs through imbalances in antigen-presenting cell subsets that fail to express the appropriate costimulatory molecules. Recall that APCs which deliver antigen in the absence of proper costimulation, in the form of CD28 ligands, render T-cells anergic (see Chapter 8). One reason why APCs in the vicinity of tumors may fail to become activated may be due to the absence of 'danger signals' that can upregulate costimulatory molecules on APCs that encounter these signals (figure 17.6). **DCs do not exist in a state of perpetual activation** and are unable to provide proper costimulation unless they encounter appropriate molecules that possess DC-activating properties. In the context of infection, DC-activating molecules (Toll-like receptor ligands) are derived from the infectious agent and are usually structures that are shared by many pathogens but not found in the host. Endogenous danger signals, such as the ER chaperone gp96, are thought to exist and these molecules may be released from damaged cells in order to activate local DCs; the chromatin-binding protein HMGB1 has also been reported to exhibit properties of an endogenous danger signal. Tumors that release danger signals may fail to tolerize DCs and become subject to effective immune attack which may result in tumor rejection or persistence through selection of immune escape mutants (figure 17.6). Conversely, tumors that fail to release danger signals may be simply regarded as self and may fail to elicit significant immune responses.

There are also other reasons why the immune system may become tolerant to a tumor. For example, many solid tumors secrete large amounts of angiogenic factors such as **vascular endothelial cell growth factor** (VEGF) that promote the development of the new blood vessels

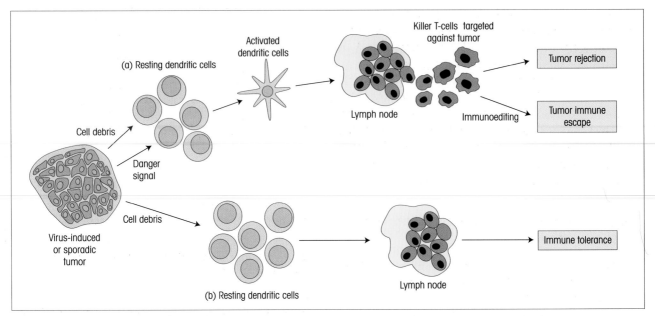

Figure 17.6. Danger signals may dictate whether dendritic cells prime for T-cell responses or induce tolerance to tumors. Growing tumors typically shed material from dead or dying cells and this debris is picked up by local dendritic cells (DCs) which transport it to the local lymph nodes for presentation to T-cells. (a) Where the tumor is shedding molecules ('danger signals') that are capable of activating DCs, maturation of the DC occurs and these cells are capable of eliciting robust immune responses from appropriate T-cells. Such tumors may then become subject to immune attack by the activated T-cells resulting either in rejection of the tumor, or 'immunoediting' of the tumor to eliminate only the cells presenting the antigen that initiated the response. (b) In the absence of signals that activate DCs, resting DCs that encounter tumor-derived material fail to become activated and any T-cells such DCs subsequently encounter may become tolerant to tumor-derived antigens presented by such DCs. (Based on Melief J.M. (2005) *Nature* **437**, 41.)

that tumors need. Evidence also suggests that VEGF can suppress the maturation of dendritic cells (DCs) and these immature or partially differentiated DCs may tolerize to antigens that they find within the vicinity of the tumor.

Tumors can also decrease their vulnerability to cytotoxic T-cell attack by expression of surface FasL (cf. p. 214) and a growth inhibitory molecule, RCAS1, which react with T-cells bearing their corresponding receptors and stop them in their tracks. Tumors have also frequently been found to secrete other immunosuppressive factors such as TGF-β and IL-10. Such factors may help to keep burgeoning immune responses at bay by inducing suppressor or regulatory T-cell populations that inhibit responses to the tumor. Natural regulatory T-cells (Tregs) that normally guard against the development of autoimmunity may also hamper robust T-cell responses against tumors. It should also be borne in mind that internal defects in the cell death machinery, that facilitated the establishment of the tumor in the first instance, may also render such cells resistant to the best efforts of cytotoxic T-cells and NK cells to eradicate them. The very existence of such 'Houdini' mechanisms builds a case in favor of the notion that the adaptive immune system has a significant role in suppressing tumor growth and provides hope that this can be exploited in the clinic.

Cancers which express neoantigens of **low immunogenicity** do not come creeping out of the woodwork when patients are radically immunosuppressed and, although T-cell responses can often be rescued from tumor-infiltrating lymphocytes or relatively high numbers of tumor-specific CD8 T-cells may be detected by the peptide–HLA tetramer technique in peripheral blood, they may be functionally deficient due perhaps to suppression by local IL-10 and TGFβ. Mutation of p53 and its overexpression are very common events in human cancer and are often associated with the production of antibodies; but while these could prove to have a diagnostic utility, it is most unlikely that they are of benefit to the patient, the current view being that *cell-mediated* responses are crucial to the attack against internal antigens expressed in solid tumors. Reluctantly, one has to accept the view that, with tumors of weak immunogenicity, we are dealing with low-key reactions which clearly play little role in curbing the neoplastic process. That is not to say that these 'weak' antigens cannot be exploited for therapeutic purposes as we shall soon see.

UNREGULATED DEVELOPMENT GIVES RISE TO LYMPHOPROLIFERATIVE DISORDERS

We should now turn our attention to the manner in

which cells involved in immune responses themselves may undergo malignant transformation, giving rise to leukemia, lymphoma or myeloma characterized by uncontrolled proliferation. An obvious example is the subset of adult human T-cell leukemia associated with **HTLV-1** (human T-cell leukemia virus type 1). After infection of the T-cell, the viral tax protein, which is constitutively expressed, stimulates transcription of *IL-2*, *IL-2R*, etc., leading to vigorous proliferation; however, only if there is a subsequent chromosome abnormality (see below) does malignant transformation take place.

Deregulation of protooncogenes is a characteristic feature of many lymphocytic tumors

The realization that viral oncogenes are almost certainly derived from normal host genes concerned in the regulation of cellular proliferation has led to the identification of many of these so-called protooncogenes. One of them, c-*myc*, appears to be of crucial importance for entry of the lymphocyte, and probably many other cells, from the resting G0 stage to the cell cycle, while shutdown of c-*myc* expression is linked to exit from the cycle and return to G0. Thus deregulation of c-*myc* expression will prevent cells from leaving the cycle and consign them to a fate of continuous replication. This is just what is seen in many of the neoplastic B-lymphoproliferative disorders, where the malignant cells express high levels of c-myc protein usually associated with a reciprocal chromosomal translocation involving the c-*myc* locus. For example, Burkitt's lymphoma is a B-cell neoplasia with a relatively high incidence among African children in whom there is an association with the EBV; in most cases studied, the c-*myc* gene, located on chromosome 8 band q24, is joined by a reciprocal translocation event to the μ heavy chain gene on chromosome 14 band q32 (figure 17.7). It is suggested that the normal mechanisms which downregulate c-*myc* can no longer work on the translocated gene and so the cell is held in the cycling mode. Less frequently, c-*myc* translocates to the site of the κ (chromosome 2) or λ (chromosome 22) loci.

Chromosome translocations are common in lymphoproliferative disorders

Most lymphomas and leukemias have visible chromosome abnormalities bound up with translocations to B-cell immunoglobulin or T-cell receptor gene loci but not necessarily involving c-*myc*. A reciprocal translocation between the μ chain gene on chromosome 14 and the *bcl*-2 oncogene on chromosome 18 has been identified in almost all follicular B-cell lymphomas, and another between the T-cell gene on chromosome 14 (q11) and

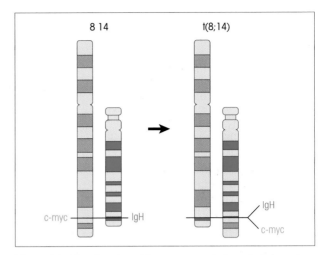

Figure 17.7. Translocation of the c-*myc* gene to the μ chain locus in Burkitt's lymphoma.

another presumed oncogene on chromosome 11 in a *T-cell acute lymphoblastic leukemia* (T ALL).

Lymphomagenesis is a multistep process. The lack of proliferative control engendered by deregulation of c-*myc* and other similar events induced by chromosomal translocations is permissive for the vulnerability to induction of neoplasia, but is not in itself sufficient to bring about malignant transformation. This appears to be due to the fact that while overexpression of proteins that drive cell-cycle entry (such as Myc) enhances the rate of cell division, this is negated by a simultaneous increase in the rate of cell death, as has been amply demonstrated by Evan and colleagues in several models. This most likely represents a safeguard against unrestrained proliferation and probably applies to most proteins that promote cell cycle entry. However, mutations that interfere with the programed cell death machinery can often synergize with lesions that promote enhanced rates of cell division. Thus, transgenic mice harboring a c-*myc* gene driven by the μ heavy chain enhancer (E$_\mu$-*myc* mice) have hyperplastic expansions of the pre-B-cell population in the bone marrow and spleen during the preneoplastic period and yet do not develop tumors until 6–8 weeks of age; and then they are monoclonal not polyclonal, suggesting that a random second event is required before autonomy is achieved. Indeed, if the E$_\mu$-*myc* transgenic mice are now infected with viruses carrying the v-*raf* oncogene, they rapidly develop lymphomas. Alternatively, crossing E$_\mu$-*myc* transgenic mice with strains overexpressing the potent cell death inhibitory protein, Bcl-2, results in the rapid development of B-cell lymphomas. Thus genes that regulate cell division and cell death can synergize in the process of malignant transformation and the associated unfettered cell proliferation.

Different lymphoid malignancies show maturation arrest at characteristic stages in differentiation

Lymphoid cells at almost any stage in their differentiation or maturation may become malignant and proliferate to form a clone of cells which are virtually 'frozen' at a particular developmental stage because of defects in maturation. The malignant cells bear the markers one would expect of normal lymphocytes reaching the stage at which maturation had been arrested. Thus, chronic lymphocytic leukemia cells resemble mature B-cells in expressing surface class II and Ig, albeit of a single idiotype in a given patient. Using monoclonal antibodies directed against the terminal deoxynucleotidyl transferase (figure 17.9a), class II MHC, Ig and specific antigens on cortical thymocytes, mature T-cells and non-T, non-B acute lymphoblastic leukemia cells, it has been possible to classify the lymphoid malignancies in terms of the phenotype of the equivalent normal cell (figure 17.8).

Susceptibility to malignant transformation is high in lymphocytes at an early stage in ontogeny. If we look at Burkitt's lymphoma, the EBV-induced translocation of the c-*myc* to bring it under control of the *IgH* gene complex is most likely to occur at the pro-B-cell stage, since the chromatin structure of the Ig locus opens up for transcription as signaled by the appearance of sterile C_μ transcripts. Furthermore, the cell is likely to escape immunological recognition because, in its undifferentiated resting form, it has downregulated its EBV-encoded antigens and MHC class I polymorphic specificities, and the adhesion molecules LFA-1, LFA-3 and ICAM-1, as mentioned above.

At one time it was thought that maturation arrest occurred at the stage when the cell first became malignant, but we now know that the tumor cells can be forced into differentiation by agents such as phorbol myristate acetate, and the current view is that cells may undergo a few differentiation steps after malignant transformation before coming to a halt. The demonstration of a myeloma protein idiotype on the cytoplasmic μ chains of pre-B-cells in the same patient certainly favors the idea that the malignant event had occurred in a pre-B-cell whose progeny formed the plasma cell tumor. However, an alternative explanation could be transfection of normal pre-B-cells by an oncogene complex from the myeloma cells, possibly through a viral vector. With the exciting discovery of retroviruses associated with certain human T-cell leukemias, this is an interesting possibility.

Immunohistological diagnosis of lymphoid neoplasias

With the availability of a range of monoclonal antibodies and improvements in immuno-enzymatic technology, great strides have been made in exploiting, for diagnostic purposes, the fact that malignant lymphoid cells display the markers of the normal lymphocytes which are their counterparts.

Leukemias

This point can be made rather well if one looks at the markers used to distinguish between the various types of leukemia (table 17.1). Whereas T ALL and B ALL cases have a poor prognosis, the patients positive for the common acute lymphoblastic leukemia antigen (CALLA; figure 17.9b), which includes most childhood leukemias, belong to a prognostically favorable group, many of whom are curable with standard therapeutic combinations of vincristine, prednisolone and L-asparaginase. Bone marrow transplantation may help in the management of patients with recurrent ALL provided that a remission can first be achieved. Expression of the lymphoid lineage markers CD2 and CD19 on leukemic blasts is an indication of good prognosis in adults with the disease.

Chronic lymphocytic leukemia is uncommon in people under 50 years and is usually relatively benign, although the 10–20% of patients with a circulating

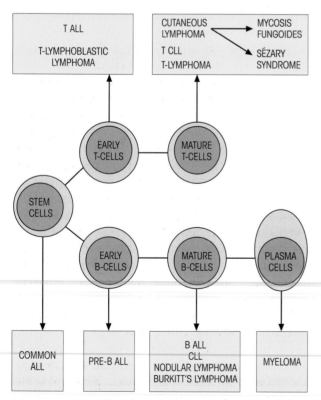

Figure 17.8. Cellular phenotype of human lymphoid malignancies. ALL, acute lymphoblastic leukemia; CLL, chronic lymphocytic leukemia. (After Greaves M.F. & Janossy G., personal communication.)

Table 17.1. Classification of lymphocytic leukemia by immuno-enzymatic staining.

Lymphocyte marker	Common ALL	Pre-B ALL	B-cell ALL	T-cell ALL	Chronic lymphocytic leukemia
*CALLA (CDIO)	+	+	−	−	−
Cytoplasmic μ	−	+	−	−	−
Surface μ	−	−	+	−	+
Surface κ or λ	−	−	+	−	+
Pan-B	−	+	+	−	+
TdT	+	+	−	+	−
CD5	−	−	−	+	+
CD2	−	−	−	+	−
HLA-DR	+	+	+	−	+

*Antigen-specific for lymphoid precursor cells and pre-B-cells.

monoclonal Ig have a bad prognosis. Excessive numbers of CLL small lymphocytes are found in the blood (figure 17.9c–e) and, being derived from a single clone, they can be stained only with anti-κ or anti-λ (table 17.1). Their weak expression of CD5 strongly suggests that they may be derived from the equivalent of the B-1 cell population, especially since they can be encouraged to make the IgM polyspecific autoantibodies typical of this subset, if pushed by phorbol ester stimulation.

Lymphomas

The extensive use of markers has greatly helped in the diagnosis of non-Hodgkin's lymphomas. In the first place, the sometimes difficult distinction between a lymphoproliferative condition and carcinoma can be made with ease by using monoclonal antibodies to the leukocyte common antigen (CD45), which will react with all lymphoid cells whether in paraffin or cryostat sections, and antibodies to cytokeratin which recognize most carcinomas (figure 17.9f). Second, the cell of origin of the lymphoma can be ascertained by panels of monoclonals which differentiate the cellular elements which form normal lymphoid tissue.

The majority of non-Hodgkin's lymphomas are of B-cell origin and the feature which gives the game away to the diagnostic immunohistologist is the synthesis of monotypic Ig, i.e. of one light chain only (figure 17.9g); in contrast, the population of cells at a site of reactive B-cell hyperplasia will stain for both κ and λ chains (figure 17.9h).

Follicle center cell lymphomas (figure 17.9g) imitating the reactive germinal center account for over 50% of the B-lymphomas. They exhibit monotypic surface Ig, and the larger centrocytes and centroblasts which make up two-thirds of the cases contain cytoplasmic Ig. They stain for MHC class II and weakly for CALLA. Morphologically similar cells make up tumors variously labeled as 'mantle zone lymphoma' or 'small cleaved cell lymphoma' but differ from follicle center cells in positive surface staining for IgM *and* IgD and CD5, and negativity for CALLA. Burkitt's lymphoma lymphoblastoid cells (figure 17.9i) exhibit the common ALL antigen and surface IgM.

The overall prognosis for patients with non-Hodgkin's lymphoma is poor, even though improved by combined chemotherapy. Transplanted patients are 35 times more likely to develop lymphoma than normals, and there are indications that this cannot necessarily be attributed to the long-term immunosuppression.

Hodgkin's disease attacks the gross architecture of lymphoid tissue and is characterized by the binucleate giant cells known as Reed–Sternberg cells (figure 17.9j) which appear to have a germinal center B-cell lineage. Therapy depends upon the stage of the disease; patients with disease localized to lymphoid tissue above the diaphragm respond well to radiotherapy, while those with more widespread disease are treated more aggressively.

Plasma cell dyscrasias

Multiple myeloma

This is defined as a malignant proliferation of a clone of plasma cells in the bone marrow secreting a monoclonal Ig. The myeloma or 'M' component in serum is recognized as a tight band on paper electrophoresis (figure 17.10) as all molecules in the clone are of course identical and have the same mobility. Since Ig-secreting cells produce an excess of light chains, free light chains are present in the plasma of multiple myeloma patients, can be recognized in the urine as Bence-Jones protein (cf. figure 15.24) and give rise to amyloid deposits (see below). The characteristic 'punched out' osteolytic lesions in bones are thought to be due to the release of osteoclastic factors such as IL-6 by the abnormal plasma cells in the marrow. If untreated, the disease is rapidly progressive. With chemotherapy, the mean survival time from diagnosis is now about 5 years.

'M' bands have been found in the sera of a number of individuals who have no clinical signs of myeloma; the comparative rarity with which invasive multiple myeloma develops in these people and the constant level of the monoclonal protein over a period of years suggest the presence of benign tumors of the lymphocyte–plasma cell series.

Amyloid. Between 10% and 20% of patients with

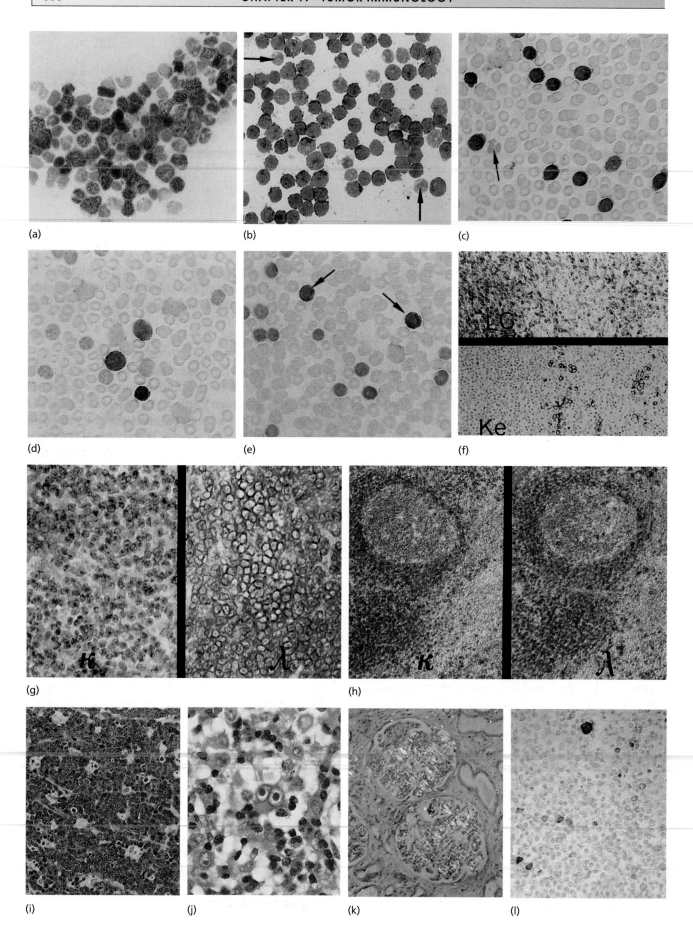

(a)

(b)

(c)

(d)

(e)

(f)

(g)

(h)

(i)

(j)

(k)

(l)

Figure 17.9. (*Opposite*) **Immunodiagnosis of lymphoproliferative disorders.** (a) Cytocentrifuged blast cells from a case of acute lymphoblastic leukemia stained by anti-terminal deoxynucleotidyl transferase (TdT) using an immuno-alkaline phosphatase method (cells treated first with mouse monoclonal anti-TdT, then anti-mouse Ig and finally with an immune complex of mouse anti-alkaline phosphatase + alkaline phosphatase before developing the enzymatic reddish-purple color reaction). Many strongly stained blast cells are seen together with unlabeled normal marrow cells. (b) Immuno-alkaline phosphatase staining of bone marrow cells from a case of acute lymphoblastic leukemia, using monoclonal antibody specific for the common acute lymphoblastic leukemia antigen (anti-CALLA; antibody J5). The majority of cells are strongly labeled. Two nonreactive cells are indicated by arrows. (c,d,e) Immuno-alkaline phosphatase labeling of blood smears from a case of chronic lymphocytic leukemia with three monoclonal antibodies (anti-HLA-DR, anti-CD3 antigen and anti-CD1 antigen): (c) HLA-DR antigen is present on all the leukemic cells seen, but absent from a polymorph (arrowed); (d) three normal T-cells are labeled for the CD3 antigen, but the leukemic cells are negative; (e) CD1 antigen is strongly expressed on two normal lymphocytes (arrowed), but also weakly expressed on the chronic lymphocytic leukemia (CLL) cells. This pattern is typical of CLL. (f) A case of gastric carcinoma (stained at the bottom using anticytokeratin, Ke) with a heavy lymphocytic infiltrate (top, stained with antileukocyte common antigen, LC). (g) Diffuse follicle center type B-cell lymphoma showing λ light chain restriction; compare with (h) a reactive lymph node staining for both κ and λ light chains. (i) Burkitt's lymphoma showing 'starry sky' appearance. (j) Hodgkin's disease showing mixed cellularity and characteristic binucleate Reed–Sternberg cell with massive prominent nucleoli in the center of the figure. (k) Birefringent amyloid deposits in kidney glomeruli visualized by Congo Red staining under polarized light. (l) A case of malignant lymphoma associated with macroglobulinemia, showing lymphoplasmacytoid cells stained by the brown immunoperoxidase reaction for cytoplasmic IgM. ((a)–(e) Very kindly provided by Professor D. Mason, and (f)–(l) by Professor P. Isaacson.)

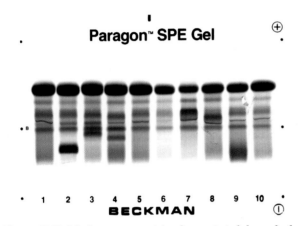

Paragon™ SPE Gel

BECKMAN

Figure 17.10. Myeloma paraprotein demonstrated by gel electrophoresis of serum. Lane 1, normal; lane 2, γ-paraprotein; lane 3, near β-paraprotein; lane 4, fibrinogen band in the γ region of a *plasma* sample; lane 5, normal serum; lane 6, immunoglobulin deficiency (low γ); lane 7, nephrotic syndrome (raised α_2-macroglobulin, low albumin and Igs); lane 8, hemolyzed sample (raised hemoglobin/haptoglobin in α_2 region); lane 9, polyclonal increase in Igs (e.g. infection, autoimmune disease); lane 10, normal serum. (Gel kindly provided by Mr A. Heys.)

myeloma develop widespread amyloid deposits which contain the variable region of the myeloma light chain. Being identical, the variable region fragments polymerize and form the characteristic amyloid fibrils which are recognizable by their birefringence on staining with Congo Red (figure 17.9k). Other components in amyloid have not yet been characterized. The fibrils are relatively resistant to digestion and accumulate in the ground substance of connective tissue where they can lead to pathological changes in the kidneys, heart and brain. Amyloid can also be formed secondarily to chronic inflammatory conditions such as rheumatoid arthritis and familial Mediterranean fever, but in this case involves the polymerization of a unique substance, Amyloid A (AA), a protein derived from the N-terminal part of a serum precursor (SAA) of molecular weight 90 kDa. SAA behaves as an acute phase protein in that its concentration increases rapidly in response to tissue injury or inflammation. Levels rise with age and the minority of individuals with high values are those most likely to develop amyloid.

Waldenström's macroglobulinemia

This disorder is produced by the unregulated proliferation of cells of an intermediate appearance called lymphoplasmacytoid cells which secrete a monoclonal IgM, the Waldenström macroglobulin (figure 17.9l). Remarkably, many of the monoclonal proteins have autoantibody activity, anti-DNA, anti-IgG (rheumatoid factor), and so on. It has been suggested that, like the CLL cells, they are of the B-1 lineage which secrete 'natural' antibodies (cf. p. 245). Since the IgM is secreted in large amounts and is confined to the intravascular compartment, there is a marked rise in serum viscosity, the consequences of which can be temporarily mitigated by vigorous plasmapheresis. The disease runs a fairly benign course and the prognosis is quite good, although the appearance of lymphoplasmacytoid tumor cells in the blood is an ominous sign.

Heavy chain disease

Heavy chain disease is a rare condition in which quantities of abnormal heavy chains are excreted in the urine — γ chains in association with malignant lymphoma and α chains in cases of abdominal lymphoma with diffuse lymphoplasmacytic infiltration of the small intestine. The amino acid sequences of the N-terminal regions of these heavy chains are normal, but they have a deletion extending from part of the variable domain through most of the C_H1 region so that they lack the structure required to form cross-links to the light chains. One idea is that the defect arises through faulty coupling of *V*- and *C*-region genes (cf. p. 54).

Immunodeficiency secondary to lymphoproliferative disorders

Immunodeficiency is a common feature in patients with lymphoid malignancies. The reasons for this are still obscure, but it seems as though the malignant cells interfere with the development of the corresponding normal cells, almost as though they were producing some cell-specific chalone (inhibitor) or transfecting suppressor factor. Thus, in multiple myeloma, the levels of normal B-cells and of nonmyeloma Ig may be grossly depressed and the patients may be susceptible to infection with pyogenic bacteria.

APPROACHES TO CANCER IMMUNOTHERAPY

Although immune surveillance seems to operate only against strongly immunogenic tumors, the identification of a range of tumor antigens is a positive step forward (table 17.2), and has set the stage for exploring how these antigens may be exploited to harness the patient's own immune system in the fight against cancer. On one point all are agreed: if immunotherapy is to succeed, it is essential that the tumor load should first be reduced by surgery, irradiation or chemotherapy, since not only is it unreasonable to expect the immune system to cope with a large tumor mass, but considerable amounts of antigen released by shedding would tend to prevent the generation of any significant response in some cases due to the stimulation of T-suppressor/regulatory cells. This leaves the small secondary deposits as the proper target for immunotherapy.

So what type of immune response is required for tumor destruction? Studies in mouse models, as well as cancer patients, over the past decade or so suggest that a number of criteria need to be fulfilled in order to obtain killing of tumor cells in sufficient numbers to positively impact on the course of disease. First, sufficient numbers of T-cells with highly avid recognition of tumor antigens must be generated. Then, these cells must be able to traffic to the site of the tumor and invade the stroma (supporting cells) associated with the tumor. Finally, these lymphocytes should become activated at the site of the tumor and be capable of engaging the tumor with cytotoxic granules or cytokines such as TNF. Experience to date suggests that fulfilling all of these criteria poses an immense challenge and that immunotherapy is unlikely to offer any 'magic bullet' cures. More realistically, immunological manipulations, in tandem with conventional chemo- and radiotherapy, is likely to be the way forward.

Table 17.2. Potential tumor antigens for immunotherapy. (Reproduced with permission from Fong L. & Engleman E.G. (2000) Dendritic cells in cancer immunotherapy. *Annual Review of Immunology* 18, 245.)

Antigen	Malignancy
Tumor specific	
Immunoglobulin V-region	B-cell non-Hodgkin's lymphoma, multiple myeloma
TCR V-region	T-cell non-Hodgkin's lymphoma
Mutant p21/ras	Pancreatic, colon, lung cancer
Mutant p53	Colorectal, lung, bladder, head and neck cancer
Developmental	
p210/bcr-abl fusion product	Chronic myelogenous leukemia, acute lymphoblastic leukemia
MART-1/Melan A	Melanoma
MAGE-1, MAGE-3	Melanoma, colorectal, lung, gastric cancers
GAGE family	Melanoma
Telomerase	Various
Viral	
Human papilloma virus	Cervical, penile cancer
Epstein–Barr virus	Burkitt's lymphoma, nasopharyngeal carcinoma, post-transplant lymphoproliferative disorders
Tissue specific	
Tyrosinase	Melanoma
gp100	Melanoma
Prostatic acid phosphatase	Prostate cancer
Prostate-specific antigen	Prostate cancer
Prostate-specific membrane antigen	Prostate cancer
Thyroglobulin	Thyroid cancer
α-fetoprotein	Liver cancer
Overexpressed	
Her-2/*neu*	Breast and lung cancers
Carcinoembryonic antigen	Colorectal, lung, breast cancer
Muc-1	Colorectal, pancreatic, ovarian, lung cancer

Antigen-independent cytokine therapy

The first clear indication that manipulation of the immune system could be beneficial came from studies that utilized antigen-independent strategies to nonspecifically boost the immune response to the tumor. Cytokines such as IL-2, IFN and TNF have pleiotrophic effects on the immune system and some of these have shown promise in animal models as well as in clinical settings. Systemic toxicity has limited the utility of TNF which exhibits rapid and severe hepatotoxicity in animal models and is therefore of limited use in cancer therapy.

Interleukin treatment

High doses of IL-2 have been administered to patients with metastatic melanoma or kidney cancer, and at least partial tumor regression was observed in 15–20% of patients, with some patients displaying complete regression. The beneficial effects of high doses of IL-2 may be due to stimulation of pre-existing tumor-responsive T-cells or due to NK activation. On activation by IL-2 or IL-12, NK cells are capable of killing a variety of fresh tumor cells *in vitro* and, on the basis of studies on mice with mammary glands carrying the HER-2/*neu* oncogene, it would not be unreasonable to conduct a trial of systematic IL-12 treatment in cancer patients with minimum residual disease in an attempt to prevent recurrence and to inhibit incipient metastases. Because of the promising results seen upon IL-2 administration, many subsequent tumor vaccine trials have been conducted in combination with this cytokine.

Interferon therapy

In trials using IFNα and IFNβ, a 10–15% objective response rate was seen in patients with renal carcinoma, melanoma and myeloma, an approximate 20% response rate among patients with Kaposi's sarcoma, about 40% positive responders in patients with various lymphomas and a remarkable response rate of 80–90% among patients with hairy cell leukemia and mycosis fungoides.

With regard to the mechanisms of the antitumor effects, in certain tumors IFNs may serve primarily as antiproliferative agents; in others, the activation of NK cells and macrophages may be important, while augmenting the expression of class I MHC molecules may make the tumors more susceptible to control by immune effector mechanisms. In some circumstances the antiviral effect could be contributory.

For diseases like renal cell cancer and hairy cell leukemia, IFNs have induced responses in a significantly higher proportion of patients than have conventional therapies. However, in the wider setting, most investigators consider that their role will be in combination therapy, e.g. with active immunotherapy or with various chemotherapeutic agents where synergistic action has been observed in murine tumor systems. IFNα and β synergize with IFNγ and the latter synergizes with TNF. IFNα acts as a radiation sensitizer and its ability to increase the expression of estrogen receptors on cultured breast cancer cells suggests the possibility of combining IFN with anti-estrogens in this disease.

Colony-stimulating factors

Normal cell development proceeds from an immature stem cell with the capacity for unlimited self-renewal, through committed progenitors, to the final lineage-specific differentiated cells with little or no potential for self-renewal. Therapy aimed at inducing tumor cell differentiation is founded on the idea that the induction of cell maturation decreases and possibly abrogates the capacity of the malignant clone to divide. Along these lines, GM-CSF has been shown to enhance the differentiation, decrease the self-renewal capacity and suppress the leukemogenicity of murine myeloid leukemias. Recombinant human products are now undergoing trials.

It is over 100 years since the physician Coley gave his name to the mixture of microbial products termed **Coley's toxin**. This concoction certainly livens up the innate immune system and does produce remission in a minority of patients. The suggestion has been made that these beneficial effects are due to the release of TNF since the vascular endothelium of tumors is unduly susceptible to damage by this cytokine and hemorrhagic necrosis is readily induced. It is questionable whether the critical levels of TNF are reached in the human since these would be very toxic, although one study involving perfusion of an isolated limb with TNF, IFNγ and melphalan provoked lesions in the tumor endothelium without affecting the normal vasculature. Opinion is coming round to the view that the Coley phenomenon may be linked more to boosting a pre-existing weak antitumor immunity.

Stimulation of cell-mediated immune responses

The current dogma is that T-cells rather than antibodies are capable of savaging solid tumors, particularly those expressing processed intracellular antigens on their surface, and, since the majority are MHC class II negative, it looks as though we are aiming at essentially CD8 cytotoxic T-cell responses, although CD4 T-cells can be involved in protective reactions against tumor-associated vasculature and are required for persistence of CD8 T-cells.

Vaccination with viral antigens

Based on the not unreasonable belief that certain forms of cancer (e.g. lymphoma) are caused by oncogenic viruses, attempts are being made to isolate the virus and prepare a suitable vaccine from it. In fact, large-scale protection of chickens against the development of Marek's disease lymphoma has been successfully achieved by vaccination with another herpes virus native to turkeys. In human Burkitt's lymphoma, work is in progress to develop a vaccine to exploit the ability of Tc cells to target **EBV-related antigens** on the cells of all Burkitt's tumors. It may be an advantage to treat the patient at the same time with cytokines to upregulate the expression of ICAM-1, LFA-3 and possibly of the virus itself.

Immunization with whole tumor cells

A variety of approaches utilizing both autologous and allogeneic whole tumor cell preparations have been tried in an effort to awaken antitumor responses. This has the advantage that we do not necessarily have to know the identity of the antigen concerned. The disadvantage is that the majority of tumors are weakly immunogenic, and do not present antigen effectively and so cannot overcome the **barrier to activation of** *resting T-cells*. Remember, the surface MHC–peptide complex on its own is not enough; costimulation with molecules such as B7.1 and B7.2 and possibly certain cytokines is required to push the G0 T-cell into active proliferation and differentiation. Once we get to this stage, however, **the activated T-cell no longer requires the accessory costimulation** to react with its target, for which it has a greatly increased avidity due to upregulation of accessory binding molecules such as CD2 and LFA-1 (cf. p. 176; figure 17.11). Whole cell immunization approaches have been largely unsuccessful in human clinical trials, possibly because of the very limited quantity of antigenic molecules present in whole cells where the majority of proteins present are nonimmunogenic.

When proper costimulation is provided encouraging results have been reported, at least in animal models. Vaccination with B7-transfected murine melanoma generated CD8+ cytolytic effectors which protected against subsequent tumor challenge; in other words, transfection enabled the melanoma cells to present their own antigens efficiently, while the untransfected cells were vulnerable targets for the cytotoxic T-cells so produced. A further telling observation was that an irradiated nonimmunogenic melanoma line which had been transfected with a retroviral vector carrying the *GM-CSF* gene stimulated potent and specific antitumor immunity, almost certainly by enhancing the differentiation and activation of host antigen-presenting cells.

A less sophisticated but more convenient approach ultimately utilizing similar mechanisms involves the administration of the irradiated melanoma cells together with BCG which, by generating a plethora of inflammatory cytokines, increases the efficiency of presentation of tumor antigens derived from necrotic cells. In a large-scale study of over 1500 patients, 26% of vaccinees were alive at 5 years compared with only 6% of those treated with the best available conventional therapy. It would be exciting to suppose that in the future we might expose a tumor surgically and then transfect it *in situ* by firing gold particles (cf. p. 147) bearing appropriate gene constructs such as B7, IFNγ (to upregulate MHC class I and II), GM-CSF, IL-2, and so on (figure 17.11). There is a real risk of inducing autoimmune responses to cryptic epitopes shared with other normal tissues which the prudent investigator will not overlook.

Therapy with subunit vaccines

The variety of potential tumor antigens thus far identified (table 17.2) has spawned a considerable investment in clinical therapeutic trials using peptides as vaccines. Because of the pioneering work in characterizing melanoma-specific antigens, this tumor has been the

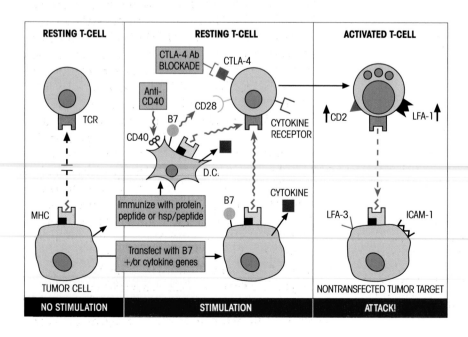

Figure 17.11. Immunotherapy by transfection with costimulatory molecules. The tumor can only stimulate the resting T-cell with the costimulatory help of B7-1 and -2 and/or cytokines such as GM-CSF, γ-interferon and various interleukins, IL-2, -4 and -7. CTLA-4 blockade enhances immunogenicity. Alternatively, the T-cell can be stimulated directly by tumor antigens presented by dendritic cells (DCs) which can themselves be activated by cross-linking their surface CD40 with antibody (see below). Once activated, the T-cell with upregulated accessory molecules can now attack the original tumor lacking costimulators.

focus of numerous studies which exploit to the full the academic background to modern immunology. Encouraging results in terms of clinical benefit, linked to the generation of cytolytic T-cells (CTLs), have been obtained following vaccination with peptides complexed with heat-shock proteins or modified at class I anchor residues to improve MHC binding. Such peptides have been delivered either alone, using recombinant viruses (fowlpox, adenovirus, vaccinia), or as naked DNA, along with adjuvant. The inclusion of accessory factors, such as IL-2 or GM-CSF, and **CTLA-4 blockade** can be crucial for success. Potentially tolerogenic peptide vaccines can be converted into strong primers for CTL responses by triggering CD40 with a cross-linking antibody which can substitute for T-cell help in the direct activation of CTLs (figure 17.12). Anti-CD40 treatment alone was also shown to partially protect mice bearing *CD40-negative* lymphoma cells, an effect attributed to the activation of endogenous dendritic antigen-presenting cells (cf. figure 17.11). However, although some promising indications of immune responses to tumors have been recorded using such approaches, a recent evaluation of multiple vaccine-based clinical trials involving 440 patients, mainly suffering from melanoma, produced an objective response rate of only 2.6%. This disappointingly poor statistic is rather sobering and suggests that we still have some way to go before optimism is warranted. It would be premature to write-off vaccination

approaches at this stage, however, as it should be borne in mind that all of the clinical trials that have been carried out using such vaccines have been conducted in patients with advanced disease. Moreover, all standard therapies have, more often than not, also failed in such individuals. Vaccination with tumor antigens may prove to be more successful where early diagnosis has occurred, or where a genetic predisposition towards a familial form of cancer exists, as a preventative measure against tumor development.

Adoptive T-cell transfer

Adoptive cell transfer (ACT) with large numbers of *ex vivo* expanded T-cells may overcome some of the barriers to effective therapy seen with conventional vaccination approaches (figure 17.13). It may even be possible to genetically engineer the adoptively transferred cells to constitutively express cytokines such as IL-2 or GM-CSF to boost their activity. The generation of cytotoxic T-cell effectors *ex vivo* has the potential to uncover responses that are not evident in an environment where tumor-derived inhibitory factors, or T-regulatory cells, may be present. The typical approach involves isolating T-cells from patients and these are then expanded *in vitro* in the presence of high concentrations of IL-2 (figure 17.13). To maximize the chances of expanding rare tumor-reactive T-cell precursors, mature DCs expressing costimulatory signals along with a source of tumor antigen are now in common use. Over a period of 2–3 weeks 1000-fold expansion of T-cells can be achieved. These *in vitro* expanded CD8 T-cells are then transferred back to the patient (up to 10^{11} cells per individual!) but can rapidly disappear if the tumor burden is high. Administration of IL-2 *in vivo* or cotransfer of CD4 T-cells can improve CD8 T-cell survival; **the presence of CD4 T-cells appear to be crucial for persistence of CD8 T-cells** and optimal cytotoxic effector function. The failure of vaccination approaches using predominantly class I-based peptides may be due to the lack of CD4 T-cell expansion and this should be perhaps borne in mind for future studies. ACT of *in vitro* expanded lymphocytes into lymphodepleted hosts can result in up to 75% of circulating T-cells with antitumor activity, way beyond the levels seen with peptide vaccines. Although the numbers of individuals that have received such ACT-based therapy are still low, very impressive objective response rates of 40–50% have been reported in lymphodepleted melanoma patients, with persistence of transferred cells for up to 4 months. Clearly some risks must be borne in mind when transferring such large numbers of activated lymphocytes into a patient, not least the possibility of generating autoimmunity to tissues other than the tumor. Careful selection of tumor antigens to favor

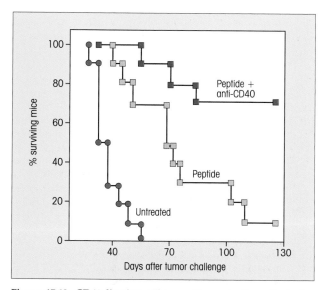

Figure 17.12. CD40 ligation enhances the protective effect of a peptide vaccine against a pre-existing tumor. Six days after injection of human papilloma virus-16 (HPV16)-transformed syngeneic cells, mice were immunized with the HPV16-E7 peptide in incomplete Freund's adjuvant with or without an anti-CD40 monoclonal, or left untreated. (Data from Diehl L. *et al.* (1999) *Nature Medicine* 5, 774, reproduced with permission.)

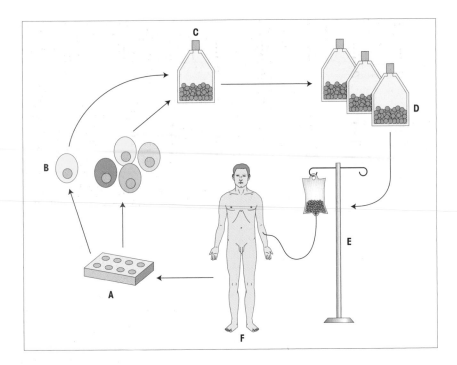

Figure 17.13. Improving the efficacy of adoptive cell transfer-based immunotherapy. A variety of strategies are being employed to enhance the efficacy of adoptive therapy using *ex vivo* expanded T-cells. A, Tumor-reactive T-cells from the patient are stimulated *in vitro* with APCs. To enhance stimulation of tumor-reactive T-cells APCs can be transfected with genes encoding tumor antigens. B, Selection of tumor-reactive T-cell clones or lines can be enhanced using peptide–MHC tetramers or bispecific antibodies to stimulate specific T-cell precursors. C,D, Tumor-specific cells are then expanded in IL-2 followed by (E) intravenous infusion of tumor-specific T-cells into the patient. F, Successful persistence of the transferred T-cells may be enhanced by prior depletion of host lymphocytes and/or administration of homeostatic cytokines (IL-2, IL-15, IL-21) post-infusion. (Based upon Riddell S.R. (2004) *Journal of Experimental Medicine* **200**, 1533.)

those that are not expressed, or are minimally expressed, on tissues other than the tumor is clearly essential in these situations.

There are some indications that lymphocyte-mediated tumor eradication may be simply a numbers game. While peptide vaccination approaches can increase circulating tumor-reactive cells five- to ten-fold, this pales in comparison with observations that up to 40% of circulating CD8 T-cells are reactive against EBV in patients with infectious mononucleosis. Early indications suggest that ACT is capable of achieving such impressive numbers of specific T-cells, especially when combined with prior lymphodepletion. The lymphopenic environment may be favorable as this may free-up space in the lymphoid compartment for the incoming T-cells and create less competition for homeostatic cytokines such as IL-7 and IL-15. Another advantage of this approach is that depletion of recipient lymphocytes can remove suppressor/regulatory T-cells that are suspected to play a significant part in damping down antitumor responses in the first place.

NK cell therapy

We have already alluded to the possible importance of NK cells in tumor surveillance and tumor killing, so it is natural to consider that *in vivo* expansion or adoptive transfer of large numbers of activated NKs may also be of clinical benefit. NK-based therapies are somewhat lagging behind T-cell-based approaches although they are not being overlooked. Clinical trials on cancer patients have assessed the effects of daily subcutaneous administration of low-dose IL-2, following high-dose cytotoxic chemotherapy, for its effects on NK cell numbers and activation status in these individuals. While NK cell expansion was seen, these cells did not appear to be maximally cytotoxic, perhaps because of inhibitory NK receptors finding the appropriate ligands on the tumor. More recent attempts involved using NK cells from related **haploidentical donors** to treat poor prognosis patients with acute myeloblastic leukemia. The idea here is to achieve a partial mismatch between the donor NKs and the recipient that may provoke NK activation and greater tumor kill as a result. Expansion and persistence of the donor NK cells was observed after high-dose immunosuppression of recipients and complete remission in five out of 19 patients was achieved; encouraging signs indeed.

Dendritic cell therapy

The sheer power of the **dendritic antigen-presenting cell (DC)** for the initiation of T-cell responses has been the focus of an ever-burgeoning series of immunotherapeutic strategies which have elicited tumor-specific protective immune responses via injection of isolated DC loaded with tumor lysates or tumor antigens or peptides derived from them. Considerable success has been achieved in animal models and increasingly with human patients (figure 17.14). The copious numbers of DCs needed for each patient's individual therapy are obtained by expansion of CD34-positive precursors in bone marrow by culture with GM-CSF, IL-4 and TNF, and sometimes with extra goodies such as stem cell

Figure 17.14. Clinical response to autologous vaccine utilizing dendritic cells pulsed with idiotype from a B-cell lymphoma. Computed tomography scans through patient's chest: (a) prevaccine and (b) 10 months after completion of three vaccine treatments. The arrow in (a) points to a paracardiac mass. All sites of disease had resolved and the patient remained in remission 24 months after beginning treatment. (Photography kindly supplied by Professor R. Levy from the article by Hsu F.J. *et al.* (1996) *Nature Medicine* **2**, 52; reproduced by kind permission of Nature America Inc.)

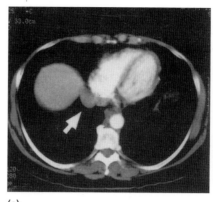
(a)

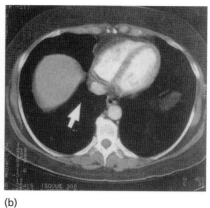
(b)

factor (SCF) and Fms-like tyrosine kinase 3 (Flt3)-ligand. CD14-positive monocytes from peripheral blood are easier to access, and generate DC in the presence of GM-CSF plus IL-4; however, they need additional maturation with TNFα which increases cost and the chance of bacterial contamination. Another approach is to expand the DCs *in vivo* by administration of Flt3-ligand. The circulating blood DCs increase in number 10–30-fold and can be harvested by leukophoresis.

Some general points may be made. First, where peptides are used to load the DC, sequences which bind strongly to a given MHC class I haplotype must be identified; sequences will vary between patients with different haplotypes and they may not include potential CD4 helper epitopes. Recombinant proteins will overcome most of these difficulties, and a mixture should be even better since it should recruit more CTLs and be more able to 'ride out' any new tumor antigen mutations. However, proteins taken up by DCs are relatively inefficient at 'cross-priming' CD8 CTLs through the class I processing pathway, although several tactics are being explored to circumvent this problem: they include conjugation to an HIV-tat 'transporter' peptide which increases class I presentation 100-fold and transfection with RNA and recombinant vectors such as fowlpox. Second, the procedure is cumbersome and costly but, if it becomes common, it will be streamlined and, anyway, the costs must be set against the expenses of conventional therapy and the immeasurable benefit to the patient. Third, why does the administration of small numbers of antigen-pulsed DCs induce specific T-cell responses and tumor regression in patients in whom both the antigen and DCs are already plentiful? The suggestion has been made that DCs in or near malignant tissues may be defective or immature, perhaps due to vascular endothelium growth factor (VEGF) or IL-10 secretion by the tumor which may arrest DC maturation to generate immature 'tolerogenic' DCs. Such immature DCs may smother tumor-reactive T-cell responses at

birth rather than nurture them. Alternatively, immature DCs that capture antigen in the vicinity of a tumor, in the absence of appropriate Toll receptor ligands or danger signals, may simply not function as effective antigen-presenting cells (figure 17.6). It will certainly be interesting to see whether direct treatment of patients with Flt3-ligand plus accessory cytokines or intratumoral transfection with MIP-3α (CCL20) (cf. p. 196), which attracts immature DCs, can initiate an antitumor response through maturation and activation of endogenous DCs.

Vaccination against neovascularization

Solid tumors are composed of malignant cells as well as a variety of nonmalignant cell types such as endothelial cells and fibroblasts. Because solid tumors cannot grow to any appreciable size without a blood supply, tumors stimulate the production of new blood vessels by secreting angiogenic factors, such as VEGF, that stimulate endothelial cell proliferation. Because growing tumors are highly reliant on their blood supply, attacking the tumor vasculature by targeting antigens selectively expressed on these blood vessels may deprive the tumor of oxygen and nutrients; provoking regression one would hope. VEGF, one of a family of angiogenic factors, exerts its effects through interaction with its cognate receptor, VEGF-R2 (also known as KDR in humans and Flk-1 in the mouse), which provides signals that promote proliferation, survival and motility of endothelial cells. Antibodies directed against VEGF-R2, or indeed VEGF itself, can block tumor angiogenesis in murine tumor models but translation into the clinic has been hampered due to problems relating to delivery of sufficient amounts of these agents to fully block VEGF-R2 activity. An alternative strategy involves **breaking immune tolerance** to VEGF-R2-positive endothelial cells by pulsing *in vitro* generated DCs with soluble VEGF-R2 followed by transferring these cells back into the animal. A major advantage of this approach is that the tumor endothelium, unlike the tumor itself, is genetically stable as it represents nontransformed tissue, and this makes it unlikely that mutant cells will arise that have lost VEGF-R2 expression. This strategy has been reported to generate VEGF-R2-specific neutralizing antibody as well as cytotoxic T-cells capable of effectively destroying endothelial cells.

Treatment of leukemia

Radical cytoablative treatment of leukemia patients using radiochemotherapy will destroy bone marrow stem cells. These can be removed prior to treatment, purged of any leukemic cells with cytotoxic antibodies, and reinfused subsequently to 'rescue' the patient (figure 17.15). However, not all leukemic cells are eliminated by this treatment, and a more effective strategy is transplantation of *allogeneic* bone marrow from reasonably MHC-compatible donors which exerts an important, albeit not completely understood, graft-vs-leukemia effect. Purging the bone marrow of T-cells to prevent graft-vs-host (g.v.h.) disease, which is a serious complication of such transplants, would at the same time remove the prized antileukemic activity. A dilemma. 'Suicide gene therapy' could provide a solution as illustrated in figure 17.16. Stem cells from the T-cell-purged allogeneic bone marrow are given together with donor T-cells transfected with herpes simplex virus thymidine kinase. The T-cells provide factors which facilitate engraftment, defense against viral infection and the graft-vs-leukemia action at a time when the recipient patient will have a low tumor burden. With time, as graft-vs-host disease develops, the dividing aggressor donor T-cells can be switched off

by administration of ganciclovir through the mechanism explained in the legend to figure 17.16.

An alternative which avoids g.v.h. disease altogether is to inject the purged bone marrow together with an allogeneic cytotoxic T-cell clone specific for a leukemia-associated peptide presented by the MHC allele of

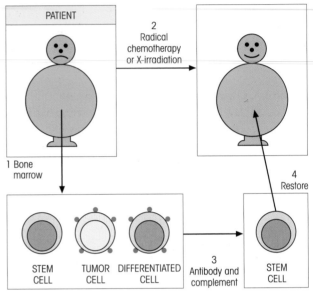

Figure 17.15. Treatment of leukemias by autologous bone marrow rescue. By using cytotoxic antibodies to a differentiation antigen (●) present on leukemic cells and even on other normal differentiated cells, but absent from stem cells, it is possible to obtain a tumor-free population of the latter which can be used to restore hematopoietic function in patients subsequently treated radically to destroy the leukemic cells. Another angle is positive selection of stem cells utilizing the CD34 marker.

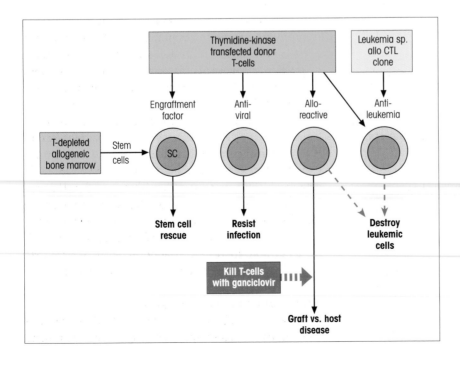

Figure 17.16. Treatment of leukemia with allogeneic bone marrow transfer. T-depleted allogeneic marrow provides the stem cells to 'rescue' the patient treated with cytoablative therapy. T-cells from the donor, transfected with thymidine kinase (TK), help engraftment, provide protection against infection and eliminate residual tumor cells by a graft-vs-leukemia effect. The alloreactive cells eventually produce graft-vs-host disease and can be eliminated by administration of ganciclovir. This is converted by the TK into a nucleoside analog which ultimately becomes toxic for dividing cells. The alternative shown is to destroy leukemic cells by supplementing purged allogeneic marrow with a leukemia peptide-specific CTL clone produced in third party T-cells. (Based on articles by Cohen J.L., Boyer O. & Klatzmann D. (1999) *Immunology Today* **20**, 172; and Stauss H.J. (1999) *Immunology Today* **20**, 180.)

the prospective recipient patient. This usually works because the residues on the MHC helices which contact the T-cell receptor are relatively conserved (unlike those within the groove), so that the allo-T-cells can recognize the MHC–peptide complex from the leukemia. Potential targets are cyclin-D1 and mdm-2 which are overexpressed in tumor cells and, in leukemic cells in particular, the transcription factors WT-1 and GATA1 and the differentiation antigens myeloperoxidase and CD68, which are expressed exclusively in hematopoietic cells and are likely to have established tolerance in the patient but not in the allogeneic CTL donor (who will have been exposed to different processed peptides) (cf. p. 368). A rather masterful development would be to transfect the recipient with the genes encoding the T-cell receptor of the allo-CTL clone. Again, looking to the future, transfection of T-cells *in vitro* with a humanized scFv–Fcγ–transmembrane segment–CD3ζ construct has been shown to render them cytotoxic for cells expressing the surface antigen.

Table 17.3. Selected mAbs approved or in late-stage clinical trials for cancer therapy. (From data of Adams G.P. & Weiner L.M. (2005) *Nature Biotechnology* **23**, 1147.)

Target antigen	Format	Indication	Status
HER2/neu	Unconjugated	Breast cancer	Approved for therapeutic use
CD20	Unconjugated	Lymphoma	Approved for therapeutic use
CD20	^{90}Y- and ^{131}I-conjugates	Lymphoma	Approved for therapeutic use
EGF receptor	Unconjugated	Colorectal cancer	Approved for therapeutic use
VEGF	Unconjugated	Colorectal and lung cancer	Approved for therapeutic use
CD52	Unconjugated	Chronic lymphocytic leukemia	Approved for therapeutic use
CD33	Drug-conjugate	Acute myelogenous leukemia	Approved for therapeutic use
GD2	Unconjugated	Neuroblastoma	In late-stage clinical trials
CTLA-4	Unconjugated	Melanoma	In late-stage clinical trials
MHC Class II	Unconjugated	Non-Hodgkin's lymphoma	In late-stage clinical trials

Passive immunotherapy with monoclonal antibodies

After many false dawns, monoclonal antibodies are finally delivering on their early promise and some of the most promising results from immunotherapeutic approaches to cancer treatment have been achieved with humanized monoclonal antibodies. As detailed earlier (see Chapter 6), early attempts to use mouse monoclonal antibodies for therapeutic purposes were severely hampered by strong immune responses against the foreign sequences within the mouse antibody; the so-called *h*uman *a*nti-*m*ouse *a*ntibody (HAMA) response. These early difficulties have now been overcome and numerous 'humanized' monoclonal antibodies have now entered clinical trials and several have been approved for therapeutic use (table 17.3). Antibodies reacting with antigens on the surface of tumor cells can protect the host by complement-mediated opsonization and lysis (modified by host complement regulatory proteins) and through recruitment of macrophage and NK ADCC function by engagement of FcγRIII receptors, although for macrophages this is partially countered by inhibitory FcγRII signals. These FcR-bearing cells serve not only as cytotoxic effectors but also as multivalent surfaces which hyper-cross-link antibody-coated target cells so providing, in many cases, a transmembrane signal which leads to apoptosis or premature exit from the cell cycle. This effect appears to sensitize neoplastic cells to irradiation and DNA-damaging chemotherapy and holds out the exciting prospect of novel synergistic treatments whose efficacy may be enhanced by the increased immunogenicity of the dying cells.

Immunologists have long been entranced by the idea of eliminating tumor cells by specific antibody linked to a killer molecule and there is a truly impressive array of ingenious initiatives. It is axiomatic that multimeric fragments bind much more avidly than monomeric fragments due principally to the lower off-rates (cf. p. 92), and that constructs in the 60–120 kDa range are optimal for targeting solid tumors—too large and penetration is difficult, too small and kidney secretion is excessively fast. Monovalent fragments include Fv, scFv selected by antigen from phage libraries (cf. p. 150) and V_H domains based on the large CDR loops of the camels and llamas. For polymers we have bivalent and bispecific (think about the difference) diabodies (cf. p. 117), trivalent and trispecific triabodies, even tetrabodies, and Fabs have been linked into dimers or trimers.

Therapeutic immunoconjugates

While antibody alone is sometimes effective, immunoconjugates are where the most exciting developments have been made, particularly with respect to solid tumors. Therapeutic immunoconjugates consist of a tumor-targeting antibody linked with a toxic effector component, which can be either a radioisotope, a toxin or a small drug molecule. Initial attempts to treat tumors with such immunoconjugates proved disappointing, mainly because the cytotoxic payloads that were conjugated to antibody were conventional chemotherapeutic drugs (such as doxorubicin) which are not sufficiently toxic when delivered in small doses. Dosimetry studies using **radioimmunoconjugates** indicate that very modest amounts, between 0.01% and 0.001% of the administered antibody per gram of solid tumor, actually reach the tumor site. This effectively means that the effector drug or toxin has to work in the picomolar range. The nature of the problem can be grasped when one considers that many conventional chemotherapeutics are effective in the micromolar or high nanomolar range.

This limitation prompted a search for much more toxic molecules to act as conjugates and toxins seemed to fit the bill initially. Protein toxins such as pseudomonas exotoxin and diphtheria toxin are highly toxic *in vitro* and display activity in animal models, but they also proved to be highly immunogenic in humans and rapidly induce neutralizing antibody responses which limit their efficacy and the ability to administer repeated doses: a problem known as the *human anti-toxin antibody* (HATA) response. In some cases, practically 100% of patients developed HATA responses by their second treatment with a toxin immunoconjugate. Quite apart from HATA, another disadvantage of **immunotoxin conjugates** is a syndrome that appears to result from nonspecific toxin-induced damage to endothelium, called **vascular leak syndrome,** which also reduces the maximum tolerated doses of such conjugates that can be used. However, where patients are severely immunosuppressed, in the case of hematologic malignancies for example, immunotoxin conjugates are of benefit; very impressive complete remission rates approaching 70% have been recorded for patients with Hairy cell leukaemia using an anti-CD22-pseudomonas toxin conjugate.

Another approach that has been pursued for several years now aims to exploit the cytotoxic properties of radionuclides, such as iodine-131 and yttrium-90, to irradiate the tumor in a highly precise manner. Several clinical trials have been conducted with such radioimmunoconjugates, and while there have been some notable successes, ^{90}Y and ^{131}I anti-CD20 conjugates for non-Hodgkin's lymphoma for example, the results have been generally disappointing. It has proved difficult to achieve therapeutic efficacy with many radioimmunoconjugates without exceeding the **maximum tolerated dose**, and side-effects such as myeloablation are frequently seen. Attempts have been made to reduce these nonspecific toxic effects by using α particle emitters, such as astatine-211, that have much shorter path lengths than β-emitters which reduces collateral damage to other cells. Such manipulations have the desired effect, with up to 1000-fold higher absorbed dose ratios in target organs with α-emitters relative to their β-emitter counterparts. But every silver lining has a cloud, or so it seems; the α particle radioimmunoconjugates have half-lives ranging from 60 minutes to a few hours or so, making them impractical for routine clinical use.

The search for toxic molecules in the high picomolar range eventually paid off with the discovery of inhibitors of tubulin polymerization such as auristatin and molecules that cause DNA double-strand breaks such as calicheamicin and esperamicin. One very attractive feature of these agents is that conjugation of the drug to the antibody frequently converts it into a **pro-drug** which requires removal from the antibody to regain activity. Because the linker between drug and antibody is stable in the blood, the conjugate exhibits virtually no toxicity until it becomes bound and internalized by an antigen-positive target cell. Many such **drug immunoconjugates** are currently in clinical trials or have been approved for a range of cancers, including: acute myeloid leukemia (anti-CD33-calicheamycin), colorectal and pancreatic cancer (anti-CanAg-DM1), small cell lung carcinoma (anti-CD56-DM1) and several other malignancies (anti-Her2/neu-DM1). Considerable effort is also underway to develop even more potent cytotoxic compounds for the preparation of drug immunoconjugates. Because of their stability, potency and clinical utility, small drug immunoconjugates are likely to rule the roost within a short time.

Attack on the tumor blood supply

For solid tumors, the focus is upon two main targets. The first would be **minimal residual micrometastases in the bone marrow** which occur in one-third to one-half of patients with epithelial cancer after curative radical treatment of the primary lesion. The second would be the **reactive tissue evoked by the malignant process**, such as stromal fibroblasts expressing the F19 glycoprotein and newly formed blood vessels.

As we discussed earlier, tumors generally cannot grow beyond 1 mm in diameter without the support of blood vessels which the tumor promotes formation of by secreting angiogenic factors such as VEGF. New blood vessels are biochemically and structurally different from normal resting blood vessels and so provide differential targets for therapeutic monoclonal antibodies, even though the cancer cells themselves in a solid tumor are less vulnerable to antibodies directed to specific antigens on their surface. Thus, receptors for VEGF and Eph, oncofetal fibronectin, matrix metalloproteases MMP-2 and MMP-9 and the pericyte markers aminopeptidase A and the NG2 proteoglycan are all highly and selectively expressed in vasculature undergoing angiogenesis. Consequently, considerable effort has been expended in the direction of angiogenesis inhibitors such as humanized monoclonal antibodies against VEGF and its main receptor VEGF-R2.

A noteworthy maneuver, which is unexpectedly successful, is to identify peptides that home specifically to the endothelial cells of certain tumors by injecting peptide phage libraries *in vivo*. One of the panel of peptide motifs which has emerged from this probing strategy includes RGD in the cyclic peptide CDCRGD-CFC, a selective binder of the $\alpha_V\beta_3$- and $\alpha_V\beta_5$-integrins known to be upregulated in angiogenic tumor endothelial cells. For therapeutic exploitation, these peptides can be linked to appropriate drugs, such as doxorubicin, or a pro-apoptotic peptide. Overall, there are undoubtedly a substantial number of targets for the 'magic bullets'.

IMMUNODIAGNOSIS OF SOLID TUMORS

Circulating and cellular tumor markers

Analysis of blood for the oncofetal antigens, α-fetoprotein in hepatoma and carcinoembryonic antigen in tumors of the colon, has provided valuable diagnostic information, but enthusiasm has been slightly curtailed by the knowledge that there is a high incidence of so-called 'false positives'. Reappearance of these proteins after surgical removal of the primary is strongly indicative of fresh tumor growth. A hefty increase in the ratio of free to bound prostate-specific antigen (PSA) in the blood may signal cancer of the prostate. The GM1 monosialoganglioside has been demonstrated in the blood of 96% of patients with pancreatic carcinoma and 64% of patients with colorectal carcinomas, as against 2% in normal subjects.

Identification of the cell type by monoclonal antibodies is of value for the diagnosis and treatment of an increasing number of tumors, including the lymphoproliferative disorders as discussed earlier (see p. 394).

Tumor imaging *in vivo*

The same principles which govern the localization of monoclonal antibodies for tumor therapy apply equally to imaging. Maximizing the binding to tumor relative to normal tissue and surrounding fluids is the name of the game. For example, the use of a bifunctional antibody which targets the tumor and an isotope chelator can be followed 24–120 hours later with the chelate-containing radionuclide which allows clearance of uncombined antibody.

The Thomson–Friedenreich (T) antigen (Galβ1-3-GalNAcα-O-Ser), expressed in the mucins of various types of epithelial cancer, has proved to be a highly successful target for antibody imaging. So has the F19 glycoprotein associated with proliferating fibroblasts in the stroma of many carcinomas, as presumably the many antigens associated with tumor angiogenesis will prove to be.

Detection of micrometastases in bone marrow

Because of the difficulty in detecting individual tumor cells in distant organs, the diagnosis of early disseminated cancer has not been possible, and attempts to identify earlier stages and to monitor the immunotherapy of early disease have been hindered. A major advance was made when micrometastases were demonstrated by immunocytochemistry in the bone marrow of patients with colorectal cancer and were related to more widespread disease (table 17.4) and a high relapse rate. The method involves scanning pelvic crest bone marrow aspirates taken at surgery for epithelial cells by staining for cytokeratin (cf. figure 17.9f) and proliferation markers such as the Ki67 nuclear antigen and receptors for transferrin and epidermal growth factor. Detection of micrometastases in the marrow of patients with small cell lung carcinoma also predicted early relapse.

Table 17.4. Detection of bone marrow micrometastases by staining for epithelial cytokeratin in colorectal cancer patients. (From data of Schlimok G. *et al.* (1990) *Journal of Clinical Oncology* **8**, 831.)

Dukes' Stage		Positive reaction with mAb CK2 for cytokeratin in bone marrow aspirate	
		No. patients	% Positive
A	Limited to mucosa	3	0
B	Extending into muscularis propria	58	14
C	Involving local nodes	62	34
D	With distant metastatic spread	33	39

SUMMARY

Cellular transformation

- Cancer is typically caused by genetic lesions that affect genes that promote proliferation in tandem with lesions that interfere with the elimination of cells through apoptosis.
- Transformed cells are not usually highly immunogenic.

Tumor antigens

- Many candidate tumor antigens have now been identified but most are specific to an individual tumor and are not shared between individuals.
- Processed peptides derived from oncogenic viruses are powerful MHC-associated transplantation antigens.
- Some tumors express genes which are silent in normal tissues: sometimes they have been expressed previously in embryonic life (oncofetal antigens).
- Many tumors express weak antigens associated with point mutations in oncogenes such as *ras* and *p53*. Peptides presented by heat-shock proteins 70 and 90 represent the unique chemically induced tumor antigens. The surface Ig on chronic lymphocytic leukemia (CLL) cells is a unique tumor-specific antigen.
- Dysregulation of tumor cells frequently causes structural abnormalities in surface carbohydrate structures.
- The v6 and v10 exons of CD44 are intimately involved with metastatic potential. Loss of blood group A determinants leads to a poor prognosis.

Immune response to tumors

- T-cells generally mount effective surveillance against tumors associated with oncogenic viruses or UV induction which are strongly immunogenic.
- More weakly immunogenic tumors are not controlled by T-cell surveillance, although sometimes low-grade responses are evoked.
- NK cells probably play a role in containing tumor growth and metastases. They can attack MHC class I-negative tumor cells because the class I molecule imparts a negative inactivation signal to NK cells. The A-NK subset, which expresses high levels of adhesion molecules, is more cytolytic for fresh tumor cells.
- Tumors utilize a variety of mechanisms to escape host immune responses which suggests that the immune system exerts selective pressure on tumors.

Unregulated development gives rise to lymphoproliferative disorders

- Deregulation of the c-*myc* protooncogene is a characteristic feature of many B-cell tumors.
- Chromosome translocations that create chimeric genes and result in deregulated expression of oncogenes or other genes that can affect cell division/cell death are common.

- Lymphoid malignancies show maturation arrest at characteristic stages in differentiation.
- The surface markers of leukemias and lymphomas identified by monoclonal antibodies are important aids in diagnosis. Most non-Hodgkin's lymphomas are of B-cell origin, are associated with EBV and express a monoclonal surface Ig.
- Multiple myeloma represents a malignant proliferation of a single clone of plasma cells producing a single 'M' band on electrophoresis. 10–20% have widespread amyloid deposits containing the variable region of the myeloma light chain.
- Waldenström's macroglobulinemia is produced by unregulated proliferation of a clone producing monoclonal IgM causing a marked rise in serum viscosity.
- Malignant lymphoid cells produce secondary immunodeficiency by suppressing differentiation of the corresponding normal lineage.

Approaches to cancer immunotherapy

- Immunotherapy is only likely to work after a tumor mass has been debulked.
- Innate immune mechanisms can be harnessed. High concentrations of IL-2 can enhance responses to malignant melanoma and other tumors, systemic IL-12 may be effective against minimal residual disease. IFNγ and β are very effective in the T-cell disorders, hairy cell leukemia and mycosis fungoides, less so but still significant in Kaposi's sarcoma and various lymphomas; they may be used in synergy with other therapies. GM-CSF enhances proliferation and decreases leukemogenicity of murine myeloid leukemias.
- Cancer vaccines based on oncogenic viral proteins are likely to be effective and will provide a prophylactic measure against virus-induced cancers, such as cervical cancer.
- Weakly immunogenic tumors provoke anticancer responses if given with an adjuvant, such as BCG, or if transfected with costimulatory molecules, such as B7 and cytokines IFNγ, IL-2, -4 and -7.
- CD8 CTLs are favored for the attack on solid tumors, and CD4 T helper cells are likely to be required for persistence and optimal effector function of CD8 T-cells.
- A variety of potential tumor antigens have been identified and intense effort is being expended in the investigation of peptides as subunit vaccines. Their immunogenicity can be enhanced by complexing with heat-shock proteins and by accessory factors such as GM-CSF, CTLA-4 blockade and anti-CD40 stimulation.
- Clinical trials using peptide-based vaccines have been disappointing but adoptive cell transfer-based

(Continued p.409)

immunotherapy using *in vitro* expanded CD8 T-cells has shown more promise.

• Powerful immunogens have been created by pulsing dendritic antigen-presenting cells with peptides from melanoma antigens and framework regions of CLL Ig.

• A graft-vs-leukemia effect is achieved by allogeneic CTLs or by allogeneic bone marrow transplantation with measures to limit graft-vs-host disease.

• Monoclonal antibodies conjugated to drugs, toxins or radiolabels can target tumor cells or antigens on new blood vessels or the reactive stromal fibroblasts associated with malignancy. Encouraging, even impressive, therapeutic results have been obtained with antibodies to CD20 in B-cell lymphoma, CD33 in myeloid leukemia, anti-MUC-1 in ovarian cancer and c-erbB2 overexpressed on breast cancers. Bifunctional antibodies can bring effectors such as NK and Tc close to the tumor target.

Immunodiagnosis of solid tumors

• Many circulating tumor markers are diagnostic, e.g. α-fetoprotein in hepatic carcinoma and carcinoembryonic antigen in colorectal carcinoma.

• Monoclonal antibody to tumor surfaces can provide a basis for imaging. Certain tumor mucins, the F19 glycoprotein on reactive stromal fibroblasts and VEGF on new blood vessels around the tumor are good targets.

• Detection of micrometastases in bone marrow by immunocytochemistry provides valuable information on prognosis and the efficacy of new therapies.

See the accompanying website (**www.roitt.com**) for multiple choice questions.

FURTHER READING

Banchereau J. & Palucka A.K. (2005) Dendritic cells as therapeutic vaccines against cancer. *Nature Reviews Immunology* **5**, 296–306.

Begent R.H.J. *et al.* (1996) Clinical evidence of efficient tumor targeting based on single-chain Fv antibody selected from a combinatorial library. *Nature Medicine* **2**, 979–984.

Forbes I.J. & Leong A.S.-Y. (1987) *Essential Oncology of the Lymphocyte.* Springer-Verlag, Berlin.

Ho W.Y. *et al.* (2003) Adoptive immunotherapy: engineering T-cell responses as biologic weapons for tumor mass destruction. *Cancer Cell* **3**, 431–437.

Lake R.A. & Robinson B.W.S. (2005) Immunotherapy and chemotherapy: a practical partnership. *Nature Reviews Cancer* **5**, 397–405.

Leonard R.C.F., Duncan L.W. & Hay F.G. (1990) Immunocytological detection of residual marrow disease at clinical remission predicts metastatic relapse in small cell lung cancer. *Cancer Research* **50**, 6545–6548.

Mannel D., Murray C., Risau W. & Clauss M. (1996) Tumor necrosis: factors and principles. *Immunology Today* **17**, 254–256.

Morton D.L. & Barth A. (1996) Vaccine therapy for malignant melanoma. *CA: A Cancer Journal for Clinicians* **46**, 225–244.

Murphy A. *et al.* (2005) Gene modification strategies to induce tumor immunity. *Immunity* **22**, 403–414.

Payne G. (2003) Progress in immunoconjugate cancer therapeutics. *Cancer Cell* **3**, 207–212.

Rafii S. (2002) Vaccination against tumor neovascularization: promise and reality. *Cancer Cell* **2**, 429–431.

Rosenberg S.A., Yang J.C. & Restifo N.P. (2004) Cancer immunotherapy: moving beyond current vaccines. *Nature Medicine* **10**, 909–915.

Ruoslahti E. & Rajotte D. (2000) An address system in the vasculature of normal tissues and tumors. *Annual Review of Immunology* **18**, 813–827.

Smyth M.J. Godfrey D.I. & Trapani J.A. (2001) A fresh look at tumor immunosurveillance and immunotherapy. *Nature Immunology* **2**, 293–299.

Srivastava P.K. (2000) Immunotherapy of human cancer: lessons from mice. *Nature Immunology* **1**, 363–366.

Stein H. & Mason D.Y. (1985) Immunological analysis of tissue sections in diagnosis of lymphoma. In Hoffbrand A.V. (ed.) *Recent Advances in Haematology*, Vol. 4, p. 127. Churchill Livingstone, Edinburgh.

Tumor Immunology (2006) *Current Opinion in Immunology* **18**(2). (Critical overviews of the whole field appearing annually, which are well-worth reading.)

Zou W. (2005) Immunosuppressive networks in the tumor environment and their therapeutic relevance. *Nature Reviews Cancer* **5**, 263–274.

18 Autoimmune diseases

INTRODUCTION

The monumental repertoire of the adaptive immune system has evolved to allow it to recognize and ensnare virtually any shaped microbial molecules, either at present in existence or yet to come, and in so doing, has been unable to avoid the generation of lymphocytes which react with the body's own constituents. This is abundantly so for T-cells which actually depend upon a degree of self-recognition for positive selection to operate during their development within the thymus (p. 234). We have already discussed the tolerance mechanisms which exist to prevent these self-components from provoking an adaptive immune response but, as with all machinery, there is always a chance that these systems might break down, and the older the individual, the greater the chance of this happening. Notwithstanding the IgM low affinity **autoantibodies** (i.e. antibodies capable of reacting with 'self'-components) produced by CD5$^+$ B-1 cells as part of the 'natural' antibody spectrum which we will discuss later, we are here concerned more with autoimmune phenomena which appear in relation to certain defined human diseases. Ideally, we wish to apply the term '**autoimmune disease**' to those cases where it can be shown that the **autoimmune process contributes to the pathogenesis of the disease** rather than situations where apparently harmless autoantibodies are formed following tissue damage, e.g. heart antibodies appearing after a myocardial infarction. Yet the role of autoimmunity in many disorders is still not clearly defined, and it is as a matter of convenience that we will refer to all maladies firmly associated with autoantibody formation as 'autoimmune diseases', except where it can be shown that the immunological phenomena are purely secondary findings.

THE SCOPE OF AUTOIMMUNE DISEASES

The spectrum of autoimmune diseases

These disorders may be looked upon as forming a spectrum. At one end we have '**organ-specific diseases**' with organ-specific autoantibodies. **Hashimoto's disease** of the thyroid is an example: there is a specific lesion in the thyroid involving infiltration by mononuclear cells (lymphocytes, macrophages and plasma cells), destruction of follicular cells and germinal center formation, accompanied by the production of circulating antibodies with absolute specificity for certain thyroid constituents (Milestone 18.1).

Moving towards the center of the spectrum are those disorders where the lesion tends to be localized to a single organ but the antibodies are nonorgan-specific. A typical example would be **primary biliary cirrhosis** where the small bile ductule is the main target of inflammatory cell infiltration but the serum antibodies present—mainly mitochondrial—are not liver-specific.

At the other end of the spectrum are the '**nonorgan-specific or systemic autoimmune diseases**' broadly belonging to the class of rheumatological disorders, exemplified by **systemic lupus erythematosus (SLE)**, where both lesions and autoantibodies are not confined to any one organ. Pathological changes are widespread and are primarily lesions of connective tissue with fibrinoid necrosis. They are seen in the skin (the 'lupus' butterfly rash on the face is characteristic), kidney glomeruli, joints, serous membranes and blood vessels. In addition, the formed elements of the blood are often affected. A bizarre collection of autoantibodies is found, some of which react with the DNA and other nuclear constituents of all cells in the body.

An attempt to fit the major diseases considered to be

associated with autoimmunity into this spectrum is shown in table 18.1.

Autoantibodies in human disease

At this stage in the discussion it may be of value to have a more precise account of the major autoantibodies detected in the different diseases to provide a frame-work for reference. Table 18.2 documents a list of these antibodies and the methods employed in their detection. The notes accompanying the table amplify specific points, while some of the tests are illustrated in figures 6.8, 6.29, 6.30 and 18.1. As antigens are characterized and become available in purified form, the convenient ELISA and its development into protein microarray technology is becoming a dominant technique.

Milestone 18.1—The Discovery of Thyroid Autoimmunity

Although Dacie's studies on red cell autoantibodies in certain forms of hemolytic anemia were amongst the earliest to implicate autoimmunity in the pathogenesis of disease, a direct link to disorders affecting whole organs was not established until 1956 when three major papers on thyroid autoimmunity appeared.

In an attempt to confirm Paul Ehrlich's concept of 'horror autotoxicus'—the body's dread of making antibodies to self—Rose and Witebsky immunized rabbits with rabbit thyroid extract in complete Freund's adjuvant. To what one might hazard was Witebsky's dismay and Rose's delight, this proce-dure resulted in the production of thyroid autoantibodies and chronic inflammatory destruction of the thyroid gland archi-tecture (figure M18.1.1a,b).

Having noted the fall in serum γ-globulin which followed removal of the goiter in Hashimoto's thyroiditis and the simi-larity of the histology (figure M18.1.1c) to that of Rose and Witebsky's rabbits, Roitt, Doniach and Campbell tested the hypothesis that the plasma cells in the gland might be making an autoantibody to a thyroid component, so causing the tissue damage and chronic inflammatory response. Sure enough, the sera of the first patients tested had precipitating antibodies

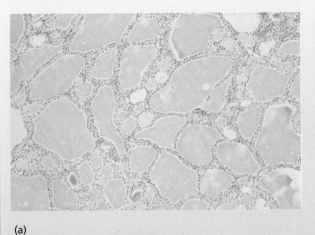

(a)

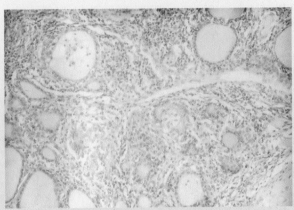

(b)

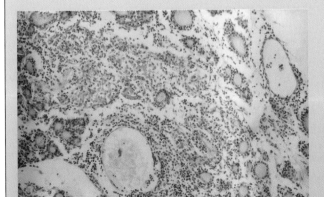

(c)

Figure M18.1.1. Experimental autoimmune thyroiditis. (a) The fol-licular architecture of the normal thyroid. (b) Thyroiditis produced by immunization with rat thyroid extract in complete Freund's adjuvant; the invading chronic inflammatory cells have destroyed the follicular structure. (Based on the experiments of Rose N.R. & Witebsky E. (1956) Studies on organ specificity. V. Changes in the thyroid gland of rabbits following active immunization with rabbit thyroid extracts. *Journal of Immunology* **76**, 417.) (c) Similarity of lesions in spontaneous human autoimmune disease to those induced in the experimental model. Other features of Hashimoto's disease such as the eosinophilic meta-plasia of acinar cells (Askenazy cells) and local lymphoid follicles are not seen in this experimental model, although the latter occur in the spontaneous thyroiditis of Obese strain chickens.

(Continued p.412)

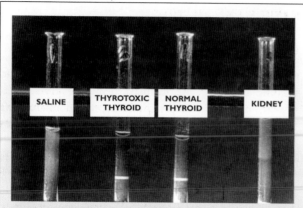

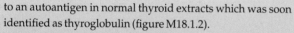

Figure M18.1.2. **Thyroid autoantibodies in the serum of a patient with Hashimoto's disease demonstrated by precipitation in agar.** Test serum is incorporated in agar in the bottom of the tube; the middle layer contains agar only, while the autoantigen is present in the top layer. As serum antibody and thyroid autoantigen diffuse towards each other, they form a zone of opaque precipitate in the middle layer. Saline and kidney extract controls are negative. (Based on Roitt I.M., Doniach D., Campbell P.N. & Hudson R.V. (1956) Autoantibodies in Hashimoto's disease. *Lancet* ii, 820.)

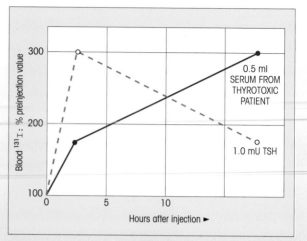

Figure M18.1.3. **The long-acting thyroid stimulator in Graves' disease.** Injection of TSH causes a rapid release of ^{131}I from the prelabeled animal thyroid in contrast to the prolonged release which follows injection of serum from a thyrotoxic patient. (Based on Adams D.D. & Purves H.D. (1956) Abnormal responses in the assay of thyrotrophin. *Proceedings of the University of Otago Medical School* **34**, 11.)

to an autoantigen in normal thyroid extracts which was soon identified as thyroglobulin (figure M18.1.2).

In far off New Zealand (depending on your geographical location!), Adams and Purves, in seeking a circulating factor which might be responsible for the hyperthyroidism of Graves' thyrotoxicosis, injected patient's serum into guinea-pigs whose thyroids had been prelabeled with ^{131}I, and followed the release of radiolabeled material from the gland with time. Whereas the natural pituitary thyroid-stimulating

hormone (TSH) produced a peak in serum radioactivity some 4 hours or so after injection of the test animal, serum from thyrotoxic patients had a prolonged stimulatory effect (figure M18.1.3). The so-called *long-acting thyroid stimulator* (LATS) was ultimately shown to be an IgG mimicking TSH through its reaction with the TSH receptor but differing in its time-course of action, largely due to its longer half-life in the circulation.

Overlap of autoimmune disorders

There is a tendency for more than one autoimmune disorder to occur in the same individual and when this happens the association is often between diseases within the same region of the autoimmune spectrum (cf. table 18.1). Thus patients with autoimmune thyroiditis (Hashimoto's disease or primary myxedema) have a much higher incidence of pernicious anemia than would be expected in a random population matched for age and sex (10% as against 0.2%). Conversely, both thyroiditis and Graves' disease are diagnosed in pernicious anemia patients with an unexpectedly high frequency. Other associations are seen between Addison's disease and autoimmune thyroid disease and occur in the rare cases of juveniles with pernicious anemia and polyendocrinopathy which includes Addison's disease, hypoparathyroidism, diabetes and thyroiditis.

There is an even greater overlap in serological findings. Thirty per cent of patients with autoimmune thyroid disease have concomitant parietal cell antibodies in their serum. Conversely, thyroid antibodies have been demonstrated in up to 50% of pernicious anemia patients. It should be stressed that these are not cross-reacting antibodies. The thyroid-specific antibodies will not react with stomach and vice versa. When a serum reacts with both organs it means that two populations of antibodies are present, one with specificity for thyroid and the other for stomach.

At the nonorgan-specific end of the spectrum, systemic autoimmune disease such as SLE is clinically associated with rheumatoid arthritis and several other disorders which are themselves uncommon: hemolytic anemia, idiopathic leukopenia and thrombocytopenic purpura, dermatomyositis and Sjögren's syndrome. Antinuclear antibodies and antiglobulin (rheumatoid) factors are a general feature.

Sjögren's syndrome occupies an interesting position;

Table 18.1. Spectrum of autoimmune diseases.

ORGAN SPECIFIC	
	Hashimoto's thyroiditis
	Primary myxedema
	Graves' disease
	Pernicious anemia
	Autoimmune atrophic gastritis
	Addison's disease
	Premature menopause (few cases)
	Male infertility (few cases)
	Myasthenia gravis
	Lambert–Eaton syndrome
	Insulin-dependent diabetes mellitus
	Goodpasture's syndrome
	Pemphigus vulgaris
	Pemphigoid
	Sympathetic ophthalmia
	Phacogenic uveitis
	Multiple sclerosis
	Autoimmune hemolytic anemia
	Idiopathic thrombocytopenic purpura
	Idiopathic leukopenia
	Primary biliary cirrhosis
	Active chronic hepatitis HBsAg − ve
	Ulcerative colitis
	Sjögren's syndrome
	Rheumatoid arthritis
	Scleroderma
	Wegener's granulomatosis
	Poly/dermatomyositis
	Discoid lupus erythematosus
NONORGAN SPECIFIC	Systemic lupus erythematosus (SLE)

aside from the clinical and serological features associated with systemic disease mentioned above, characteristics of an organ-specific disorder are evident. Antibodies reacting with salivary ducts are demonstrable and there is an abnormally high incidence of thyroid autoantibodies; histologically the affected lacrimal and salivary glands reveal changes of a similar nature to those seen in Hashimoto's disease, namely a replacement of the glandular elements by patchy lymphocytic and plasma cell granulomatous tissue. Associations between diseases at the two ends of the spectrum have been reported, but, as might be predicted from the serological data, they are not common.

Patients with organ-specific disorders are slightly more prone to develop cancer in the affected organ, whereas generalized lymphoreticular neoplasia shows up with uncommon frequency in nonorgan-specific disease.

Animal models of autoimmune disease

Both spontaneous and induced animal models have given tremendous insights into the nature of human autoimmune disease and, to assist our discussions, we felt it would be helpful to list them (table 18.3).

NATURE AND NURTURE

Genetic factors in autoimmune disease

Autoimmune phenomena tend to aggregate in certain families. For example, the first degree relatives (sibs, parents and children) of patients with Hashimoto's disease show a high incidence of thyroid autoantibodies and of overt and subclinical thyroiditis. Parallel studies have disclosed similar relationships in the families of pernicious anemia patients, in that gastric parietal cell antibodies are prevalent in the relatives who are wont to develop achlorhydria and atrophic gastritis. Turning to SLE, the degree of familial clustering measured by comparing the risk of a sibling with the risk in the population as a whole, varies between 20 and 40.

These familial relationships could be ascribed to environmental factors such as infective microorganisms, but there is powerful evidence that important genetic components must be involved. The data on **twins** is unequivocal. When thyrotoxicosis or insulin-dependent diabetes mellitus (IDDM) occurs in twins, there is a far greater concordance rate (i.e. both twins affected) in identical than in nonidentical twins. Second, we have already noted that lines of animals have been bred which spontaneously develop autoimmune disease. In other words, **the autoimmunity is genetically programed**. There is an Obese line of chickens with autoimmune thyroiditis, the Nonobese diabetic (NOD) mouse modeling human IDDM and the New Zealand Black (NZB) strain succumbing to autoimmune hemolytic anemia. The hybrid of NZB with another strain, the New Zealand White (B×W hybrid), actually develops antinuclear antibodies including anti-dsDNA and a fatal immune complex-induced glomerulonephritis, key features of human SLE.

These diseases are **genetically complex**. Genome-wide searches for mapping the genetic intervals containing genes for predisposition to disease by linkage to the many thousand microsatellite markers (polymorphic variable numbers of tandem repeats, VNTR) have so far identified 20 such regions for IDDM in NOD mice and some 25 for murine SLE. Generally speaking, a genetic predisposition to sustained inflammatory responses and loss of tolerance to self are major contributory factors.

Dominant amongst the genetic associations with autoimmune diseases is **linkage to the major histocompatibility complex (MHC)**; of the many examples are the increased risk of IDDM for DQ8 individuals, and the higher incidence of DR3 in Addison's disease and of DR4 in rheumatoid arthritis (table 18.4). Figure 18.2 shows a multiplex family with IDDM in which the

Table 18.2. Autoantibodies in human disease.

DISEASE	ANTIGEN	DETECTION OF IMMUNOLOGICAL REACTIVITY
Hashimoto's thyroiditis	Thyroglobulin	Precipitins; passive hemagglutination; ELISA
Primary myxedema	Thyroid peroxidase: Cytoplasmic	IFT on unfixed thyroid; passive hemagglutination; ELISA
	Cell surface	IFT on viable thyroid cells; C'-mediated cytotoxicity
Graves' disease	Cell surface TSH receptors	Bioassay—stimulation of mouse thyroid *in vivo*; blocking combination TSH with receptors; stimulation adenyl cyclase
	'Growth' receptors	Induction of cell division in thyroid fragments
Pernicious anemia	Intrinsic factor	Neutralization; blocking combination with vit-B_{12}; binding to intrinsic factor-B_{12} by coprecipitation
	Parietal cell H^+–K^+ ATPase	IFT on unfixed gastric mucosa
Addison's disease	Cytoplasm adrenal cells (17α-/21-hydroxylase)	IFT on unfixed adrenal cortex
Premature onset of menopause[1]	Cytoplasm steroid-producing cells	IFT on adrenal and interstitial cells of ovary and testis
Male infertility (some)[2]	Spermatozoa	Sperm agglutination in ejaculate
Insulin-dependent diabetes[3]	Cytoplasm of islet cells	IFT on unfixed human pancreas
	Insulin, GAD and ICA512	ELISA
Type B insulin resistance with acanthosis nigricans	Insulin receptor	Block hormone binding to receptor
Atopic allergy (some)	β-Adrenergic receptor	Blocking radioassay with hydroxybenzylpindolol
Myasthenia gravis	Skeletal and heart muscle	IFT on skeletal muscle
	Acetylcholine receptor	Blocking or binding radioassay with α-bungarotoxin
Lambert–Eaton syndrome	Ca^{2+} channels in nerve endings	IgG produces neuromuscular defects in mice
Multiple sclerosis[4]	Brain incl. MBP	MBP-reactive T-cells
Goodpasture's syndrome	Glomerular and lung basement membrane	Linear staining by IFT of kidney biopsy with fluorescent anti-IgG
		Radioimmunoassay with purified Ag; ELISA
Pemphigus vulgaris	Desmosomes between prickle cells in epidermis (cadherin)	IFT on skin
Pemphigoid	Basement membrane	IFT on skin
Phacogenic uveitis	Lens	Passive hemagglutination
Sympathetic ophthalmia	Uvea	(Delayed skin reaction to uveal extract)
Autoimmune hemolytic anemia[5]	Erythrocytes	Coombs' antiglobulin test
Idiopathic thrombocytopenic purpura	Platelets	Shortened platelet survival *in vivo*
Primary biliary cirrhosis	Mitochondria (pyruvate dehydrogenase)	IFT on mitochondria-rich cells (e.g. distal tubules of kidney)
Active chronic hepatitis (HBV & HCV —ve)	Smooth muscle/nuclear lamins/nuclei	IFT (e.g. on gastric mucosa)
	Kidney/liver microsomes (cyt P450)	IFT (kidney)
Ulcerative colitis	Colon 'lipopolysaccharide'	IFT; passive hemagglutination (cytotoxic action of lymphocytes on colon cells)
	Colon epithelial cell surface protein	ADCC on colon cancer cell line
		Ab data in this disease not universally accepted
Sjögren's syndrome[6]	SS-A(Ro) SS-B(La)	IFT; gel precipitation; ELISA
	Ducts/mitochondria/nuclei/thyroid	IFT
	IgG	Antiglobulin (rheumatoid factor) tests
Rheumatoid arthritis[7]	IgG	Antiglobulin test; latex agglutination; sheep red cell agglutination test (SCAT; commercial product, RAHA test) and ELISA; agalacto-glycoform
	Collagen	Passive hemagglutination
Discoid lupus erythematosus	Nuclear/IgG	IFT/antiglobulin test
Scleroderma[8]	Nuclear/IgG/centromere	IFT
	Nuclear/IgG/Scl-70	IFT; countercurrent electrophoresis; ELISA
Dermatomyositis[9]	Nuclear/IgG/Jo-1	IFT; countercurrent electrophoresis; ELISA
Mixed connective tissue disease[10]	Extractable nuclear	IFT; countercurrent electrophoresis; ELISA
Systemic lupus erythematosus	DNA[11]	ELISA; IFT on Crithidia
	snRNP (Sm & ribonucleoprotein)	IFT; gel precipitation techniques; ELISA
	Nucleoprotein	IFT
	Array of other Ag including formed elements of blood/IgG	
	Cardiolipin/β2-glycoprotein1	Radioimmunoassay
Wegener's granulomatosis	Neutrophil cytoplasm (ANCA; myeloperoxidase/serine proteinase)[12]	IFT on alcohol fixed polymorphs; ELISA

IFT, immunofluorescent test (cf. figure 18.1). ELISA, enzyme-linked immunosorbent assay (cf. figure 6.30).

disease is closely linked to a particular HLA haplotype. Another pointer to the central role of class II structure in determining T-cell responsiveness to self derives from the inability of the NOD mouse to develop pancreatic autoimmunity when just a single amino acid residue in the α-helix of the H-2 β chain is altered by introduction of a transgene. The close relationship to MHC is not altogether unexpected given that, as we shall see, autoimmune diseases are T-cell dependent and most T-cell responses are MHC restricted.

Amongst the plethora of non-MHC-linked loci may be genes responsible for the editorial control of rearranged Ig variable region genes encoding high avidity anti-DNA. Others may control the pattern of cytokine secretion affecting the milieu in early SLE which permits polyclonal B-cell activation, or influence the balance of Th1/Th2 subsets which could enhance susceptibility to IDDM or lead to resistance in otherwise predisposed subjects. Mice lacking the *p21* gene, which is a cell cycle regulator in the immune system, develop antibodies to dsDNA and other features of SLE. The gene maps within a recently defined MHC susceptibility locus with strong evidence for disease linkage. A mutation in the *IL-2* gene not affecting its functional ability to produce proliferation may be a candidate for *Idd-3* contributing to spontaneous diabetes in the NOD mouse. Polymorphism at a candidate locus identified in more than one autoimmune disease is interesting, a good example being *CTLA-4*, recently linked to IDDM and Graves' disease (figure 18.3). CTLA-4 mediates antigen-specific apoptosis capable of clonally deleting previously activated T-cells, and other 'apoptotic genes' such as *Fas*, *FasL* and *Bcl-2* are all involved in different autoimmune disorders. With so many cells dying naturally from apoptosis, it is clearly desirable for them to be immunologically inert, a state that may be achieved by the activation of transglutaminase which causes protein cross-linking and increased phagocytic removal.

Appropriate breeding experiments disclose that the genes predisposing to aggressive autoimmunity, on the one hand, are distinct from those which determine which autoantigens are involved, on the other. The **'autoimmunity genes'** contribute the common element underlying the overlaps in autoantibodies and disease discussed above, although within this group the genes which predispose to organ-specific disease must be different from those in nonorgan-specific disorders (as judged by the minimal overlap between them).

Notes to table 18.2

1 Antibodies occur in the minority of patients with associated Addison's disease of the adrenal and are directed to the 17α/21-hydroxylase, the cholesterol side-chain cleavage enzyme and a 51 kDa gonadal antigen.

2 Only a small percentage show agglutinins. Spermatozoa may be agglutinated head to head, tail to tail or joined through their midpiece. Seen also in a small percentage of infertile women.

3 Most if not all insulin-dependent diabetics have islet cell antibodies at some stage during the first year of onset but these tend to decline progressively. In contrast, islet cell antibodies in diabetic patients with an associated autoimmune polyendocrinopathy persist for many years. GAD (glutamic acid decarboxylase) Ab also occur in Stiff man syndrome. ICA512 is a protein tyrosine kinase.

4 MBP, myelin basic protein.

5 The Coombs' test involves the demonstration of bound antibody on the washed red cell by agglutination with an antiglobulin (cf. figure 15.17). Erythrocyte autoantibodies, which bind well over the temperature range 0–37°C ('warm' Ab), are mostly IgG; approximately 60% of cases are primary, the remainder being associated with other autoimmune disorders, e.g. SLE and ulcerative colitis. 'Cold' Ab, which react best over the range 0–20°C, are mostly IgM, and red cells coated with this Ab can often be agglutinated by anticomplement serum; approximately half are primary, the others being associated with *Mycoplasma pneumoniae* infection or generalized neoplastic disease of the lymphoreticular tissues.

6 Antibodies specifically reacting with the epithelium of salivary gland excretory ducts are demonstrable by immunofluorescence in over half the cases of secondary Sjögren's associated with RA or SLE. SS-A and SS-B antibodies give a speckled nuclear fluorescence pattern.

7 The main antiglobulin factors react with the Fc portion of IgG which is usually adsorbed on to latex particles (human IgG) or present in an antigen–antibody complex (sheep red cells coated with a subagglutinating dose of rabbit antibody). In the ELISA test, rabbit IgG is bound to a plastic tube, patient's serum added and the antiglobulin bound assessed by subsequent binding of labeled anti-human IgG or IgM (cf. figure 6.30). Rheumatoid factors specific for human IgG can be detected by this test using human Fcγ to coat the tubes and labeled anti-human Fdγ (the portion of the heavy chain in the Fab fragment) or IgM for the final stage.

8 In scleroderma (progressive systemic sclerosis) antinucleolar antibodies are frequently found. Scl-70 is topoisomerase 1.

9 Jo-1 is histidine tRNA synthetase.

10 This syndrome combines features of scleroderma, RA, SLE and dermatomyositis. The antigens are extractable from the nucleus and give a speckled fluorescence pattern.

11 Antibodies to single- or double-stranded DNA are assayed by a DNA-coated tube test.

12 Component of primary granule, probably serine proteinase III, gives cytoplasmic staining. In periarteritis nodosa, antibodies to myeloperoxidase give perinuclear staining in alcohol-fixed polymorphonuclear neutrophils (PMNs). Some sera react with azurocidin, a potent antibiotic. ANCA (antineutrophil cytoplasmic antibody) directed against bactericidal/permeability increasing protein is a marker for inflammatory bowel disease and primary sclerosing cholangitis.

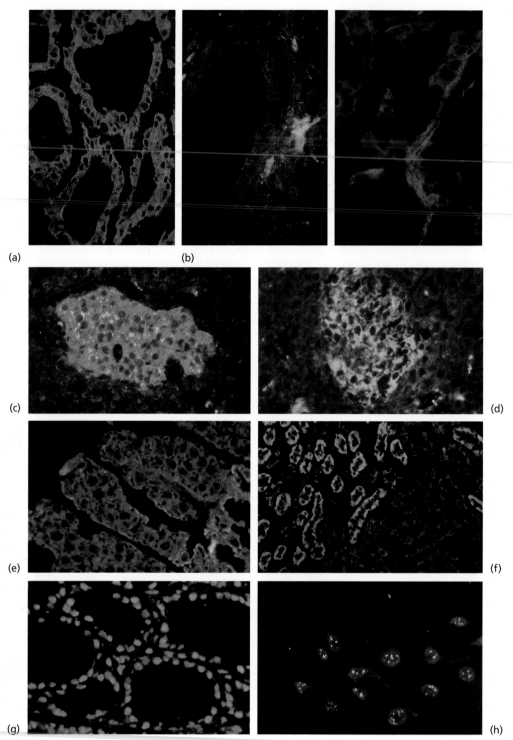

Figure 18.1. Fluorescent antibody studies in autoimmune diseases.
(a) Thyroid peroxidase (thyroid microsomal) antibodies staining cytoplasm of acinar cells. (b) Human thyroid sections stained for MHC class II: *left*—normal thyroid with unstained follicular cells and an isolated strongly MHC class II-positive dendritic cell; *right*—Graves' disease (thyrotoxic) thyroid with abundant cytoplasmic MHC class II indicative of active synthesis. (c) Fluorescence of cells in the pancreatic islets of Langerhans' stained with serum from insulin-dependent diabetic. (d) The same, showing cells stained simultaneously for somatostatin (the yellow cells are stained with rhodamine anti-somatostatin and fluorescein anti-human IgG which localizes the patient's bound autoantibody). (e) Serum of patient with Addison's disease staining cytoplasm of monkey adrenal granulosa cells. (f) Fluorescence of distal tubular cells of the kidney after reaction with mitochondrial autoantibodies. (g) Diffuse nuclear staining on a thyroid section obtained with nucleoprotein antibodies from a SLE patient. (h) Serum of a scleroderma patient staining the nucleoli of SV40-transformed human keratinocytes (K14) in monolayer culture. ((a), (c), (d), (e), (f) and (g) kindly provided by Prof. F. Bottazzo; (b) by Professor R. Pujol-Borrell; and (h) by Dr F.T. Wojnarowska.)

Table 18.3. Spontaneous and induced animal models of autoimmune disease.

		MODEL	AUTOIMMUNE DISEASE
ORGAN-SPECIFIC	SPONTANEOUS	Nonobese diabetic (NOD) mouse; BB rat NOD.H2^{h4} congenic Obese strain (OS) chicken; Buffalo rat	Insulin-dependent diabetes *Thyroiditis Thyroiditis
	INDUCED	**Complete Freund's adjuvant (CFA) incorporating brain CFA incorporating thyroid, adrenal, sperm, type II collagen, ACh-R, retinal S1 protein or g.b.m. Mouse bearing IFN-γ-insulin promoter transgene Cross reaction: heterologous with autologous r.b.c. Coxsackie B with myosin Thymectomy in 2–4 day old mice Neonatal thymectomy + X-irradiation in rats HgCl$_2$ in rats	Autoimmune encephalomyelitis Destruction of cell/tissue bearing relevant antigen Diabetes Anemia Myocarditis Widespread organ-specific Thyroiditis 'Goodpasture's'
SYSTEMIC	SPONTANEOUS	New Zealand Black (NZB) mouse strain NZB x W, BXSB p21 Knockout mouse MRL/*lpr* Motheaten mouse strain	Autoimmune hemolytic anemia SLE SLE SLE, arthritis Widespread fatal systemic disease
	INDUCED	Parent bone marrow into F1 mice CFA incorporating anti-DNA idiotype CFA incorporating TB hsp	G.v.h., pseudo SLE SLE Adjuvant arthritis

*Fed high iodine diet.

**Antigen emulsified in water/oil mixture containing killed tubercle bacilli or derivative.

ACh-R, acetyl choline receptor; r.b.c., erythrocytes; g.b.m., glomerular basement membrane.

Table 18.4. Association of HLA with autoimmune disease.

DISEASE	HLA ALLELE	RELATIVE RISK
a Class II associated		
Hashimoto's disease	DR5	3.2
Primary myxedema	DR3	5.7
Graves' disease	DR3	3.7
Insulin-dependent diabetes mellitus	DQ8	14
	DQ2 + DQ8	20
	DQ6	0.2
Addison's disease	DR3	6.3
Goodpasture's syndrome	DR2	13.1
Rheumatoid arthritis	DR4	5.8
Sjögren's syndrome	DR3	9.7
Autoimmune hepatitis	DR3	13.9
Multiple sclerosis	DR2	3
Narcolepsy	DR2	130
Dematitis herpetiformis	DR3	17
Celiac disease	DR3 + DR7	7
b Class I associated		
Ankylosing spondylitis	B27	87.4
Anterior uveitis	B27	14.6
Amyloidosis in rheumatoid arthritis	B27	8.2
Psoriasis vulgaris	Cw6	8
Myasthenia gravis	B8	3

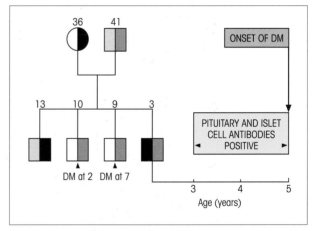

Figure 18.2. HLA haplotype linkage and onset of insulin-dependent diabetes (DM). Haplotypes: ☐ A3, B14, DR6; ■ A3, B7, DR4; ▨ A28, B51, DR4; and ▨ A2, B62, C3, DR4. Disease is linked to possession of the A2, B62, C3, DR4 haplotype. The 3-year-old brother had complement-fixing antibodies to the islet cell surface for 2 years before developing frank diabetes indicative of the lengthy pathological process preceding disease. (Data provided by Prof. G.F. Bottazzo.)

Evidence for '**autoantigen and tissue selection**' genes derives not only from breeding experiments with NZB×W mice showing separate control of red cell and nuclear antibodies, but also from genetic analysis of Obese chickens which has delineated an influence of the MHC, abnormalities in regulatory T-cell control *and a*

defect in the thyroid gland expressed as an abnormally high uptake of [131]I. Unlike normal thyroid cells, Hashimoto thyrocytes in culture display Fas molecules on their surface and, since FasL is constitutively expressed, this leads of course to mutual apoptotic homicidal death. However, since destruction of the gland during the course of disease is a prolonged process, it seems likely that, *in vivo*, this catastrophic sce-

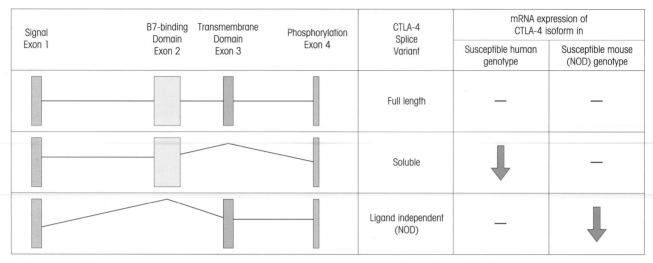

Figure 18.3. CTLA-4 linked single nucleotide polymorphism associated with autoimmune disease. The CT60 SNP variant in the noncoding 6.1 kb 3′ region of *CTLA-4* is responsible for the association of autoimmune disease with lower messenger RNA levels of the soluble splice forms of *CTLA-4*. (Data adapted from Ueda H. *et al. Nature* 2003, **423**, 506).

nario may be tempered by anti-apoptotic factors such as bcl-2. In the family studies described above (figure 18.2), there must be additional genes which are organ-related, in that relatives of patients with pernicious anemia are more prone to gastric autoimmunity than are members of Hashimoto kindreds. Further to this point, analysis has mapped the *IDDM-2* diabetes susceptibility gene to a VNTR lying 5′ to the insulin gene, which affects the transcriptional activity for insulin production and influences the level of thymic expression of insulin during a critical period in the development of self-tolerance. Susceptible strains have a low level of *thymic* but a high level of *pancreatic* insulin mRNA compared with their resistant counterparts which could foster the insulin autoreactivity often seen in the early stages of IDDM. Indeed, quite unexpectedly, it does look as though mRNA for a number of 'organ-specific' antigens can be detected in the fetal thymus and their expression is controlled by the *Aire* protein transcription factor, an E3 ubiquitin ligase present at high concentration in medullary thymic epithelial cells. Mutations in the *Aire* gene give rise to faulty negative selection of thymic organ-specific lymphocytes linked to the autoimmune polyendocrinopathy syndrome type I alluded to above, and knockout mice develop organ-specific autoimmunity so tying the threads together in a very satisfactory manner. Mutations in yet another transcription factor, Foxp3, which controls the differentiation of Tregs (cf. p. 217), lead to a common set of autoimmune conditions including IDDM and thyroiditis in mice (X-linked *scurfy* mutation) and humans (IPEX syndrome).

Unraveling complex polygenic conditions is a very tough assignment. If we may take murine

SLE as archetypal, genetic analysis of the predisposition to disease is most compatible with a threshold liability model requiring additive, or epistatic, contributions of multiple susceptibility genes probably linked to different stages of disease pathogenesis (figure 18.4).

Hormonal influences in autoimmunity

There is a general trend for autoimmune disease to occur far more frequently in women than in men (figure 18.5) probably due, in essence, to differences in hormonal patterns. There is a suggestion that higher estrogen levels are found in patients and administration of male hormones to mice with SLE reduces the severity of disease. Pregnancy is often associated with amelioration of disease severity, particularly in rheumatoid arthritis (RA), and there is sometimes a striking relapse after giving birth, a time at which there are drastic changes in hormones such as prolactin, not forgetting the loss of the placenta. We should also note the frequent development of postpartum hypothyroidism in women with pre-existing thyroid autoimmunity.

In Chapter 10, we dwelt on the importance of the neuroendocrine immune feedback encompassing the cytokine–hypothalamic–pituitary–adrenal control circuit. Abnormalities in this feedback loop have now been revealed in several autoimmune disorders. Patients with mild RA have lower corticosteroid levels than normals or patients with osteoarthritis or osteomyelitis despite the presence of inflammation. Moreover, RA patients undergoing surgery manifest grossly inadequate cortisol secretion in the face of high

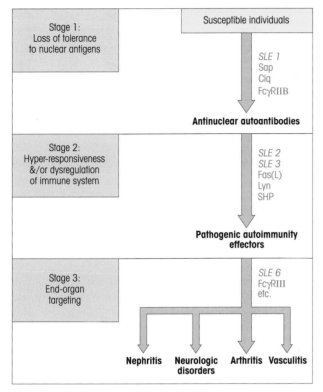

Figure 18.4. Possible stages in development of SLE in susceptible individuals. Genes or gene products are in red. A variety of genes are involved in end-organ targeting. Epistatic interactions between *SLE 1* and *3*, derived from the NZW strain, produce severe lupus when introduced together into an otherwise resistant B6 strain as a double congenic, even though neither alone causes severe disease. The NZW strain itself, which contains both genes, is resistant to disease because it has a genetic suppressor region, four of which have been identified in various murine lupus strains.

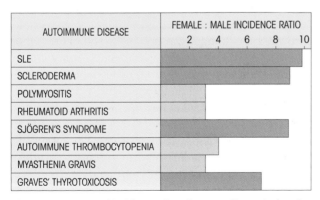

Figure 18.5. Increased incidence of autoimmune disease in females.

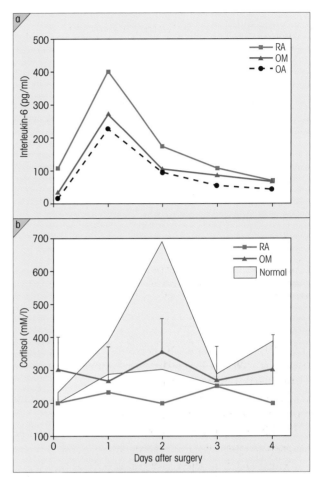

Figure 18.6. Failure of feedback control of cortisol production in rheumatoid arthritis (RA). After surgery (a) RA patients have even higher levels of plasma IL-6 than osteoarthritis (OA) and osteomyelitis (OM) controls. Nonetheless, (b) they have profoundly deficient production of cortisol which is evidence of faulty feedback control. (Data kindly provided by Professor G. Panayi from Chikanza I.C. *et al.* (1992) Defective hypothalamic response to immune and inflammatory stimuli in patients with rheumatoid arthritis. *Arthritis and Rheumatism* **35**, 1281, with permission from the publishers.)

steroid-induced apoptosis. This would imply that the feedback cycle is not operating at the lymphocyte level and could cause dysregulated immune function; the ability of IL-1 injections to delay the onset of diabetes would accord with this view.

Does the environment contribute?

Twin studies

Although the 50% concordance rate for the development of the autoimmune disease insulin-dependent diabetes mellitus (IDDM) in identical twins is considerably higher than that in dizygotic twins and suggests a strong genetic element, there is still 50% unaccounted for. This is not necessarily all due to environment, since although monozygotic twins have identical germ-line

levels of plasma IL-1 and IL-6 (figure 18.6), a phenomenon now attributed to defective hypothalamic control. The OS chicken, several strains of lupus mice and the Lewis rat, which is abnormally susceptible to the induction of autoimmunity, all show blunted IL-1-induced corticosteroid responses. Both T- and B-cells from NOD mice survive for abnormally long periods in culture and their thymocytes are relatively resistant to cortico-

immunoglobulin and T-cell receptor (TCR) genes, the processes of diversification of receptors and of internal anti-idiotype interactions are so complex that the resulting receptor repertoires will be extremely variable and unlikely to be identical. Nonetheless, a later study on concordance rates for IDDM in monozygotic twins gave the extraordinarily high figure of 70% if they were DR3/DR4 heterozygotes, but only 40% if they were not. Thus, in the same disease, the genetic element can be almost completely dominant or be a significant but minor factor in determining the outcome. As we turn to the nonorgan-specific diseases, such as SLE, we find an even lower genetic contribution with a concordance rate of only 23% in same-sex monozygotic twins, compared with 9% in same-sex dizygotic twins. There are also many examples where clinically unaffected relatives of patients with SLE have a higher incidence of nuclear autoantibodies if they are household contacts than if they live apart from the proband. However, within a given home, the spouse is less likely to develop autoantibodies than blood relatives. Summing up, in some disorders the major factors are genetic, whereas in others environmental influences seem to dominate.

Nonmicrobial factors

What environmental agents can we identify? Diet could be one—fish oils containing long-chain, highly polyunsaturated ω-3 fatty acids are reputed to be beneficial for patients with RA; someone must know whether rheumatologists in Greenland are underworked! Sunshine is an undisputed trigger of the skin lesions in SLE. Exposure to organic solvents can initiate the basement membrane autoimmunity which results in Goodpasture's syndrome—witness the high incidence of this disease in HLA-DR2 individuals who work in dry-cleaning shops or siphon petrol from other people's petrol tanks. A more contrived situation is the production of a similar disease in Brown Norway rats by the injection of mercuric chloride, but it makes its point, and there are several drug-induced diseases such as SLE, myasthenia gravis, autoimmune hemolytic anemia, and so on.

Microbes

Of course everyone's favorite environmental agent has to be an infectious microorganism and we do have some clear-cut examples of autoimmune disease following infection, usually in genetically predisposed individuals: acute rheumatic fever follows group A streptococcal pharyngitis in 2–3% of patients with a hereditary susceptibility and B3 coxsackie virus produces autoimmune myositis in certain mouse strains.

In most cases of human chronic autoimmune disease, the problem is the long latency period which makes it difficult to track down the initiating event (cf. figure 18.2) and, secondly, viable organisms usually cannot be isolated from the affected tissues.

There has been a breakthrough in the HLA-B27-related **reactive arthritis** provoked by infection with *Chlamydia*, *Yersinia* or *Salmonella*, in that T-cell responses to bacterial fragments or perhaps to cross-reacting self-epitopes present in affected joints can now be demonstrated years after the primary infection. These studies and the ability of EB virus and *Chlamydia* DNA probes to hybridize to a not insignificant proportion of synovial tissues from rheumatoid arthritis patients raises important questions regarding the cellular localization and molecular status of the 'microbial' nucleic acid in these cells.

Further complexity is injected by the knowledge that environmental microbes may sometimes **protect** against spontaneous autoimmune disease; the incidence of diabetes is greatly increased if NOD mice are kept in specific pathogen-free conditions, while Sendai virus inhibits the development of arthritis in the MRL/*lpr* strain. The extraordinary variation in incidence of diabetes in NOD colonies bred in a wide variety of different animal houses (figure 18.7) testifies to the dramatic influence of environmental flora on the expression of autoimmune disease.

AUTOREACTIVITY COMES NATURALLY

Tolerance mechanisms do not destroy all self-reactive lymphocytes. Processing of an autoantigen will lead to certain (dominant) peptides being preferentially expressed on *a*ntigen-*p*resenting *c*ells (APCs) while others (cryptic) only appear in the MHC groove in very low concentrations which, although capable of expanding their cognate T-cells in the context of thymic positive selection (cf. p. 234), may nonetheless fail to provide a sufficiently powerful signal for negative selection of these cells. As a consequence, autoreactive T-cells specific for **cryptic epitopes** will survive in the repertoire which will therefore be biased towards weak self-reactivity.

Because conventional B-2 cells are less susceptible than T-cells to tolerization by low concentrations of circulating autoantigens such as thyroglobulin (figure 11.16), autoreactive B-cells specific for such antigens will circulate albeit unaccompanied by their cognate helper T-cells (figure 11.17) despite the mechanism of receptor editing which eliminates many naturally occurring autoreactive B-cells through continued V(D)J recombination. The reader will also recall the B-1 cell population, which starts off early in life by forming a network connected by germ-line idiotypes. The cells are

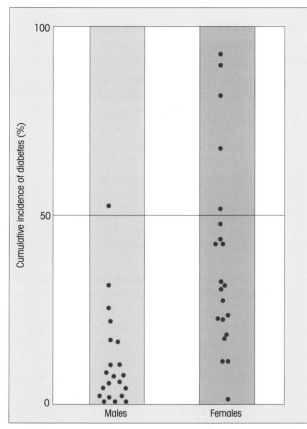

Figure 18.7. The incidence of spontaneous diabetes in geographically dispersed colonies of NOD mice at 20 weeks of age. Each point represents a single colony. The extreme spread of values is not attributable to genetic drift to any significant extent. The lower incidence in males is particularly evident. (Data adapted from Pozzilli P., Signore A., Williams A.J.K. & Beales P.E. (1993) NOD mouse colonies around the world. *Immunology Today* **14**, 193.)

stimulated, presumably by T-independent type 2 idiotypic interactions, to produce so-called '**natural antibodies**', a term applied to those serum antibodies thought to be present before external antigen challenge and therefore arising independently of conventional antigen stimulation. These are germ-line antibodies, mostly IgM, although a proportion belong to the IgG and IgA classes. They include a basic set of autoantibodies with low affinity reactivity for multiple specificities and cross-reactivity with common bacterial antigens usually of a carbohydrate nature. One can see this as a strategy which ensures that preliminary excitation of cells by these internal network interactions will provide bacterial protection, especially since the polymeric nature of the carbohydrate antigens ensures that the IgM antibodies, even though of low affinity, can bind with high avidity to the microbes.

These natural antibodies might also act as transporting agents responsible for scavenging effete body components or as regulators which actually prevent stimulation of autoreactive cells in the conventional B-2 cell population either by masking autoantigen epitopes or by overall idiotype regulation. The latter view receives some encouragement from a report that the IgM fraction of normal serum can block binding of autologous IgG F(ab')$_2$ fragments to a range of autoantigens. These natural autoantibodies presumably make a contribution to the so-called 'nonspecific' Ig binding of otherwise normal sera to test autoantigens, but slightly stronger reactions are evident in a small proportion of younger people and the incidence increases with age. Although not associated with clinically apparent tissue damage, it should be noted that, in the case of the thyroid and stomach at least, biopsy has linked the presence of raised titers of antibody, especially of the IgG class, with minor thyroiditis or gastritis lesions (as the case may be), and postmortem examination has identified 10% of clinically normal middle-aged women with significant but limited degrees of lymphadenoid change in the thyroid, similar in essence to that characteristic of Hashimoto's disease.

As enthusiasts for symmetry and order might have predicted, there appears to be an analogous T-cell population, of phenotype CD3$^+$ CD4$^-$8$^-$ bearing the B-cell marker B220, containing large internally activated cells which react strongly with self-T-cells and are expanded in early life. It is possible that they connect to the CD5$^+$ B-cell network through idiotype interactions with cells of this lineage present in the thymus. The reader may be surprised to learn that, in generating T-cell lines, it is not an uncommon experience to isolate cells which proliferate and release IL-2 in response to autologous class II-positive feeder cells; even allowing for the fact that the presence of these feeders in the cultures will tend to select for such autoreactive cells, it would not have been predicted that cells with these specificities would be permitted to roam around freely in the body unless constrained in some way. In this connection it has been suggested that there is an 'immunological homunculus' in which dominant autoantigens in the body are imprinted on the immune system and the T-cells which recognize them are heavily controlled by regulatory T-cells (cf. p. 216).

Although precursors of the effector cells of autoimmune disease are present in normal individuals, abnormal conditions must be required for their stimulation. In experimental models of organ-specific disease, such as that induced in the thyroid by injection of thyroglobulin in complete Freund's adjuvant, the effector T-cells and the plasma cells making high affinity IgG autoantibodies are generated in normal animals. Complete Freund's will not produce antibodies to double-stranded DNA, Sm or other autoantigens typical of nonorgan-specific disorders and this may be telling us that the relevant antigen-specific helper T-cells are not available in the normal repertoire. However, if T-cells are stimulated by radically different approaches, nonorgan-specific antibodies can be coaxed out of normal animals; in one system, allogeneic T-cells inducing a graft-vs-host (g.v.h.) reaction are stimulated by, and thence polyclonally activate, class II-bearing B-cells, while another involves immunization with a public anti-DNA idiotype (16/6) in complete Freund's.

IS AUTOIMMUNITY DRIVEN BY ANTIGEN?

This is not such a silly question as it might appear since lymphocytes can be stimulated not only by antigens but also by anti-idiotypes and by superantigens as well as other polyclonal activators. And if the answer is in the affirmative, is the self-molecule an autoimmunogen or just an autoantigen, i.e. does it drive the autoimmune response or is it merely recognized by its products?

Organ-specific disease

First, some direct evidence straight from the shoulder. The Obese strain (OS) chicken spontaneously develops precipitating IgG autoantibodies to thyroglobulin and a chronic inflammatory antithyroid response which destroys the gland so causing hypothyroidism. If the source of antigen is removed by neonatal thyroidectomy, no autoantibodies are formed. Injection of these animals with normal thyroglobulin then induces antibodies. Thyroidectomy of OS chickens with established thyroiditis is followed by a dramatic fall in antibody titer. Conclusions: the spontaneous antithyroglobulin immunity is initiated and maintained by autoantigen from the thyroid gland. Furthermore, since the response is completely T-cell dependent, we can infer that both B- and T-cells are driven by thyroglobulin in this model. An entirely parallel study in NOD mice showed that destruction of the β-cells in the pancreas by alloxan switched off the stimulus to autoantibody production.

As usual, human disease is a tougher nut to crack and one has to rely on more indirect evidence. T-cell lines have been established from thyrotoxic glands and it has been possible to show direct stimulation by whole thyroid cells. Removal of the putative antigen source by thyroidectomy of Hashimoto patients is followed by a fall in serum γ-globulins, one of the clues which led to the discovery of thyroid autoimmunity (cf. Milestone 18.1); incidentally, this accords well with the data from OS chickens quoted above. The production of high affinity IgG autoantibodies accompanied by somatic mutation is taken as powerful evidence for the selection of B-cells by antigen in a T-dependent response. The

reason for this, simply, is that high affinity IgG antibodies only arise through mutation and selection by antigen within germinal centers (cf. p. 205). Suffice it to say that ample evidence for somatic mutation and high affinity antibodies has been reported. More indirect is the argument that, when antibodies are regularly formed against a cluster of epitopes on a single molecule (e.g. thyroglobulin) or of antigens within a single organ (e.g. thyroglobulin plus thyroid peroxidase), it is difficult to propose a hypothesis which does not depend finally on stimulation by antigen.

Systemic autoimmunity

The question is even harder to answer here, particularly since antigen removal is impossible. With respect to B-cells, the same arguments marshaled for organ-specific disease obtain, i.e. high affinity mutated IgG autoantibodies directed often to antigen clusters such as the constituents of the nucleosome. (Readers who like delving into mechanisms should consult figure 18.10b.5 and then figure 18.11c to follow the manner in which an activated B-cell, specific for one component in a complex, can present epitopes on a second constituent of the same complex to an activated T-helper.)

T-cells are critical for such responses and, indeed, depletion of CD4 T-cells in NZB or NZB×W mice abrogates autoantibody production. Fine so far, but from there on we are in black box territory since we are woefully ignorant of the antigen specificity of the T-cells. So much so that more radical hypotheses are tendered. One of these postulates that we are really dealing with T-helper responses to the antigenic legacy of an earlier microbial infection (see above). Another view which has been seriously mooted is that the T-cells do not see conventional antigen at all, clearly the case with DNA responses, but instead are devoted to the recognition of idiotype; SLE for example would be an **'idiotype disease'** resulting from network breakdown. Conceivably, the network may break down spontaneously or be 'hacked' into by microbes (cf. figure 18.12). We may notice that immunization of mice with monoclonal autoantibodies to DNA, ribonucleoprotein (RNP) and Sm has stimulated production of the corresponding antibody bearing the original idiotype; this must have involved an internal network.

Is autoantigen available to the lymphocytes?

Our earliest view, with respect to organ-specific antibodies at least, was that the antigens were sequestered within the organ, and through lack of contact with the lymphoreticular system failed to establish immunological tolerance. Any mishap which caused a release of the antigen would then provide an opportunity for autoantibody formation. For a few body constituents this holds true, and in the case of sperm, lens and heart for example, release of certain components directly into the circulation can provoke autoantibodies. But, in general, the experience has been that injection of *unmodified* extracts of those tissues concerned in the organ-specific autoimmune disorders does not readily elicit antibody formation. Indeed, detailed investigation of the thyroid autoantigen, thyroglobulin, has disclosed that it is not completely sequestered within the gland but gains access to the extracellular fluid around the follicles and reaches the circulation via the thyroid lymphatics (figure 18.8). Even in the brain, the ability of systemically injected T-cell clones specific for myelin basic protein to induce encephalitis (cf. p. 443) reveals the exposure of the target antigen. In fact, in the majority of cases—e.g. red cells in autoimmune hemolytic anemia, RNP and nucleosome components present as blebs on the surface of apoptotic cells in SLE, and surface receptors in many cases of organ-specific autoimmunity—the autoantigens are readily accessible to circulating lymphocytes.

Presumably, antigens present at adequate concentrations in the extracellular fluid will be processed by professional APCs, but for autoantigens associated with cells, the derivative peptides will only interact 'meaningfully' with specific T-cells if there are appropriate MHC surface molecules, if the concentration of processed peptide associated with them is significant and, for resting T-cells, if costimulatory signals can be given. As we shall see, these are important constraints.

CONTROL OF THE T-HELPER CELL IS PIVOTAL

The message then is that we are all sitting on a minefield of self-reactive cells, with potential access to their respective autoantigens, but since autoimmune disease is more the exception than the rule, the body has homeostatic mechanisms to prevent them being triggered under normal circumstances. Accepting its limitations,

figure 18.9 provides a framework for us to examine ways in which these mechanisms may be circumvented to allow autoimmunity to develop. It is assumed that the key to the system is control of the autoreactive T-helper cell since the evidence heavily favors the T-dependence of virtually all autoimmune responses; thus, interaction between the T-cell and MHC-associated peptide becomes the core consideration. We start with the assumption that these cells are normally unresponsive because of clonal deletion, clonal anergy, T-suppression or inadequate autoantigen presentation. Immediately, one could conceive of an *abnormal* degree of responsiveness to self-antigens as a result of relatively low

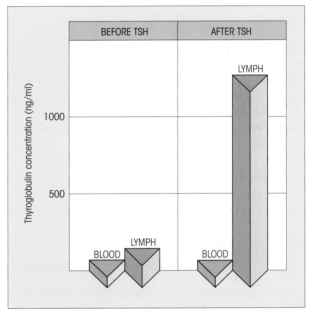

Figure 18.8. Thyroglobulin in the cervical lymph draining the thyroid in the rat. The concentration of thyroglobulin is increased after injection of pituitary thyroid-stimulating hormone (TSH), showing that the release from thyroid follicles is linked to the physiological activity of the acinar cells. Colloid is taken up at the apical margin and thyroglobulin cleaved proteolytically to thyroid hormones which are released together with undegraded protein from the base of the cell. (From Daniel P.N., Pratt D.E., Roitt I.M. & Torrigiani G. (1967) *Quarterly Journal of Experimental Physiology* **52**, 184.)

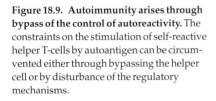

Figure 18.9. Autoimmunity arises through bypass of the control of autoreactivity. The constraints on the stimulation of self-reactive helper T-cells by autoantigen can be circumvented either through bypassing the helper cell or by disturbance of the regulatory mechanisms.

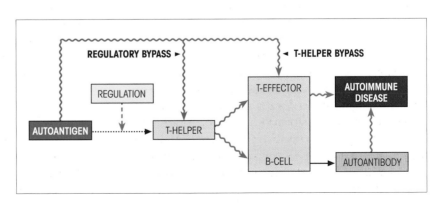

intrathymic expression of a particular molecule (cf. p. 418). Abnormalities in the signaling pathways affecting the thresholds for positive and negative selection in the thymus would also affect subsequent responsiveness to peripheral autoantigens. So might defects in apoptotic cell death. It would be interesting to know whether the innate resistance of the NZB mouse to tolerization by a protein antigen such as bovine serum albumin can be nailed to one of these causes or whether it is a consequence of defects in regulatory cells (see below).

AUTOIMMUNITY CAN ARISE THROUGH BYPASS OF T-HELPERS

Provision of new carrier determinant

Allison and Weigle argued independently that, if autoreactive T-cells are tolerized and thereby unable to collaborate with B-cells to generate autoantibodies (figures 18.10a and 18.13), provision of new carrier determinants to which no self-tolerance had been established would bypass this mechanism and lead to autoantibody production (figures 18.10b and 18.13).

1 Modification of the autoantigen

A new carrier could arise through post-translational modification to the molecule (figure 18.10b.1), seen for example in the low galactosylation of Fcγ sugar chains and citrullination of vimentin in rheumatoid arthritis. Iodination of thyroglobulin may create important T-cell neo-epitopes since the fetal protein lacks iodine and it is of interest that the severity of autoimmune thyroiditis is ameliorated in Obese strain chickens when the birds are put on a low iodine diet.

Modification can also be achieved through combination with a drug (figure 18.10b.3). In one example of many, the autoimmune hemolytic anemia associated with administration of α-methyldopa might be attributable to modification of the red cell surface in such a way as to provide a carrier for stimulating B-cells which recognize the rhesus antigen. This is normally regarded as a 'weak' antigen and would be less likely to induce B-cell tolerance than the 'stronger' antigens present on the erythrocyte.

2 Cross-reactions with B-cell epitopes

Many examples are known in which potential human autoantigenic B-cell epitopes are present on a microbial exogenous cross-reacting antigen which provides the new carrier that provokes autoantibody formation (figure 18.10b.2). The mechanism is spelt out in more detail in figure 18.11a. Two low molecular weight envelope proteins of *Yersinia enterolytica* share epitopes with the extracellular domain of the human thyroid-stimulating hormone (TSH) receptor; in rheumatic

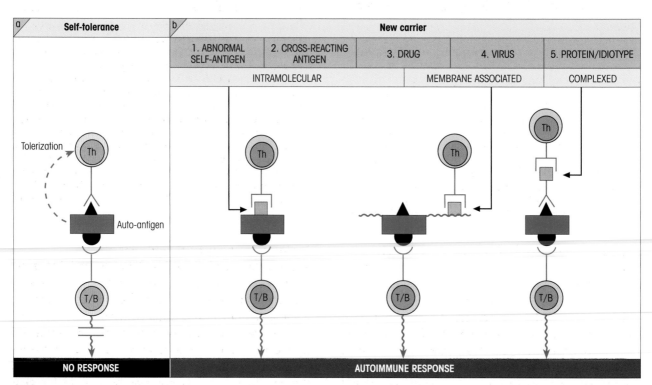

Figure 18.10. T-helper bypass through new carrier epitope (▢) generates autoimmunity. For simplicity, processing for MHC association has been omitted from the diagram, but is elaborated in figure 18.11. (a) The pivotal autoreactive T-helper is unresponsive either through tolerance or inability to see a cryptic epitope. (b) Different mechanisms providing a new carrier epitope.

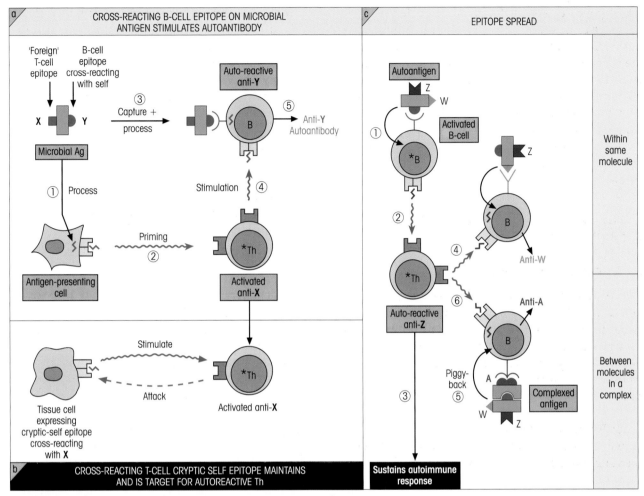

Figure 18.11. Mechanisms of microbial induction of autoimmunity and epitope spread. (This is a complex mouthful but digestion is recommended because these ideas are crucial. The more faint-hearted may require an ice-pack and persistence, but following the numbers should help.) (a) A microbial antigen bearing an epitope Y which cross-reacts with self and a foreign T-cell epitope X is (1) processed by an antigen-presenting cell, (2) activates the T-helper which (3) recognizes the processed X after capture by an anti-Y B-cell and (4) stimulates the B-cell to secrete anti-Y autoantibody. (b) The *activated* anti-X T-helper, as distinct from the *resting* cell, may recognize and be stimulated by a cross-reacting cryptic T-cell epitope expressed by a tissue cell. This will maintain the autoimmune response even after elimination of the microbe, because of the persistence of the self-epitope. The tissue expressing the epitope will also be a target for immunological attack. Note also that a T-helper primed nonspecifically by a polyclonal super-

antigen activator could also fulfil the same function of responding to a cryptic epitope. (c) If the autoantigen is soluble or capable of uptake and processing after capture by the activated autoreactive B-cell (1) (either from (a) or through nonspecific polyclonal activation), a new epitope can be presented on the B-cell class II which now stimulates an autoreactive (anti-Z) T-helper (2) which can now sustain an autoimmune response entirely through autoantigen stimulation (3). It can also produce epitope spread within the same molecule through helping a B-cell which captures the autoantigen through a new epitope W (4). It can also permit epitope spread to another component in an intermolecular complex such as nucleosomal histone–DNA or idiotype-positive (Id$^+$) anti-DNA–DNA which is 'piggy-backed' into the B-cell (5) which presents processed antigen to the T-helper (6) in the cases cited, specific for histone or Id, respectively. *Denotes activation.

fever, antibodies produced to the *Streptococcus* also react with heart, and the sera of 50% of children with the disease who develop Sydenham's chorea give neuronal immunofluorescent staining which can be absorbed out with streptococcal membranes. Colon antibodies present in ulcerative colitis have been found to cross-react with *Escherichia coli* 014. There is also some evidence for the view that antigens common to *Trypanosoma cruzi*, cardiac muscle and the peripheral nervous system provoke some of the immunopathological lesions seen in Chagas' disease.

3 Molecular mimicry of T-cell epitopes

The drawback with the Allison–Weigle model of cross-reaction of B-cell epitopes and the provision of a new T-cell carrier is that, once the cross-reacting agent is eliminated from the body, and with it the T-cell epitope, the only way that the autoimmunity can be sustained is for the activated B-cell to capture circulating autoantigen and, after processing, present it to the T-helper (figure 18.11c). This is not readily feasible for **cell-associated antigens** but their special link with T-cell recognition puts them in a totally different ballpark.

In this case, if an infecting agent mimics an autoantigen by producing a **cross-reacting T-cell epitope**, the resulting T-cell autoimmunity could theoretically persist even after elimination of the infection. The autoantigen will normally be presented to the resting autoreactive T-cell as a **cryptic epitope** and by definition will be unable to provide an activating signal. The cross-reacting infectious agent will provide abundant antigen on professional APCs which can prime the T-cell and upregulate its adhesion molecules so that it now has the **avidity** to bind to and be persistently activated by the cryptic self-epitope presented on the target tissue cell provided that it is associated with the appropriate MHC molecule (figure 18.11b). Remember the transgenic cytotoxic T-cells (Tc) which could only destroy the pancreatic β-cells bearing a viral transgene when they were **primed** by a real viral infection (cf. figure 11.10). Recall also the tumor cells that could only be recognized by primed not resting T-cells (cf. figure 17.11). Theoretically, the resting T-cell could also be primed in a nonantigen-specific manner by a microbial **superantigen**.

Although we have ascribed the dominant role of MHC alleles as risk factors for autoimmune diseases to their ability to present key antigenic epitopes to autoreactive T-cells, they might also operate in a quite distinct way. We may recollect that, during intrathymic ontogeny, T-cells are positively selected by weak interaction with self-peptides complexed with MHC. Now since around **50% of the class II peptides are MHC derived** (figure 5.21), then the mature T-cells leaving the thymus will have been selected with a strong bias to weak recognition of self-MHC peptides presented by class II. There must therefore be a major pool of self-reactive T-cells vulnerable to stimulation by exogenously derived cross-reacting epitopes which mimic these MHC peptides. Just so. The critical sequence QKRAAVDTY of the rheumatoid arthritis susceptibility allele HLA-DRB1*0401 is closely similar to the QKRAAYDQY of the dnaJ heat-shock protein of *E. coli*, and this peptide presented by DQ causes proliferation of synovial T-cells from RA patients. In fact, a large number of microbial peptide sequences with varying degrees of homology with human proteins have been identified (table 18.5), although it should be emphasized at this stage that they only provide clues for further study. The mere existence of a homology is no certainty that infection with that organism will necessarily lead to autoimmunity because everything depends on several contingencies, including the manner in which the proteins are processed by the APCs, and we cannot predict, as yet, which peptides will be presented and in what concentration.

Table 18.5. Molecular mimicry: homologies between microbes and body components as potential cross-reacting T-cell epitopes.

Microbial molecule	Body component
Bacteria:	
Arthritogenic *Shigella flexneri*	HLA-B27
Klebsiella nitrogenase	HLA-B27
Proteus mirabilis urease	HLA-DR4
Mycobact. tuberculosis 65 kDa hsp	Joint (adjuvant arthritis)
E.coli DNAJ hsp	RA shared DRB1 T-cell epitope
Viruses:	
Coxsackie B	Myocardium
Coxsackie B	Glutamic acid decarboxylase
EBV gp110	RA shared DRB1 T-cell epitope
HBV octamer	Myelin basic protein
HSV glycoprotein	Acetylcholine receptor
Measles hemagglutinin	T-cell subset
Retroviral gag p32	U-1 RNA

4 'Piggy-back' T-cell epitopes and epitope spread

One membrane component may provide help for the immune response to another (associative recognition). In the context of autoimmunity, a new helper determinant may arise through drug modification as mentioned above, or through the insertion of viral antigen into the membrane of an infected cell (cf. figure 18.10b.4). That this can promote a reaction to a pre-existing cell component is clear from the studies in which infection of a tumor with influenza virus elicited resistance to uninfected tumor cells. The appearance of cold agglutinins often with blood group I specificity after *Mycoplasma pneumoniae* infection could have a similar explanation. In a comparable fashion, T-cell help can be provided for a molecule such as DNA, which cannot itself form a T-cell epitope, by complexing with a T-dependent carrier, in this example a histone, or an anti-DNA idiotype to which T-cells were sensitized. For this mechanism to work, the helper component must still be physically attached to the fragment bearing the B-cell epitope. When this is recognized by the B-cell receptor, the helper component will be 'piggy-backed' into the B-cell, processed and presented as an epitope for recognition by T-cells (figure 18.11c). By the same token, the autoimmune response can spread to other epitopes on the same molecule. Think about it.

Idiotype bypass mechanisms

We have argued the evidence for internal regulated idiotype networks involving self-reactivity at some length. This raises the possibility of involving autoreactive lymphocytes with responses to exogenous agents through idiotype network connections, particularly since some autoimmune diseases are characterized by major cross-reactive idiotypes.

Thus, knowing that T-helpers with specificity for the

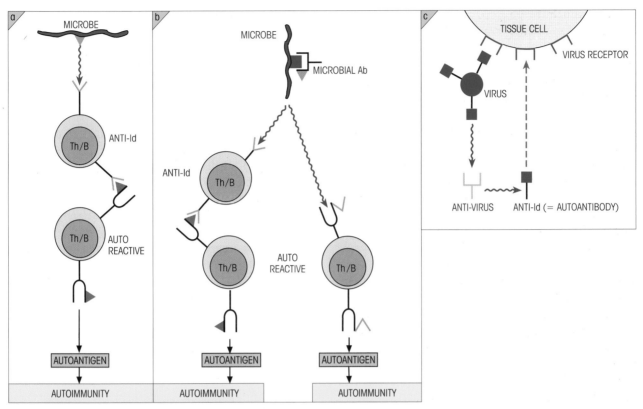

Figure 18.12. Idiotypic mechanisms leading to autoimmunity. (a) Microbial antigen cross-reacts with autoreactive lymphocyte Id. (b) Microbial antibodies either share Ids with or are anti-Id to autoreactive lymphocytes. (c) Anti-virus generates anti-Id which is autoantibody to viral receptor (Plotz).

idiotype on a lymphocyte receptor can be instrumental in the stimulation of that cell, it is conceivable that an environmental agent such as a parasite or virus, which triggered antibody carrying a public idiotype (cross-reactive idiotype, CRI), which happened to be shared with the receptor of an autoreactive T- or B-cell, could provoke an autoimmune response (figure 18.12b). Similarly, if it is correct that the germ-line idiotypes on autoantibodies generate a whole range of anti-idiotypes which mediate the response to exogenous antigens, then, by the same token, it is conceivable that antibodies produced in response to an infection may react with the corresponding idiotype on the autoreactive lymphocyte (figure 18.12a). For example, a hybridoma from a myasthenia gravis patient secreted an anti-Id to an acetylcholine receptor autoantibody; this anti-Id was found to react with the bacterial product 1,3-dextran. Finally, it is possible for Id network interactions to allow a viral infection to give rise to autoantibodies reacting with the viral receptor (figure 18.12c). Since viruses all bind to specific complementary receptors on the cells they infect, this sequence of events may have serious consequences; we note for example that β-adrenergic receptors are the surface targets for certain reoviruses and that rabies virus binds to the acetylcholine receptor.

Polyclonal activation

Microbes often display adjuvant properties through their possession of polyclonal lymphocyte activators such as bacterial endotoxins, which act by providing nonspecific inductive signals that bypass the need for specific T-cell help, either by stimulation of CD8 T-cells through upregulation of dendritic cell CD40 or by direct interaction with B-cell mitogen receptors (cf. p. 178). This can occur by direct interaction with the B-lymphocyte or indirectly through stimulating the secretion of nonspecific factors from T-cells or macrophages. The variety of autoantibodies detected in cases with infectious mononucleosis must surely be attributable to the polyclonal activation of B-cells by the Epstein–Barr (EB) virus. Curiously, lymphocytes from many patients with SLE and from mice with spontaneous lupus produce abnormally large amounts of IgM when cultured *in vitro* as if they were under polyclonal activation. Nevertheless, it is difficult to see how a pan-specific polyclonal activation could give rise to the patterns of autoantibodies characteristic of the different autoimmune disorders without the operation of some antigen-directing factor. We have already hinted at scenarios in which polyclonally activated B- or T-cells might contribute to a sustained autoimmune response (see legend to figure 18.11b,c).

AUTOIMMUNITY CAN ARISE THROUGH BYPASS OF REGULATORY MECHANISMS

Regulatory cells try to damp down autoimmunity

It should be emphasized that these T-helper bypass mechanisms for the induction of autoimmunity do not by themselves ensure the continuation of the response, since normal animals have been shown to be capable of damping down autoantibody production through CD4 regulatory T-cell interactions as, for example, in the case of red cell autoantibodies induced in mice by injection of rat erythrocytes (figure 18.13). When regulatory T-cell activity is impaired by low doses of cyclophosphamide, or if strains like the SJL which have prematurely aging regulators are used, induced autoimmunity is prolonged and more severe. Much work has focused on the CD4$^+$ CD25$^+$ Foxp3$^+$ regulatory T-cell (cf. figure 10.10) which has been shown to suppress many different autoimmune phenomena. However, cellular control

mechanisms are never straightforward and it is important to appreciate that CD25$^-$ T-cells have proved to be effective in controlling T-cell mediated disease in certain circumstances. Interestingly, TGFβ can convert these CD4$^+$, CD25$^-$, Foxp3$^-$ cells to the CD4$^+$, CD25$^+$, Foxp3$^+$ Tr1 phenotype (cf. figure 10.10) characteristic of the mucosal regulatory cells which mediate oral tolerance; they produce IL-10 on activation and promote the differentiation of T-cells that secrete TGFβ (Th3) and skew responses towards the Th2-type pole. Yet another player in the field is the NKT-cell which is deficient in NOD mice, but can prevent the development of diabetes if transferred from F1(Balb/c×NOD) donors. Patients with a variety of autoimmune diseases have been reported to have reduced numbers of this cell type. From quite a different tack, small numbers of an encephalitogenic T-cell clone **vaccinated** normal recipients against the pathogenic consequences of a subsequent higher dose, hinting strongly at anti-idiotypic control. The interrelationships between this panoply of antigen-, idiotype-, hsp- and possibly nonspecific regulators (figure 18.14) need sorting.

Defects in regulation contribute to spontaneous autoimmunity

A relationship between self-regulators and the control of autoimmunity is revealed by the startling effect of thymectomy carried out within a narrow window of 2–4 days after birth in the mouse which gives rise to widespread organ-specific autoimmune disease affecting mainly the stomach, thyroid, ovary, prostate and sperm; circulating antibodies are frequently detected and deposits of Ig and complement are often seen around the basement membranes. We have alluded earlier to the evidence for intrathymic promiscuous expression of mRNA for a whole set of nominally organ-specific antigens such as insulin, thyroglobulin and myelin basic protein. These are expressed in rare large medullary cells often at the center of lymphocyte rosettes, presumably guiding the formation of potential organ-specific suppressive regulators such as the *Aire* transcription factor described earlier between days 2 and 4, the time at which thymectomy upsets the balance between autoreactive and suppressor cells.

Peripheral T-cell responses are controlled by dendritic cells. IL-4 prevents maturation of dendritic cells, and subsequent interaction of these immature cells with cognate T-cells results in peripheral tolerization. Interaction between dendritic cell CD30 and its ligand is important for peripheral deletion of self-reactive T-cells; thus, deletion of pancreatic islet reactive CD8 T-cells failed to occur in CD30 knockout mice and these cells were highly aggressive, as few as 150 provoking dia-

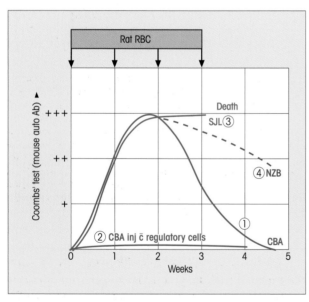

Figure 18.13. Regulation of self-reactivity. When CBA strain mice (1) are injected with rat red cells, autoantibodies are produced by this cross-reacting antigen (see figure 18.11a) which coat the host erythrocytes and are detected by the Coombs' antiglobulin test (see p. 439). Despite repeated injections of rat erythrocytes, the autoantibody response is switched off by the expansion of CD4 mouse red cell-specific regulatory cells which do not affect antibody production to the heterologous erythrocyte determinants. When these regulatory cells are injected into naive CBA mice (2), rat red cells cannot induce autoantibodies. The SJL strain (3), in which suppressor activity declines rapidly with age, is unable to regulate the autoimmune response and develops particularly severe disease. The response is also prolonged in the autoimmune NZB strain (4). (Based on data of Cooke A. & Hutchings P., e.g. *Immunology* 1984, **51**, 489.)

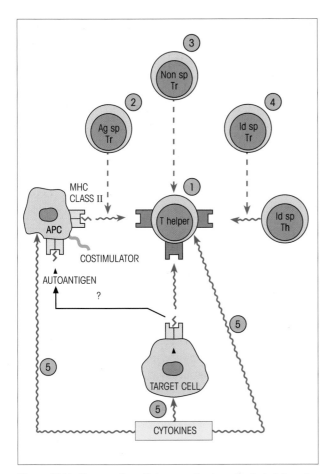

Figure 18.14. Bypass of regulatory mechanisms leads to triggering of autoreactive T-helper cells through defects in (1) tolerizability or ability to respond to or induce T-regulators (Tr), or (2) expression of antigen-specific, (3) hsp and other nonspecific or (4) idiotype-specific T-regulators, or (5) through imbalance of the cytokine network, producing derepression of class II genes with inappropriate cellular expression of class II and presentation of antigen on target cell, stimulation of APC, and possible activation of anergic T-helper. The beneficial effect of pooled whole Ig in certain human autoimmune diseases, such as idiopathic thrombocytopenic purpura, and of T-cell vaccination in experimental autoimmune encephalomyelitis (EAE) and adjuvant arthritis in rats lends weight to the idea of idiotype control mechanisms. Evidence for a regulatory CD4 subset comes from studies reporting inflammatory infiltrates in liver, lung, stomach, thyroid and pancreas in athymic rats reconstituted with CD45RB^{hi}/CD4 T-cells but not with unfractionated or CD45RB^{lo} CD4 cells (presumably the regulators).

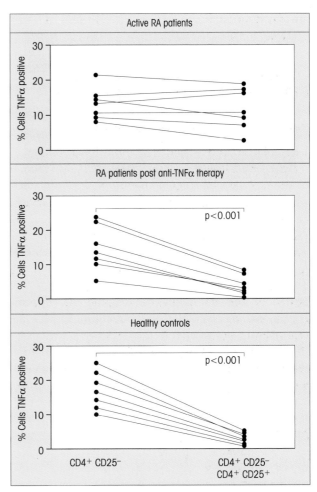

Figure 18.15. Reversal of compromised regulatory T-cell function in rheumatoid arthritis (RA) patients by anti-TNF therapy. CD4$^+$CD25$^-$ cells isolated from peripheral blood were stimulated with a mixture of anti-CD3 and anti-CD28 alone or after adding back the CD4$^+$CD25$^+$ putative regulatory T-cells. Activation of the T-cells was assessed by staining for intracellular TNFα. The lines join values for individual patients after adding back regulatory CD4$^+$CD25$^+$ T-cells. The regulatory T-cells were dysfunctional in active RA but were able to suppress activation of the CD25$^-$ population after successful anti-TNFα therapy. (Data from Ehrenstein M.R. *et al.* (2004) *Journal of Experimental Medicine* **200**, 277–285.)

betes in adoptive recipients. The numbers of dendritic cells in humans at risk for diabetes and in NOD mice are grossly reduced, which would accord with a critical role in preventing disease by promoting autoregulatory responses. Another curious feature is that macrophages from diabetic patients and relatives with the susceptible HLA haplotype constitutively express high levels of the COX-2 enzyme responsible for the synthesis of prostanoids. Something interesting is simmering here and should break surface soon.

A progressive loss of regulatory cells with age would account for the inability of the NZB mouse to normalize the experimental induction of red cell autoimmunity (figure 18.13) and for the increasing resistance to the induction of tolerance to soluble proteins in elderly NZB mice, apparently associated with a sudden fall in the plasma concentration of the thymic peptide thymulin before the onset of disease (note: thymulin is said to inhibit the autoreactive response of spleen cells to syngeneic fibroblasts in culture). Recent findings have identified compromised apparently nonspecific regulatory T-cell function in rheumatoid arthritis patients and, fascinatingly, its normalization after successful therapy with anti-TNF monoclonals (figure 18.15).

Do abnormalities in apoptotic mechanisms also

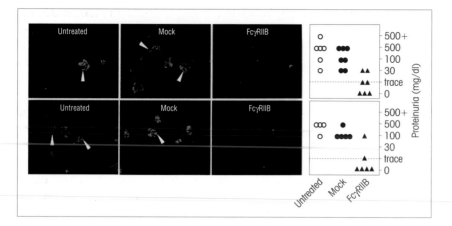

Figure 18.16. Retroviral transduction of the regulatory IgG receptor on B-cells (FcγRIIB) in spontaneous lupus prone mice. Six months after the bone marrow transfer, immune complex deposition is reduced and kidney function is improved. Kidney sections were examined for the presence of IgG complexes with direct immuno-fluorescence (×40). Arrowheads indicate subendothelial complexes indicative of active lupus. (Excerpted with permission from McGaha T.L., Sorrentino B. & Ravetch J.V. (2005) *Science* **307**, 591, Copyright 2005 AAAS).

contribute to these regulatory defects? T- and B-cells of NOD mice are resistant to apoptosis, as are lymphocytes of the MRL/*lpr* lupus mouse strain which has a *fas* gene mutation. This mutation produces the characteristic lymphoproliferation, and possibly failure to limit the expansion of self-reactive T- and B-cell clones by apoptosis. The *gld* lupus model complements this situation with mutations in the *fas ligand*.

Unexpectedly, attention has now turned to yet another facet of the processes of immune regulation, namely the regulatory IgG receptor on B-cells whose function is feedback control through surface immune complex signaling (cf p. 212). Evidently, dysfunction in the FcγRIIB B-cell receptor in lupus-prone mice can be corrected by retroviral transduction of a normal gene (figure 18.16).

We have previously drawn attention to the distinctive properties of the B-1 population with respect to its propensity to synthesize IgM autoantibodies and its possible intimate relationship to the setting up of the regulatory idiotype network (cf. p. 421), and one must seriously entertain the hypothesis that unregulated activity by these cells could be responsible for certain autoimmune disorders. The pitifully named motheaten strain is heavily into autoimmunity, and the mice make masses of anti-DNA and anti-polymorphs and die with intense pneumonitis, often before they have tasted the fruits of life. They exhibit reduced catalytic activity of their protein tyrosine phosphatase 1C due to mutation. Their IgM levels rise to a staggering 25–50 times normal and—this is quite bizarre—their B-cells are nearly all CD5+, i.e. B-1. This population is also raised in the NZB mouse and largely accounts for the production of the IgM autoantibodies in this strain. Now here is a persuasive experiment. When transgenes encoding an NZB red cell autoantibody were introduced into normal mice, no B-2 cells were present and 50% developed autoimmune disease. Intraperitoneal injection of erythrocytes deleted the B-1 cells and prevented disease.

This tells us that the NZB hemolytic anemia is due to red blood cell autoantibodies produced by B-1 cells, that this population is only tolerized properly when the antigen gains access to the peritoneum where they develop, and that some (around 50%), but not all, animals can control the autoreactive clones. Whether B-1 cells escape regulatory control and undergo an unrestrained isotype switch to the pathogenic IgG antibodies responsible for disease in other models, such as the NZB×W mouse, is still a question on which the jury's verdict is awaited, although depletion of B-1 lymphocytes greatly reduces the immune complex glomerulonephritis. The IdD-23 idiotype characteristic of natural autoantibodies has been identified on a monoclonal IgG anti-DNA—but one idiotype doesn't make a summer, if we can misquote a well-known saying!

In humans, a high proportion of B-1 cells make IgM rheumatoid factors (anti-Fcγ) and anti-DNA using germline genes. In rheumatoid arthritis patients, although there are increased numbers of circulating B-1 cells, the polyclonal rheumatoid factors synthesized do not, by and large, bear the public idiotypes of this subset. SLE could be different because the 16/6 public idiotype associated with germ-line genes encoding anti-DNA is found on a significant fraction of the IgG anti-DNA in patients' serums. Gene sequencing would help to establish the relationship between B-1 cells and IgG autoantibody synthesis.

Upregulation of T-cell interaction molecules

The majority of organ-specific autoantigens normally appear on the surface of the cells of the target organ in the context of class I but not class II MHC molecules. As such they cannot communicate with T-helpers and are therefore immunologically silent. Pujol-Borrell, Bottazzo and colleagues reasoned that, if the class II genes were somehow derepressed and class II molecules were now synthesized, they would endow the surface molecules with potential autoantigenicity (figure 18.14). Indeed, they have been able to show that human thyroid cells in tissue culture can be persuaded to express HLA-DR (class II) molecules on their surface after stimulation with γ-interferon (IFNγ), and, further, that the cytoplasm of epithelial cells from the glands of patients with Graves' disease (thyrotoxicosis) stains strongly with anti-HLA-DR reagents, indicating active synthesis of class II polypeptide chains (figure 18.1b). Inappropriate class II expression has also been reported on the bile ductules in primary biliary cirrhosis and on endothelial cells and some β-cells in the diabetic pancreas both in the human and in the BB rat model.

Whether adventitious expression of class II on these cells through activation by something like virally induced IFN is responsible for *initiating* the autoimmune process by priming autoreactive T-helpers, or whether reaction with *already activated* T-cells induces class II by release of IFNγ and makes the cell a more attractive target for provoking subsequent tissue damage, is still an unresolved issue. However, transfection of mice with the class II *H-2A* genes linked to the insulin promoter led to expression of class II on the β-islet cells of the pancreas but did *not* induce autoimmunity. Lack of B7 costimulatory molecules seems to be responsible for the failure of these class II-positive β-cells to activate naive T-cells, a job which may have to be left to the professional dendritic APCs.

Cytokine imbalance may induce autoimmunity

By contrast, transfection with the *IFNγ* gene on the insulin promoter under the same circumstances produced a local inflammatory reaction in the pancreas with aberrant expression of class II *and* diabetes; this must have been a result of autoimmunity since a normal pancreas grafted into the same animal suffered a similar fate. This implies that unregulated cytokine production producing a local inflammatory reaction can initiate autoimmunity, probably by enhancing the presentation of islet antigen by recruiting and activating dendritic cells, by increasing the concentration of processed intracellular autoantigen available to them, and by increasing their avidity for naive T-cells through upregulation of adhesion molecules; perhaps previously anergic cells may be made responsive to antigen (figure 18.14). Once primed, the T-cells can now interact with the islet β-cells which will be displaying increased amounts of class II and adhesion molecules for T-cells on their surface.

This all seems very straightforward but, although other proinflammatory cytokines, IL-12 and TNF as well as IFNγ, can promote the induction of organ-specific autoimmune disease at an early time by priming pathogenic Th1 responses, late expression of the same cytokines can drive the terminal differentiation and death of autoreactive T-cells. Thus we can in fact correct some spontaneous models of autoimmune disease by the injection of cytokines: IL-1 cures the diabetes of NOD mice, *tumor necrosis factor* (TNF) prevents the onset of SLE symptoms in NZB×W hybrids and *transforming growth factor-β1* (TGFβ1) is known to protect against collagen arthritis and relapsing *experimental autoimmune encephalomyelitis* (EAE). The pleiotropic effects of the cytokines on different cell types involved at different stages in these diseases, and their positive and negative networking interactions with each other, add some uncertainty to the analysis and prediction of these complex events.

Turning to human disorders, a window on cytokine activity in SLE has been provided by analysis showing expression of a number of genes known to be upregulated by interferon-α (figure 18.17) and elevated levels of the cytokine which correlate with more severe disease. Conceivably, this results from stimulation of leukocytes by chromatin-containing immune complexes.

AUTOIMMUNE DISORDERS ARE MULTIFACTORIAL

We must come back to this. Undoubtedly, the autoimmune diseases have a multifactorial etiology combining

Figure 18.17. The IFN-α signature in a major subset of SLE patients. Expression patterns of IFN-induced genes in the blood of lupus patients and controls (Red = highly expressed). The black bar indicates 22 of the IFN-upregulated genes which delineate the 'signature pattern'. (Reproduced from Baechler E.C., Gregersen P.K. & Behrens T.W. (2004) *Current Opinion in Immunology* **16**, 803, with permission of the authors and publishers.)

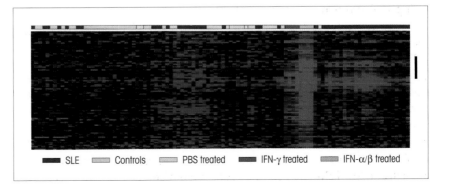

polygenic traits and environmental influences. Many of the defects we have discussed, individually not necessarily uncommon, may contribute in various combinations to different disorders. No one gene is sufficient or required for disease onset and in any individual, disease susceptibility, presentation in terms of target organ severity and prognosis reflect additive or epistatic effects of several fortuitously inherited alleles, many of which may be shared with other autoimmune diseases. Even in a disease-prone strain of mice expressing an identical array of susceptibility genes, the proportion of animals developing autoimmune pathology (penetrance) increases with age and suggests that the expression of these complex traits requires an internal stochastic or environmental triggering of events, the probability of which increases with time. Thus, superimposed upon a genetically complex susceptibility, we might be dealing with some aging process affecting the thymus or the lymphoid stem cells and their internal control of self-reactivity. Sex hormones and defective pituitary–adrenal feedback loops may contribute. Now throw into this melange a panoply of dietary and other environmental factors, particularly microbial agents, which could have a variety of effects on the target organs, the lymphoid system and the cytokine network.

PATHOGENIC EFFECTS OF HUMORAL AUTOANTIBODY

We should now look at the evidence which helps to uncover the mechanisms by which autoimmunity, however it arises, plays a **primary pathogenic role** in the production of tissue lesions within the group of diseases labeled as 'autoimmune'. Let us look first at autoantibody effectors.

Blood cells

The erythrocyte antibodies play a dominant role in the destruction of red cells in **autoimmune hemolytic anemia**. Normal red cells coated with autoantibody eluted from Coombs' positive erythrocytes (cf. figure 15.17) have a shortened half-life after reinjection into the normal subject, essentially as a result of their adherence to Fcγ receptors on phagocytic cells in the spleen.

Some children with immunodeficiency associated with very low white cell counts have a serum lymphocytotoxic factor which requires complement for its activity. Lymphopenia occurring in patients with systemic lupus erythematosus (SLE) and rheumatoid arthritis (RA) may also be a direct result of antibody, since nonagglutinating antibodies coating the white cells have been reported in such cases.

Platelet antibodies are apparently responsible for **idiopathic thrombocytopenic purpura** (ITP). IgG from a patient's serum when given to a normal individual causes a depression of platelet counts and the active principle can be absorbed out with platelets. The transient neonatal thrombocytopenia which may be seen in infants of mothers with ITP is explicable in terms of transplacental passage of IgG antibodies to the child.

The primary **antiphospholipid syndrome** is characterized by recurrent venous and arterial thromboembotic phenomena, recurrent fetal loss, thrombocytopenia and cardiolipin antibodies. Passive transfer of such antibodies into mice is fairly devastating, resulting in lower fecundity rates and recurrent fetal loss. The effect seems to be mediated through reaction of the autoantibodies with a complex of cardiolipin and β_2-glycoprotein 1 which inhibits triggering of the coagulation cascade. The placental trophoblast is a primary target of these antibodies since the villous cytotrophoblast is one of the few cell types which externalizes phosphatidyl serine during development.

Surface receptors

Thyroid

Under certain circumstances antibodies to the surface of a cell may stimulate rather than destroy (cf. 'stimulatory hypersensitivity'; Chapter 15). This would seem to be the case in **Graves' disease** (thyrotoxicosis or Basedow's disease) where a direct link with autoimmunity came with the discovery by Adams and Purves of thyroid-stimulating activity in the serum of these patients (Milestone 18.1), ultimately shown to be due to the presence of antibodies to TSH receptors (TSH-Rs), which seem to act in the same manner as TSH itself (cf. p. 412). Both operate through the adenyl cyclase system as indicated by the potentiating effect of theophylline, and both produce similar changes in ultrastructural morphology in the thyroid cell, but it is one of Nature's 'passive transfer experiments' which links TSH-R antibodies most directly with the pathogenesis of Graves' disease. When thyroid-stimulating antibodies (TSAbs) from a thyrotoxic mother cross the placenta, they cause the production of neonatal hyperthyroidism (figure 18.18), which resolves after a few weeks as the maternal IgG is catabolized.

There is reason to believe that enlargement of the thyroid in Graves' disease is due to the action of antibodies which react with a 'growth' receptor and directly stimulate cell division as distinct from metabolic hyperactivity. By contrast, sera from patients with **primary myxedema** (atrophic thyroiditis) contain antibodies capable of blocking the stimulation of growth by TSH, thereby preventing the regeneration of follicles which is

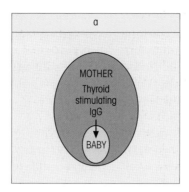
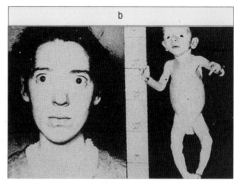

Figure 18.18. Neonatal thyrotoxicosis.
(a) The autoantibodies which stimulate the thyroid through the TSH receptors are IgG and cross the placenta. (b) The thyrotoxic mother therefore gives birth to a baby with thyroid hyperactivity which spontaneously resolves as the mother's IgG is catabolized. (Photograph courtesy of Professor A. MacGregor.)

a feature of the enlarged **Hashimoto goiter**. Graves' disease is often associated with exophthalmos which might be due to cross-reaction of antibodies to a 64 kDa membrane protein present on both thyroid and eye muscle.

Muscle and nerve

The transient muscle weakness seen in a proportion of babies born to mothers with **myasthenia gravis** calls to mind neonatal thrombocytopenia and hyperthyroidism and would certainly be compatible with the transplacental passage of an IgG capable of inhibiting neuromuscular transmission. Strong support for this view is afforded by the consistent finding of antibodies to muscle acetylcholine receptors (ACh-Rs) in myasthenics and the depletion of these receptors within the motor endplates. In addition, myasthenic symptoms can be induced in animals by injection of monoclonal antibodies to ACh-R or by active immunization with the purified receptors themselves. Nonetheless, the majority of babies with myasthenic mothers do not display muscle disease and it may be that they are protecting themselves through production of antibodies directed to idiotypes on the maternal autoantibodies.

Neuromuscular defects can also be elicited in mice injected with serum from patients with the **Lambert–Eaton** syndrome containing antibodies to presynaptic calcium channels. Autoantibodies to sodium channels which cross-react with *Campylobacter* bacilli have been identified in **Guillain–Barré syndrome**, a self-resolving peripheral polyneuritis. Rather more wayout is **Rasmussen's encephalitis**, a childhood disease of relentless and intractable focal seizures with an inflammatory histopathology in the brain; these patients have antibodies which act as agonists and kill kainic acid-responsive neurons through overstimulation of type 3 glutamine receptors. Would one uncover yet more phenomena of this kind in other neurological disorders if the search was widened and intensified?

Stomach

The underlying histopathological lesion in **pernicious anemia** is an atrophic gastritis in which a chronic inflammatory mononuclear invasion is associated with degeneration of secretory glands and failure to produce gastric acid. The development of achlorhydria is almost certainly accelerated by the inhibitory action of antibodies to the gastric proton pump, an H^+,K^+-dependent ATPase located in the membranes of the secretory canaliculi, and possibly also the gastrin receptors.

The idea that some cases of gastric ulcer may result from the stimulation of acid secretion by activation through antibodies to histamine receptors is appealing and we still await the further work required to establish its validity.

Other cellular receptors

Some patients with **atopic allergy** have serum blocking antibodies to β-adrenergic receptors and these may represent just one of many different types of factor which could alter the baseline sensitivity of mast cells and make the individual more at risk for the development of disease. The flip side of the coin is revealed in the cardiomyopathy of Chagas' disease where antibodies to these receptors act as agonists and increase the heart rate. Antibodies which block insulin receptors are a rare exotic species found in patients with acanthosis nigricans (type B) and ataxia telangiectasia associated with insulin resistance.

Other tissues

Gut

Some patients with **autoimmune atrophic gastritis** diagnosed by achlorhydria and parietal cell antibodies (see table 18.2) just meander on year after year without developing the vitamin B_{12} deficiency which precipitates **pernicious anemia**. It is probable that autoimmune destruction is roughly balanced by regeneration of mucosal cells, an explanation which could account for the observation that high doses of steroids may restore gastric function in certain patients with pernicious anemia. However, the balance would be upset were the patient now to produce antibodies to intrinsic factor in the lumen of the gastrointestinal tract; these would neutralize the small amount of intrinsic factor still available and the body would move into negative balance for B_{12}. The symptoms of B_{12} deficiency, pernicious anemia and sometimes subacute degeneration of the cord, would then appear some considerable time later as the liver stores became exhausted (figure 18.19).

The normally acquired tolerance to dietary proteins seems to break down in **celiac disease** where T-cell sensitivity to wheat gluten in the small intestine can be demonstrated. Since gluten can bind strongly to the extracellular matrix protein, endomysium, one could hypothesize that uptake of the complex by IgA B-cells specific for endomysium would 'piggy-back' the gluten into the B-cell for processing and presentation on MHC class II to gluten-specific T-helpers (cf. figure 18.11). Stimulation of the B-cell would now follow with secretion of the IgA endomysial antibodies which are exclusive to patients with celiac disease. Together with the increased expression of Fcα receptors in the lamina propria and evidence of complement and eosinophil activation, it is conceivable that antibody-mediated mechanisms could be pathogenic.

Skin
An antibody pathogenesis for **pemphigus vulgaris** is

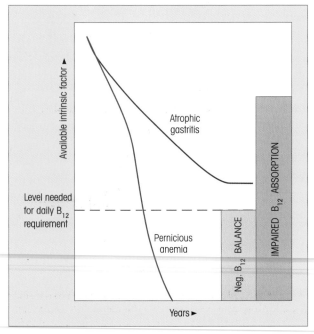

Figure 18.19. Pathogenesis of pernicious anemia. Patients with longstanding atrophic gastritis having parietal cell but no intrinsic factor antibodies do not go into negative B_{12} balance. Pernicious anemia develops when intrinsic factor antibodies become superimposed upon the atrophic gastritis. (After Doniach D. & Roitt I.M. (1964) *Seminars in Hematology* **I**, 313.)

favored by the recognition of a 130 kDa autoantigen on stratified squamous epithelial cells which is a member of the cadherin family of Ca^{2+}-dependent adhesion molecules. Likewise, antibodies to desmoglein 1 probably mediate the blistering of the epidermis in **pemphigus foliaceus**.

Sperm
In some **infertile males**, agglutinating antibodies cause aggregation of the spermatozoa and interfere with their penetration into the cervical mucus.

Glomerular basement membrane (g.b.m.)
With immunological kidney disease, the experimental models preceded the finding of parallel lesions in the human. Injection of cross-reacting heterologous g.b.m. preparations in complete Freund's adjuvant produces glomerulonephritis in sheep and other experimental animals. Antibodies to g.b.m. can be picked up by immunofluorescent staining of biopsies from nephritic animals with anti-IgG. The antibodies are largely, if not completely, absorbed out by the kidney *in vivo* but they appear in the serum on nephrectomy and can passively transfer the disease to another animal of the same species.

An entirely analogous situation occurs in humans in certain cases of glomerulonephritis, particularly those associated with lung hemorrhage (**Goodpasture's syndrome**). Kidney biopsy from the patient shows *linear* deposition of IgG and C3 along the basement membrane of the glomerular capillaries (figure 15.18a). After nephrectomy, g.b.m. antibodies can be detected in the serum. Lerner and his colleagues eluted the g.b.m. antibody from a diseased kidney and injected it into a squirrel monkey. The antibody rapidly fixed to the g.b.m. of the recipient animal and produced a fatal nephritis (figure 18.20). It is hard to escape the conclusion that the lesion in the human was the direct result of attack on the g.b.m. by these complement-fixing antibodies. The lung changes in Goodpasture's syndrome are attributable to cross-reaction with some of the g.b.m. antibodies.

Curiously, mercuric chloride produces anti-g.b.m. glomerulonephritis in Brown Norway rats and, *pari passu*, as the disease remits, there is an upsurge in anti-idiotype suppressors. Nonsusceptible strains produce suppressors rather promptly.

Heart
Neonatal lupus erythematosus is the most common cause of permanent **congenital complete heart block**. Almost all cases have been associated with high maternal titers of anti-La/SS-B or anti-Ro/SS-A. The mother's

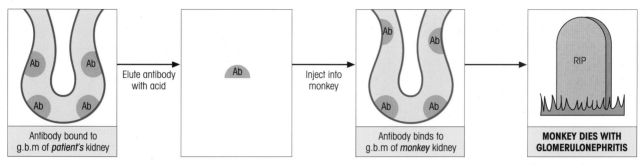

Figure 18.20. Passive transfer of glomerulonephritis to a squirrel monkey by injection of antiglomerular basement membrane (anti-g.b.m.) antibodies isolated by acid elution from the kidney of a patient with Goodpasture's syndrome. (After Lerner R.A., Glascock R.J. & Dixon F.J. (1967) *Journal of Experimental Medicine* **126**, 989.)

heart is unaffected. The key observation was that anti-Ro bound to neonatal rather than adult cardiac tissue and altered the transmembrane action potential by inhibiting repolarization (figure 18.21). IgG anti-Ro reaches the fetal circulation by transplacental passage but, although maternal and fetal hearts are exposed to the autoantibody, only the latter is affected. Anti-La/SS-A also binds to affected fetal hearts reacting with laminin in the basement membrane.

PATHOGENIC EFFECTS OF COMPLEXES WITH AUTOANTIGENS

Systemic lupus erythematosus (SLE)

Where autoantibodies are formed against soluble components to which they have continual access, complexes may be formed which can give rise to lesions similar to those occurring in serum sickness, especially when defects in the early classical complement components prevent effective clearance. Thus, although homozygous complement deficiency is a rare cause of SLE (cf. figure 15.25), the archetypal immune complex disorder, it represents the most powerful disease susceptibility genotype so far identified; more than 80% of cases with homozygous C1q and C4 deficiency have SLE. Up to one-half of the patients carry autoantibodies to the collagenous portion of C1q, but in truth there are a rich variety of different autoantigens in lupus (cf. table 18.2), some of them constituents of the nucleosome (cf. figure 18.1g), with the most pathomnemonic being **double-stranded DNA** (dsDNA). Anti-dsDNA is enriched in cryoglobulins and acid eluates of renal tissue from patients with lupus nephritis where it can be identified, presumably in complexes containing complement, by immunofluorescent staining of kidney biopsies from patients with evidence of renal dysfunction. The staining pattern with a fluorescent anti-IgG or anti-C3 is punctate or 'lumpy-bumpy' as once described (figure

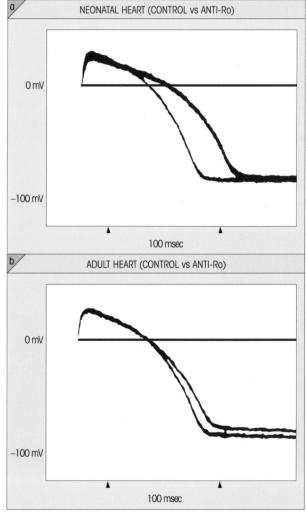

Figure 18.21. Anti-Ro affects conduction in neonatal but not adult heart. (a) Action potential of neonatal NZW rabbit cardiac fiber before and 20 minutes after superfusion with serum containing anti-Ro/SS-A; the repolarization phase of the action potential is reduced by 30%. (b) The same with an adult cardiac fiber showing only 5% reduction. (Reproduced from Alexander E. *et al.* (1992) *Arthritis and Rheumatism* **35**, 176.) Anti-La/SS-B can be eluted from the fetal cardiac tissue of infants with congenital heart block. It reacts with fetal but not adult laminin in the basement membrane.

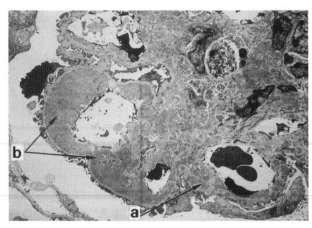

Figure 18.22. Renal biopsy of an SLE patient with severe immune complex glomerulonephritis and proteinuria. Electron micrograph showing irregular thickening of glomerular capillary walls by subepithelial complexes (a) and subendothelial complexes (b). The mesangial region shows abundant (probably phagocytosed) complexes. (Courtesy of Dr A. Leatham.)

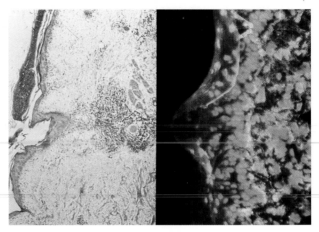

Figure 18.23. The 'lupus band' in SLE. *Left*—section of skin showing slight thickening of the dermo-epidermal junction with underlying scattered inflammatory cells and a major inflammatory focus in the deeper layers. Low power H & E. *Right*—green fluorescent staining of a skin biopsy at higher power showing deposition of complexes containing IgG (anti-C3 gives the same picture) on the basement membrane at the dermo-epidermal junction. (Kindly provided by Professor D. Isenberg.)

15.18b), in marked contrast with the linear pattern caused by the g.b.m. antibodies in Goodpasture's syndrome (figure 15.18a). The complexes grow in size to become large aggregates visible in the electron microscope as amorphous humps on both sides of the g.b.m. (figure 18.22). During the active phase of the disease, serum complement levels fall as components are affected by immune aggregates in the kidney and circulation. Deposition of complexes is widespread as the name implies and, although 40% of patients *eventually* develop kidney lesions, the corresponding figures for organ involvement are 98% for skin (figure 18.23), 98% for joints/muscle, 64% for lung, 60% for blood, 60% for brain and 20% for heart.

Spontaneous production of anti-dsDNA is also a dominant feature of the animal models of SLE, NZB×W, MRL/*lpr*, BXSB and the *p21* single gene knockout mice, which involve fatal immune complex disease. Cationic anti-DNA, with arginines strategically positioned in locations of paratopic significance, emerges strongly as the disease progresses. The high affinity and IgG class of these antibodies, and the amelioration of symptoms and reduction of renal glomerular immune complexes by treatment of NZB×W mice with DNase I or anti-CD4, provide convincing evidence for a T-dependent antigen-driven complex-mediated pathology. But since DNA itself is not a thymus-dependent antigen and the SLE autoantibodies include a cluster directed to the physically linked antigens constituting the nucleosome, one might envisage a 'piggy-back' mechanism of the type portrayed in figure 18.11. Knowing that nucleosome 'blebs' appear on the surface of apoptotic cells and that a spontaneous expansion of nucleosome-specific T-cell populations precedes the clinical onset of SLE, a

likely scenario would involve the internalization of nucleosome material captured on the surface receptors of anti-DNA B-cells, presentation of processed histone peptide–MHC class II complex to the histone-specific T-helper cells, and clonal proliferation of DNA antibody-forming cells (figure 18.24). Complexes of anti-DNA with circulating nucleosome material are demonstrable, and these will bind through the histone (and presumably cationic anti-DNA) to extracellular heparan sulfate where they can accumulate and damage end-organ targets such as the kidney glomerulus.

There is yet another 'piggy-back' pathway. The possible involvement of idiotypes was mooted earlier by reference to experiments in which immunization of mice with human monoclonal antinuclear antibodies gave rise to the production of new anti-bodies of similar idiotype and specificity—in biblical terms, 'antibody begets antibody'. Suppose a major public idiotype network is kicked into action by a microbial infection (cf. figure 18.12); for example, the 16/6 idiotype on a human anti-DNA circulating as a natural autoantibody is also carried on a germ-line antibody to *Klebsiella*. A T-helper cell recognizing processed 16/6 Id could stimulate anti-DNA B-cells which had captured a complex of DNA with the Id-positive natural autoantibody (cf. figure 18.12 and p. 426).

Rheumatoid arthritis

Morphological evidence for immunological activity

The joint changes in RA are in essence produced by the **malign growth of the synovial cells** as a pannus

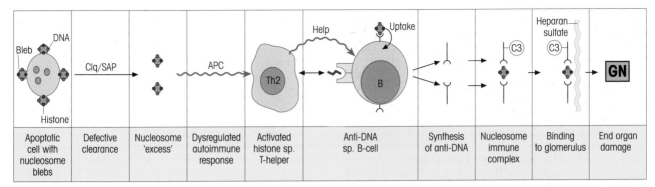

Apoptotic cell with nucleosome blebs	Defective clearance	Nucleosome 'excess'	Dysregulated autoimmune response	Activated histone sp. T-helper	Anti-DNA sp. B-cell	Synthesis of anti-DNA	Nucleosome immune complex	Binding to glomerulus	End organ damage

Figure 18.24. Conceivable pathogenetic pathway leading to end-organ damage in SLE. Nucleosomes derived from apoptotic cells can stimulate anti-DNA production by a 'piggy-back' mechanism in susceptible hosts. The resulting complexes bind to heparan sulfate in the glomerular basement membrane where they induce glomerulonephritis. The high incidence of lupus in C1q deficient individuals and the susceptibility of lupus patients to skin rashes on exposure to UV in sunlight, which induces apoptosis in skin cells, are well known. SAP, serum amyloid precursor; APC, antigen-presenting cell; GN, glomerulonephritis.

overlaying and destroying cartilage and bone (figure 18.25a–f). The synovial membrane which surrounds and maintains the joint space becomes intensely cellular as a result of considerable immunological hyper-reactivity, as evidenced by large numbers of T-cells, mostly CD4, in various stages of activation, usually associated with dendritic cells and macrophages (figure 18.25l); clumps of plasma cells are frequently observed and sometimes even secondary follicles with germinal centers are present as though the synovium had become an active lymph node (figure 18.25g–i). Indeed, it has been estimated that the synthesis of immunoglobulins by the synovial tissue ranks with that of a stimulated lymph node. There is widespread expression of surface HLA-DR (class II); T- and B-cells, dendritic and synovial lining cells and macrophages are all positive, indicative of some pretty lively action (figure 18.25k). The thesis is that this fiery immunological reactivity provides an intense stimulus to the synovial lining cells which undergo a Dr Jekyll to Mr Hyde transformation into the invasive pannus which brings about joint erosion through the release of destructive mediators.

IgG autosensitization and immune complex formation

Autoantibodies to the IgG Fc region (figure 18.27a), known as **antiglobulins** or **rheumatoid factors**, are the hallmark of the disease, being demonstrable in virtually all patients with RA. The majority have IgM antiglobulins which react in the classical latex and sheep cell agglutination tests (table 18.2, note 7), and both they and the 'seronegative' patients who fail to react in these tests can be shown to have elevated levels of **IgG antiglobulins** detectable by solid-phase immunoassay (cf. p. 136; figure 18.26).

We must take into account a strange and unique feature of IgG antiglobulins; because they are both antigen and antibody at the same time (figure 18.27a), they are capable of **self-association** (figure 18.27b) to form what are in effect 'hermaphroditic' immune complexes. IgG aggregates can be regularly detected in the synovial tissues and in the joint fluid where they give rise to typical acute inflammatory reactions with fluid exudates. Analysis shows them to consist almost exclusively of immunoglobulins and complement, while a major proportion of the IgG is present as self-associated antiglobulin as shown by binding to an Fcγ immunosorbent after treatment with pepsin.

What is extraordinary is that the percentage of Fcγ sugars completely lacking galactose in the IgG of both juvenile and adult RA patients is nearly always higher than in the controls and can be as high as 60%. This abnormal glycosylation might increase the autoantigenicity of the Fc region, strengthen the self-association of IgG rheumatoid factor, enhance the interaction with inflammatory mediators such as mannose-binding protein through exposure of N-acetylglucosamine in the agalacto-IgG glycoform with activation of the classical complement pathway (cf. p. 23) and stimulation of macrophages through binding of TNF, and finally it might increase autoantibody production through defective feedback control mediated by FcγRIIB regulatory B-cell receptors. It is well established that pregnant women with RA have a remission of their disease as they approach term, but an exacerbation postpartum; as the arthritis remits, the agalacto-IgG values fall but, as the disease worsens after birth, agalacto-IgG becomes abnormal again suggesting intimate involvement with the disease process. Long-term studies in closed communities of Pima Indians, who have an unusually high incidence of RA, have shown that changes in IgG galactose provide an early marker of future clinical disease and we know they can be of **prognostic value** in patients with early RA.

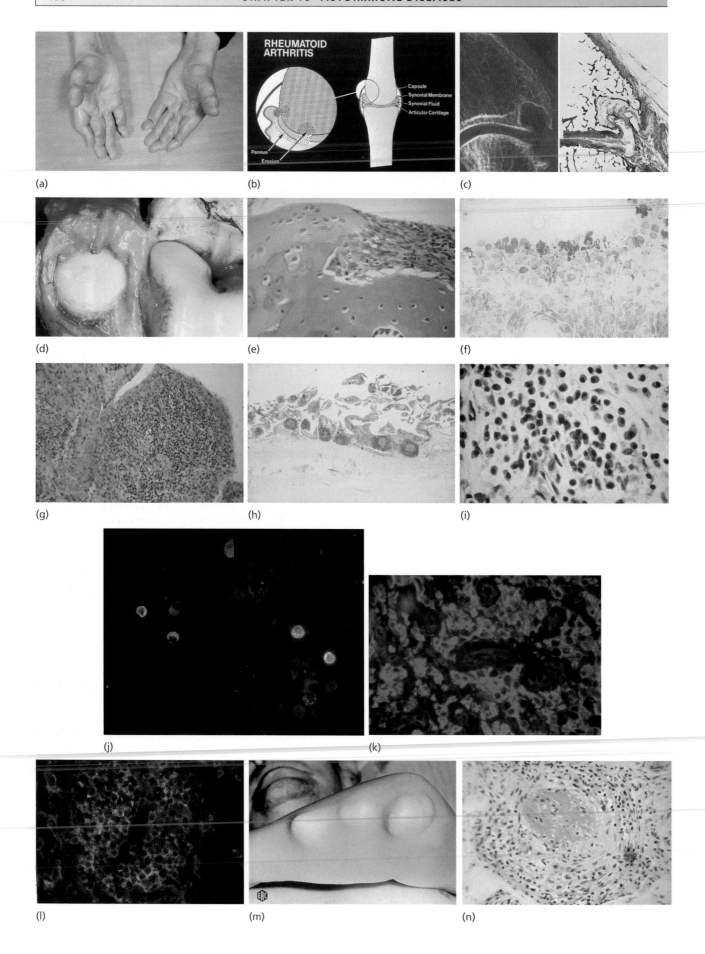

(a)

(b)

(c)

(d)

(e)

(f)

(g)

(h)

(i)

(j)

(k)

(l)

(m)

(n)

Figure 18.25. (*Opposite*) **Rheumatoid arthritis (RA).** (a) Hands of a patient with chronic RA showing classical swan-neck deformities. (b) Diagrammatic representation of a diarthrodial joint showing bone and cartilagenous erosions beneath the synovial membrane-derived pannus. (c) Proximal interphalangeal joint depicting marked bony erosion and marginal erosion of the cartilage. (d) Early pannus of granulation tissue growing over the patella. (e) Histology of pannus showing clear erosion of bone and cartilage at the cellular margin. (f) Histology of the pannus stained for macrophage nonspecific esterase; note long, stained dendritic processes. (g) Chronic inflammatory cells in the deeper layers of the synovium in RA. (h) A hypervillous synovium revealing well-formed secondary follicles with germinal centers (relatively rare occurrence). (i) A high power view of an area of diseased synovium showing collections of classical plasma cells. (j) Plasma cells isolated from a patient's synovial tissue stained simulta-neously for IgM (with fluorescein-labeled F(ab')₂ anti-μ) and rheumatoid factor (with rhodamine-labeled aggregated Fcγ). Two of the four IgM-positive plasma cells appear to be synthesizing rheumatoid factors. (k) Rheumatoid synovium showing large numbers of cells stained by anti-HLA-DR (anti-class II). (l) Rheumatoid synovium showing class II-positive accessory cells (green) in intimate contact with CD4⁺ T-cells (orange). (m) Large rheumatoid nodules on the forearm. (n) Granulomatous appearance of the rheumatoid nodule with central necrotic area surrounded by epithelioid cells, macrophages and scattered lymphocytes. Plasma cells making rheumatoid factor are often demonstrable and the lesion probably represents a response to the formation of insoluble anti-IgG complexes. (Kindly given by (a) Professor D. Isenberg; (c), (d), (e), (g), (h) and (i) Dr L.E. Professor Glynn; (f) Professor J. Edwards; (j) Professors P. Youinou and P. Lydyard; and (k) and (l) Professor G. Janossy.)

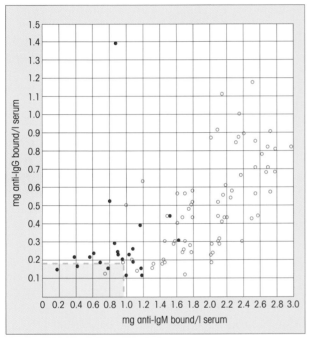

Figure 18.26. **IgM and IgG antiglobulins** determined by tube radioassay in patients with seropositive (open circles) and seronegative (filled circles) rheumatoid arthritis. The dashed lines indicate the 95% confidence limits (mean ± 2 SD) of the normal group. (From Nineham L., Hay F.C. & Roitt I.M. (1976) *Journal of Clinical Pathology* **29**, 1121.)

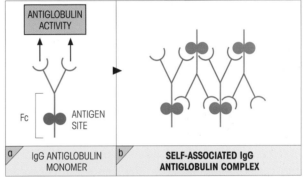

Figure 18.27. **Self-associated complexes of IgG antiglobulins.** Although of relatively low affinity, the strength of binding is boosted by the 'bonus effect' of the mutual attachment and, furthermore, such complexes in the joint may be stabilized by IgM antiglobulin and C1q which have polyvalent binding sites for IgG. Degradation of the Fc regions by pepsin releases the 'hidden' binding sites involved in the self-association. X-ray analysis of a complex of IgG Fc with two Fab fragments, isolated from a monoclonal IgM rheumatoid factor derived from an RA patient, showed binding of the Fab paratopes using the outer rather than the inner residues of the conventional antigen combining site CDRs; this suggests a novel form of cross-reactivity by allowing simultaneous binding to another antigen. (Sutton B. *et al.* (2000) *Immunology Today* **21**, 177.)

The production of tissue damage

As explained in the legend to figure 18.27, the complexes can be stabilized by the multivalent Fcγ-binding molecules, IgM rheumatoid factor and C1q, and when present in the joint space they may initiate an Arthus reaction leading to an influx of polymorphs with which they react to release *reactive oxygen intermediates* (ROIs) and lysosomal enzymes. These include neutral proteinases and collagenase which can **damage the articular cartilage** by breaking down proteoglycans and collagen fibrils. More damage results if the complexes are adherent to the cartilage, since the polymorph binds but is unable to internalize them ('frustrated phagocytosis'); as a result, the lysosomal hydrolases are released extracellularly into the space between the cell and the cartilage where they are protected from enzyme inhibitors such as α₂-macroglobulin.

The aggregates may also stimulate the macrophage-like cells of the synovial lining, either directly through their surface receptors or indirectly through phagocytosis and resistance to intracellular digestion. At this point we should acknowledge that the release of cytokines such as TNF and GM-CSF from activated T-cells (see below) provides further potent macrophage stimulation.

The activated synovial cells grow out as a malign pannus (cover) over the cartilage (figure 18.25d) and, at the margin of this advancing granulation tissue, breakdown can be seen (figure 18.25e), almost certainly as a result of the release of enzymes, ROIs and especially of IL-1, 6 and TNF. Activated macrophages also secrete plasminogen activator and the plasmin formed as a consequence activates a latent collagenase produced by synovial cells. Sensitization to partially degraded collagen may occur and this could lead secondarily to amplification of the lesion. The secreted products of the stimulated macrophage can activate chondrocytes to exacerbate **cartilage breakdown**, and osteoclasts to bring about **bone resorption** which is a further complication of severe disease (figure 18.25c). Subcutaneous nodules are granulomas (figure 18.25m,n) possibly formed through local production of insolubilized self-associating antiglobulins.

T-CELL-MEDIATED HYPERSENSITIVITY AS A PATHOGENIC FACTOR IN AUTOIMMUNE DISEASE

Rheumatoid arthritis again

The chronically inflamed synovium is densely crowded with activated T-cells and their critical role in the disease process is emphasized by the beneficial effects of cyclosporin and anti-CD4 treatments, and by the increased risk of disease associated with the 'shared epitope' sequences Q(R)K(R)RAA from residues 70–74 on the DRβ chain of DR1 and certain DR4 alleles. High levels of IL-15 within the synovial membrane can recruit and activate T-cells whose secretion of cytokines and ability to induce macrophage synthesis of TNF and further IL-15 will drive pannus development powerfully with consequent erosion of cartilage and bone (figure 18.25e.). Chondrocytes themselves may also be disease targets.

Just as in SLE, the antigenic specificity of these T-cells is still unknown. An appealing clue has come from the finding that the QKRAA shared epitope sequence, which lies within a polymorphic region of HLA-DR4/1 subtypes, is also present in the dnaJ heat-shock proteins from *E. coli*, *Lactobacillus lactis* and *Brucella ovis*, as well as the Epstein–Barr virus gp110 protein. This already provides an opportunity for priming of T-cells with autoreactive specificity for a processed peptide containing QKRAA presented by another HLA molecule, as discussed previously (p. 426). The plot deepens with the realization that QKRAA binds to a second *E. coli* heat-shock protein dnaK and that HLA-DR containing the QKRAA sequence binds the *self* analogue of dnaK, namely hsp73, which targets selected proteins to lysosomes for processing. What this all means remains to be resolved but note the involvement of the hsp family yet again. Suspicion of previous microbial encounters is engendered by the discovery by PCR amplification of nucleotide sequences characteristic of *Mycoplasma fermentans*, *Chlamydia* and Epstein–Barr virus in a substantial proportion of synovial tissues removed from RA patients. Further work on the intracellular location, molecular status and possible expression of this material is awaited with interest.

The antigenic history of **reactive arthritis** is more amenable to study since it is triggered by an infection either of the urogenital tract by *Chlamydia trachomatis* or of the enteric tract with *Yersinia*, *Salmonella*, *Shigella* or *Campylobacter*. The synovial tissue in reactive arthritis remarkably still retains antigenic descendants or memorials of the initiating bacteria many years after infection which can drive local T-cells. All the microbes are either obligate or facultative intracellular bacteria and so may escape the immune system by hiding inside cells, probably aided by high local production of IL-4. However, we may be dealing with molecular mimicry. Natural infection with *Salmonella typhimurium* generates CD8 cytotoxic T-cells which recognize an immunodominant epitope of the GroEL molecule presented by the class Ib Qa-1 and cross-react with a peptide from mouse hsp60, so permitting a reaction with stressed macrophages. HLA-B27 individuals are particularly at risk and the importance of the microbial component is emphasized by experiments on mice bearing the B27 transgene; if reared in a germ-free environment, lesions are restricted to the skin, but in the microbiological wilderness of the normal animal house, the skin, gut and joints are all affected. Why, as in RA, are the joints targeted and what does B27 do? Only one in 300 of the T-cells in the reactive arthritis synovium is CD8 and therefore class I restricted. It could be that a cross-reactive B27 sequence functions as a cryptic epitope perpetuating a gentle microbial stimulus with an amplifying autoimmune response.

Before leaving the subject, one should not overlook the curious behavior of fibroblasts isolated from synovial tissue in established rheumatoid arthritis. In culture, they secrete collagenase which would contribute to cartilage breakdown, but more ominously they proliferate spontaneously due to unrestrained control of the cell cycle by cyclin-dependent kinases 4 and 6 and their respective D-cyclins. This implies that they would be refractory to conventional therapies and might be a cause of apparently intractable disease.

Organ-specific endocrine disease

To make a fairly sweeping statement, inflammatory organ-specific diseases are generally linked to T-helper-

1 (Th1) responses. Clones producing EAE or transferring diabetes from NOD mice produce IL-2 and γ-interferon (IFNγ), while in collagen arthritis IL-12 can be substituted for the mycobacteria in the complete Freund's adjuvant. By contrast, Th2 CD4s are responsible for the polyclonal activation in murine lupus, the glomerulonephritis and necrotizing vasculitis induced in Brown Norway rats by mercuric chloride, and the chronic autoimmunity generated during graft-vs-host disease. However, the Th1/Th2 polarization is not apparent in diseases such as myasthenia gravis, Graves' thyrotoxicosis, Sjögren's syndrome and primary biliary cirrhosis.

Autoimmune thyroiditis

The inflammatory infiltrate in autoimmune thyroiditis is usually essentially mononuclear in character (see figure M18.1.1c) and, although not an infallible guide, this has been taken as an expression of T-cell-mediated hypersensitivity. Firm evidence for a direct participation of T-lymphocytes has yet to be provided, although the demonstration of class II molecules on patients' thyrocytes and the presence of antigen-specific Th1 cells in the thyroid would accord with an involvement of these cells.

We must turn to the animal models for further evidence albeit indirect. Draconian stamping out of T-cells in the Obese strain chicken prevented the spontaneous development of atrophic autoimmune thyroiditis and, at the target cell level, the threshold for induction of MHC class II on OS thyrocytes by IFNγ is far lower than that reported for normal thyroid cells, further reinforcing the notion that a thyroid abnormality is a contributory factor to the susceptibility phenotype. The other model, in which thyroiditis is induced by thyroglobulin in complete Freund's adjuvant (see figure M18.1.1b), can be transferred to naive histo-compatible recipients with CD4+ T-cell clones specific for peptides containing thyroxine established from immunized animals. We see now that there is considerable diversity in the autoimmune response to the thyroid leading to tissue destruction, metabolic stimulation, growth promotion or mitotic inhibition which in different combinations account for the variety of forms in which autoimmune thyroid disease presents (figure 18.28).

Insulin-dependent diabetes mellitus (IDDM)

Just as in autoimmune thyroiditis, IDDM involves chronic inflammatory infiltration and destruction of the specific tissue, in this case the insulin-producing β-cells of the pancreatic islets of Langerhans. The delay in onset of disease achieved by early treatment with cyclosporin, at levels which have little effect on antibody production,

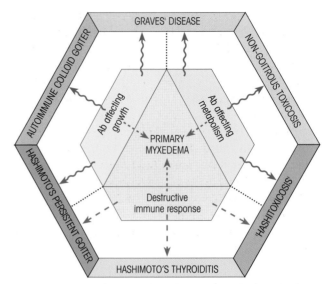

Figure 18.28. Relationship of different auto-reactive responses to the circular spectrum of autoimmune thyroid diseases. Responses involving thyroglobulin and the thyroid peroxidase (microsomal) surface microvillous antigen lead to tissue destruction, whereas autoantibodies to TSH (and other ?) receptors can stimulate or block metabolic activity or thyroid cell division. 'Hashitoxicosis' is the down-to-earth term used by our Scots colleagues to describe a gland showing Hashimoto's thyroiditis and thyrotoxicosis simultaneously. (Courtesy of Professors D. Doniach and G.F. Bottazzo.)

points an accusing finger at effector T-cells as the agents of destruction, since this drug targets T-cell cytokine synthesis so specifically. *In vitro* T-cell responses to islet cell antigens including glutamic acid decarboxylase (GAD) directly reflect the risk of progression to clinical IDDM. The strength of the risk factors associated with certain HLA-DQ alleles also has a strong whiff of T-cell action although, quite mysteriously, monocytes (and dendritic APCs?) constitutively expressing cyclooxygenase-2 (COX-2), the inducible enzyme responsible for the synthesis of prostaglandin E_2 and other prostanoids, were present in relatives (of IDDM patients) bearing these alleles and in the patients themselves.

To obtain further insight into the cellular siege and destruction of the islet β-cells, one has to turn to the **Nonobese diabetic (NOD) mouse** which spontaneously develops diabetic disease closely resembling human IDDM in its range of autoimmune responses and the association of islet breakdown with a chronic infiltration by T-cells and macrophages (figure 18.29). T-cells infiltrating the islets in diabetic mice had a Th1-type cytokine profile and could transfer disease to NOD recipients congenic for the severe combined immunodeficiency (*SCID*) mutation. Just as in the human disease, MHC class II alleles hold a pivotal controlling position and introduction of a transgene, in which residues at position 56 or 57 of the H-2Aβ chain

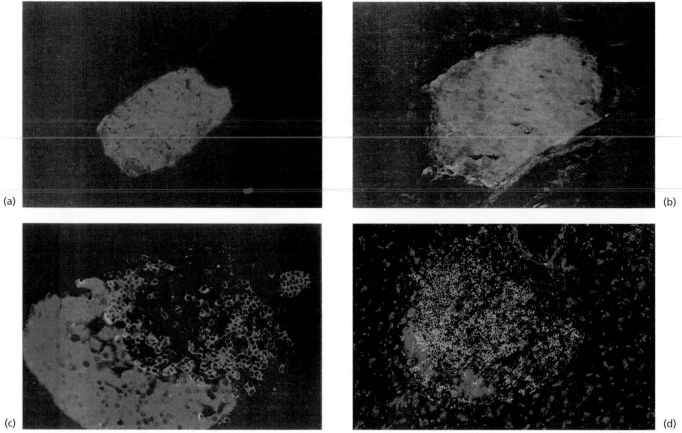

(a)

(b)

(c)

(d)

Figure 18.29. Destruction of pancreatic islet β-cells by infiltrating T-cells in the Nonobese diabetic (NOD) mouse. (a) Normal intact islet. (b) Early peri-islet infiltration. (c) Penetration of the islet by infiltrating T-cells. (d) Almost complete destruction of insulin-producing cells with replacement by invading T-cells. Insulin stained by rhodamine-conjugated antibodies and T-cells by fluoresceinated anti-CD3. (Data reproduced from Quartey-Papafio R., Lund T., Cooke A. *et al.* (1995) *Journal of Immunology* **154**, 5567; photographs kindly provided by Dr Jenny Phillips.)

are altered, drastically inhibits the development of diabetes. One of the non-MHC susceptibility loci in NOD which mapped to the *IL-1R* and *Bcg* genes on chromosome 1 was associated with natural resistance to infection by intracellular parasites. As a result, the NOD mouse is resistant to *Mycobacterium avium*, but after recovery from infection the onset of diabetes is prevented. That responses to hsp60 may be involved is implied by reports that a 24-amino acid peptide from this protein is the target of diabetogenic T-cells in both patients and the NOD mouse, and treatment with this peptide downregulates spontaneous disease. Cohen has interpreted this as a result of dysregulation of idiotypic networks and notes that the level of a particular idiotype associated with a TCR CDR3 consistently falls prior to the onset of diabetes, while mice reared under germ-free conditions which might inhibit the development of a natural idiotype network are more susceptible to IDDM. Time will test the validity of this hypothesis. Notwithstanding this evidence relating to hsp and idiotypes, in the final analysis, one has to take into account the following: up to 50% of the infiltrating T-cells isolated from pre-

diabetic NOD islets are insulin-specific and can transfer disease to young NOD mice; GAD-specific T-cells can also be recovered and are also diabetogenic; and tolerance to either insulin or GAD prevents the onset of disease. Presumably the latter can be accommodated by an organ-related bystander tolerance mechanism described below (p. 451). Overall, the data seem to be consistent with the necessity for two pathogenic pathways, one dependent on hsp and the other on an organ-specific response, operating either synergistically or serially, to achieve the final destruction of the pancreatic β-cells.

GAD in the central and peripheral nervous system produces γ-aminobutyric acid (GABA), a major inhibitory neurotransmitter, from glutamine. Autoantibodies to GAD are seen not only in early diabetes, but also in **Stiff man syndrome** (sounds like a cue for a Western) where the GABA-ergic pathways controlling motor neuron activity are defective. The antibodies cannot be pathogenic because GAD is present on the inner surface of the plasma membrane, but T-cells could be. How the brain as distinct from the pancreatic islet

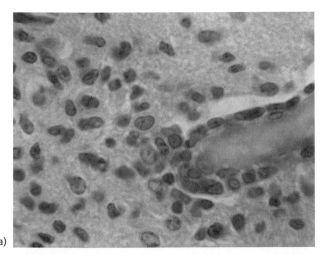

(a)

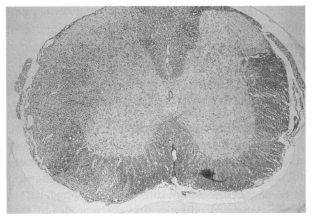

(b)

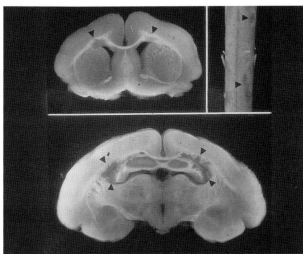

(c)

Figure 18.30. Experimental autoimmune encephalomyelitis (EAE), a demyelinating model for multiple sclerosis induced by immunization with brain antigens in complete Freund's adjuvant (CFA). (a) Early lesion of EAE in the rat at 9 days after immunization with rat spinal cord homogenate in CFA. The lesion in brain white matter, which is probably a few hours old, shows perivenous infiltration of lymphocytes and monocytes (a pure mononuclear inflammation) with cells invading the nervous parenchyma. Myelin is not stained. (b) Lumbar spinal cord of rat with chronic EAE after immunization with myelin proteolipid protein. Large demyelinating lesions in dorsal columns, in both left (large) and right (small) columns, as well as on lower left. Also gray matter involved with ongoing inflammation, in particular affecting left dorsal horn. Normal myelin is stained brown. (c) Chronic relapsing EAE in guinea-pig. Large demyelinated plaques in brain white matter (arrows) closely similar to plaques of multiple sclerosis. (Legend and slides provided by Dr B. Waksman; (b) originally from Dr Trotter and (c) from Drs Lassmann and Wisniewski.)

could be specifically targeted is a conundrum but 30% of patients do develop IDDM.

Multiple sclerosis (MS)

The idea that MS could be an autoimmune disease has for long been predicated on the morphological resemblance to *e*xperimental *a*utoimmune *e*ncephalomyelitis (EAE), a demyelinating disease leading to motor paralysis (figure 18.30) produced by immunization with myelin, usually *m*yelin *b*asic *p*rotein (MBP) in complete Freund's. T-cell clones specific for MBP will transfer disease but this can be exacerbated by injection of a monoclonal antibody to Theiler's virus, a murine encephalomyelitis virus, cross-reacting with an epitope on myelin and oligodendrocytes. Presumably the T-cell incites a local inflammation affecting the endothelial cells at the blood–brain barrier which opens the gate for antibody to penetrate the brain tissue.

How much of this is relevant to human disease? First, the serologically determined Caucasian DR2 phenotype (DRB1*1501, DQA1*0102, DQB1*0602) is strongly asso-

ciated with susceptibility to MS. At least 37% of activated T-cells responsive to IL-2/4 in cerebrospinal fluid were specific for myelin components, compared with a figure of 5% for subjects with other neurological disturbances. A Leu.Arg.Gly. amino acid sequence motif found in around 40% of TCR Vβ5.2 N(D)N rearrangements in T-cells from MS lesions was present in a Vβ5.2 clone from an MS patient cytotoxic towards targets containing the MBP 89–106 peptide and in encephalitogenic rat T-cells specific for MBP peptide 87–99. One is greatly encouraged to continue with attempts to induce tolerance.

Psoriasis

Given the evidence for T-cell-mediated pathogenesis (p. 359), the isolation of clones specific for group A β-hemolytic streptococci from guttate skin lesions has fostered the thought that pathology is initiated by exotoxin (i.e. superantigen) recruited T-cells and is maintained by specific cells reacting both with streptococcal M protein and a cryptic skin epitope, possibly a keratin variant presented by cytokine-activated keratinocytes. There is

Table 18.6. Autoimmunity tests and diagnosis.

DISEASE	ANTIBODY	COMMENT
Hashimoto's thyroiditis	Thyroid	Distinction from colloid goiter, thyroid cancer and subacute thyroiditis Thyroidectomy usually unnecessary in Hashimoto goiter
Primary myxedema	Thyroid	Tests +ve in 99% of cases. If suspected hypothyroidism assess 'thyroid reserve' by TRH stimulation test
Graves' disease	Thyroid	High titers of cytoplasmic Ab indicate active thyroiditis and tendency to post-operative myxedema: anti-thyroid drugs are the treatment of choice although HLA-B8 patients have high chance of relapse
Pernicious anemia	Stomach	Help in diagnosis of latent PA, in differential diagnosis of non-autoimmune megaloblastic anemia and in suspected subacute combined degeneration of the cord
Insulin-dependent diabetes mellitus (IDDM)	Pancreas	Insulin Ab early in disease. GAD Ab standard test for IDDM. Two or more autoAb seen in 80% of new onset children or prediabetic relatives but not in controls
Idiopathic adrenal atrophy	Adrenal	Distinction from tuberculous form
Myasthenia gravis	Muscle ACh receptor	When positive suggests associated thymoma (more likely if HLA-B12), positive in >80%
Pemphigus vulgaris and pemphigoid	Skin	Different fluorescent patterns in the two diseases
Autoimmune hemolytic anemia	Erythrocyte (Coombs' test)	Distinction from other forms of anemia
Sjögren's syndrome	Salivary duct cells, SS-A, SS-B	
Primary biliary cirrhosis	Mitochondrial	Distinction from other forms of obstructive jaundice where test rarely +ve Recognize subgroup within cryptogenic cirrhosis related to PBC with +ve mitochondrial Ab
Active chronic hepatitis	Smooth muscle anti-nuclear and 20% mitochondrial	Smooth muscle Ab distinguish from SLE Type 1 classical in women with Ab to nuclei, smooth muscle, actin and asialoglycoprotein receptor (these Ab disappear on remission indicating reduction in steroids) Type 2 in girls and young women with anti-LKM-1 (cyt P450)
Rheumatoid arthritis	Antiglobulin, e.g. SCAT and latex fixation	High titer indicative of bad prognosis
	Antiglobulin + raised agalacto-Ig	Prognosis of rheumatoid arthritis
	Perinuclear	V.sp. for early RA. Dominant residue citrulline (post-translational modification of arginine)
SLE	High titer antinuclear, DNA	DNA antibodies present in active phase Ab to double-stranded DNA characteristic; high affinity complement-fixing Ab give kidney damage, low affinity CNS lesions
	Cardiolipin/β2 glycoprotein 1	Thrombosis, recurrent fetal loss and thrombocytopenia
Scleroderma	Nucleolar + centromere Scl-70	Characteristic of the disease
Wegener's granulomatosis	Neutrophil cytoplasm	Antiserine protease closely associated with disease; treatment urgent

specific for the proteolipid (PLP) brain antigen, delivered a platelet-derived growth factor (PDGF-A) transgene to the inflamed brain of an animal with EAE; contact with antigen stimulated the clone and the secreted growth factor induced proliferation of the oligodendrocyte pro-genitor cells involved in remyelination. This would be a highly customized therapy only suitable for the well-heeled, but a cheaper gambit is to inject a plasmid DNA coding for Fas ligand in liposomes directly into the organ under attack. This manipulation, carried out in an experimental autoimmune thyroiditis model, induced persisting expression of FasL on thyroid follicular cells and total abrogation of antithyroglobulin cytotoxic T-lymphocytes.

The reader may recall the spontaneous proliferation of RA synovial fibroblasts when placed in culture. These cells undergo irreversible cell cycle arrest if subjected to γ-irradiation, which induces the synthesis of the p16^{INK4a} senescence protein. This is a tumor suppressor which blocks the stable association of cyclin-dependent kinases 4 and 6 with their respective D-cyclins and inhibits their ability to mastermind the passage of cells

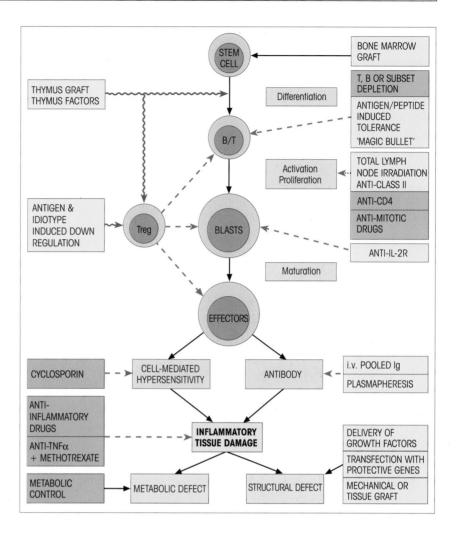

Figure 18.33. The treatment of autoimmune disease. Current conventional treatments are in dark orange; some feasible approaches are given in lighter orange boxes. (In the case of a live graft, bottom right, the immunosuppressive therapy used may protect the tissue from the autoimmune damage which affected the organ being replaced.)

into the G1 phase of the cell growth cycle. Injection of the RA fibroblasts with a recombinant adenovirus encoding the $p16^{INK4a}$ gene halted their growth and reduced synovial cell hyperplasia in the adjuvant arthritis model. If focus on expression of this gene fosters a new therapeutic approach to RA, it might also find utility in other disorders such as atherosclerosis, scleroderma and possibly late stage asthma. Conceivably, the benefit of adding methotrexate to anti-TNF therapy in RA (see below) might be partly attributable to an effect on fibroblast proliferation in addition to its inhibition of anti-idiotype synthesis.

Based on the possibility that multiple sclerosis is virally driven, patients have been treated with IFNβ; relapse rates were reduced by a third in relapsing–remitting disease, but there was only a modest effect on progressive disease. Note, however, that IFNβ influences some T-cell functions in addition to its effect on viral proliferation.

Anti-inflammatory drugs

Patients with severe myasthenic symptoms respond

well to high doses of steroids and the same is true for serious cases of other autoimmune disorders, such as SLE and immune complex nephritis, where the drug helps to suppress the inflammatory lesions.

In RA, steroids are very effective, but the recognition of a defective pituitary–adrenal feedback loop in these patients has inspired a novel approach aiming to restore normal corticosteroid levels by a depot of methylprednisolone (Depomedrone) which delivers a low daily dose—the earlier in the disease the better. This treatment accelerates the induction of remission and decreases the side-effects of second-line agents such as gold salts. Selectins and adhesion molecules on endothelial cells and leukocyte integrins appear to be downregulated and this would seriously impede the influx of inflammatory cells into the joint. Anti-inflammatory drugs such as salicylates, innumerable synthetic prostaglandin inhibitors and metalloproteinase poisons are widely used. The so-called second-line drugs, sulfasalazine, penicillamine, gold salts and antimalarials such as chloroquine, all find an important place in therapy but their mode of action is unknown.

An outstanding advance in therapy has been the

finding that neutralizing TNF with a humanized monoclonal antibody is most effective, so revealing the pathogenetic role of this cytokine. Most significantly, synergistic administration with methotrexate does seem to offer more lasting benefit (figure 18.34) essentially through suppression of a response to the monoclonal antibody, but possibly also through an effect on fibroblasts (see above). This therapy has ramifications deeper than might be expected from merely blocking a component of the inflammatory process since the treatment normalizes the compromised T-cell regulatory function seen in RA patients (cf. figure 18.15).

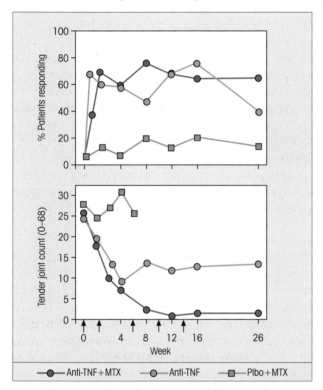

Figure 18.34. Synergy of anti-TNF and methotrexate in the treatment of rheumatoid arthritis. Top panel: Duration of response to therapy as defined by 20% Paulus criteria at three doses of monoclonal chimeric anti-TNF (infliximab) with and without methotrexate (MTX) and placebo (Plbo) plus MTX. Results shown are the proportion (%) of patients responding at weeks 1, 2, 4, 8, 12, 16 and 26. The Paulus response is achieved by 20% improvement in four out of six of the following: tender joint and swollen joint scores, duration of morning stiffness, erythrocyte sedimentation rate and a two grade improvement in the patient's and observer's assessment of disease severity. Lower panel: Serial measurements (median values) of the tender joint count, before (day 0), during (weeks 1–14) and after (weeks 14–26) treatment. Results are included only up to the point at which ≥50% of patients remained in the trial (up to week 6 for the placebo plus MTX group). Arrows indicate the timing of infusions of infliximab at weeks 0, 2, 6, 10 and 14. Methotrexate was given weekly and virtually eradicated the production of antibodies to the human chimeric antibody. Note the normalization of defective regulatory T-cell function by this treatment (cf. figure 18.15). (Data kindly provided by Professors R.N. Maini, M. Feldmann *et al.*, see Maini R.N. *et al.* (1998) reproduced with permission from Lippincott, Williams & Wilkins, MD, USA, *Arthritis and Rheumatism* **41**, 1552.)

Immunosuppressive drugs

In a sense, because it blocks cytokine secretion by T-cells, cyclosporin is an anti-inflammatory drug and, since cytokines like IL-2 are also obligatory for lymphocyte proliferation, cyclosporin is also an antimitotic drug. It is of proven efficacy in uveitis, early type I diabetes, nephrotic syndrome and psoriasis and of moderate efficacy in idiopathic thrombocytopenic purpura, SLE, polymyositis, Crohn's disease, primary biliary cirrhosis and myasthenia gravis. In a double-blind randomized control trial, cyclosporin demonstrated significant though not complete disease suppression over 12 months in a group of previously refractory rheumatoid arthritis (RA) patients. Unfortunately, high toxic doses were used but the synergy with rapamycin is a strong indication for a trial of combined therapy. Leflunomide is a promising new agent for treatment of RA. Its active metabolite inhibits *de novo* rUMP synthesis leading to G1 arrest of cycling lymphocytes.

While awaiting more selective therapy, conventional nonspecific antimitotic agents such as azathioprine, cyclophosphamide and methotrexate, usually in combination with steroids, have been used effectively in SLE, RA, chronic active hepatitis and autoimmune hemolytic anemia for example. High-dose i.v. cyclophosphamide plus adrenocorticotropic hormone (ACTH) or total lymph node irradiation through its effect on the peripheral immune system either slowed or stopped the advance of disease in approximately two-thirds of progressive multiple sclerosis (MS) patients for 1–2 years, a strong indication that the disease is mediated by immune mechanisms. This is further supported by the unfortunate finding that IFNγ exacerbates disease in the majority.

Immunological control strategies

Cellular manipulation

It should one day be practical to correct any relevant defects in stem cells or in thymus processing by gene therapy, bone marrow or thymus grafting or perhaps, in the latter case, by thymic hormones. Many centers are trying out autologous stem cell transplantation following hemato-immunoablation by cytotoxic drugs in severe cases of autoimmune disease. Around two-thirds of a series of difficult cases of SLE, scleroderma, juvenile and adult RA and so on, stabilized or improved. Transplant-related mortality risk at 2 years was 8±6%, comparable to that seen with cancer patients.

If defects in programed cell death in antigen-activated T-cells contribute in any way to the development of certain autoimmune diseases, bisindolylmaleimide, which potentiates weak and moderate apoptotic signals, might be therapeutic.

Because T-cell signaling is so pivotal, it is the target for many strategies. Injection of monoclonal anti-MHC class II and anti-CD4 successfully fends off lupus in spontaneous mouse models, and it is relevant to record the preliminary clinical observations that injection of immunoglobulins eluted from placentas, and shown to contain anti-allo-class II, significantly ameliorates the symptoms of RA. Immunization with a cyclic peptide from a polymorphic region of the β chain of the Nonobese diabetic (NOD) class II molecule protected a large proportion of the mice from disease. It is unclear whether the mechanism involves a block on MHC antigen presentation or relates to the MHC mimicry hypothesis (cf. p. 426).

Some take the anti-IL-2 receptor approach to deplete activated T-cells, but we would like to refer back to our discussion of the long-lasting effect of *nondepleting* anti-CD4 for the induction of tolerance (figure 16.13 (2) and (3)), particularly when reinforced by repeated exposure to antigen (cf. p. 375). Antigen reinforcement of course is an obvious continuing feature in autoimmune disease, so that anti-CD4 should be ideal as a therapy in disorders where the natural 'switch-off' tolerogenic signals are still accepted by the CD4 cells. Ongoing trials in RA still look promising. Excellent remissions have been recorded in patients with Wegener's granulomatosis who were refractory to normal treatment, following sequential injection of anti-CD52 (Campath-1H) and nondepleting anti-CD4 monoclonals.

Pulsing MS patients with the antileukocyte humanized monoclonal Campath-1H (anti-CD52) produced a brutal and surprisingly persistent reduction in T-cell numbers. Over a 2-year period virtually no new lesions were detected, although in half the patients there was progression of pre-existing lesions. A startling 33% developed Graves' disease (wow!), although this disturbing statistic was not a feature of many other disorders, including RA, where Campath-1H has been used.

Now, if one takes the view that rheumatoid factor immune complexes are major players in the pathogenesis of the RA joint lesions, logic suggests the radical approach of B-cell ablation with monoclonal anti-CD20 as used in the treatment of B-cell leukemia. Results to date are most encouraging (figure 18.35). There looks to be a good future for similar therapy in SLE.

Manipulation of regulatory mediators

We can correct some spontaneous models of autoimmune disease by injection of cytokines: IL-1 cures the diabetes of NOD mice; TNF prevents the onset of SLE symptoms in NZB×W hybrids; and transforming growth factor-β1 (TGFβ1) is known to protect against collagen arthritis and relapsing EAE. We have already reminded ourselves of the maintenance doses of steroids to restore the defective adrenal feedback control on leukocytes in RA.

Could transfection of the target organ with a protective cytokine like TGFβ prove to be a good bet (visions of firing a biolistic gun at islets pretransplantation?)?

Idiotype control with antibody

The powerful immunosuppressive action of anti-idiotype antibodies has led to much rumination on the feasibility of controlling autoantibody production by provoking appropriate interactions within the immune network. There are intimate network interactions between hormone receptors, hormones and their respective antibodies and it might be that the autoimmune disorders involving these receptors are especially amenable to idiotype control. There is a growing

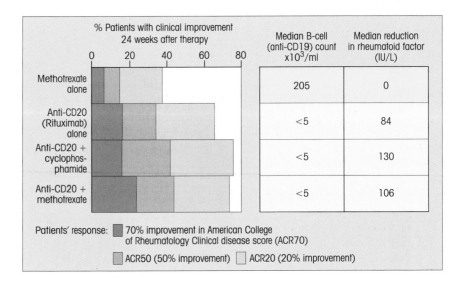

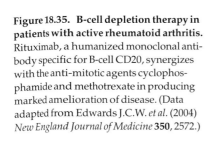

Figure 18.35. B-cell depletion therapy in patients with active rheumatoid arthritis. Rituximab, a humanized monoclonal antibody specific for B-cell CD20, synergizes with the anti-mitotic agents cyclophosphamide and methotrexate in producing marked amelioration of disease. (Data adapted from Edwards J.C.W. *et al.* (2004) *New England Journal of Medicine* **350**, 2572.)